A Companion to the Anthropology of Environmental Health

The *Blackwell Companions to Anthropology* offers a series of comprehensive syntheses of the traditional subdisciplines, primary subjects, and geographic areas of inquiry for the field. Taken together, the series represents both a contemporary survey of anthropology and a cutting edge guide to the emerging research and intellectual trends in the field as a whole.

1. *A Companion to Linguistic Anthropology*, edited by Alessandro Duranti
2. *A Companion to the Anthropology of Politics*, edited by David Nugent and Joan Vincent
3. *A Companion to the Anthropology of American Indians*, edited by Thomas Biolsi
4. *A Companion to Psychological Anthropology*, edited by Conerly Casey and Robert B. Edgerton
5. *A Companion to the Anthropology of Japan*, edited by Jennifer Robertson
6. *A Companion to Latin American Anthropology*, edited by Deborah Poole
7. *A Companion to Biological Anthropology*, edited by Clark Larsen
8. *A Companion to the Anthropology of India*, edited by Isabelle Clark-Decès
9. *A Companion to Medical Anthropology*, edited by Merrill Singer and Pamela I. Erickson
10. *A Companion to Cognitive Anthropology*, edited by David B. Kronenfeld, Giovanni Bennardo, Victor C. de Munck, and Michael D. Fischer
11. *A Companion to Cultural Resource Management*, edited by Thomas King
12. *A Companion to the Anthropology of Education*, edited by Bradley A. Levinson and Mica Pollock
13. *A Companion to the Anthropology of the Body and Embodiment*, edited by Frances E. Mascia-Lees
14. *A Companion to Paleopathology*, edited by Anne L. Grauer
15. *A Companion to Folklore*, edited by Regina F. Bendix and Galit Hasan-Rokem
16. *A Companion to Forensic Anthropology*, edited by Dennis Dirkmaat
17. *A Companion to the Anthropology of Europe*, edited by Ullrich Kockel, Máiréad Nic Craith, and Jonas Frykman
18. *A Companion to Border Studies*, edited by Thomas M. Wilson and Hastings Donnan
19. *A Companion to Rock Art*, edited by Jo McDonald and Peter Veth
20. *A Companion to Moral Anthropology*, edited by Didier Fassin
21. *A Companion to Gender Prehistory*, edited by Diane Bolger
22. *A Companion to Organizational Anthropology*, edited by D. Douglas Caulkins and Ann T. Jordan
23. *A Companion to Paleoanthropology*, edited by David R. Begun
24. *A Companion to Chinese Archaeology*, edited by Anne P. Underhill
25. *A Companion to the Anthropology of Religion*, edited by Janice Boddy and Michael Lambek
26. *A Companion to Urban Anthropology*, edited by Donald M. Nonini
27. *A Companion to the Anthropology of the Middle East*, edited by Soraya Altorki
28. *A Companion to Heritage Studies*, edited by William Logan, Máiréad Nic Craith and Ullrich Kockel
29. *A Companion to Dental Anthropology*, edited by Joel D. Irish and G. Richard Scott
30. *A Companion to the Anthropology of Environmental Health*, edited by Merrill Singer

A Companion to the Anthropology of Environmental Health

Edited by
Merrill Singer

WILEY Blackwell

This edition first published 2016

Registered Office
John Wiley & Sons, Ltd, The Atrium, Southern Gate, Chichester, West Sussex, PO19 8SQ, UK

Editorial Offices
350 Main Street, Malden, MA 02148-5020, USA
9600 Garsington Road, Oxford, OX4 2DQ, UK
The Atrium, Southern Gate, Chichester, West Sussex, PO19 8SQ, UK

For details of our global editorial offices, for customer services, and for information about how to apply for permission to reuse the copyright material in this book please see our website at www.wiley.com/wiley-blackwell.

Library of Congress Cataloging-in-Publication Data

Names: Singer, Merrill, editor of compilation.
Title: A companion to the anthropology of environmental health / edited by Merrill Singer.
Description: Chichester, UK ; Malden, MA : John Wiley & Sons, 2016. | Includes bibliographical references and index.
Identifiers: LCCN 2015044829 (print) | LCCN 2015050092 (ebook) | ISBN 9781118786994 (cloth) | ISBN 9781118786925 (ePub) | ISBN 9781118787137 (Adobe PDF)
Subjects: LCSH: Environmental health. | Public health–Anthropological aspects.
Classification: LCC RA565.A3 C66 2016 (print) | LCC RA565.A3 (ebook) | DDC 362.1–dc23
LC record available at http://lccn.loc.gov/2015044829

A catalogue record for this book is available from the British Library.

Cover image: Getty/greg0070

Set in 10/12.5pt Galliard by SPi Global, Pondicherry, India

1 2016

Contents

Notes on Contributors

Joseph S. Alter teaches anthropology at the University of Pittsburgh and has published a number of books, including *The Wrestler's Body*, *Knowing Dil Das*, *Gandhi's Body*, *Asian Medicine and Globalization*, *Yoga in Modern India*, and *Moral Materialism: Sex and Masculinity in Modern India*. His research is based in South Asia and is currently focused on the cultural history of nature cure as a globalized system of medicine, biosemiotics and social theory, and the natural history of animals in the human imagination.

Mary K. Anglin is an associate professor in the Department of Anthropology at the University of Kentucky, where she recently completed a term as department chair. Through long-term ethnographic research, based in urban northern California, she has examined breast cancer as a public health problem and a social crisis, with attention to the role of social activism in challenging biomedical views of "risk" as well as approaches to treatment. Her recent work explores differences of ethnicity, race, nationality, and social class among women diagnosed with breast cancer, and the implications of such differences for quality of life and survival. Future plans include a return to ethnographic work on issues of environmental contamination in Appalachia, with attention to their impact on communities and human health. The theme that unites these various projects is an abiding interest in health inequities and social justice and the potential uses of a critically applied anthropology.

George J. Armelagos (1936–2014) was a globally known biological anthropologist, and Goodrich C. White Professor of Anthropology at Emory University. Armelagos's work had a significant impact on paleopathology, skeletal biology, the anthropology of infectious diseases, and bioarchaeology. His many publications have been honored for their contributions to the theoretical and methodological understanding human disease, diet, and biosocial variation, including the social interpretation of race, within an evolutionary context. His accolades include the Viking Fund Award from the Wenner-Gren Foundation for Anthropological Research, the Franz Boas Award from the American Anthropological Association, and the Charles Darwin Award for Lifetime Achievement from the American Association of Physical Anthropologists.

Hans A. Baer is associate professor/honorary research fellow in the School of Social Political Sciences at the University of Melbourne. He has published 19 books and some 180 book chapters and refereed articles on a diversity of research topics, including Mormonism, African American religion, sociopolitical life in East Germany, critical medical anthropology, medical pluralism in the United States, United Kingdom, and Australia, the critical anthropology of climate change, and Australian climate politics. He is coauthor, along with Merrill Singer and Ida Susser, of *Medical Anthropology and the World System: A Critical Perspective* (3rd edition, 2013).

Nicola Bulled, PhD, is a medical anthropologist on the faculty of the Interdisciplinary and Global Studies program at Worcester Polytechnic Institute, Worcester, MA. Her research has focused on the biopolitics of global infectious disease prevention and management efforts, working with disadvantaged and vulnerable populations in the United States, Lesotho, and South Africa. She also has worked on public health programming projects with the Colorado Department of Public Health and Environment, Boston Medical Center, Boston University, Institute for Community Health in Cambridge, Boston Public Health Commission, Massachusetts State Laboratory Institute, and the Centers for Disease Control. Her current research examines public resistance to health interventions, especially what drives it, the forms it takes, and how contemporary global public health architecture might be restructured to address this issue.

Maryann Cairns is a doctoral candidate in anthropology at the University of South Florida (USF). Her research focuses on issues of water, sanitation, and wastewater treatment in Latin America and the Caribbean. Her dissertation research was funded through a grant from the National Science Foundation. She has also received funding from the American Water Works Association, USF's Institute for the Study of Latin America and the Caribbean, and the University of South Florida Challenge Grant Program.

Elizabeth Cartwright is professor in the Department of Anthropology and is the director of the Hispanic Health Projects and the Latino Studies Program at Idaho State University. She has published widely on structural vulnerability and health among immigrant and ethnic populations and has worked in Mexico, Peru, and Bolivia. She focuses on systematic ethnographic methodologies that use text-based narratives and visual data. She has extensive experience in obstetric nursing and publishes in the fields of anthropology, nursing, and women's health. In addition to her academic work, Cartwright is the cofounder of Crescendos Alliance, a nonprofit organization that uses community-based, participatory research to improve the lives of farmworkers in the United States and South America. She is an associate editor for the journal *Medical Anthropology.*

Melissa Checker is the Hagedorn Professor of Urban Studies at Queens College, and associate professor of Anthropology and Environmental Psychology at the CUNY Graduate Center. Her research focuses on environmental justice activism in the United States, urban sustainability, and environmental gentrification. She is coeditor of *Sustainability in the Global City: Myth and Practice* (2015), as well as the author of *Polluted Promises: Environmental Racism and the Search for Justice in a Southern Town* (2005) and the coeditor of *Local Actions: Cultural Activism, Power, and Public Life* (2004). She has published numerous articles in academic journals as well as mainstream publications.

Ajiang Chen is professor of sociology at Hohai University, where he chairs the Environment and Society Research Centre. He holds a PhD in sociology from the Chinese Academy of Social Sciences. He has carried out research on environmental sociology and rural development in several fieldsites in China. His books include *Secondary Anxiety: A Social Interpretation of Pollution in the Taihu Basin* and *Cancer Village Research: Understanding and Responding to Environmental Health Risks.*

Abigail Dumes received her PhD in sociocultural anthropology from Yale University. She is a lecturer in the Department of Anthropology at the University of Michigan and is currently working on a book manuscript entitled *Divided Bodies: The Practice and Politics of Lyme Disease in the United States.*

Laura Eichelberger is assistant professor of anthropology at the University of Texas at San Antonio, and a former cancer prevention fellow at the National Cancer Institute (National Institutes of Health) in the Division of Cancer Epidemiology and Genetics. Her research focuses on water, sustainability, and health to explore how political, economic, and ecologic factors intersect to shape disease risks historically and throughout the life course.

Chris Degeling is a veterinarian, health social scientist, and field philosopher whose interests include the social and cultural dimensions and ethics of human–animal interactions. His work is interdisciplinary and appears in public health, social science, philosophy, and veterinary journals. He is a Research Fellow at the Centre for Values, Ethics and the Law in Medicine at the University of Sydney, and a member of the Sydney Environment Institute and the Marie Bashir Institute for Infectious Disease and Biosecurity.

Lisa L. Gezon has been doing research in Madagascar on issues of human–environmental relationships since 1990, with a focus on drugs and health since 2004. Her recent book is entitled *Drug Effects: Khat in Biocultural and Socioeconomic Perspective* (2012). She has been teaching at the University of West Georgia since 1996 and is currently professor and chair of the Department of Anthropology. Her current research is on holistic health and wellness in Guatemala and in the United States.

Hannah Graff is senior policy researcher at the UK Health Forum, an international nongovernmental organization focused on the primary prevention of noncommunicable diseases. Hannah holds a BA (Hons) in Anthropology from the College of Wooster (USA) where she focused on disease understanding and experience cross-culturally. She went on to read for an MPhil in Medical Anthropology at the University of Oxford with a focus on place, disease etiology and burden, and the influences of policy. Hannah has experience in international public health policy research and development with particular work on obesity, HIV/AIDS, the built environment, and health in all policies.

Kristin N. Harper is a science writer and editor. She earned her MPH in global epidemiology and her PhD in population biology, ecology, and evolution from Emory University, performed research at Columbia University as a Robert Wood Johnson Health & Society Scholar, then founded Harper Health & Science Communications. Her area of expertise is infectious diseases, and she employs genomics, epidemiology, and paleopathology to better understand pathogen evolution and the impact of microbes on human history.

José E. Hasemann Lara has an MA in anthropology and an MPH in global infectious diseases, both from the University of South Florida. He currently is a doctoral student in anthropology at the University of Connecticut, focusing on citizenship, derogation, urbanization, political ecology, infectious diseases, and public health. His dissertation research is being carried out in Brownsville, Texas and Tegucigalpa, Honduras on dengue fever.

Kirsten Hastrup is professor of anthropology at the University of Copenhagen. She has a long-term interest in the entwinement of environmental and social history, notably in Iceland, where she has done extensive historical and ethnographic research and published several monographs spanning the period from the Middle Ages to modern times. Over the past eight years she has studied and published on the development in High Arctic Greenland, where a community of hunters has to reorient themselves as the dramatically changing sea ice makes their livelihood increasingly precarious, aggravated also by marine pollution. Among her recent publications is the edited volume *Anthropology and Nature* (2014).

G. Derrick Hodge is an economic anthropologist whose work has focused on how material logics condition cultural systems and public ethics. He has maintained a 15-year field presence in Havana, where he works with youth in the post-socialist transformations. He is currently the director of research at the General Commission on Religion and Race, and Affiliated Research Faculty at George Mason University.

Stephanie C. Kane is a professor in the School of Global and International Studies at Indiana University. Her research on environmental and social justice dimensions of urban water ecology and infrastructure has been published as a book, *Where the Rivers Meet the Sea: The Political Ecology of Water* (2013), as articles, in *Human Organization*, *PoLAR*, *Journal of Folklore Research*, *Crime Media Culture*, *Social Text*, and book chapters.

Helen Kopnina (PhD, Cambridge University, 2002) is a researcher in the fields of environmental education and environmental social sciences. Helen is currently employed at both at the Leiden University and at The Hague University of Applied Science (HHS) in The Netherlands. At the Leiden Institute of Cultural Anthropology and Development Sociology she is an assistent professor of environmental anthropology. At the HHS, she is a coordinator and lecturer on the Sustainable Business program. Kopnina is the author of over 60 peer-reviewed articles and (co)author and (co)editor of 12 books, including *Sustainability: Key Issues* (2015), *Culture and Conservation: Beyond Athropocentrism* (2015), and *Handbook of Environmental Anthropology* (2016).

Gina Larsen is a researcher at the University of South Florida. Her research focuses on the links between environmental destruction and human health and well-being. Her master's thesis research was funded by the National Science Foundation. She has also worked on National Science Foundation and Environmental Protection Agency funded projects focused on water politics and the human dimensions of climate change.

Peter C. Little is an assistant professor in the Department of Anthropology at Rhode Island College. He earned his PhD in applied anthropology from Oregon State University and is author of *Toxic Town: IBM, Pollution, and Industrial Risks* (2014). Little's interests in anthropology are focused largely on environmental and medical anthropology, with a strong focus on political ecology and science and technology studies. Fascinated by the complexities of human–environment relations and the neoliberal and biopolitical dimensions of public health, ecology, and economy, Little has published on the health and environmental justice dimensions of high-tech industrial pollution. He is currently developing an ethnographic research project on the political ecology of electronic waste (e-waste) in Accra, Ghana, exploring how high-tech donations and the global e-waste economy invoke environmental health disaster.

Anna Lora-Wainwright is associate professor in the human geography of China at the University of Oxford. Her research concerns development, health, and environmental issues in rural China. She recently published a special issue of the journal *The China Quarterly* titled "Dying for Development: Pollution, Illness and the Limits of Citizens' Agency in China" (2013) and a monograph, *Fighting for Breath: Living Morally and Dying of Cancer in a Chinese Village.*

Olivia Marcus received her MPH from Columbia University and is currently working toward a PhD in applied medical anthropology at the University of Connecticut. She has done extensive work concerning HIV prevention, health-seeking behavior among people living with HIV/AIDS, and sexual health promotion. She is concerned with sustainable intervention design. Her current fieldwork for her doctoral dissertation concerns healing practices in the Peruvian Amazon and the implications of health syncretism and medical pluralism on tourism and rights to intangible heritage.

Megan Mauger is a graduate of the University of Delaware, where she majored in environmental science within the College of Earth, Ocean, and the Environment and completed minors in anthropology and environmental humanities. Megan has a variety of experiences volunteering on organic farms, relating sustainable agriculture to watershed management, and working with environmental outreach and advocacy groups.

Amy McLennan is a postdoctoral associate at the School of Anthropology and Museum Ethnography at the University of Oxford. She has a BMedSci from Flinders University, a BSc(Hons) in Anatomical Sciences from the University of Adelaide, and MPhil and DPhil degrees in Medical Anthropology from the University of Oxford. Her doctoral research was based on long-term ethnographic fieldwork in the Republic of Nauru. She investigated historical and contemporary political ecological changes, local sociocultural changes, and the iterative links between these, changing food practices, and obesity emergence in the small Pacific island nation. She is currently involved in interdisciplinary research projects focusing on the social, political, and historical aspects of food and nutrition, diet-related noncommunicable diseases, and health governance.

Melissa K. Melby is an assistant professor in the Department of Anthropology at the University of Delaware, with a joint appointment in Behavioral Health and Nutrition. She holds degrees in chemistry, environment and development, and anthropology, and spent over 10 years conducting research on menopause and soy, developmental origins of childhood obesity, and cultural consensus analysis of dietary problems in Japan. Research interests include how biophysical and sociocultural environmental factors influence human health.

Ivo Ngade, PhD is currently an Andrew Mellon postdoctoral fellow in the Department of Anthropology, Rhodes University in South Africa. After receiving a Master of Cultures and Development Studies (Anthropology) and the Certificate of Advanced Studies in Social and Cultural Anthropology at Leuven University, he received a PhD from the Department of African Languages and Cultures at Ghent University (Belgium) in 2014. His research domains include HIV-related sexual risk behaviors among youth, technology usage and social relationships, transactional sex, youth culture, and transnational migration. Currently, he is working on local responses to fear of emergent infectious diseases, especially Ebola, in Cameroon.

Anja Olsen has an MSc in nutrition and a PhD in cancer epidemiology. She has worked within nutritional epidemiology since 2000 and is author and coauthor of more than 200 peer-reviewed scientific articles. Her primary focus has been on cohort studies (the Diet, Cancer and Health cohort and the European Investigation into Cancer and Nutrition) where she has studied associations between dietary habits (wholegrain, fruits and vegetables, alcohol, meat) and cancer incidence. She has a special interest in biomarker studies, including studies on hormonal factors (enterolactone and estrogen metabolites), studies on biomarkers of wholegrain intake (alkylresorcinols), and substances with potential negative effects (acrylamide). She is affiliated as senior researcher at the Danish Cancer Society Research Center.

Anne Marie Rieffestahl has an MSc in anthropology from the University of Copenhagen. She also holds an MSN degree in nursing and has extensive international experience in health work with Médicins sans Frontières. In her recent research, she has been part of a multidisciplinary Nordic collaboration investigating health effects of whole grains, especially in relation to noncommunicable diseases. Her primary focus has been on the agency regarding food habits and health among different groups of people in the Nordic countries. A number of publications are forthcoming on these topics. She is affiliated as project manager at the Centre for Clinical Education, the Capital Region of Copenhagen.

Melanie Rock is an anthropologist and social worker whose research program focuses on the implications for public health, public policy, and mental health promotion arising from human coexistence with nonhuman animals, especially companion animals or pets. Melanie is based at the University of Calgary, Canada, where she holds appointments in the Faculty of Medicine (Department of Community Health Sciences), the Faculty of Veterinary Medicine (Department of Ecosystem and Public Health), the Faculty of Social Work, and the Faculty of Arts (Department of Anthropology). Also at the University of Calgary, she co-directs the Population Health & Inequities Research Centre within the Institute for Public Health.

Gabriela M. Sheets is a PhD candidate at Emory University and her dissertation focuses on the microbial ecology of early childhood in semi-rural El Salvador.

Funding from the US Fulbright Foundation, Wenner-Gren Foundation, and the Earth Microbiome Project has supported her longitudinal study, which investigates the ecological, cultural, and political economic forces that shape the early development of the infant gut microbiome. Gabriela also teaches courses at Emory that creatively engage intersections of sustainability, development, microbiology, epigenetics, and human health. George Armelagos was her childhood hero and she is honored to have her name next to his.

Merrill Singer, PhD, a medical and cultural anthropologist, is a professor in the Departments of Anthropology and Community Medicine at the University of Connecticut. The central focus of his work is the social origins and maintenance of health inequality. Over his career, his research and writing have addressed HIV/AIDS in highly vulnerable and disadvantaged populations, illicit drug use and drinking behavior, community and structural violence, and the political ecology of health including the health consequences of climate change. His current research focuses on community health impacts of climate change and epidemics of fear in response to infectious disease. Dr. Singer has published over 275 journal articles and book chapters, and with this volume has authored or edited 30 books. He is a recipient of the Rudolph Virchow Professional Prize, the George Foster Memorial Award for Practicing Anthropology, the AIDS and Anthropology Paper Prize, the Prize for Distinguished Achievement in the Critical Study of North America, the Solon T. Kimball Award for Public and Applied Anthropology from the American Anthropological Association, and the AIDS and Anthropology Research Group's Distinguished Service Award.

Eleanor S. Stephenson (BA Victoria, MSc Oxford) is a PhD student in the Department of Geography at McGill University, Montreal, Canada with research interests in environmental justice and governance. Her doctoral work focuses on nonrenewable resource development in the Eastern Canadian Arctic. Her past research has addressed environmental change and food security in Western Nepal; shale gas development in Western Canada, published in *Energy Policy*, *Canadian Political Science Review*, and *Sustainability*; and environmental change in circumpolar and upland regions, published in *WIREs*, *Climate Change*, *Regional Environmental Change*, and *Climatic Change*.

Peter H. Stephenson (BA Arizona, MA Calgary, PhD Toronto) is emeritus professor of anthropology and in the School of Environmental Studies at the University of Victoria, British Columbia, Canada. He is a founding fellow of the Canadian Anthropology Society and recipient of the Weaver Tremblay award for applied Canadian anthropology. He has done research, especially among "vulnerable" populations including Vietnamese refugees, First Nations, frail seniors and Hutterites in Canada and among migrants and seniors in the Netherlands. His major publications include *The Hutterian People* (1991), *A Persistent Spirit: Towards Understanding Aboriginal Health in British Columbia* (1995), *Zombie Factory: Culture, Stress & Sudden Death* (with M. Korovkin, 2010), and

Contesting Aging and Loss (with J. Graham, 2010), and many journal articles and book chapters.

Stanley Ulijaszek is professor of human ecology and director of the Unit for Biocultural Variation and Obesity at the University of Oxford, and vice-master of St Cross College Oxford. He graduated from the University of Manchester in Biochemistry, and took his PhD at the University of London (King's College). His work on nutritional ecology and anthropology has involved fieldwork and research in Papua New Guinea, the Cook Islands, and South Asia. He presently conducts multidisciplinary research into the political ecology of obesity globally, using anthropological, public health, epidemiological, political, and economic historical frameworks.

Linda M. Whiteford is a medical anthropologist and professor of anthropology at the University of South Florida, She has degrees in anthropology and public health and is an internationally recognized researcher, lecturer, and author who consults for the World Bank, WHO, and PAHO. Her recent books include *Global Health in Times of Violence*, *Primary Health Care in Cuba: The Other Revolution*, *Anthropological Ethics for Research and Practice*, and *Globalization, Water and Health: Resource Management in Times of Scarcity.*

Rebecca K. Zarger is an associate professor in the Department of Anthropology at the University of South Florida. Her research focuses on human–environment relationships and has been funded by the US National Science Foundation, Inter-American Foundation, and the Spencer Foundation. Dr. Zarger is coeditor-in-chief of the *Journal of Ecological Anthropology*, coeditor of the book *Ethnobiology and Biocultural Diversity*, and has published in *Current Anthropology*, *Ecology and Society*, *Annals of Anthropological Practice*, and *Landscape and Urban Planning.*

Introduction

Merrill Singer

"Climate change is the biggest global health threat of the 21st century." This is the jarring opening line of a report issued by the Commission on Climate Change that was jointly sponsored by *The Lancet* and University College of London's Institute for Global Health (2009). As stressed by the Intergovernmental Panel on Climate Change (IPCC), there has been a 1.6 °F rise in global average temperature since the beginning of the twentieth century and the rate of warming is expected to continue to increase as the current century unfolds. The 2014 IPCC report highlights the fact that in addition to a change in the global average temperature, other health, social, and environmental climate change impacts that have occurred to date have hit all regions of the world and have affected everything from access to food and water to exposure to extreme weather. "In view of these impacts, and those that we have projected for the future, no one on this planet is going to be untouched by climate change," commented Rajendra Pachauri, the chairman of the IPCC during the release of the newest report's conclusions (quoted in Thompson 2014).

While climate change has emerged as a mounting multidimensional influence on health, it does not act alone in the consequential interface of humans

A Companion to the Anthropology of Environmental Health, First Edition. Edited by Merrill Singer.

with the physical and climatic environment. As examined in close detail in this volume, there are numerous, complex, and often interlocked environmental threats to health, and many of them, like climate change, are of anthropogenic origin or at least are significantly influenced by human actions in the world. What climate change does bring to the fore, however, is the growing urgency of environmental health in the array of factors that produce human sickness, loss of well-being, suffering, and death. Environment health, which the World Health Organization (WHO) defines as all of the health-related physical, chemical, and biological factors external to a person, and all the related factors impacting behavior, in short, arguably has become the most important contemporary determinant of human health. Environmental factors shape both infectious and non-infectious diseases, access to adequate diet, exposure to chronic stress, and even, going beyond the WHO definition, the impact of genetics on health. It can fairly be argued that the global health discourse on environmental health, despite its urgent tone at times, fails to fully acknowledge how fundamental the ways humans interact with their environments, built and "natural," are (and always have been) a key influence on the quality of human life. Today, with climate change among other disruptions of the environment produced by human actions, the stakes have risen considerably; indeed, in the eyes of some, the very sustainability of our species hangs in the balance.

This volume in the Companion series focuses on the examination – from the viewpoint especially of the subdiscipline of medical anthropology – of the diverse and consequential ways health and the environment intersect. Anthropology has a long history of developing an understanding of the human condition in light of the pressures and opportunities presented by local and more regional environments. Beginning in the 1950s, however, a distinct environmental anthropology (or ecological anthropology) emerged, and has undergone various changes and theoretical developments ever since. This trajectory in anthropology began to touch base with an emergent medical anthropology during the 1960s. Medical anthropology has had its own internal debates concerning the role of the environment in human health, but in recent years the field has moved toward a broadly shared political ecology of health perspective that is informed by a grounded ethnographic methodology, awareness of the centrality of culture to human experience and action; recognition of the growing health impact of a plethora of anthropogenic ecological crises; an understanding of health as a biosocial process that reflects the interdependence of humanity and the environment; and a recognition of the interconnection of social structure and environmentally mediated political economy on health production. The chapters in this edited volume exhibit and extend the state of knowledge of environmental health in medical anthropology, and in related disciplines, and point to needed future directions in this rapidly growing field of inquiry and application. In short, these chapters provide a political ecological foundation for modern medical anthropology.

Three Big Challenges for the Anthropology of Environmental Health

As anthropologists, epidemiologists, and other social science researchers seek to address the growing problem of environmental health, they are hampered by three vexing challenges:

1. *Challenge of attribution*: It is difficult to definitively show that particular aspects or changes in the environment, including anthropogenic transformations, cause specific health consequences.
2. *Challenge of the elite contrarians*: There are economically and politically powerful elite polluters and environmental disruptors who aggressively question undesirable research findings and actively resist regulation of contaminating and environmentally destructive behaviors.
3. *Challenge of partisan governance*: Policy makers under the sway of elite polluters tend not to respond effectively or promptly to anthropogenic environmental health risks even when they are confirmed by extensive scientific research.

Each of these points can be illustrated by the case of the Eagle Ford shale area of South Texas, one of the least publicized yet most active oil and gas drilling sites in the United States (Morris, Song, and Hasemyer 2014). Shale gas has been rapidly increased as a source of energy in recent years, driven by demand and rising oil prices, aggressive profit seeking, declines in production from conventional gas reservoirs, government support, and the introduction of new technologies like hydraulic fracturing ("fracking") and horizontal drilling. The Eagle Ford "play" – a term used in the oil and gas industry to refer to a geographic area that has come *into play* because of energy discoveries – is the largest individual economic development initiative in Texas history and ranks as the most significant oil and gas development project in the world based on capital investment (about $30 billion). Energy sources at the Eagle Ford are distributed over a 400-mile-long, 50-mile-wide expanse that was formed approximately 145 to 65 million years ago during the Cretaceous period when the region lay below a warm shallow sea. Organic-rich sediments of fossiliferous marine shales that were deposited during this period, and now are found 4000–14,000 feet below the ground surface, have turned the area around the Texas town of Eagle Ford into a contemporary energy hot bed that is being tapped by over 7000 oil and gas wells, with many more rigs on the drawing boards. As announced by the Texas Railroad Commission (2013), a state body that issues drilling permits and regulates oil and gas production in the state (although, despite its name, no longer oversees railroad issues): "The shale revolution is sweeping the country and revolutionizing energy and the economy, with Texas and the Eagle Ford Shale leading the way."

The various petrochemical facilities at the Eagle Ford have the state's permission to release hundreds of tons of chemicals per year into the environment, including nitrogen oxides, carbon monoxide, sulfur dioxide, benzene, formaldehyde, particulate matter, and hydrogen sulfide (Morris, Song, and Hasemyer 2014). While the federal Clean Air Act was designed specifically to restrict polluting facilities, the law is enforced at the state level, and lawmakers in Texas – the nation's biggest oil producer – tend to be energy industry-friendly; indeed, many top lawmakers in the state are themselves involved in the industry and profit personally from it. A technical study commissioned by the state of Texas and conducted by environmental scientists through the Alamo Area Council of Governments in San Antonio (2013) assessed the emissions impact of increased oil and gas production in the Eagle Ford Shale. The study projected a steady and significant rise of nitrogen oxides (NO_x) and volatile organic compounds (VOC) emissions in the play. NO_x is known to react with VOCs in the presence of sunlight to create ground-level or tropospheric ozone, a significant health risk.

Epidemiological studies have provided evidence that air pollutants, including tropospheric ozone, are associated with adverse long- and short-term health damage, including increased mortality. Long-term exposure to tropospheric ozone is linked to excess respiratory and cardiovascular morbidity and mortality, including incidence of asthma, diminishment in lung function growth in children, and lung cancer (Katsouyanni 2003). Short-term exposure to tropospheric ozone has been linked to an array of adverse health effects, including increased rates of hospital admissions and emergency department visits, exacerbation of chronic respiratory conditions, and decreased lung function (Lippmann 1993; Bell *et al.* 2004). Tropospheric ozone also impairs immune response to respiratory pathogens by limiting the clearance of microbes from the respiratory tract and by degrading the activity of macrophages (Jakab 1988). The macrophage phagocytic system, which includes cells in the lungs that destroy invading pathogens, foreign particles, cancerous or diseased cells, and cellular debris, is the defense component of the lungs most susceptible to the adverse effects of air pollutants and thus increased air pollution is linked to rising rates of respiratory tract infections (Schmitzberger *et al.* 1993).

Despite these identified connections, debates over the science of environmental health are considerable and often intense. Complications include the fact that "The science base is rarely complete. For any given exposure, data may not be available about specific health effects, about health effects of exposures at specific dose levels ..., about responses among specific subgroups of the population, or about effects of concomitant exposures to other substances" (Johnson 2005: 976). Moreover, levels of exposure to environmental risks are often uncertain or unknown because of limitation in the availability of detailed monitoring and inevitable variations of across local settings and population groups. Exposures can involve diverse pathways and processes. Further, while specific pollutants may be implicated in a range of health outcomes, few diseases are easily or directly attributable to single environmental pollutants (Little 2014). Often, as Lora-Wainwright and Chen discuss in their chapter, there is an "evidence gap" between sufferer experiences and the narrow parameters used in official records or set by prevailing law. Additionally, prolonged "latency times, the effects of cumulative exposures, and multiple exposures to different pollutants which might act synergistically all create difficulties in unravelling associations between environmental pollution and health" (Briggs 2003: 1). Consequently, ascribing particular health problems to specific industry-caused air, land, and water pollution in places like the Eagle Ford is tricky. The challenge is exacerbated because

> Scientists "really haven't the foggiest idea" how oil and gas development affects public health, [according to] Aaron Bernstein, associate director of the Center for Health and the Global Environment at Harvard University. Bernstein blames the information gap on a lack of monitoring and research, particularly in the rural, less affluent communities where most … drilling occurs. (Morris, Song, and Hasemyer 2014)

The Texas Commission on Environmental Quality (TCEQ), which is charged in oil and gas drilling areas with regulating emissions and ensuring air quality, firmly maintains that

> monitoring data provides evidence that overall, shale-play activity does not significantly impact air quality or pose a threat to human health. This conclusion is based on several million air-monitoring data points for volatile organic compounds (VOCs) and other air pollutants that the TCEQ has collected since 2000, in both the Eagle Ford and Barnett shales. While improperly operated facilities can result in temporary, local, unauthorized emissions, there are no indications that these emissions are of sufficient concentration or duration to harm residents of the Eagle Ford or Barnett shales. (TCEQ 2013)

This stance reflects the consistent discounting of adverse public health impacts of oil and gas industry operations by commissioners on the TCEQ, including the routine anti-EPA (Environmental Protection Agency) stance of Commission chair Bryan Shaw (e.g., Shaw 2011). An eight-month joint investigation by the Center for Public Integrity, InsideClimate News, and The Weather Channel (Morris, Song, and Hasemyer 2014), however, concluded that

- The air monitoring system in Texas is so limited that the state actually knows almost nothing about the extent of the pollution in the Eagle Ford region.
- Only five permanent air monitors exist in the 20,000-square-mile Eagle Ford play, and all of these are located on the fringes of the area, at considerable distance from the heavy drilling areas where emissions are the greatest.
- Thousands of oil and gas facilities are permitted to self-audit their emissions and do not report findings to the state.
- Enforcement is weak; of the 284 oil and gas industry-related complaints that were filed with the TCEQ by residents in the Eagle Ford area from Jan. 1, 2010 until Nov. 19, 2013, only two led to companies being modestly fined, despite 164 documented violations.
- The Texas legislature cut the TCEQ's budget by a third since the beginning of the Eagle Ford boom.
- The amount specifically budgeted for air monitoring equipment dropped from $1.2 million to $579,000 between 2008 and 2014.

- Although commissioners of the TCEQ declined to be interviewed in study by the Center for Public Integrity (CPI) and its collaborators, it issued a statement affirming that air pollution is not a problem in the Eagle Ford area.

In the view of Texas State Representative Harvey Hilderbran, "I believe if you're anti-oil and gas, you're anti-Texas" (quoted in Morris, Song, and Hasemyer 2014). Echoing this sentiment, Commissioner David Porter of the Texas Railroad Commission rejected the finding of the CPI-led study, on the grounds that the research team was "strictly anti-oil and gas," and arguing that investigators were guilty of "using – or perhaps I should say misusing – whatever facts or statistics they can find to make their case" (quoted in Everley 2014). On its web site, the Independent Petroleum Association of American (IPAA), a trade group representing oil and natural gas producers, vigorously attacked the report point by point, arguing, for example, that while pollutants like benzene (which is used in fracking) have been linked to cancer, attribution of a benzene-related health risk produced by oil and gas drilling is questionable:

> [The link] is based on a variety of factors, including long-term exposure at elevated levels. The InsideClimate/CPI team was basing its health scare on short-term samples that actually fall well below the short-term health threshold. The largest sources of benzene exposure in the United States, according to the Environmental Protection Agency, are automobiles and roads. (Everley 2014)

In short, the IPAA asserted that "there is no credible threat to air quality or public health associated with shale development" (Everley 2014).

The existence of a close connection between the energy industry and Texas governmental regulatory bodies is a central theme of the CPI-led report. Indeed, in recent years Texas Railroad Commission leaders have been described as acting "more as [industry] cheerleaders than regulators" (Cortez-Neavel 2013). Craig McDonald, director of Texans for Public Justice, a non-governmental organization that tracks money in politics, critically refers to the Commission as the "The Oil and Gas Protection Institute" and describes it as "the poster child for being a captured agency" because of its hands-off approach to the industry it regulates (quoted in Price 2012). The tenor of this relationship is inscribed in the intensity of a response to the announcement by the US Fish and Wildlife Service of its plan to place the dwindling lesser prairie chicken population, a bird found in Texas among other states, on the list of "threatened species" in May 2014. Texas Railroad Commissioner David Porter reacted to the report saying:

> I am extremely disappointed in the U.S. Fish and Wildlife Service's decision to list the Lesser Prairie Chicken as threatened under the Endangered Species Act ... It appears the federal agency has been influenced heavily by the environmentalist agenda, which has very little to do with preservation of this species and more with the eradication of the oil and gas industry. Unfortunately, this is another prime example of how the Endangered Species Act is seldom used for its intended purposes, but is being used as a political tool in the Obama administration's war on fossil fuels. (Quoted in Price 2014)

Texas Railroad Commissioner Christi Craddick added to Porter's umbrage, asserting: "This kind of federal intrusion creates unworkable difficulties for Texas businesses and landowners ... The result will undoubtedly impact Texas energy production in the chicken's range area throughout the Panhandle and in the heart of the Permian Basin, with damaging effects on operators who produce more than one-third of this nation's crude oil" (quoted in Price 2014).

In fact, it is sometimes difficult in Texas to specify the actual boundary separating oil and gas regulators and the energy industry. Members of the Texas Commission on Environmental Quality, appointees of the governor, for example, have close ties to the private energy sector. After three of the last four commissioners completed their terms, they began working as lobbyists for oil and gas concerns, and together have been paid hundreds of thousands of dollars in fees since 2010. Jeffrey Saitas, the TCEQ's executive director, during the period from 1998 to 2002, earned between $635,000 and $1.3 million in fees in 2013, primarily from energy companies (Hasemyer, Wieder, and Suderman 2014). Likewise, John Hall, chairman of the Texas Natural Resource Conservation Commission, a TCEQ predecessor, earned $225,000 in 2008 for his lobbying efforts from utilities, landfill companies, and oil companies, according to data filed with the state Ethics Commission. Former TCEQ Commissioner Robert Huston helped to found Espey Huston, which lobbies government to relax environmental regulations. Kathleen Hartnett White, who served as chairwoman of the Commission between 2003 and 2007, went on to direct the Center for Natural Resources at the Texas Public Policy Foundation, a group that advocates for deregulation and receives some of its income from the companies TCEQ is charged with regulating (Price 2009).

Members of the Texas Railroad Commission are elected officials who serve six-year terms. Before successfully running for the Commission in 2010, David Porter headed a CPA company in Midland Texas that provided accounting and tax services to oil and gas producers, royalty owners, oil field service companies, and other small businesses and individuals. Barry Smitherman, Chairman of the Commission, and a 2014 candidate for Texas attorney general, filed campaign information on January 15, 2014 indicating that he had raised more than $2 million for his election campaign, with employees of energy companies being among his top contributors. Before being elected to the Commission in 2012, Christi Craddick worked as an attorney specializing in oil and gas, water, tax issues, electric deregulation, and environmental policy. In her election bid to the Commission, Craddick raised more than $1 million in campaign contributions, 25 percent from the energy industry. Both Porter and Craddick have ties to the oil-rich Permian Basin area of Texas. Christi Craddick's father, State Representative Tom Craddick, owns stock in nine oil companies (with a value of $1.5 million), five of which are active in the Eagle Ford. Tom Craddick has received significant levels of campaign donations from employees of the oil and gas industry (Hasemyer, Wieder, and Suderman 2014). Overall, 42 of the 181 members of the Texas legislature or their spouses own stock or receive royalties from energy companies active in the Eagle Ford, while the Governor of Texas, Rick Perry, has received over $11.5 million in campaign contributions from energy companies since the year 2000. Lon Burnam, a member of the Texas state legislature who has emerged as the most outspoken critic of oil and gas industry dominance over energy and environmental policy in Texas, refers to the state's government as "a wholly owned subsidiary of the oil and gas industry" (quoted in Hasemyer, Wieder, and Suderman 2014).

In light of this complex of Three Big Challenges, and as explored in this book through multiple cases from around the world, building a rigorous and effective anthropology of environmental health must combine the development of a theory-guided evidence base, which includes sensitive investigation of the lived experiences of environmental health sufferers, with an active commitment to engagement and application. This effort is likely to have significant impact only if it is strengthened through its collaboration with citizen and other democratic efforts to challenge corporate and governmental opposition to making the protection of environmental health a central value within society.

Themes Articulated in This Volume

This volume brings together a significant set of new essays by anthropologists concerned with the often contested but undeniably consequential intersection of human health and the environment. While varied in their specific topics and regions of focus, the authors who contributed to this work seek to expand the growing trend in environmental consciousness in the health arena by bringing to bear the global sweep, local depth, holistic understanding, and ecobiosocial framework of twenty-first-century medical anthropology (Baer and Singer 2014). Focused on expanding the theoretical foundation and evidence base of environmental health, this book is organized around six integrated core themes.

First, it has become increasingly clear that humans are portentously reshaping the ecological systems of Earth, including both the chemical and biological features of the planet. The scale of our impact as a global forcing agent has led to the recommendation that the current geological epoch, beginning with the Industrial Revolution, be designated as the Anthropocene. This suggestion has been taken seriously enough by environmental scientists that an Anthropocene Working Group has been organized as part of the Subcommission on Quaternary Stratigraphy, the scientific body charged with proposing recent geological ages by the International Union of Geological Sciences. At the heart of this initiative is recognition of the dramatic changes being ushered in by the sharp rise in atmospheric CO_2 to over a third above the level that characterized the preindustrial period (as well as increases in other greenhouse gases like methane, as well as black carbon). These developments, including both their contribution to the steady heating up of the planet as well as the human role driving in this process, "ha[ve] been demonstrated beyond reasonable doubt … by systematic measurements since the 1950s … and by the record of atmospheric composition, now nearly a million years long, preserved in Antarctic ice" (Zalasiewicz *et al.* 2010).

Beyond, but often entwined with climate change, are a wide range of other environmental transformations and ecological crises that also are tied to the impact of humans on the planet, as seen in the following three examples. Deforestation, which has accelerated over time, drives climate change by destroying an important site of carbon sequestration and adding carbon to the atmosphere, which, in turn, leads to droughts that further damage forests in a downward spiral. Notably, in 2012 the UN Development Program reported that the Peruvian Amazon rainforest had become a net emitter of carbon dioxide rather than oxygen (Collyns 2013). Similarly, the massive dosing of Earth in ever more powerful pesticides, herbicides, industrial fertilizers, and other older and novel chemicals, diminishes soil quality as a growing medium, pollutes rivers and lakes, feeds toxic algae blooms, and injures coral reefs, degradations that are further enhanced by global warming. Release of toxins (oxides of nitrogen and volatile organic compounds) into the atmosphere through manufacturing, gasoline vapors, chemical solvents, and the ever expanding vehicular load on the roadways that now crisscross most regions of the world, leads to chemical reactions in the presence of sunlight to produce the air pollutant known as photochemical smog (or ground-level ozone). Atmospheric ozone is a greenhouse gas that traps heat and warms the earth, but new research shows that at ground level it adds to global warming by destroying the ability of plants to use and hence sequester extra carbon dioxide. Increasing smog, it is believed, will additively prevent over 260 billion metric tons of carbon from being removed from the atmosphere by plants through the twenty-first century. At the same time, it reduces plant primary productivity and crop yields (Sitch *et al.* 2007). As these examples indicate, human actions, and their consequences, contribute to global warming and cause an array of other adverse environmental modifications, and these, in turn, both contribute to and are enhanced by climate change, resulting in the further significant reshaping of planetary biochemistry and ecosystems. At the geographic level, the magnitude and varied expressions of our impact on the planet lie quite literally beneath our feet:

> The Anthropocene is represented physically by the sediment layers that have accumulated in recent years. Some of these layers are human-made – the concrete and bricks of our cities. Others are heavily modified – the soils of our fields, and the polluted muds of estuaries. Yet others have formed bereft of measurable [but not less significant] human influence – the recent sand dunes of the Sahara or the Empty Quarter of Arabia. (Zalasiewicz *et al.* 2010: 2230)

The second theme is the ecobiosocial conception of health, namely the idea that health is a product of the interaction of environmental factors, biological factors, and social factors. Human health reflects relations among various species in any local environment, as seen in the significant role of zoonotic disease in human health, the importance of animal reservoirs, and human/animal interaction patterns. Many of the changes we have triggered in environmental conditions rebound upon us, often in quite unexpected ways, adversely affecting the quality of human well-being. This rebound loop connects the health of humans and the health of the environment, including nonhuman animal and plant health. Consequently, this book mobilizes an anthropological perspective to examine the diverse ways the activities of human communities, and of the globalizing societies of the contemporary world, impact the environment, often adversely, and, in turn, are impacted by a changed environment in terms of health issues. This process reveals the fundamental ways in which human beings are "not simply agents of environmental change … [but] are also objects of that change" (Nash 2006: 7).

It is now well established, for example, that human activities (e.g., burning fossil fuels extracted from the environment), especially since the beginning of the Industrial Revolution, have significantly and negatively impacted the environment, including being the primary driver of global climate change. The heating up of the environment, and the diverse other environmental changes, local and regional, caused by a heating planet, in turn are beginning to have significant impacts on human health, from the spread of infectious disease vectors to rises in respiratory problems, and from heat-related illnesses like heat stroke to the varied health consequences of extreme weather and flooding (and drought). Of equal importance, social movements emerge and have impact around issues of anthropogenic environmental threats. This behavior too is of critical importance in understanding complex patterns of human/environment interaction in health. Indeed anthropogenic environmental diseases have become primary shapers of global health in the contemporary era, as reported in the chapters of this book and in other available research literature. The World Health Organization (Prüss-Üstün and Corvalán 2006) maintains that one-quarter of the global health burden is due to modifiable environmental factors, with children bearing the highest disease and death toll from environmentally mediated sources. Of the 102 major diseases identified by the WHO, environmental risk factors are reported to contribute to disease burden in 85 categories. The specific fraction of disease attributable to the environment by the WHO varies considerably across disease conditions. Yet, even WHO estimates do not include the full measure of the health consequences of climate change, environmental pollution, and the degradation of ecological systems.

A recent assessment by the Pure Earth/Blacksmith Institute (2014), based on new data from the World Health Organization and other sources, concludes that the scale of the problem is much greater than suggested by the World Health Organization. Analyses by the Institute suggest that air, water, and chemical pollution has developed into one of the biggest threats to health in the developing world, where it is responsible for over 10 million deaths per year, more than any of the world's major infectious diseases. The human casualties of pollution are now three times the combined total of the big three infectious killers: malaria, HIV/AIDS, and tuberculosis. Even the 2014 Ebola epidemic, despite the level of global panic that it has sparked, has not had anything near the level of actual health impact as anthropogenic environmental pollution.

The third theme is political ecology, or the ways the unequal structural relations within and across societies leave their deep footprints on the environment, including the creation of cases of environmental injustice, like the building of hazardous and polluting manufacturing facilities in poorer communities or the abandonment of communities after they have been severely polluted (Checker 2005; Auyero and Swistun 2009). It is not possible to understand the nature of anthropocentric environmental change and its health consequences independent of an analysis of the structures of social power and social inequality that drive our technological engagement with the planet, deeply influence the distribution of the environmental and health outcomes of this engagement, and organize the degree and kinds of access to health care available for environmental (and other) diseases. Like other consequences of a global system structured by extensive social inequalities, the lion's share of pollution-related deaths are found among the poor in low- and middle-income countries, places populated by people who have the least resources to respond to a life threat they were not primarily responsible for creating. In essence, the poor of the world have become "the poisoned poor." Consequently, the chapters of this book examine the social determinants of gross environmental health inequalities, including both stark expressions of environmental racism and resulting social suffering and social struggles for environmental justice in diverse settings. Of particular importance, to adapt Rose's (1992) expression, is the excavation of the "causes of the causes" of environmental health inequality.

The World Health Organization estimates that the infant death rate from environmental causes is 12 times greater in developing than in developed countries. Moreover, although 25 percent of all deaths in developing regions are attributable by the WHO to environmental causes, in developed regions only 17 percent of deaths are attributed to such causes (Prüss-Üstün and Corvalán 2006). The issue often is not poor environments in developing countries, however, but the fact that environmental health in poor countries is a consequence of economic development in rich ones. Beyond rich and poor countries, a nation's specific location and roles in the world economic system are critical determinants of environmental health. At the same time, even in wealthy nations, marginalized populations suffer considerably higher environmental health burdens just as the elite of poor nations escape the environmental health burden found in local populations (Baer, Singer, and Susser 2013).

The social mechanisms and activities employed and engaged by the powerful that result in increased and disproportionate environmental health problems among the poor and less powerful are manifold. Exemplary are the ways corporate actions make it difficult for people to make good health choices. This pattern is illustrated by Dietrich (2013) in her ethnographic account of environmental pollution and the pharmaceutical industry in Puerto Rico. Government public health education in the region where she worked ignored environmental damage caused by industry and focused instead on "lifestyles," including household diets high in fat and alcohol. In an interview with a pro-industry local deputy mayor who was in charge of health, Dietrich reported that he lamented that it was extremely unfortunate that people did not understand that nutrition and exercise were the keys to public health. "Absent from the conversation about obesity and its role as a risk factor for heart disease," Dietrich (2013: 171) comments, "were questions about the role of both environmental and occupation health considerations." Embedded in this view of the causes of ill health is the assumption that the individual is almost completely responsible for personal health – especially so if information is provided and someone fails to act in a healthy manner. Social barriers to "compliance," including financial costs, the benefits of specific behavior configurations (e.g., peer support and acceptance), and the existence of alternative cultural frameworks, are routinely overlooked. Moreover, surveys on health-related behavior, in the absence of measures of ambient air or water quality, industrial toxins dumped into the local environment, harmful chemicals in everyday consumer products, the quality of food grown in chemically restructured soils, job-related exposures to carcinogens, and a range of other anthropogenic impacts on the environments of human experience, are "virtually guaranteed to find a relationship between any number of [individual behaviors] and participants' reported health problems" (Dietich 2013: 172).

A different type of example of the role of social structure and inequality in environmental health involves increases in food insecurity produced when families are forced off the land and then are alienated from direct production. As Oxfam International (2014a) reports with reference to the growing crisis of land grabs by banks and private investors in various locations around the world,

> Demand for land has soared as investors look for places to grow food for export, grow crops for biofuels, or simply buy-up land for profit. But in many cases, land sold as "unused" or "undeveloped" is actually being used by poor families to grow food. These families are often forcibly kicked off the land. Promises of compensation are broken. Often people are violently evicted by hired thugs.

This pattern is seen, for example, in the state of Mato Grosso do Sul, Brazil where agribusiness expansion, particularly of sugar cane (from 160,000 hectares in 2007 to 570,000 hectares between in 2012) has been linked to a significant jump in the level of violence against indigenous people (Oxfam International 2014b). Demand for sugar in developed nations, leading to rising international sugar prices, has enhanced agribusiness commitment to acquiring additional land for sugar production in a Brazilian state in which land title often is not registered and indigenous food producers cannot match the legal and other resources, including the use of violence, employed by agribusinesses seeking to expand their acreage. Indigenous people and Quilombolas (descendants of slaves who escaped and established communities in rural and forested areas) represent over 25 percent of all people in Brazil enmeshed in such land conflicts. For these people, access to land for immediate for production is critical to the dietary health and well-being of their families, while forced or "legal" eviction pushes them into overcrowded urban slums where they face a new set of environmental threats to health.

In Mato Grosso do Sul, as elsewhere, those who face environmental health injustice resist at both individual and collective levels, and the pattern of social response, what might be called struggles for environmental health, is also of vital importance to the understanding being developed by anthropologists engaged in work at the intersections of health and the environment. On October 16, 2013, hundreds of indigenous women, many in traditional ethnic clothing, marched through the streets of Lima, Peru with signs bearing messages like "Climate change is affecting our harvests and food for our children" (Oxfam

America 2014). Taking to the streets to demand government action is prompted by the growing impact of climate change being experienced in Peru. Already the country has lost 39 percent of its tropical glaciers due to rising temperatures in the Andes. The UN Development Program projects a temperature rise of up to 6 °C in many parts of the Andes by the end of this century, a scenario that will have significant harmful impacts on health as a result of arable land and potable water losses (Collyns 2013). In addition to indigenous responses, groups like Movimiento Ciudando Frente al Cambio Climático, Peru (Citizen's Movement Against Climate Change) have formed to challenge current patterns of environmentally unsustainable economic growth based on maximizing profits and consumption while putting the planet and people's health at grave risk. The emergence of social movements like this is contributing to the growth of a critical medical anthropology of climate change that analyzes vast environmental degradation in terms of the rise of global capitalism with its focused emphasis on profit making, treadmill of production and consumption, heavy reliance on fossil fuels, and commitment to ever ongoing economic expansion (Baer 2012; Baer and Singer 2014).

The fourth theme emerges from the fact that anthropogenic changes to the environment are themselves interactive (e.g., the interaction of climate change and burnt fossil fuel, paint, and solvent gases in the creation of respiratory disease-causing ground-level ozone). This kind of interface, termed *pluralea interaction* (multiple harms), and its effects on human health can be seen in populations of traditional anthropological interest like indigenous peoples. Among the Inuit, for example, this pattern is seen in the rise of new dietary risks that stem from the consumption of raw or undercooked beluga whale meat. As Tocasie Burke of Nunavut, the largest and northernmost Canadian territory, observes:

> When someone catches [a beluga,] everyone gathers to have a feast ... It's like a welcoming of spring, kind of .... Also, whatever is left over is usually aged ... Nothing goes in the garbage ... It means a lot. People celebrate it ... It is part of our culture ... Everyone prefers to eat it raw with soy sauce ... People don't expect it until [they] try it. It's got an oily taste to it. (Quoted in Eustace 2008)

Recent research, however, has shown that despite the cultural and dietary appeal of beluga meat the whales are now being parasitized by *Toxoplasma gondii*, a pathogen commonly associated with cats that presents a particular danger to pregnant women and individuals with weakened immune systems. The appearance of *T. gondii* in the Arctic beluga is a somewhat unexpected finding as ice and cold water temperatures have served as ecological barriers for many microorganisms.

One hypothesis is that the pathogen was brought to the region by cats that are now kept as pets by Arctic-dwelling families, was washed into the ocean in cat feces, and survived there long enough to infect belugas because of warming ocean waters. This process is facilitated by the level of parasite shedding by infected cats (up to 100 million *T. gondii* oocysts – minuscule egg-like structures – in a 10-day period) and the hardy nature of the microorganism.

The term "pollutagen" (polluting pathogens) has been developed to describe land-based infectious agents that are now infecting marine mammals in the time of global warming (Solomon 2013). In response to the discovery of beluga infection with a pathogen that can cause blindness, be fatal to fetuses and immunocompromised individuals, and is linked to schizophrenia and other bipolar disorders, University of British Columbia researchers issued a health advisory to Inuit families in the region to avoid eating raw whale meat.

Multiple other ways that human activity remodels the environment and produces health consequences include the dietary impacts of overfishing and global warming contribution to lake shrinkage, human destruction of animal habitats and resulting loss of biodiversity and increases in the spread of infectious diseases, ocean dumping of plastics and the ensuing entry of toxins from plastic into the food chain, and increased exposure to environmental carcinogens in the workplace, in home consumer products, and as a result of industrial release by petrochemical and other manufacturing facilities.

A final theme is ecosyndemics, the adverse interactions among diseases that are mediated by the environment. For example, global warming has contributed to the movement of the disease leishmaniasis into Europe, by making the continent more climatically hospitable to the sandfly vector of the disease. In Europe, leishmaniasis is interacting with HIV/AIDS (especially among injection drug users), resulting in the accelerated progression of both diseases and consequent negative health outcomes. Human communities, and the individuals who compose them, live with multiple and potentially interacting diseases, often shaped by the ways the structure of social relations finds expression in environmental health. Human impact on the world, intended and unintended, is increasing the likelihood that previously unlinked and geographically dispersed diseases are developing overlapping distributions. This creates the potential for diseases for historically independent disease to cluster in a population, often with unexpected and sometimes lethal consequence. In Spain, for example, visceral leishmaniasis has contributed to a diminishment of the life expectancy of HIV-infected individuals. At the same time, HIV infection increases the risk of developing by 10–1000 times in endemic areas. Overall in southern Europe 25 to 70 percent of adult visceral leishmaniasis cases are related to HIV infection while between 1.5 and 9 percent of AIDS cases suffer from newly acquired or reactivated visceral leishmaniasis. Both of these infectious diseases, one of which is highly sensitive to environmental conditions because it can be vector-borne, decrease cellular immune response by attacking similar components of the immune system (Paredes *et al.* 2003).

These themes are developed in environmental health assessments carried out in varied sociocultural contexts around the world based on ethnographically informed multimethod, holistic, and micro–macro relational approaches common to contemporary anthropological and related analyses. Among the key questions addressed in the book are:

- Why do human pollute and degrade their environments?
- What specific threats to health are a consequence of such behavior and how?

- How are environmental health problems distributed (across and within societies) and why?
- How do human communities perceive, understand, and seek to limit environmental health problems?
- What is the future of human health?

Without question, human health today, in the past, and in the future is strongly influenced by interactions with on the environment of multiple and diverse kinds that play out on various scales. Importantly, the environments that impact human health today, and increasingly in the future, are and will be significantly and adversely shaped by human activity. Environmental health, and our role in creating it, is central to contemporary human health, and hence to the ongoing forging of an anthropology of health and illness.

REFERENCES

Alamo Area Council of Governments in San Antonio. 2013. *Oil and Gas Emission Inventory, Eagle Ford Shale.* https://www.documentcloud.org/documents/1109217-aacog-oil-and-gas-emission-inventory-april-4-2014.html.

Auyero, J. and Swistun, D. 2009. *Flammable. Environmental Suffering in an Argentine Shantytown.* Oxford: Oxford University Press.

Baer, H. 2012. *Global Capitalism and Climate Change: The Need for an Alternative World System.* Lanham, MD: AltaMira.

Baer, H. and Singer, M. 2014. *The Anthropology of Climate Change: An Integrated Critical Perspective.* New York: Routledge, Earthscan.

Baer, H., Singer, M., and Susser, I. 2013. *Medical Anthropology and the World System.* Westport, CT: Greenwood.

Bell, M., McDermott, A., Zeger, S., Samet, J., and Dominici, F. 2004. "Ozone and Short-term Mortality in 95 US Urban Communities, 1987–2000." *Journal of the American Medical Association*, 292(19): 2372–2378.

Briggs, D. 2003. "Environmental Pollution and the Global Burden of Disease." *British Medical Bulletin*, 68(1): 1–24.

Checker, M. 2005. *Polluted Promises: Environmental Racism and the Search for Justice in a Southern Town.* New York: New York University Press.

Collyns, D. 2013. "Why Climate Change Threatens Peru's Poverty Reduction Mission." Povertymatters blog. http://www.theguardian.com/global-development/poverty-matters/2013/dec/13/undp-climate-change-peru-poverty-reduction (accessed February 16, 2014).

Cortez-Neavel, B. 2013. "Anti-Federal Sentiment Dominates Discussion of Texas Oil and Gas Industry." *Observer*, January 10. http://www.texasobserver.org/anti-federal-sentiment-dominates-discussion-of-texas-oil-and-gas-industr/ (accessed November 23, 2015).

Detrich, A. 2013. *The Drug Company Next Door: Pollution, Jobs, and Community Health in Puerto Rico.* New York: New York University Press.

Eustace, C. 2008. "Belugas both Beautiful and Tasty for Canada's Inuit." *Vancouver Sun*, October 2. http://www.canada.com/story.html?id=ff0e0fd5-04a5-45ce-accc-859b9c754296 (accessed February 15, 2014).

Everley, S. 2014. "Activism and Deception Underlie Weather Channel's Eagle Ford Shale Report." Energy Indepth. Available at http://energyindepth.org/texas/activism-deception-weather-channel-eagle-ford-shale-report/ (accessed November 23, 2015).

Hasemyer, D., Wieder, B., and Suderman, A. 2014. "Saturated with Oil Money, Texas Legislature Saved Industry from Pollution Rule." The Center for Public Integrity. http://www.publicintegrity.org/2014/02/18/14240/saturated-oil-money-texas-legislature-saved-industry-pollution-rule (accessed November 23, 2015).

Jakab, G. 1988. "Modulation of Pulmonary Defense Mechanisms against Viral and Bacterial Infections by Acute Exposures to Nitrogen Dioxide." *Research Report of the Health Effects Institute*, 20: 1–38.

Johnson, B. 2005. "Environmental Health Policy." In H. Frumkin (Ed.), *Environmental Health from Global to Local* (pp. 961–987). San Francisco, CA: Jossey-Bass.

Katsouyanni, K. 2003. "Ambient Air Pollution and Health." *British Medical Bulletin*, 68(1): 143–156.

Lippmann, M. 1993. "Health Effects of Tropospheric Ozone: Review of Recent Research Findings and Their Implications to Ambient Air Quality Standards." *Journal of Exposure Analysis and Environmental Epidemiology*, 13: 103–129.

Little, P. 2014. *Toxic Town: IBM, Pollution and Industrial Risks.* New York: New York University Press.

Morris, J., Song, L., and Hasemyer, D. 2014. *Big Oil, Bad Air: Fracking the Eagle Ford Shale of South Texas.* Washington, DC: Center for Public Integrity.

Nash, L. 2006. *Inescapable Ecologies: A History of Environmental Disease, and Knowledge.* Berkeley: University of California Press.

Oxfam America. 2014. "Connecting the Two Perus." *Oxfam Closeup*, 14(1): 9.

Oxfam International. 2014a. "Land Grabs." http://www.oxfam.org/en/grow/landgrabs (accessed February 16, 2014).

Oxfam International. 2014b. "The Human Side of the Sugar Rush in Brazil." https://www.oxfam.org/en/multimedia/photos/human-side-sugar-rush-brazil (accessed November 23, 2015).

Paredes, R., Munoz, J., Diaz, I., Domingo, P., Gurgui, M., and Clotet, B. 2003. "Leishmaniasis in HIV Infection." *Journal of Postgraduate Medicine*, 49: 39–49.

Price, A. 2009. "Environmental Regulators Find Higher-Paying Jobs in Industry." *American-Statesman.* http://texasnuclearsafety.org/downloads/aas_011809.pdf (accessed November 23, 2015).

Price, A. 2012. "Public Hearing at Capitol on Name, Enforcement of Texas Railroad Commission." *Statesman.* http://www.statesman.com/news/news/state-regional/public-hearing-at-capitol-on-name-enforcement-of-t/nTZdf/ (accessed November 23, 2015).

Price, B. 2014. "Feds Push Anti-Oil Environmentalist Agenda Over Prairie Chicken." http://www.breitbart.com/Breitbart-Texas/2014/03/30/Feds-Cave-to-Environmentalist-Agenda-Lesser-Prairie-Chicken-Added (accessed November 23, 2015).

Prüss-Üstün, A. and Corvalán, C. 2006. *Preventing Disease through Health Environments: Towards an Estimate of the Environmental Burden of Disease.* Geneva: WHO Press.

Pure Earth/Blacksmith Institute. 2014. "The Poisoned Poor: Toxic Chemicals Exposures in Low- and Middle-Income Countries." Global Alliance on Health and Pollution. http://www.gahp.net/new/wp-content/uploads/2013/09/GAHPPoisonedPoor_Report-Sept-2013.pdf (accessed November 23, 2015).

Rose, G. 1992. *Strategy of Preventive Medicine.* Oxford: Oxford University Press.

Schmitzberger, R., Rhomberg, K., Buchele, H., Puchegger, R., Schizberger-Natzmer, D., Kemmler, G., and Panosch, B. 1993. "Effects of Air Pollution on the Respiratory Tract of Children." *Pediatric Pulmonology*, 152: 68–74.

Shaw, B. 2011. Testimony of Dr. Bryan W. Shaw, Chairman of the Texas Commission on Environmental Quality. US Senate Committee on Environment and Public Works, Subcommittee on Clean Air and Nuclear Safety hearing entitled, "Oversight: Review of EPA Regulations Replacing the Clean Air Interstate Rule (CAIR) and the Clean Air Mercury Rule (CAMR)." http://www.epw.senate.gov/public/index.cfm?FuseAction=Files.View&FileStore_id=eedf7d18-3b2f-4a1c-b267-713eca4fc1cd (accessed November 23, 2015).

Sitch, S., Cox, P., Collins, W., and Huntingford, C. 2007. "Indirect Radiative Forcing of Climate Change through Ozone Effects on the Land-Carbon Sink." *Nature*, 448: 791–794.

Solomon, C. 2013. "How Kitty Is Killing the Dolphins." *Scientific American*, 308(5). http://eds.b.ebscohost.com.ezproxy.lib.uconn.edu/ehost/detail?sid=a97b9ddd-1655-44ef-8129-7f7e7ff2c46c%40sessionmgr112&vid=5&hid=106&bdata=JnNpdGU9ZWhvc3QtbGl2ZSZzY29wZT1zaXRl#db=sch&AN=87376562 (accessed February 15, 2014).

Texas Commission on Environmental Quality. 2013. "Maintaining Air Quality in the Eagle Ford Shale." http://www.tceq.texas.gov/publications/pd/020/2013-NaturalOutlook/maintaining-air-quality-in-the-eagle-ford-shale (accessed November 23, 2015).

Texas Railroad Commission. 2013. *Eagle Ford Shale Task Force Report*. http://www.rrc.state.tx.us/commissioners/porter/reports/Eagle_Ford_Task_Force_Report-0313.pdf.

The Lancet and University College of London's Institute for Global Health. 2009. "Commission on Climate Change." *The Lancet*, 373(9676): 1659.

Thompson, A. 2014. "IPCC Says Climate Change Is Here, World Needs to Adapt." Climate Central. http://www.climatecentral.org/news/climate-changes-impacts-are-here-will-worsen-without-adaptation-ipcc-says-1 (accessed November 23, 2015).

Zalasiewicz, J., Williams, M., Steffen, Wil., and Crutzen, P. 2010. "The New World of the Anthropocene." *Environmental Science and Technology*, 44: 2228–2231.

PART I

Theories, Methods, and Anthropological Perspectives on Key Issues in Environment and Health

CHAPTER 1

Ecosocial and Environmental Justice Perspectives on Breast Cancer: Responding to Capitalism's Ill Effects

Mary K. Anglin

> With nearly 80,000 chemicals on the market in the United States, many of which are used by millions of Americans in their daily lives and are un- or understudied and largely unregulated, exposure to potential environmental carcinogens is widespread. One such ubiquitous chemical, bisphenol A (BPA), is still found in many consumer products and remains unregulated in the United States, despite the growing link between BPA and several diseases, including various cancers.
>
> LaSalle D. Leffall, Jr. and Margaret L. Kripke, Preface to *Reducing Environmental Cancer Risk*

In a manner evocative of Rachel Carson's *Silent Spring* (1962), Leffall and Kripke (2010) recently called attention to the massive number of synthetic chemicals circulating throughout the United States, as well as globally, and whose impact on human health and the environment remain largely unknown. While the American Cancer Society criticized the report for being "provocative" and representing "hypothesis" as "consensus" (Sampson 2010), it was based on

A Companion to the Anthropology of Environmental Health, First Edition. Edited by Merrill Singer.

the limited scientific evidence available – and this was precisely the concern identified by Leffall and Kripke. Among other things, their analysis raised the questions: Why has so little cancer research focused on the interaction of environmental factors with human physiology, and what is known or knowable at this juncture? Is it possible to talk meaningfully about breast cancer "prevention" in the absence of such information? One might add: Which interests are served when the proprietary claims of industry outweigh the public's right to know about the various effects of the familiar and not-so-familiar chemicals dispersed throughout our world? Whose voices are authoritative; which are left out of official discussions; and where is there room for popular dissent? And what does any of this mean for an understanding of the links between health and environmental conditions, much of which have been altered by human commerce in its regional and global forms?

With breast cancer as its focus, this chapter provides an account of a controversy in medicine – and its gendered and racialized terms – as well as an exploration of how forms of activism and shifts in paradigms about cancer have opened up new avenues for investigating social and environmental parameters of illness and health. In conjunction with ecosocial approaches articulated by public health researchers, the present analysis draws upon anthropological views concerning the relationship between political economy, health, and the environment, and the use of ethnographic methods to document their interplay through the spaces of daily life. Central to such a discussion has been the development of an anthropology of cancer, with attention to breast cancer specifically, and to which Leo Chavez, Holly Mathews, Juliet McMullin, Diane Weiner, Maren Klawiter, and others have contributed (Klawiter 2008; McMullin and Weiner 2008; Mathews, Burke, and Kampriani 2015). Finally, I draw upon my own ethnographic work in northern California (1992–) on breast cancer, activism, and racial/ethnic inequalities, in conjunction with writings and testimony by and about women living with cancer.

As Rachel Carson argued more than 50 years ago, the pivotal issue is whether and how such knowledge might be employed to reconfigure environmental and related policies for the United States, as well as elsewhere in the global North:

> The choice, after all, is ours to make. If, having endured much, we have at last asserted our "right to know," and if, knowing, we have concluded that we are being asked to take senseless and frightening risks, then we should no longer accept the counsel of those who tell us that we must fill our world with poisonous chemicals; we should look about and see what other course is open to us. (Carson 1962: 277–278)

When *Silent Spring* was first published, Carson did not disclose her own diagnosis of advanced breast cancer, lest the conclusions of long-term scientific research appear to be limited by personal bias. However, breast cancer activists and others articulating the need for environmental justice draw upon both dimensions of Carson's life and work to address matters of equity, health, and sustainability on multiple fronts.

Environmental organizations have for some time argued that the approach of government agencies in the United States is to be "inconclusive by design" in investigating potential hazards associated with synthetic chemicals, and non-interventionist about their production, distribution, or usage (Russell, Lewis, and Keating 1992). Passage of the US Toxics Substances Control Act (TSCA) in 1976 mandated the registration of chemical compounds prior to their widespread manufacture or importation; by 2006, over 82,000 chemicals had been registered through the TSCA Inventory (Environmental Protection Agency/EPA 2007). However, the 1000–1500 applications received each year from prospective manufacturers include "little or no toxicity or fate data" about the compounds themselves, since this is not a formal requirement (EPA 2007: 4). Furthermore, synthetic chemicals existing prior to 1976 were automatically included as part of the TSCA Inventory.[1] To cite a review conducted on behalf of the nonprofit organization, the Breast Cancer Fund, "Complete toxicological screening data are available for just 7 percent of these chemicals and more than 90 percent have never been tested for their effects on human health" (Gray 2010: 14).

In the aftermath of TSCA's passage, regulatory agencies have continued to prioritize economic considerations, with "scientific certainty" about harm as "the only justification for advocating active protective policy measures" (Silverstein 2012: 1; see also Brown 2011; Clapp 2012). Additionally, some manufacturing interests have demonstrated their willingness to forcefully dispute and/or restrict access to scientific data on the toxicities associated with particular compounds (Michaels 2008; Morris and Hamby 2013; Aviv 2014). As a result, the continued viability of chemicals such as bisphenol A (BPA) is not regarded as surprising, despite evidence of health effects and a presumptive link to cancer (National Toxicology Program 2008).

What distinguished the commentary by Leffall and Kripke, then, was not the originality of their argument or muckraking tone. Rather, it was the status of being the *2008–2009 Annual Report from the President's Cancer Panel*, the advisory board established in 1971 to monitor cancer policy and provide guidance to the President of the United States. Reasoning that "the grievous harm from this group of carcinogens has not been adequately addressed by the National Cancer Program," Leffall and Kripke (2010) ended their prefatory letter to President Barack Obama with an appeal for radical change:

> The American people – even before they are born – are bombarded continually with myriad combinations of these dangerous exposures. The Panel urges you most strongly to use the power of your office to remove the carcinogens and other toxins from our food, water, and air that needlessly increase health care costs, cripple our Nation's productivity, and devastate American lives.

Cancer prevention, they argued, requires more than biomedicine's current "narrow focus" on individual decision making and behavior as the principal source of disease risk (Leffler and Kripke 2010: vii). Greater emphasis must be placed on protecting human health and the ecosphere from unwarranted, often unidentified exposures to harmful substances – with the burden of proof shifted toward determining the *safety* of chemical compounds and with much stricter regulation.[2] In short, expert testimony before the 2008–2009 President's Cancer Panel and the Panel's own conclusions recorded the need for "a comprehensive, cohesive policy agenda" reflecting the precautionary principle.[3]

The Panel's report has been described as "a fundamental shift toward a winning strategy" in the "war on cancer," a much-needed "call to action," "an integrated and comprehensive critique," and, conversely, "unbalanced" for the lesser attention given "modifiable risk factors" at the level of individual behavior (Rizzo 2010; Clapp cited in Cone 2010; Schettler cited in Cone 2010; Thun cited in Sampson 2010; Cooney 2010). For the purposes of the present essay, the *2008–2009 Annual Report from the President's Cancer Panel* represents a watershed moment in a decades-old debate over the role of environmental factors in the etiology of chronic diseases, with cancer as the preeminent example. Of particular interest are the various entities and resources that helped to shape its findings. These include the history and different forms of breast cancer advocacy, the efforts of environmental justice advocates, the collaborative activities of lay or citizen science, decades of public health and clinical studies on breast cancer etiology, ongoing research on the health effects of environmental contaminants, development of international law concerning the precautionary principle, and passage of "green" municipal and state ordinances within the United States.

Beyond Pink Ribbon Marketing: Rethinking the Models of Breast Cancer

One in eight: for women living in twenty-first-century United States, these are the odds of being diagnosed with breast cancer over the course of a lifetime (SEER 2014). During the late twentieth century, the likelihood of a breast cancer diagnosis increased sharply – with breast cancer incidence rising from 101.92 (per 100,000) in 1976, to 141.47 in 1999, and declining slightly to 126.02 in 2010 (Howlader *et al.* 2013). Thus, despite President Nixon's signing of the National Cancer Act in 1971 and proclamation of a "war on cancer," the incidence of invasive breast cancer rose by 36 percent between 1973 and 2000 (Howe and Clapp 2012: 131, 134). In the early 1990s, recognition of that trend inspired a social movement to address the rising rates of mortality from the disease, and the limited diagnostic and treatment options then available.

To quote the web site for Silent Spring Institute, a nonprofit research organization drawing its inspiration from Rachel Carson, "women today are more likely to develop breast cancer than any previous generation" (Silent Spring Institute 2014a). According to estimates in December 2012, 2.9 million women in the United States were living and contending with invasive breast cancer, at all stages of disease, and with some women in remission from cancer. An additional 232,340 women received new diagnoses of invasive breast cancer during 2013, and 39,620 women died from this disease (American Cancer Society 2013; SEER/Surveillance Epidemiology, and End Results 2014). Irrespective of media coverage of October as "Breast Cancer Awareness Month" in the United States and the promotion of what has been termed "pink ribbon culture," breast cancer remains a significant public health problem and contributor to mortality (Ehrenreich 2001; King 2006; Brenner 2007; Sulik 2011; Howe and Clapp 2012; Anglin 2013). As Ruthann Rudel and colleagues report, "the global economic costs of premature death and disability from breast cancer" are estimated to be $88 billion annually, with the costs of treatment reaching $17 billion per year in the United States alone (Rudel *et al.* 2014: 3; see also ACS 2010; IBCERCC 2013).

Grass-roots organizations in the United States have, for more than two decades, pursued various means to delineate the human costs of this disease. Linda Reyes, cofounder of one such organization, described the growth of a social movement from women's participation in cancer support groups to the initiation of national conversations for which the narratives, histories, and demands of women with breast cancer have a central role: "All that most people with cancer have to count on is each other. That's why it will be people with cancer who take the leadership in challenging the cancer establishment by dragging cancer out into the open as a social and political issue" (1991: 245).

One example comes from testimony given at the 1995 public hearing on "Women, Health and the Environment," before a panel composed of representatives from the EPA, the Food and Drug Administration (FDA), the federal cancer registry (SEER), the American Cancer Society, the California State Legislature, city/county departments of health, the Indigenous People's Network, and the Human Rights Commission. The panel likewise included the Honorable Bella Abzug of the Women's Environmental and Development Organization (WEDO) and representatives from Greenpeace, as sponsors/coordinators of the event and a series of related conferences nationwide. At this hearing, convened in San Francisco, the first speaker translated rates of cancer incidence and mortality into the losses occurring like clockwork to families throughout the country:

> You've heard the numbers. Every three minutes somewhere in the United States a woman is diagnosed with breast cancer and every twelve minutes a woman dies from breast cancer. That's five women every hour, 120 women every day across the U.S. What does that mean in human terms ...? It means that we're losing our mothers, our sisters, our daughters, our friends. (Testimony #1, Women, Health and the Environment 1995)

"The numbers" themselves were regarded as indisputable; the primary point of contention was whether they indicated biomedicine's successes or the failure to recognize a health crisis with far-reaching consequences. For similar reasons, a coalition established on Long Island in 1990 took the eponymous, if quickly outdated, name of *1 in 9* (One in Nine 2014) to denote their firsthand knowledge of the breast cancer epidemic and the mission of an advocacy organization that even now continues to operate from the grass roots.

In one sense, it was the apparent simplicity of health statistics, as well as their application in a dominant explanatory framework, which the membership of regional coalitions and nationally focused advocacy organizations sought to destabilize. Life stories and accounts of health practices illustrate the range of experience which did not neatly correspond with prevailing interpretations of risk and/or prevention: examples of how diagnostic technologies, at times, produced ambiguous or even misleading results; and the many instances in which biotech modalities have fallen short in the treatment of advanced or aggressive cancer (reversing the conventional logic which assigns such failings to cancer patients themselves). As Reyes (1991: 245) noted, "Other people rarely see how defenseless cancer patients are, especially those who are very sick." Activism brought those accounts and experiences to the forefront.

From the outset, grass-roots organizations and women dealing with cancer questioned biomedical accounts that attribute the rise in breast cancer cases to the efficacy of population-based cancer screening. Equally significant have been the limitations of mid- and late-twentieth-century theories regarding breast cancer etiology, and the continued emphasis on "traditional risk factors" for the disease. Listed as traditional or established risks for breast cancer are factors such as a woman's chronological age, family history of breast cancer, benign breast disease, age at menarche, maternal age at birth of first child, nulliparity or childlessness, age at menopause, genetic influence (with the recently discovered breast cancer genes, BRCA 1 and BRCA 2, as preeminent examples), ethnicity, race, and socioeconomic status (Kelsey and Berkowitz 1988; Kelsey and Gammon 1990; Newman, Millikan, and King 1997). The list of "possible," or likely, risks for breast cancer includes obesity (as measured by body mass index), diet and physical exercise, consumption of alcohol, use of oral contraceptives and, more recently, also hormone replacement therapy (HRT).[4]

In short, epidemiologic research has concentrated on family/personal histories of breast and ovarian cancer and benign breast disease; forms of genetic inheritance that are considered significant, if relatively rare (present in 7–10% of diagnosed cases); women's reproductive health strategies, viewed as lifestyle considerations; other behaviors which are understood to be "modifiable"; and parameters of social stratification. Central to the biomedical argument has been the notion that endogenous (or internally produced) estrogens play a crucial role in the development of invasive breast cancer. Childbearing, along with other forms of reproductive decision making, influences a woman's exposure to estrogens and thereby amplifies risk. Insofar as they are comprised of *exogenous* estrogens, oral contraceptives and HRT would likewise elevate breast cancer risk; such effects are seen as magnified by the addition of progestin (Writing Group for the Women's Health Initiative 2002).

From the standpoint of women diagnosed with breast cancer and others involved in advocacy, one of the biggest concerns with the risk factors approach has been the almost exclusive attention to individual-level characteristics. To quote Dianne Dillon-Ridgley, keynote presenter for the Raleigh, NC conference on "Cancer and the Environment" (1995), the line of reasoning can be summarized as "whatever has caused [breast cancer], you did it." Situated within this nexus of multiple and ambiguously defined etiologic factors is "a particular violence of neglect and indifference," as the eco- and cancer activist

Adele Friedman observed in a posthumously published essay (1991: 52). In apparently reprimanding cancer patients for ways of living adopted in the United States over the course of the twentieth century, the risk factors approach, in Friedman's words (1991: 52), echoes "our national disregard for women's lives."

Added to the critiques of biomedical individualism and disregard for women is the point that roughly 70 percent of breast cancer cases in the US do *not* correlate with the list of "established" risks, undermining their explanatory value beyond quite specific instances (Kelsey and Berkowitz 1988; Kelsey and Gammon 1990; ACS 2014). Indeed, for more than 20 years, clinicians/researchers such as Samuel Hellman (1993) have warned against reliance on the risk factors paradigm in the face of contradictory evidence, characterizing this as a form of "dogma."

Virginia Lewiston, a participant in the initial ethnographic interviews I conducted (1991–1994) and thereafter, commented that it was impossible to "make sense" of her own breast cancer diagnosis by "looking inward," so as to locate the causal forces through her life history and/or strategies for raising a family:

> I had been a political activist for more than ten years and had enough of a political perspective to know that it didn't make sense for me to have breast cancer. There was nothing that made sense for me to have it. Therefore it wasn't a question I could answer by looking inward, the "why question." I had to look outward …
>
> [I shouldn't have had the disease] for all the reasons that 80% [*sic*] of the women diagnosed with breast cancer shouldn't have had it. It was not in my family. I had done all the right things. I had kids at the right age; I had nursed kids at the right age for the right length of time. Being an academic household, there was enough money for a good diet and enough understanding of the food groups and stuff like that. There was just *no* reason of any of the acknowledged risk factors. They weren't there. Therefore, I shouldn't have had the disease, *but I did.* (Anglin, Interview 0–14, emphasis in original).

Lewiston relied upon an explicitly feminist perspective to examine the logic of the predominant model and to dismiss, on empirical as well as political grounds, its gendered assumptions. At the same time, she recognized the class privileges associated with being part of "an academic household," affecting both her ability to "do all the right things" as well as her health before and after the cancer diagnosis.

Following Lewiston, Dillon-Ridgley, and others, one might argue that if traditional risk factors have not readily explained the cases of middle-class, "White non-Hispanic" women over the age of 50 – the demographic group in the United States for which the rate of breast cancer incidence remains highest (ACS 2013) – still less would this framework account for the experiences of women who are neither Euro-American nor elite. Within the realm of public health research, Krieger, Chen, and Waterman (2010: S132) reported on racial/ethnic differences for the recent (post-1999) and modest decline in breast cancer incidence attributed to decreasing HRT use. As those authors explained, given the fact of unequal access to high-tech medicine in the United States, HRT was rarely a treatment option and thus would not constitute a risk factor for women from African American, Hispanic, Asian/Pacific Islander, Native American/Alaska Native, and low-income populations.

Likewise, McKenzie and Jeffrys (2009) concluded from their meta-analysis of clinical studies and epidemiologic research that "lifestyle"-related factors and "socioeconomic position" jointly contribute to racial/ethnic disparities in breast cancer mortality, albeit in ways that had yet to be ascertained.[5] Exploring the foundation of these inequalities would require an intersectional approach attuned to multiple facets of social location, as Harold Freeman (2014) noted in his recent commentary for the *New York Times.* From the vantage point of a cancer surgeon who had spent much of his career working in Harlem and the former director of the National Cancer Institute's Center to Reduce Cancer Health Disparities, Freeman wrote: "I began to see that cancer's invasiveness was deeply rooted in human conditions, and began asking questions such as: What does it mean to be black in America? What does it mean to be poor? And what does it mean to be black and poor and at the same time to have cancer?" (Freeman 2014: A27).

That African American women have the highest rate of mortality from breast cancer in the United States – a gap that emerged in the late 1980s and continues to widen – is, by all accounts, indicative of racism's synergistic effects combined with gender-based discrimination, the stress of living in poverty, and difficulty in obtaining timely, appropriate health care and other resources.[6] More difficult to explain through the emphasis on risk factors or even an awareness of barriers to health care is the finding that, among US women under 40, African American women have the highest incidence of breast cancer. Likewise, African American women are at much greater risk of being diagnosed with the "triple negative" subtype of breast cancer, which does not respond well to chemotherapy or the current forms of biological treatment.[7] From the standpoint of biomedicine, the prevailing explanations have pointed to variation at the level of oncogenes, cancer cells, and subtypes of breast cancer: a contemporary reading of race as biologically based.

By way of contrast, ecosocial perspectives in public health have advanced the argument that *all* biological phenomena, including diseases, are dynamic entities and not solely determined by a combination of genetic and behavioral factors (Krieger *et al.* 1997; Krieger, Chen, and Waterman 2011; Krieger 2013: 22, 23; see also Gilbert and Epel 2009; Piersma and van Gils 2010; Smith 2012). Consistent with the work of anthropologists on "local biologies," the aim of ecosocial perspectives has been to examine "embodied histories" as reflections of societal and ecological forces, cellular pathologies, and particular constellations of the life course.[8] Thus, for example, a critically important biomarker of breast cancer such as estrogen receptor (ER) status is no longer considered the "fixed trait of tumors," as the risk factors paradigm might suggest. Instead, it is understood to be a "flexible characteristic of cells" responding to shifts in hormonal levels and, equally importantly, to *nonhormonal* exposures.[9] As with health inequities generally, racial/ethnic disparities in breast cancer are thus viewed as emergent and mutable: outcomes of socioeconomic and health-related policies, rather than "innate differences." The key, as Lewiston once noted, is in looking outward.

"Hot Spots": Place, Environment, and Breast Cancer

In the early 1990s, cancer activists articulated the need for "real prevention," by which they meant a departure from short-term trajectories of containment (through early diagnosis) and a concerted effort to resolve this health crisis for successive generations. Public debates on mammography, such as those aired at the 1994 San Francisco hearing, concerned ways of interpreting shifts in the patterns of disease over time; only secondarily did they address the value of a particular technology for population-based screening or the ascertainment of individual cases.[10] Equally important, activists began calling attention to a newly evident *geography of risk*: metropolitan areas and regions with well-documented and precipitous growth in the incidence of breast cancer, sometimes described as cancer clusters or "hot spots" (Anglin 1998; see also Farmer 2006 [1992]). At the same time, they posed questions about the environmental factors or other conditions that might account for those differences. Notions about personal responsibility for a cancer diagnosis were in this way dislodged by increasing public awareness that, as Judy Brady put it (1991: 27), "we are, in fact, victims of a social crime, the crime of poisoning our environment." As Sandra Steingraber explained from her dual position as cancer survivor and field biologist, to engage in such activities was no simple matter because it "mean[t] learning to get beyond the silence of reprieve in order to challenge the social and economic structures that allow cancer to lay claim to a third of us" (1991: 41, 39; see also 1997).

Thus, in the 1990s, the membership of One in Nine responded to state reports of increased breast cancer incidence on Long Island through their own community-based, participatory research on local cancer clusters; protests convened at the Nassau County courthouse; a public demand for research on environmental links to breast cancer (culminating in the multi-year, federally funded Long Island Breast Cancer Study Project); and the call for more extensive monitoring of pesticides and other contaminants within New York State.[11] Similarly, members of the Massachusetts Breast Cancer Coalition (MBCC), formed in 1991, called upon their state legislature "to declare breast cancer an epidemic" and to fund scientific research investigating the elevated rates of incidence documented for Cape Cod (MBCC 2014). Three years later, with financial support made available through the Massachusetts Department of Public Health, MBCC "founded 'a laboratory of their own' and named it Silent Spring Institute in tribute to Rachel Carson" (Silent Spring 2014b; see also MBCC 2014). In California, cancer activists worked with a state advocacy network (California Breast Cancer Organizations or CABCO), other constituent groups, and members of the state assembly on 1993 legislation to establish a statewide research institute – the California Breast Cancer Research Program, or CBCRP – with funding derived from a $.02 increase (per pack of cigarettes) to the state tobacco tax, along with taxpayer contributions.[12] As has been the case for Silent Spring Institute, from its inception, CBCRP focused on developing a national model for collaborative and groundbreaking scientific research with practical application; "the identification and elimination of environmental causes of breast cancer" remains one of its priorities (California Breast Cancer Research Program 2014b; Milliken 2004; McPartland, Dantzker, and Portier 2015).

At the national level, WEDO and Greenpeace launched their 1994 campaign bringing together representatives from environmental justice organizations and "grassroots and national women's groups," along with "leading scientific experts," in a series of meetings whose ultimate goals were to influence US health policy as well as shape the recommendations ensuing from the UN's Fourth World Conference on Women (Women Health and Environment: Action for Cancer Prevention 1994, United Nations 1995).[13] One could make the case that another byproduct, eight years later, was the convening of an "International Summit on Breast Cancer and the Environment": the outcome of collaborative planning by environmental justice advocates, representatives from breast cancer organizations, and public health researchers from the University of California, Berkeley. Consensus findings from the International Summit, subsequently presented to a joint hearing of the California state legislature, included the call for innovative scientific research "that mirrors real-world exposures to environmental agents" and implementation of the precautionary principle in "public health/prevention" policies (Buffler 2002; Buffler *et al.* 2003; see also Joint Informational Hearing 2002; Milliken 2004).

In her ethnography of breast cancer organizations in the Bay Area of California, Maren Klawiter (2008) presented a quite different perspective on the role of science in "cultures of action." Bay Area organizations, in this rendering, largely eschewed scientific research – and especially that of cancer epidemiology – as delaying tactics and looked, instead, to political action as a strategy for reducing toxic exposures and thereby preventing breast cancer. An example of the latter was the annual "Toxic Tour of the Cancer Industry," whose purpose was to "stop cancer where it starts" (Klawiter 2008: 203, see also 204–211). Using the devices of street theatre, activists picketed the headquarters of companies that were alleged to produce carcinogens and/or profit from an ever-increasing market for cancer therapies. By way of contrast, the "institutional domains of public health and medicine," including the aforementioned International Summit on Breast Cancer and the Environment, were regarded as "colonizing new domains of risk" and legitimating biopolitical regimes (Klawiter 2008: 256–257).

Klawiter's account might be viewed as a presentation of "the politics of skepticism" regarding the limitations and cultural biases inherent to Western scientific methods, as well as the manipulation of technical expertise throughout the regulatory process, as Melissa Checker (2012) and other scholars of environmental justice have argued (see also Brulle and Pellow 2006; Brodkin 2009; Wilson 2010; Johnson and Ranco 2011; Cohen and Ottinger 2011). Thus, the widespread use of risk assessment methodologies to evaluate environmental hazards has been soundly criticized on a variety of grounds. Among the problems noted are the potential for miscalculating the toxicities of specific chemicals, given the limits of testing to date; the tendency to underestimate both the means and levels of community exposures (dose); limitations in accounting for the synergistic and cumulative effects of repeated exposure to multiple chemicals; the under-rating of health effects due to the long latency period for many chronic diseases, including cancer; and the requirement of absolute proof of harm before remedial actions are undertaken (Checker 2007; Johnson and Ranco 2011; Rudel and Perovich 2012). In the 1995 "Cancer and the Environment" conference, risk assessment techniques were denounced as bureaucratic practices whereby "I decide how much poison you're going to get" (Anglin 1998: 195).

Furthermore, breast cancer activists have been vocal in their criticism of the early epidemiologic work investigating potential linkages between exposure to environmental contaminants and breast cancer. Studies by Nancy Krieger and colleagues at Kaiser (1994) and David Hunter and colleagues from Harvard (1997: 1253), for example, did not support the hypothesis of a link between "'environmental estrogens' such as organochlorines in pesticides and industrial chemicals" and increased breast cancer risk, as had previously been reported by Wolff *et al.* (1993). Their findings – along with the published responses of a segment of clinicians and researchers who took "reassurance" from them (Key and Reeves 1994: 1520; see also Anderson 1994; MacMahon 1994; Sternberg 1994; Taubes 1994) – were described by witnesses at the San Francisco hearing as evidence of a conservative trend in science (Anglin 1998: 193–196).

On a similar note, the membership of One in Nine and other activists who pressed for the Long Island Study Project (LIBCSP) found that institutional procedures for peer review effectively precluded "lay" involvement in the $31 million research program (1992–2002), and that decisions about study design or the chemical contaminants to be investigated were the province of researchers. The end result, according to Baralt and McCormick (2010: 1669), was that "advocates questioned whether the research methods and the variables selected by the scientists advanced the knowledge of possible carcinogeneity [*sic*] of environmental exposures," in particular, their decision to study a chemical that had long been outlawed in the United States. On the other hand, the investigators received criticism about the undue influence of the public over their work (McCormick *et al.* 2004). Yet, if this example of "community-initiated breast cancer and environment studies" did not fully adhere to the principles of participatory research, it nonetheless served as a landmark in the development of alternative approaches to the research process (Gammon *et al.* 2002; Brody, Tickner, and Rudel 2005; Winn 2005).

Thus, "science as usual" was disrupted by activist calls for "different science" and the promotion of models for the "democratization of science" (Anglin 1998; McCormick *et al.* 2004).[14] Perhaps the most radically inclusive orientation has been that taken by Silent Spring Institute, where community interests are treated as formally as the criteria of biological plausibility and (preliminary) scientific evidence in determining research priorities. "Including community concern as a decision-making criterion helps avoid studies that, although elegantly designed, do not answer relevant questions," as Brody *et al.* (2005: 923) have observed. A further elaboration of this model is illustrated by the NIEHS-funded Northern California Household Exposure Study of 2006, through its efforts to combine "exposure assessment science" with the concerns of environmental justice and breast cancer advocacy (Brody *et al.* 2009). Congruent with the emphasis of NIEHS on community-based participatory research, the latter research team evaluated its own implementation of "community science" as a framework for investigating specific exposures to endocrine-disrupting compounds and other pollutants.[15]

That such approaches produce "good science" is attested by their records of publication on topics including the body burden of specific chemicals; reviews of the epidemiologic literature on environmental pollutants and breast cancer, with attention to methodologic problems and their potential resolution; new exposure biomarkers which could be implemented in breast cancer research; and the use of animal data to create "new directions for epidemiology, chemicals testing, and risk assessment for breast cancer prevention" (Rudel *et al.* 2007; see also Wolff *et al.* 2005; Brody *et al.* 2007; Zota *et al.* 2008; Rudel *et al.* 2014). In effect, they combine the insights of traditional approaches to breast cancer – namely, the emphasis on estrogenic exposures as increasing risk – with the multi-decade documentation of pesticides and other environmental contaminants as endocrine disruptors and, finally, the attention given by ecosocial perspectives to societal forces, ecological conditions, and the dynamism of local biologies over the life course.[16]

Then, again, "in mobilizing science for their own ends, grassroots groups have been creating alternative methods for knowing about and representing the health effects of pollution" (Cohen and Ottinger 2011: 8). While Cohen and Ottinger refer specifically to the US environmental justice movement, their argument extends to breast cancer organizations and cancer activists who have been strongly influenced – as has the American public, in general – by the transformative practices of that movement (Wilson 2010). Thus, in the midst of equivocation regarding the impact of environmental contaminants on human health, the Breast Cancer Fund produced its own version of "clear science": a series of monographs (2002–2010) summarizing "The State of the Evidence" about everyday exposures to radiation and chemicals and their potential connection to breast cancer (Breast Cancer Fund 2015a, 2015b). In her introduction to the 2010 edition, Janet Gray (2010: 10) characterized the report's primary objective as that of "provid[ing] the groundwork for economic and political changes that can lower the future incidence of breast cancer for our children and grandchildren" and noted that "we also join the collective effort to turn the tide on a number of other diseases."

Equally important, activists have brought their own life stories and specialized knowledge into scientific proceedings such as the International Summit on Breast Cancer and the Environment. Karen Holly's presentation, "as an 'at risk' African American female who was 34 years old when diagnosed with an aggressive stage III breast cancer," illustrated the complexities of embodied history and, more than this, altered the terms of subsequent discussion.[17] Thus, she concluded with the following series of questions:

> So I ask you: if the air is polluted and the waters are tainted, if economics only allow me to afford to live in Richmond near chemical plants, and if my fruits and veggies are being sprayed and my beef and chicken are hormonally being enhanced, just what else can I do? What exposures, or combinations of exposures, must be looked at and studied? What are the studies being conducted to protect our future? Is poverty a carcinogen? (Holly 2002)

Holly well understood the synergies of race, class, gender, and cancer; the issue was whether scientists or policy makers would recognize or apply intersectional approaches in their approaches to environmental risk. In posing questions about "economics," she connected practices which target low-income communities of color as a "dumping ground" for toxic industry with the increased incidence of breast cancer among African American women under 40 (see also Pierce 2002). For those attending the International Summit, it was a powerful moment.

From a greater remove, perhaps the most noteworthy contributions of grassroots groups and advocacy organizations have been their articulation of the need for "real prevention" through the precautionary principle and continued support for publicly accountable, innovative science on environmental health. The precautionary principle shifts the focus away from the need for strong evidence of harm, in the form of adverse health effects, to the primacy of safety in regulatory procedures (Raffensperger and Tickner 1999). Kriebel *et al.* (2001: 871) summarize this logic as: "If a clearly safer alternative exists, why accept even a small, highly uncertain risk?"

In the context of breast cancer activism, "precautionary thinking" has meant the emphasis on health, as measured by the well-being of successive generations of women and their communities, and an expanded view of the research endeavor as a form of advocacy (Brody *et al.* 2005: 921). Thus, passage of the Breast Cancer and Environmental Research Act of 2008 – a bill that had previously been introduced, debated, and defeated over the course of nine years – is as much a testament to the doggedness of the grass roots and the partnerships formed with progressive scientists, as it is a reflection of the federal commitment to collaborative and groundbreaking environmental science (see also Platner *et al.* 2002; IBCERCC 2013). And it is in this context that we might place the findings from the President's Cancer Panel convened in 2008–2009, and the renewal of Rachel Carson's call for "our 'right to know.'"

NOTES

1 EPA (2007). Valerie Brown (2011: A485) makes note of the fact that TSCA has not been revised since its passage in 1976, "due in part to legislative gridlock and lack of consensus among stakeholders." At best, TSCA is viewed as an "ineffective and obsolescent" vehicle of regulation that has served to obstruct progress toward the creation and use of safer chemicals (Brown 2011: A485–A486; see also Scientific Understanding Work Group, The National Conversation on Public Health and Chemical Exposures 2011). Congressional efforts began in 2015 to modify or "reform" TSCA.

2 See McPartland, Dantzker, and Portier (2015) for their recommendations for developing a more "robust" chemical testing program at the EPA.

3 Leffall and Kripke (2010: vii, xi). The precautionary principle emphasizes "the assurance of safety" and preventative measures, where the threat exists for substantial harm and "even in the face of scientific uncertainty" (Goldstein 2001: 1358, Kriebel *et al.* 2001: 871; see also Cameron and Abouchar 1991; Raffensperger and Tickner 1999; Foster, Vecchia and Repacholi 2000; Grandjean 2004; Rabinowitz and Conti 2013). In summarizing results from the 2009–2011 *National Conversation on Public Health and Chemical Exposures*, Brown notes that a precautionary approach could include "a shift toward reintegrating environmental and occupational health with public health" (2011: a485; Leadership Council 2011).

4 On the relationship between HRT use and breast cancer incidence, see Clarke *et al.* (2006); Glass *et al.* (2007); Ravdin *et al.* (2007); Stewart *et al.* (2007).

5 Among other concerns, McKenzie and Jeffrys (2009: 57) observe that, "It is very common for studies to adjust for many factors simultaneously, which does not enable investigation of which specific factors could be important determinants of ethnic inequalities in survival." Furthermore, given the failure of cancer registries in the United States to routinely collect socioeconomic data, analyses of the relationship between social class and breast cancer incidence (or mortality) are, at best, speculative (see Krieger and Fee 1994; Krieger *et al.* 1999; Isaacs and Schroeder 2004; Anglin 2006; Clegg *et al.* 2009).

6 See ACS (2009, 2014). The negative impact on health has been variously described as the "weathering effect" (Geronimus 2001); "the Sojourner Truth Syndrome" (Mullings and Wali 2000; Mullings 2006); and the state of being "sick and tired of being sick and tired," as the civil rights activist Fannie Lou Hamer observed of her community and her own unsuccessful battle with breast cancer (DeMuth 1964).

7 Triple negative breast cancer is defined as a rare subtype of breast cancer that does not present or "express" receptors for estrogen, progesterone, or the epidermal growth factor, HER2/neu. See especially Carey *et al.* 2006 for their report on the Carolina Breast Cancer Study that examined racial differences in breast cancer subtypes and the higher prevalence of triple negative breast cancer among premenopausal African American women. While Tamimi, Colditz, and Hazra (2012) argue for a relationship between traditional risk factors and some molecular subtypes of breast cancer, it is with an important caveat. They note (2012: 159): "Identifying risk factors for less common subtypes such as luminal B, HER2-type and basal-like tumors [e.g., triple-negative breast cancers] has important implications for prevention of these more aggressive subtypes."

8 See Gaines (1992); Lindenbaum and Lock (1993); Lock (1995); Lock and Nguyen (2010).

9 See Krieger (2013: 23, 25); Carey *et al.* (2006).

10 At the San Francisco hearing, for example, Abzug noted that no specific evidence was provided for the contention that the secular trend of increased breast cancer incidence could be attributed to women's greater access to mammography screening in the United States (Chair's Remarks, Comment Period, Women, Health, and the Environment). See also Anglin (1998: 185–186, 197, note 3 on p. 204); Anglin unpublished field notes (1995).

It should be noted that there are other important dimensions of this critique of mammography – namely, that it relies on ionizing radiation, which is carcinogenic and to which breast tissue is especially sensitive; that it is an imprecise technology which produces both false negative and false positive laboratory results; and that far too many diagnoses have been made of precancerous conditions that would not have developed into invasive breast cancer. See, for example, Fletcher's (2011) review of the impact of 35 years of mammography screening.

11 McQuiston (1992); One in Nine (2014); see also Gammon *et al.* (2002); Winn (2005); Osuch *et al.* (2012).

12 See the California Breast Cancer Research Program (2014a). See also the California Health and Safety Code Section 104145, and the California Revenue and Taxation Codes Section 30461-30462.1 and Section 18791-18796 (amended AB-28 Oct 11, 2007). In the most recent "Annual Report to the State of California Legislature," Kavanaugh-Lynch, Croughan, and Beckwith (2010) report that the California Breast Cancer Research Program (CBCRP) provided $16,872,114 for California-based research projects during 2010, and $215 million in grants since the inception of the program. Subsequent to 2010, reports from the CBCRP to the State of California Legislature are submitted every five years, rather than annually.

13 The San Francisco hearing was selected as the inaugural event, partly as the result of a report from the Northern California Cancer Center (1995) documenting the rate of breast cancer incidence in San Francisco Bay Area as the highest in the world.

14 For example, the National Institute of Environmental Health Sciences (NIEHS) and the National Cancer Institute (NCI) have jointly funded four Breast Cancer and Environmental Research Centers (BCERC) that have, as one of their aims, the fostering of partnerships between scientists and advocates in environmental health research. See Baralt and McCormick (2010), Wolff and Barlow (2011), and Osuch *et al.* (2012) for divergent views about the success of the BCERC as form of research collaboration and especially the impact of advocates' views on studies undertaken by the Centers.

15 See Brown *et al.* (2012); Adams *et al.* (2011). One of the issues the research collaborative addressed, ultimately with success, was the reluctance of one university institutional review board (IRB) to accept the full partnership of community organizations, especially regarding access to and use of study data (Brown *et al.* 2010).

16 As Birnbaum (2013: 321) has argued, human exposure to persistent organic pollutants may function like a kind of "uncontrolled medicine" disrupting the endocrine system and "resulting in a staggering increase in several diseases." Looking at specific periods of human development, or windows of exposure, helps to account for differences in body burden of persistent organic pollutants. Moreover, attention to the impact of particular chemicals on breast development, during these sensitive periods, may explain increased breast cancer risk. See also Wolff *et al.* (2005), Brody, Rudel, and Kavanaugh-Lynch (2011), and Pestana *et al.* (2013).

17 I am drawing here from Karen Holly's later testimony as part of "Breast Cancer and the Environment: Second Informational Hearing," a Joint Informational Hearing of the Senate Health and Services Committee and the Assembly Health Committee, San Francisco, October 23, 2002. This is identical to her presentation for the International Summit on Breast Cancer and the Environment.

REFERENCES

Adams, C. Brown, P., Morello-Frosch, R., Brody, J.G. Rudel, R., Zota, A., Dunagan, S., Tovar, J., and Patton, S. 2011. "Disentangling the Exposure Experience: The Roles of Community Context and Report-back of Environmental Exposure Data." *Journal of Health and Social Behavior*, 52: 180–196.

ACS (American Cancer Society). 2009. *Cancer Facts and Figures for African Americans, 2009–2010.* Atlanta, GA: American Cancer Society.

ACS (American Cancer Society). 2010. *Breast Cancer Facts and Figures, 2009–2010.* Atlanta, GA: American Cancer Society.

ACS (American Cancer Society). 2013. *Breast Cancer Facts and Figures, 2013–2014.* Atlanta, GA: American Cancer Society.

ACS (American Cancer Society). 2014. *Breast Cancer Facts and Figures, 2013–2014.* Atlanta, GA: American Cancer Society.

Anderson, L.F. 1994. "DDT and Breast Cancer: The Verdict Isn't In." *Journal of the National Cancer Institute*, 86: 576–577.

Anglin, M.K. 1998. "Dismantling the Master's House: Cancer Activists, Discourses of Prevention, and Environmental Justice,." *Identities: Global Studies in Culture and Power*, 5: 183–218.

Anglin, M.K. 2006. "Whose Health? Whose Justice? Examining Quality of Care and Breast Cancer Activism through the Intersections of Gender, Race, Ethnicity, and Class." In A. Schulz and L. Mullings (Eds.), *Health at the Intersections of Gender, Race, and Class* (pp. 313–341). New York: Jossey-Bass/Pfeiffer.

Anglin, M.K. 2013. "Learning Social Justice and Activist Ethnography from Women with Breast Cancer." In C. Craven and D.-A. Davis (Eds.), *Feminist Activist Ethnography: New Priorities for Feminist Methods & Activism* (pp. 39–52). Lanham, MD: Lexington Books.

Aviv, R. 2014. "A Valuable Reputation: After Tyrone Hayes Said a Chemical Was Harmful, Its Makers Pursued Him." Annals of Science, *The New Yorker*, February 10. http://www.newyorker.com/magazine/2014/02/10/a-valuable-reputation (accessed June 1, 2014).

Baralt, L.B. and McCormick, S. 2010. "A Review of Advocate-Scientist Collaboration in Federally Funded Environmental Breast Cancer Research Centers." *Environmental Health Perspectives*, 118: 1668–1675.

Birnbaum, L.S. 2013. "When Environmental Chemicals Act Like Uncontrolled Medicine." *Trends in Endocrinology and Medicine*, 24: 321–323.

Brady, J. (Ed.) 1991. *One in Three: Women with Cancer Confront an Epidemic.* Pittsburgh, PA: Cleis Press.

Breast Cancer Fund. 2015a. "Clear Science." http://www.breastcancerfund.org/clear-science/ (accessed January 1, 2015).

Breast Cancer Fund. 2015b. "Breast Cancer and Our Environment." http://www.breastcancerfund.org/clear-science/environmental-breast-cancer-links/ (accessed January 1, 2015).

Breast Cancer and Environmental Research Act of 2008, Pub L. No. 110-354, 122 Stat. 3984 (October 8, 2008). http://www.gpo.gov/fdsys/pkg/PLAW-110publ354/pdf/PLAW-110publ354.pdf.

Brenner, B. 2007. "Think Before You Buy Pink." The Burrill Report (October 1, 2007). http://www.burrillreport.com/article-think_before_you_buy_pink.html (accessed February 7, 2014).

Brodkin, K. 2009. *Power Politics: Environmental Activism in South Los Angeles.* New Brunswick, NJ: Rutgers University Press.

Brody, J.G., Morello-Frosch, R., Zota, A., Brown, P., Perez, C., and Rudel, R.A. 2009. "Linking Exposure Assessment Science with Policy Objectives for Environmental Justice and Breast Cancer Advocacy: The Northern California Household Exposure Study." *American Journal of Public Health*, 99, Supplement 3: S600–S609.

Brody, J.G., Moysich, K.B., Humblet, O., Attfield, K.R., Beehler, G., and Rudel, R.A. 2007. "Environmental Pollutants and Breast Cancer." *Environmental Factors in Breast Cancer* Supplement to Cancer 109 # 12: 2667–2711.

Brody, J.G., Rudel, R., and Kavanaugh-Lynch, M. 2011. "Testing Chemicals for Effects on Breast Development, Lactation, and Cancer." *Environmental Health Perspectives*, 119: A326–A327.

Brody, J.G., Tickner, J., and Rudel, R.A. 2005. "Community-Initiated Breast Cancer and Environmental Studies and the Precautionary Principle." *Environmental Health Perspectives*, 113: 920–925.

Brown, P., Brody, J.G., Morello-Frosch, R., Tovar, J., Zota, A.R., and Rudel, R.A. 2012. "Measuring the Success of Community Science: The Northern California Household Exposure Study." *Environmental Health Perspectives*, 120: 326–331.

Brown, V.J. 2011. "Are We on the Same Page? Action Agenda of the National Conversation on Public Health and Chemical Exposures." *Environmental Health Perspectives*, 119: a484–a487.

Brulle, R.J. and Pellow, D.N. 2006. "Environmental Justice: Human Health and Environmental Inequalities." *Annual Review of Public Health* 27: 103–124.

Buffler, P. 2002. "Report from the U.S. Centers for Disease Control and Prevention International Summit on Breast Cancer and the Environment." Testimony to the Senate and Senate Health and Human Services Committee and Assembly Health Committee, Joint Informational Hearing on Breast Cancer and the Environment, San Francisco, CA: San Francisco City Hall, October 23, 2002.

Buffler, P. *et al.* 2003. "International Summit on Breast Cancer and the Environment: Research Needs." May 22–25, 2002, Santa Cruz, CA.

California Breast Cancer Research Program. 2014a. "About Us." http://cbcrp.org/about/index.html (accessed October 20, 2014).

California Breast Cancer Research Program. 2014b. "Special Research Initiatives." http://cbcrp.org/priorities/sri/index.html.

Cameron, J. and Abouchar, J. 1991. "The Precautionary Principle: A Fundamental Principle of Law and Policy for the Protection of the Global Environment." 14 *Boston College International and Comparative Law Review*.

Carey, L.A., Perou, C.M., Livasy, C.A., Dressler, L.G., Cowan, D., Conway, K., Karaca, G., … Millikan, R.C. 2006. "Race, Breast Cancer Subtypes and Survival in the Carolina Breast Cancer Study." *Journal of the American Medical Association* 294: 2492–2502.

Carson, R. 1962. *Silent Spring*. Boston, MA: Houghton Mifflin.

Checker, M. 2007. "'But I Know It's True': Environmental Risk Assessment, Justice, and Anthropology." *Human Organization*, 66: 112–124.

Checker, M. 2012. "'Make Us Whole': Environmental Justice and the Politics of Skepticism." *Capitalism Nature Socialism*, 23: 35–51.

Clapp, R.W. (Ed.) 2012. *From Critical Science to Solutions: The Best of Scientific Solutions*. Amity, NY: Baywood Publishing.

Clarke, C.A., Glaser, S.L., Uratsu, C.S., Selby, J.V., Kushi, L.H., and Herrinton, L.J. 2006. "Recent Declines in Hormone Therapy Utilization and Breast Cancer Incidence: Clinical and Population-based Evidence." Letter to the Editor. *Journal of Clinical Oncology*, 24: e49–50.

Clegg, L.X., Reichman, M.E., Miller, B.A., Hankey, B.F., Singh, G.K., Lin, Y.D., Goodman, M.T., … Edwards, B.K. 2009. "Impact of Socioeconomic Status on Cancer Incidence and Stage at Diagnosis: Selected Findings from the Surveillance, Epidemiology, and End Results: National Longitudinal Mortality Study." *Cancer Causes and Control*, 20: 417–435.

Cohen, B. and Ottinger, G. 2011. "Introduction: Environmental Justice and the Transformation of Science and Engineering." In G. Ottinger and B.R. Cohen (Eds.), *Technoscience and Environmental Justice: Expert Cultures in a Grassroots Movement* (pp. 1–18). Cambridge, MA: MIT Press.

Cone, M. 2010. "President's Cancer Panel: Environmentally Caused Cancers Are 'Grossly Underestimated' and 'Needlessly Devastate American Lives'." *Environmental Health News*, May 6. http://www.environmentalhealthnews.org/ehs/news/presidents-cancer-panel (accessed February 1, 2014).

Cooney, C.M. 2010. "Research Issues and Initiatives: Cancer Report Examines Environmental Hazards." *Environmental Health Perspectives*, 118 (8): A336.

DeMuth, J. 1964. "'Tired of Being Sick and Tired.'" *The Nation, June* 1: 549.

Ehrenreich, B. 2001. "Welcome to Cancerland: A Mammogram Leads to a Cult of Pink Kitsch." *Harper's Magazine* (November): 43–53.

Environmental Protection Agency (EPA). 2007. Office of Pollution Preventions and Toxics: OPPT Accomplishments Report 2005–2006. http://epa.gov/oppt/ar/oppt_ar_20052006.pdf (accessed February 1, 2014).

Farmer, P. 2006 [1992]. *AIDS and Accusation: Haiti and the Geography of Blame.* Berkeley: University of California Press.

Fletcher, S.A. 2011. "Breast Cancer Screening – A 35-Year Perspective." *Epidemiologic Reviews*, 33: 165–175.

Foster, K., Vecchia, P., and Repacholi, M.H. 2000. "Risk Management: Science and the Precautionary Principle." *Science* 288 (May 12): 979–981.

Freeman, H.P. 2014. "Why Black Women Die of Cancer." The Opinion Pages. *New York Times*, March 13. http://www.nytimes.com/2014/03/14/opinion/why-black-women-die-of-cancer.html?_r=0 (accessed March 14, 2014).

Friedman, A. 1991. "Cancer as Violence Against Women." In J. Brady (Ed.), *One in Three: Women with Cancer Confront an Epidemic* (pp. 51–57). Pittsburgh, PA: Cleis Press.

Gaines, A.D. (Ed.) 1992. *Ethnopsychiatry: The Cultural Construction of Professional and Folk Pyschiatries.* Albany, NY: State University of New York Press.

Gammon, M., Neugut, A.I., Santarella, R.M., Teitlebaum, S.L., *et al.* 2002. "The Long Island Breast Cancer Study Project: Description of a Multi-Institutional Collaboration to Identify Environmental Risk Factors for Breast Cancer." *Breast Cancer Research and Treatment*, 74: 235–254.

Geronimus, A.T. 2001. "Understanding and Eliminating Racial Inequalities in Women's Health in the United States: The Role of the Weathering Conceptual Framework." *Journal of the American Women's Medical Association*, 56(4): 133–136.

Gilbert, S.F. and Epel, D. 2009. *Ecological Developmental Biology: Integrating Epigenetics, Medicine, and Evolution.* Sunderland, MA: Sinauer Associates.

Glass, A.G., Lacey, J.V. Jr., Carreon, J.D., and Hoover, R.N. 2007. "Breast Cancer Incidence, 1980–2006: Combined Roles of Menopausal Hormone Therapy, Screening Mammography, and Estrogen Receptor Status." *Journal of the National Cancer Institute*, 99: 1152–1161.

Goldstein, B.D. 2001. "The Precautionary Principle also Applies to Public Health Actions." *American Journal of Public Health*, 91: 1358–1361.

Grandjean, P. 2004. "Implications of the Precautionary Principle for Primary Prevention and Research." *Annual Review of Public Health*, 25: 199–223.

Gray, J. 2010. *State of the Evidence: The Connection between Breast Cancer and the Environment*, 6th ed. San Francisco, CA: Breast Cancer Fund.

Hellman, S. 1993. "Dogma and Inquisition in Medicine." *Cancer*, 71: 2430–2433.

Holly, K. 2002. "Personal Testimony Regarding Breast Cancer and the Environment." Testimony to the Senate and Senate Health and Human Services Committee and Assembly Health Committee, Joint Informational Hearing on Breast Cancer and the Environment. San Francisco, CA: San Francisco City Hall, October 23, 2002.

Howe, G.K. and Clapp, R.W. 2012. "Are We Winning or Losing the War on Cancer? Deciphering the Propaganda of the NCI's 33-Year War." In R.W. Clapp (Ed.), *From Critical Science to Solutions: The Best of Scientific Solutions* (pp. 131–146). Amity, NY: Baywood Publishing.

Howlader, N. Noone, A.M., Krapcho, M., Garshell, J., Neyman, N., Altekruse, S.F., Kosary, C.L., ... Cronin, K.A., eds. 2013. "4. Breast." In SEER Cancer Statistics

Review, 1975–2010, National Cancer Institute, Bethesda, MD. http://seer.cancer.gov/csr/1975_2010/, based on November 2012 SEER data submission, posted to the SEER web site, April 2013.

Hunter, D.J., Hankinson, S.E., Laden, F., Colditz, G.A., Manson, J.E., Willett, W.C., Speizer, F.E., and Wolff, M.S. 1997. "Plasma Organochlorine Levels and the Risk of Breast Cancer." *New England Journal of Medicine*, 337: 1253–1258.

IBCERC / Interagency Breast Cancer and Environment Coordinating Committee. 2013. *Breast Cancer and the Environment: Prioritizing Prevention*. Research Triangle Park, NC: National Institute of Environmental Health Sciences.

Isaacs, S.L. and Schroeder, S.A. 2004. "Class – The Ignored Determinant of the Nation's Health." *New England Journal of Medicine*, 351: 1137–1142.

Johnson, J.R. and Ranco, D.J. 2011. "Risk Assessment and Native Americans at the Cultural Crossroads: Making Better Science or Redefining Health?" In G. Ottinger and B.R. Cohen (Eds.), *Technoscience and Environmental Justice: Expert Cultures in a Grassroots Movement* (pp. 179–199). Cambridge, MA: MIT Press.

Joint Informational Hearing of the Senate Health and Human Services Committee and Assembly Health Committee: "Breast Cancer and the Environment: Second Informational Hearing," Senator Deborah Ortiz and Assemblyman Dario Frommer, Chairs, October 23, 2002, Sacramento, CA.

Kavanaugh-Lynch, M.H.E., Croughan, M., and Beckwith, S. 2010. "*California Breast Cancer Research Program: Annual Report to the State of California Legislature*," Office of the President, University of California, Oakland, CA.

Kelsey, J.L. and Berkowitz, G.S. 1988. "Breast Cancer Epidemiology." *Cancer Research*, 48: 5615–5623.

Kelsey, J.L. and Gammon, M.D. 1990. "Epidemiology of Breast Cancer." *Epidemiologic Reviews*, 12: 228–240.

Key, T. and Reeves, G. 1994. "Organochlorines in the Environment and Breast Cancer." *British Medical Journal*, 308: 1520–1521.

King, S. 2006. *Pink Ribbons, Inc.: Breast Cancer and the Politics of Philanthropy*. Minneapolis, MN: University of Minnesota Press.

Klawiter, M. 2008. *The Biopolitics of Breast Cancer: Changing Cultures of Disease and Activism*. Minneapolis, MN: University of Minnesota Press.

Kriebel, D., Tickner, J., Epstein, P., Lemons, J., Levins, R., Loechler, E., Quinn, M., … and Stoto, M. 2001. "The Precautionary Principle in Environmental Science." *Environmental Health Perspectives*, 109: 871–876.

Krieger, N. 2013. "History, Biology, and Health Inequities: Emergent Embodied Phenotypes and the Illustrative Case of the Breast Cancer Estrogen Receptor." *American Journal of Public Health*, 103: 22–27.

Krieger, N., Chen, J.T., and Waterman, P.D. 2010. "Decline in the U.S. Breast Cancer Rates after the Women's Health Initiative: Socioeconomic and Racial/Ethnic Differentials." *American Journal of Public Health* 100, S1: S132–139.

Krieger, N., Chen, J.T., and Waterman, P.D. 2011. "Temporal Trends in the Black/White Breast Cancer Case Ratio for Estrogen Receptor Status: Disparities are Historically Contingent, Not Innate." *Cancer Causes and Control*, 22: 511–514.

Krieger, N. and Fee, E. 1994. "Social Class: The Missing Link in US Health Data." *International Journal of Health Services*, 24: 25–44.

Krieger, N., Quesenberry, C., Peng, T., *et al.* 1999. "Social Class, Race/Ethnicity, and Incidence of Breast, Cervix, Colon, Lung, and Prostate Cancer among Asian, Black, Hispanic, and White Residents of the San Francisco Bay Area, 1988–92 (United States)." *Cancer Causes and Control*, 10: 525–537.

Krieger, N., van der Eden, S.K., Zava, D., *et al.* 1997. "Race/Ethnicity, Social Class, and Prevalence of Breast Cancer Prognostic Biomarkers: A Study of White,

Black, and Asian Women in the San Francisco Bay Area." *Ethnicity and Disease*, 7: 137–149.

Krieger, N., Wolff, M.S., Hiatt, R.A., Rivera, M., Vogelman, J., and Orentreich, N. 1994. "Breast Cancer and Serum Organochlorines: A Prospective Study among White, Black, and Asian Women." *Journal of the National Cancer Institute*, 86: 589–599.

Leadership Council. 2011. *Addressing Public Health and Chemical Exposures: An Action Agenda.* http://www.nationalconversation.us/wp-content/uploads/2014/05/national-conversation-action-agenda.pdf (accessed November 24, 2015).

Leffall, D.L. Jr. and Kripke, M.D. 2010. "Preface." In S.H. Reuben (Ed.), *Reducing Environmental Cancer Risk: What We Can Do Now*, 2008–2009. Annual Report of the President's Cancer Panel, Washington, DC: US Department of Health and Human Services, National Institutes of Health, National Cancer Institute.

Lindenbaum, S. and Lock, M. (Eds.) 1993. *Knowledge, Power, and Practice: The Anthropology of Medicine and Everyday Life.* Berkeley, CA: University of California Press.

Lock, M. 1995. *Encounters with Aging: Mythologies of Menopause in Japan and North America.* Berkeley, CA: University of California Press.

Lock, M. and Nguyen, V.-K. 2010. *An Anthropology of Biomedicine.* Malden, MA: Wiley-Blackwell.

Mathews, H.F., Burke, N., and Kampriani, E. (Eds.) 2015. *Anthropologies of Cancer in Transnational Worlds.* New York: Routledge.

MBCC / Massachusetts Breast Cancer Coalition. 2014. http://mbcc.org/breast-cancer-prevention/ (accessed February 1, 2014).

McCormick, S., Brody, J., Brown, P., and Polk, R. 2004. "Public Involvement in Breast Cancer Research: An Analysis and Model for Future Research." *International Journal of Health Services*, 34: 625–646.

McKenzie, F. and Jeffreys, M. 2009. "Do Lifestyle or Social Factors Explain Ethnic/Racial Inequalities in Breast Cancer Survival?" *Epidemiologic Reviews*, 31: 52–66.

McMahon, B. 1994. "Pesticides and Breast Cancer?" *Journal of the National Cancer Institute*, 86: 572–573.

McMullin, J. and Weiner, D. (Eds.) 2008. *Confronting Cancer: Metaphors, Advocacy, and Anthropology.* Santa Fe, NM: School for Advanced Research Press.

McPartland, J., Dantzker, H.C., and Portier, C.J. 2015. "Building a Robust 21st Century Chemical Testing Program at the U.S. Environmental Protection Agency: Recommendations for Strengthening Scientific Engagement." *Environmental Health Perspectives*, 123: 1–5.

McQuiston, J.T. 1992. "Citing Breast Cancer Rates in Nassau and Suffolk, Group Asks for Research." *New York Times*, May 12. http://www.nytimes.com/1992/05/12/nyregion/citing-breast-cancer-rates-in-nassau-and-suffolk-group-asks-for-research.html (accessed October 19, 2014).

Michaels, D. 2008. *Doubt Is Their Product: How Industry's Assault on Science Threatens Your Health.* New York: Oxford University Press.

Milliken, R.C. 2004. "Maximizing the Impact of the California Breast Cancer Research Program: Studying Environmental Influences and Breast Cancer." White Paper, California Breast Cancer Research Program, Oakland, CA.

Morris, J. and Hamby, C. 2013. "Industry Muscle Targets Federal 'Report on Carcinogens.'" Center for Public Integrity (July 20, 2013, updated September 23, 2013). www.publicintegrity.org/print/13068 (accessed February 13, 2014).

Mullings, L. 2006. "Resistance and Resilience: The Sojourner Truth Syndrome and the Social Context of Reproduction in Central Harlem." In A.J. Schulz and L. Mullings (Eds.), *Gender, Race, Class, and Health: Intersectional Approaches* (pp. 345–370). San Francisco, CA: Jossey-Bass.

Mullings, L. and Wali, A. 2000. *Stress and Resilience: The Social Context of Reproduction in Central Harlem*. New York: Kluwer Press.

National Toxicology Program. 2008. NTP-CEHR Monograph on the Potential Human Reproductive and Developmental Effects of Bisphenol A NIH Publication No. 08-5994. http://ntp.niehs.nih.gov/ntp/ohat/bisphenol/bisphenol.pdf (accessed November 24, 2015).

Newman, B., Millikan, R.C., and King, M.-C. 1997. "Genetic Epidemiology of Breast and Ovarian Cancers." *Epidemiologic Reviews*, 19: 69–79.

One in Nine: The Long Island Breast Cancer Action Coalition. 2014. www.1in9.org.

Osuch, J., Silk, K., Price, C., Barlow, J., Miller, K., Hernick, A., and Fonfa, A. 2012. "A Historical Perspective on Breast Cancer Activism in the United States: From Education and Support to Partnership in Scientific Research." *Journal of Women's Health*, 21: 355–362.

Pestana, D., Teixeira, D., Faria, A., Domingues, V., Monteiro, R., and Calhau, C. 2013. "Effects of Environmental Organochlorine Pesticides on Human Breast Cancer: Putative Involvement on Invasive Cell Ability." *Environmental Toxicology*, August 2. doi: 10.1002/tox.21882.

Pierce, K. 2002. Presenter for "Breast Cancer: The Impact on Women's Lives." Breast Cancer and the Environment, Senator Deborah Ortiz, chair. Informational Hearing of the Senate Committee on Health and Human Services, Sacramento, CA: State Capitol, February 20, 2002.

Piersma, T. and van Gils, J.A. 2010. *The Flexible Phenotype: A Body-Centered Integration of Ecology, Physiology and Behavior*. New York: Oxford University Press.

Platner, J.H., Bennett, L.M., Millikan, R., and Barker, M.D.G. 2002. "The Partnership Between Breast Cancer Advocates and Scientists." *Environmental and Molecular Mutagenesis*, 39: 102–107.

Rabinowitz, P. and Conti, L. 2013. "Links Among Human Health, Animal Health and Ecosystem Health." *Annual Review of Public Health*, 34: 189–204.

Raffensperger, C. and Tickner, J. (Eds.) 1999. *Protecting Public Health and the Environment: Implementing the Precautionary Principle*. Washington, DC: Island Press.

Ravdin, P.M., Cronin, K.A., Howlader, N., Berg, C.D., Chlebowski, R.T., Feuer, E.J., Edwards, B.K., and Berry, D.A. 2007. "The Decrease in Breast-Cancer Incidence in 2003 in the United States." *New England Journal of Medicine*, 356: 1670–1674. doi: 10.1056/NEJMsr070105.

Reyes, L. 1991. "From the Trenches." In J. Brady (Ed.), *One in Three: Women with Cancer Confront an Epidemic* (pp. 245–254). Pittsburgh,PA: Cleis Press.

Rizzo, R. 2010. "President's Cancer Panel Calls for Fundamental Shift in Chemicals Policy." Statement from Breast Cancer Fund CEO Jeanne Rizzo, May 6, 2010. http://www.breastcancerfund.org/media/press-releases/presidents-cancer-panel.html (accessed February 1, 2014).

Rudel, R.A., Ackerman, J., Attfield, K.R., and Brody, J.G. 2014. "New Exposure Biomarkers as Tools for Breast Cancer Epidemiology, Biomonitoring, and Prevention: A Systematic Approach Based on Animal Evidence." *Environmental Health Perspectives*, 122: 881–895.

Rudel, R.A., Attfield, K.A., Schifano, J.N., and Brody, J.G. 2007. "Chemicals Causing Mammary Gland Tumors in Animals Signal New Directions for Epidemiology, Chemicals Testing, and Risk Assessment for Breast Cancer Prevention." *Environmental Factors in Breast Cancer Supplement to Cancer* 109(12): 2635–2666.

Rudel, R. and Perovich, L. (2012. "Accurate Risk-Based Chemical Screening Relies on Robust Exposure Estimates." Letter to the Editor. *Toxicological Sciences*, 128: 295–296.

Russell, D., Lewis, S., and Keating, R. 1992. "Inconclusive by Design: Waste, Fraud, and Abuse in Federal Environmental Health Research, An Investigative Study by the Environmental Health Network and the National Toxics Campaign Fund." https://archive.org/details/InconclusiveByDesignWasteFraudAndAbuseInFederalEnvironmentalHealth (accessed February 1, 2014).

Sampson, D. 2010. "Cancer and the Environment," ACS Pressroom Blog, posted May 6, 2010. http://acspressroom.wordpress.com/2010/05/06/cancer-and-the-environment/ (accessed February 1, 2014).

Scientific Understanding Work Group, The National Conversation on Public Health and Chemical Exposures. 2011. *Scientific Understanding Work Group Report.* Atlanta, GA: Centers for Disease Control and Prevention, Agency for Toxic Substances and Disease Registry (December 2010).

SEER / Surveillance, Epidemiology, and End Results. 2014. "Stat Fact Sheets: Breast Cancer." National Cancer Institute, Bethesda, MD. http://seer.cancer.gov/statfacts/html/breast.html (accessed February 1, 2014).

Silent Spring 2014a. "Breast Cancer and the Environment." http://www.silentspring.org/breast-cancer-and-environment (accessed February 15, 2014).

Silent Spring 2014b. "History of Silent Spring Institute." http://silentspring.org/history-silent-spring-institute (accessed October 20, 2014).

Silverstein, M. 2012. "Introduction: When Science Doesn't Have All the Answers." In R.W. Clapp (Ed.), *From Critical Science to Solutions: The Best of Scientific Solutions* (pp. 1–2). Amity, NY: Baywood Publishing.

Smith, G.D. 2012. "Epigenesis for Epidemiologists: Does Eco-Devo Have Implications for Population Health Research and Practice?" *International Journal of Epidemiology*, 41: 236–247.

Steingraber, S. 1991. "We All Live Downwind." In J. Brady (Ed.), *One in Three: Women with Cancer Confront an Epidemic* (pp. 36–48). Pittsburgh, PA: Cleis Press.

Steingraber, S. 1997. *Living Downstream: An Ecologist Looks at Cancer and the Environment.* Reading, MA: Addison-Wesley.

Sternberg, S.S. 1994. "Re: DDT and Breast Cancer." *Journal of the National Cancer Institute*, 86: 1094–1095.

Stewart, S.L., Sabatino, S.A., Foster, S.L., and Richardson, L.C. 2007. "Decline in Breast Cancer Incidence 1999–2003." *Morbidity and Mortality Weekly Report* 56: 549–553.

Sulik, G. 2011. *Pink Ribbon Blues: How Breast Cancer Culture Undermines Women's Health.* New York: Oxford University Press.

Tamimi, R.M., Colditz, G.A., Hazra, A., Baer, H.J. *et al.* 2012. "Traditional Breast Cancer Risk Factors in Relation to Molecular Subtypes of Breast Cancer." *Breast Cancer Research and Treatment*, 131: 159–167.

Taubes, G. 1994. "Pesticides and Breast Cancer: No Link?" *Science*, 264: 499–500.

Toriola, A.T. and Colditz, G. 2013. "Trends in Breast Cancer Incidence and Mortality in the United States: Implications for Prevention." *Breast Cancer Research and Treatment*, 138: 665–673.

United Nations. 1995. *Report of the Fourth World Conference on Women*, Beijing, China, September–15, 1995. http://www.un.org/womenwatch/daw/beijing/pdf/Beijing%20full%20report%20E.pdf (accessed November 1, 2014).

Wilson, S. 2010. "Environmental Justice Movement: A Review of History, Research, and Public Health Issues." *Journal of Public Management and Social Policy*, 16: 19–50.

Winn, D.M. 2005. "Science and Society: The Long Island Breast Cancer Study Project." *National Review of Cancer*, 5: 986–994.

Wolff, M.S. and Barlow, J. 2011. "Breast Cancer Environment Centers and Advocacy." *Environmental Health Perspectives*, 119(5): A 200–201.

Wolff, M.S., Britton, J.A., Teitelbaum, S.L., Eng, S., Deych, E., Ireland, K., Liu, Z., … Gammon, M.D. 2005. "Improving Organochlorine Biomarkers for Cancer Research." *Cancer Epidemiology, Biomarkers and Prevention*, 14: 2224–2236.

Wolff, M., Toniolo, P., Lee, E.W., Rivera, M., and Dubin, N. 1993. "Blood Levels of Organochlorine Residues and Risk of Breast Cancer." *Journal of the National Cancer Institute*, 85: 648–652.

Women and Sustainable Development. 1994. "Women, Health and the Environment: Action for Cancer Prevention, Consensus Statement, February 1994." http://www.iisd.org/women/vanhealt.htm (accessed October 1, 2014).

Writing Group for the Women's Health Initiative Investigators. 2002. "Risks and Benefits of Estrogen Plus Progestin in Healthy Postmenopausal Women: Principal Results from the Women's Health Initiative Randomized Controlled Trial." *Journal of the American Medical Association*, 288: 321–333.

Zota, A., Rudel, R.A., Morello-Frosch, R., and Brody, J.G. 2008. "Elevated House Dust and Serum Concentrations of PBDEs in California: Unintended Consequences of Furniture Flammability Standards?" *Environmental Science and Technology*, 42: 8158–8164.

CHAPTER 2

Effects of Agriculture on Environmental and Human Health: Opportunities for Anthropology

Melissa K. Melby and Megan Mauger

Let food be thy medicine and medicine be thy food.

Hippocrates

Introduction

Our goal in this chapter is to provide a synthesis of current scholarship on the interconnections between human and environmental health as mediated by agriculture, which has increasingly impacted both the environment and human health since its origin over 10,000 years ago. While environment broadly includes both physical and social domains, we focus more narrowly on the ecological health of the biophysical environment (e.g., soil, water, air). Following the WHO (World Health Organization), we define human health as "physical, mental and social well-being and not merely the absence of disease or infirmity" (WHO 1948). We broaden the usual definition of agriculture as cultivation of

A Companion to the Anthropology of Environmental Health, First Edition. Edited by Merrill Singer.

animals and plants for food to include food systems, because the "key to better nutrition, and ultimately to ensuring each person's right to food, lies in better food systems – smarter approaches, policies and investments encompassing the environment, people, institutions and processes by which agricultural products are produced, processed and brought to consumers in a sustainable manner" (UN 2013).

The effects of agriculture on the environment and human health are magnified by scale and intensity. We focus here primarily on contemporary industrialized agricultural practices and examine their effects on the environment and health. This chapter is not an exhaustive discussion of the interconnections between agriculture, environment, and health, but rather it lays out a conceptual framework and then focuses on a few illustrative topics connected by themes of "diversity" and "unintended consequences" for environmental and human health: (1) parallels and interconnections between agricultural practices and the soil and human microbiomes, emphasizing the importance of ecological diversity; (2) direct and indirect effects of pesticides, with a focus on pollinators and implications for global food security; and (3) political economics of food insecurity. Finally, we discuss a case study that exemplifies interdisciplinary approaches to creating sustainable alternatives, and conclude with a discussion of opportunities for anthropology (see Figure 2.1).

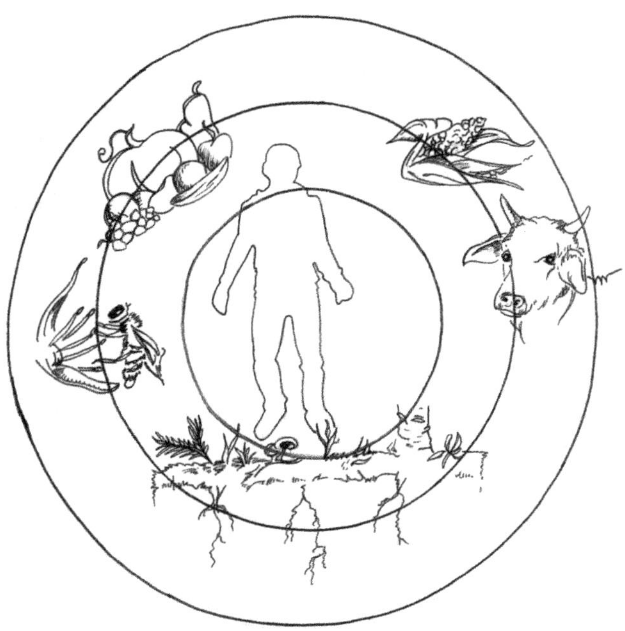

Figure 2.1 Opportunities for anthropologists to study factors influencing agriculture's effects on environmental and human health span the continuum from micro (microbiome) to macro (political economy) levels and encompass themes of ecosystem diversity and variation and unintended consequences for sustainability. Source: Drawn by Kristen Melby.

Agriculture's Impact on the Environment

> We should judge every scrap of biodiversity as priceless while we learn to use it and come to understand what it means to humanity.
>
> Edward O. Wilson, *The Diversity of Life*

The environmental effects of agriculture are a function of scale and degree of intensification (increased input per unit land and per capita). Agricultural intensification has been considered both a cause and effect of population growth, state development, centralization, and climatic or environmental change (Thurston and Fisher 2007a). Boserup proposed that population growth and pressure would tip the balance toward agricultural intensification and adoption of new agricultural technologies or strategies, thus providing an exit from the Malthusian dilemma of higher agricultural production levels leading to larger populations without resources to feed themselves (Boserup 1965). Intensification may be better understood if agriculture is viewed not only as production for subsistence but also as social production of status, prestige, and trade.

Increasing intensification, from horticulture (small-scale plots of mixed crops) to industrial agriculture (large-scale plots of single crops and increased use of technology and synthetic chemicals), appears to be a perpetual motion machine, but only because the energy inputs are often hidden from view. With increasing use of intermediaries (draft animals, machinery, and fossil fuels), energy efficiency of food production (energy out/in ratio) often decreases when analyzed from a life cycle perspective (Pimentel 1974), and environmental impact increases.

Unintended consequences of intensification include reduced biodiversity, which increases vulnerabilities to pathogens and soil nutrient deficiencies, which then require energy inputs to compensate for lost ecological services. A shift from slash-and-burn agriculture to industrial agriculture led to the replacement of crop rotations that build soil health; manure by energy-intensive ammonia-based fertilizers which acidify the soil and kill much of its living biota (O'Donnell *et al.* 2001); and natural pest control by synthetic herbicides and pesticides which diminish biodiversity. Large quantities of fossil fuels are used to produce these products as well as to power the machines that apply them. Environmental effects of current agricultural practices are summarized in Table 2.1.

Agriculture's Impact on Human Health

Agriculture has exerted significant effects on human health, not only through changes in dietary content (energy and nutrient types), but also through environmental exposure, such as zoonoses (animal-to-human transmitted diseases) (Rabinowitz and Conti 2013) and malaria (Desowitz 1991), as well as through its association with institutionalized social inequality (Price 1995), leading some to call agriculture the "worst mistake in human history" (Diamond 1987). With the Agricultural Revolution, human diets slowly began to shift away from diversity of wild foods toward a carbohydrate-based diet with domesticated grains as staple foods. This shift from food collection to food production led to negative health outcomes in many regions (Larsen 1995), as

Table 2.1 Unintended consequences and effects of agriculture on environment.

Agricultural component	*Details*	*Biodiversity*	*Unintended consequences and effects on*			
			Air	*Water*	*Soil*	*Climate change*
Monocultures		Ecosystem simplification			↓nutrients	↑Co_2
Energy Use	US avg 3:1 kcal fossil fuel energy:food energy (beef pdtn 35:1)		pollute	pollute	pollute	
Synthetic fertilizers	only 1/3-1/2 absorbed by crops			Algal blooms ↓O_2→deadzones	↑acidity, ↓biological activity and plant growth	energy use
Synthetic pesticides	99.9% may not reach targets	↓beneficial insects, birds; ↑amphibian abnormalities	pesticide drift	pollute surface and ground water		energy use
Machinery		Requires↓ biodiversity	fossil fuel pollution		↑erosion; ↓fertility	fossil fuel use
Irrigation	1/3 of food grown comes from 1/6 of irrigated cropland			↑freshwater supply	↑water logging and salinization	
Land use	↑yields Require ↑land	↓habitat			desertification	Deforestation (↑Co)
Cattle production	Resource intensive due to tropic levels: 7 kg grain → 1 kg beef	↑if moderately grazed		animal waste		↑methane

Abbreviations: ↑ = increase; ↓ = decrease; → = lead to; avg = average; pdtn = production
Source: Summarized and adapted from Horrigan, Lawrence, and Walker (2002) and McMichael *et al.* (2007).

evidenced by paleopathological data on dental caries and skeletal signs of nutritional deficiencies (Cohen and Armelagos 1984), likely mediated by increased social inequality and variable access to food and nutrition. Although evidence of declining health with increasing agriculture is common in the paleopathological record, considerable variability in geography, politics, culture, population size and nucleation, domestication, population movements, and trade influence time- and region-specific patterns (Cohen and Crane-Kramer 2007). Data from contemporary hunter-gatherers has been used to propose a "Paleolithic diet" (Eaton and Konner 1985) that provides an evolutionary context for studying human diets, but it overlooks considerable environmental variation and flexibility in human dietary behavior (Turner and Thompson 2013).

Agriculture, through nutrition, influences both infectious and chronic disease. Maternal and child undernutrition contributes not only to childhood morbidity and mortality (Black *et al.* 2008) but also to adult health problems (Victora *et al.* 2008). Undernourished children (Kuzawa 1998) and adults are more susceptible to infectious disease (Farmer *et al.* 1991). Overnutrition can lead to chronic diseases such as heart disease, stroke, cancer, and diabetes, which now account for more than 60 percent of global mortality (WHO 2011). The existence of both under- and overnutrition in many developing countries is leading to a double burden of malnutrition resulting in increased infectious and chronic disease (Tanumihardjo *et al.* 2007). The Developmental Origins of Health and Disease paradigm has linked early life undernutrition with later life chronic disease (Barker 2004; Ellison 2005), particularly among children who receive inadequate nutrition in utero but grow up in obesogenic social and physical environments characterized by energy abundance and decreased energy expenditure due to increased processed foods, fresh food deserts, and lack of opportunities for safe, healthy physical activity. Agriculture, as part of the food system influencing what is produced and what people eat, greatly affects health. "Food insecurity is now the major driver for clinical practice … [Humans] are a changing species whose ecological interface is increasingly blurred and resilience ill-defined" (Wahlqvist 2013). The concept of ecological interface is critical both in agriculture and human health and is the topic of the next section.

Ecological Interfaces: Soil and Human Microbiome

> While we live our bodies are moving particles of the earth, joined inextricably both to the soil and to the bodies of other living creatures. It is hardly surprising then that there should be some profound resemblances between our treatment of our bodies and our treatment of the earth.
>
> Wendell Berry, *The Unsettling of America*

Soil Microbiome

Soil supports food production and all terrestrial ecosystems through symbiotic relationships between bacteria, fungi, and animals. These organisms break down organic matter, which binds minerals eroded from rock to form soil. From the advent of agriculture in the Fertile Crescent to the collapse of the Roman Empire, the presence or absence of healthy soil was a driving force behind the rise and fall of civilizations (Montgomery 2007).

The food we eat, the water we drink, and the air we breathe all depend on healthy soil ecosystems, the interconnections of which we are only beginning to understand. A single gram of soil may contain as many as 100,000 cells of 6000–38,000 different species (Curtis, Sloan, and Scannell 2002). Yet, only 1 percent of bacteria have been identified and studied (Torsvik 2002). Certain types of bacteria concentrate in the rhizosphere, and defend against pests and stimulate root growth (Ramamoorthy *et al.* 2001). Plants excrete carbohydrates, glucose, and proteins that feed bacteria, completing this symbiosis.

Fungi decompose organic material into soil, recycling necessary agricultural nutrients. Their root-like extensions (mycorrhizae) facilitate communication and transport between plants and bridge connections for an estimated 80 percent of terrestrial plant communities (Smith, Read, and Harley 1997). If a sapling is shaded from the sun, fungi will respond by sending extra nutrients to the young plant. These complex systems improve ecosystem resilience to environmental disasters and disease by providing nutrients that individual plants need for optimal functioning (van der Heijden, Bardgett, and van Straalen 2008).

Supporting soil diversity appears to be key to environmental health and the future of sustainable agriculture. Healthy soil holds more water, preventing leaching of nutrients due to runoff and lessening the need for irrigation (Garrett, Ferguson, and Amaranthus 2012). Soil sequesters carbon dioxide, offsetting fossil fuel emission by 5 to 15 percent (Lal 2004), and fixes atmospheric nitrogen to produce nitrate, which along with phosphorus and potassium are the main elements limiting plant growth. Despite these myriad ecosystem services, soil is being degraded at 10–40 times the rate of replenishment (Pimentel 2006).

Soil plays an important role in human health, through its relationship with agriculture. Organic agriculture focuses on supporting microbes to create fertile soil to support plant growth. In contrast, modern industrial agricultural methods degrade soil through impaction from heavy machinery, crop monocultures that deplete soil nutrients, and synthetic chemicals that destroy biodiversity. These systems depend on high fertilizer inputs to replace nutrients fixed by microbes and large pesticide amounts to kill the remaining life. Compared to conventionally grown fruits and vegetables, organic produce has significantly higher levels of minerals, phytochemicals, and vitamin C (Heaton 2013). Thus healthy soil translates to healthier food for humans.

The long history of human influence on soil is exemplified by Amazonian anthropogenic soils *terra preta* and *terra mulata*, human-made organic-rich soils created from relatively infertile rainforest soil by addition of food and human waste as well as ash and charcoal from fires dating back several hundred or thousand years (Woods and Denevan 2009). While *terra preta* is a black soil filled with cultural debris, and thus likely unintentionally formed, *terra mulata* is more extensive and contains few artifacts, suggesting it resulted from semi-intensive cultivation, with nutrient inputs deriving from food wastes (Neves *et al.* 2003). Despite the tropical climate and frequent cultivation, these soils have maintained their high fertility, likely due to high carbon which retains nutrients and moisture, and high microbial activity (Tsai *et al.* 2009), which suggests they could be a model for sustainable agriculture in the humid tropics (Glaser and Birk 2012).

Human Microbiome

While soil microbes sustain the plants that feed us, microbes in our body break them down, providing us with health benefits. The human–environment interface is mediated by the collective genome of microbial cells inhabiting humans (human microbiome) comprised of approximately 10 times more bacterial than human cells (Lederberg 2000), most of them located in the gastrointestinal tract. With the realization that mapping of the human genome would not unlock all mysteries of human health, attention has shifted to environmental and epigenetic modifications of DNA (Jabolonka and Lamb 2005) and to symbiotic relationships with microbes which may permit humans to adapt more quickly to local changes in their environment (Dethlefsen, McFall-Ngai, and Relman 2007; Pflughoeft and Versalovic 2012).

The human gut is characterized by stable communities of microflora with high functional redundancy which may serve to limit colonization by pathogenic bacteria (Ley, Peterson, and Gordon 2006), and may influence predisposition to specific diseases. The dominant types of human gut bacteria cannot grow outside hosts, and thus likely depend on parent-to-offspring transmission. Recent evidence suggests colonization of the gastrointestinal tract may begin in utero (Funkhouser and Bordenstein 2013), possibly via the placenta. Microbiota from the vagina and feces of mothers are acquired by infants during vaginal delivery, and cesarean sections lead to different colonization patterns (Gronlund *et al.* 1999). Breast milk contains sugars that are indigestible by humans but support healthy gut microflora (Zivkovic *et al.* 2010), an example of how diet influences the composition of the microbial community (De Filippo *et al.* 2010).

Diet influences which bacteria reside in our guts and in turn which food breakdown products and metabolites are made available to us. The amount of energy available to hosts from food is modulated to a significant degree by gut microbiota (Backhed *et al.* 2005). Agriculture and domestication of animals may have selected for humans that could digest starch in the mouth (higher up in the gastrointestinal tract so bacteria in the colon receive less), and humans who produced lactase enzyme into adulthood (lactase persistence) to enable utilization of lactose without the need of gut bacteria (Wiley 2008). Humans able to break down such foods themselves would have a fitness advantage over those who required microbial fermentation, which would provide less energy because some would be used for microbial maintenance and growth. As diets have shifted toward increased carbohydrates, which are primarily absorbed in the small intestine, humans have outcompeted the microbes residing primarily in their large intestine (Walter and Ley 2011). By giving gut bacteria less fiber to break down, humans circumvent them and obtain quick and easy energy from food sources that represent a departure from evolutionary strategies.

Paralleling industrial agriculture, this increased energy efficiency may have unintended consequences.

The decreased dietary diversity of our modern food environment, characterized by increased simple sugars and fat, may change the relative abundances of various types of gut microbes which affect energy utilization and may play a role in metabolic disorders such as obesity (Ley *et al.* 2006). The importance of gut bacteria to obesity-related metabolic disorders has only recently been documented in humans (Turnbaugh *et al.* 2006), but has been harnessed in animal husbandry to increase livestock growth rates by adding antibiotics to their feed: the earlier in life they start, the greater the effect (Blaser 2011).

Heliobacter pylori provides an interesting gut microbiome-health case study. Originally thought to be caused by stress, ulcers were later blamed on *H. pylori* and treated with antibiotics. Stress may be responsible for pathogenic effects of this symbiotic bacterium, with a nearly universal distribution among humans and rarely pathogenic effects (Linz *et al.* 2007). Indeed, under less stressful conditions it may be protective against obesity by inhibiting appetite through its effects on the stomach's production of ghrelin, a hormone that stimulates food intake (Pennisi 2011).

Which bacteria are present in our bodies may also influence our health more broadly, through effects on the development of the immune system. The hygiene hypothesis (Strachan 1989) posits that increased rates of allergies and asthma may be due to an excess of hygiene and lack of appropriate exposure to microbes and parasites in contemporary society, in part due to distance from agricultural food production. Supportive evidence derives from studies where children who lived on farms had greater microbial diversity and lower rates of asthma than children in the control group (Ege *et al.* 2011); and households with a greater diversity of plants in their surrounding home had lower rates of allergies (Dunn *et al.* 2013). A driving force for the evolution of the immune system is the need to respond appropriately not only to external microbiota, but also to the diversity in host microbiota; this in turn allows the host to respond to environmental (including food) antigens and possibly self-antigens (Ley, Peterson, and Gordon 2006), suggesting that human–microbiome interactions may have far-reaching health effects.

Balance and Biodiversity: Use of Synthetic Pesticides

> To keep every cog and wheel is the first precaution of intelligent tinkering.
>
> Aldo Leopold, *A Sand County Almanac*

Just as a healthy immune system is supported by microbial diversity, an agricultural field may be more resistant to predation with greater biodiversity, where no single species is able to proliferate. Monocultures rely on synthetic pesticides for control of agricultural pests, including insects, weeds, and fungi (EPA 2014). The effects of pesticides on human health can be conceptualized on three levels: direct, indirect, and ecosystem. While correlations between agricultural pesticides and health effects exist, causal pathways are difficult to document due to (a) variations in exposure, (b) high number and variations in chemicals used, and (c) diversity of methodologies and metrics used in epidemiological studies (Dowdall and Klotz 2014). Because insects and other animals share many neurological pathways, many pesticides may be toxic to humans and other organisms that may not be pests but actually critical ecosystem organisms vital to our food system, such as pollinators (UNEP 2005). Ten of the 12 most dangerous organic chemicals are pesticides (Gilden, Huffling, and Sattler 2010). Moreover, many of these chemicals persist in the environment for years, or travel long distances through air and water, and accumulate in fatty tissue. Pesticides in the environment may have unintended consequences of damaging ecosystem services that are critical for human health and agriculture.

Pesticide effects on Human Health

The humans most vulnerable to direct effects of pesticides are those who produce and apply them: farmers and farm laborers (Villarejo 2003). An estimated 3 million acute pesticide poisonings occur annually around the globe, resulting in 250,000 deaths (WHO 2004). The majority of deaths are due to intentional exposure and suicide but data have been criticized for being conservative by not accounting for unreported cases of unintentional exposure (Jeyaratnam 1990; Murray *et al.* 2002; Dowdall and Klotz 2014). Many classes of chemicals that are unregistered or severely restricted in their (usually developed) countries of origin are exported to developing nations that have weaker restrictions or less ability to enforce existing agrochemical regulations (Smith, Kerr, and Sadripour 2008; FAO 2014). Thus poor farmers in developing countries are exposed disproportionately. In this age of globalization, much of the food in the developed world is imported from developing countries where environmental regulations are weak, thus exposing people both directly and indirectly.

Indirect exposure through ingestion of trace amounts on food receives much attention in popular discussions of reasons to buy organic produce. Use of pesticides in the global South is partly a response to demand from consumers and supermarkets in the global North for unblemished vegetables and fruit. Human health effects of pesticide residues on food are difficult to assess, but effects on reproduction and cancer among wildlife suggests concern is warranted (Jones and de Voogt 1999). While causality is difficult to demonstrate, most studies of organophosphate pesticides have found associations between exposure and increased symptom prevalence (Kamel and Hoppin 2004).

While the risks of pesticide exposure remain debated, there are documented nutritional and health benefits of avoiding pesticides. When synthetic chemicals are applied to deter pests, plants do not need to produce defensive secondary metabolites (Brandt and Mølgaard 2001), many of which may have health benefits for humans. Organic crops contain significantly more vitamin C, iron, magnesium, and phosphorus, and significantly fewer nitrates than conventional crops (Worthington 2001). Thus pesticide use may lead to an impoverishment of compounds that protect against cancer, and other lifestyle diseases (Young *et al.* 2005).

Finally, there are threats to human health that operate through ecosystem-level pathways, with the food supply put at risk by damage to pollinators and other "beneficial" organisms. About three-quarters of food crops worldwide depend on animal pollination, mostly from insects such as bees (Klein *et al.* 2007). Notably, most fruits and vegetables, sunflower, and alfalfa (used for hay to support meat and dairy production) require "pollination services" from honeybees, in contrast to soybeans and cereal grains such as corn, rice, and wheat, which are wind pollinated. Interestingly, although corn is wind pollinated, many bees now depend on corn, in the form of corn syrup, for their survival. Beekeepers often supplement bees' diets with corn syrup because loss of forage plants in monoculture-dominated landscapes means a lack of native pollen and nectar, which are more nutritious. The parallel with humans' diets, with increasing proportions of energy derived from "empty calories," is striking.

While acreage devoted to bee-pollinated crops has increased, bee numbers have decreased in North America and Europe, and in the rest of the world have not kept pace with increasing crop needs (Aizen and Harder 2009). Vulnerabilities among bee populations, and thus also bee-pollinated fruit and vegetable crops, potentially jeopardize dietary diversity and exacerbate trends in diet-related disease.

Debate continues about the cause(s) of colony collapse disorder, the syndrome resulting in bees' disappearance from their hives (Becher *et al.* 2013), but is likely due to changing agricultural practices and environments that have affected honeybees through (1) increases in the invasive *Varroa destructor* mite and pathogens; (2) the practice of transporting bees to pollinate monocultures, causing them stress during travel and increasing disease exposure with population intermixing; (3) decreased forage plants (Burkle, Knight, and Marlin 2013) due to use of nitrogen fertilizers instead of crop rotation with nitrogen-fixing plants such as clover and alfalfa which provide reliable sources of pollen and nectar for bees (Spivak *et al.* 2011); and (4) pesticides that may weaken or stress bees and other insects. While honeybees can deposit high quantities of pollen, their efficiency in terms of fruit production is only half that of wild insects (Garibaldi *et al.* 2013). By relying on a single species of pollinator for most of our bee-pollinated crops, we not only decrease efficiency but increase risk, since diversity is key to resilience.

Efforts to enhance pollinator habitats, including planting fields with flowering cover crops and planting field borders/hedgerows/grass buffer strips with native perennial or annual flowering species, not only increase pollinator population fitness but have secondary ecosystem benefits such as erosion management, nutrient runoff reduction, and pest reduction (Wratten *et al.* 2012), all of which can improve agricultural efficiency and reduce negative environmental impact. On organic farms near natural habitats, native bees are able to provide full pollination services without managed honeybees (Kremen, Williams, and Thorp 2002), thus investment in biodiversity may reduce costs and increase resilience of our food production system. Concerns about decreased yields appear unfounded, as evidenced by studies showing that organic techniques can yield the same amount of food with 20 to 40 percent less land (Badgley *et al.* 2007), and that polycultures of crops are also on average 40 percent less affected by disease (Anten 2013).

Agricultural Practices in Political Economic Perspective: Food Security

Poor health of pollinator populations may endanger the food supply, but food security goes beyond just producing adequate food. Although the developing world is producing enough food for each person to consume more than 2500 calories daily (Pinstrup-Andersen, Pandya-Lorch, and Rosegrant 1999), 842 million people suffer from chronic hunger (FAO 2013). Food security requires (1) *availability* of sufficient, safe and nutritious food; (2) physical and economic *access*; (3) *utilization* of food that meets dietary needs and food preferences for an active and healthy life; and (4) *stability* over time (FAO 2008). Food insecurity is of interest to anthropology because it allows exploration of group differences in biological (nutrition and health) outcomes, and because it is a "valuable point of entry for policy discussions on where best to focus efforts to improve biosocial outcomes mediated through food" (Hadley and Crooks 2012: 73).

Political economic factors, ranging from agricultural subsidies and conflicts of interest (e.g., US Department of Agriculture giving nutritional advice while promoting dairy and beef industries; Nestle 2002) to international agricultural policies which pressure small farmers to grow cash crops for export rather than food for their families, further result in a food production and distribution system that often leads to food insecurity. In industrialized countries, migrant farm laborers who are essential to agricultural systems are often paid so poorly that they cannot afford to buy the produce they spend hours picking each day, leading to food insecurity and poor health among farm workers (Weigel *et al.* 2007). Such ironic examples belie industrial agriculture's focus on cheap food (Appleby *et al.* 2003).

Agriculture's Contributions to Food (In)Security

Industrial agriculture has led to relatively cheap food prices, especially in the United States, but the actual price in terms of costs to the environment and human health appears to be high (Carolan 2011). Large-scale agriculture initially increases food supplies, but also drives prices (and profits) down. This increases pressure to cut costs by increasing yields, which in turn drives increased used of agrichemicals. This process makes farmers vulnerable to agribusiness and government policies, not least because of erosion of traditional crop varieties, practices, and associated knowledge (Brush 2007).

Most developed nation consumers are separated from the land – they demand low food prices at the supermarket, their only link to the food they eat. Agricultural science and technology have continually delivered higher yields at lower costs, but there are significant social and environmental costs: "farmers are forced onto an economic treadmill that decimates rural communities, and it causes serious environmental degradation" (Duram 2005: 9). As agricultural endeavors are consolidated, small family farms are made economically unsustainable due to economies of scale and government policies and subsidies. Mechanization of industrial agriculture and increasing reliance on fossil fuel leads to decreased need for human labor, and rural to urban migration. Urbanization and higher incomes often lead to changing dietary lifestyles, such as shifts from plant-based diets to grain-fed animal diets (Norton 2005) which affect food availability and access as well as the environment. Many resources used to raise animals are lost in nutrient transfer: 6 kg of plant protein are required to produce 1 kg of high-quality animal protein; fossil energy input for animal protein production averages 25 kcal per kcal protein produced, compared to 2.2 kcal of fossil energy input per 1 kcal of plant protein produced (Pimentel and Pimentel 2003). Since 37 percent of the world's grain is used to feed livestock (World Resources Institute 2002), and since growing "vast quantities of corn used to feed livestock in [the US] takes vast quantities of chemical fertilizer, which in turn takes vast quantities of oil – 1.2 gallons for every bushel ... the modern feedlot is really a city floating on a sea of oil" (Pollan 2002). Increasing demand for animal products associated with increased standards of living (for some) exacerbates food insecurity by decreasing energy efficiency, and also increases environmental impacts. Furthermore, food insecurity in low-income countries or regions may lead people to farm marginal land, with environmental impacts due to deforestation and soil erosion (Stonich 1993), while biofuel agriculture is driving farming to borderlands and buffer zones, with damaging environmental impacts (Searchinger *et al.* 2013).

Food Insecurity's Effects on Health

Strong evidence exists for associations between food insecurity and chronic diseases such as diabetes, as well as infectious diseases such as HIV/AIDS (Singer 2011; Weiser *et al.* 2011), although the direction of causality is not entirely clear. Hadley and Crooks (2012) argue that food insecurity and poor health outcomes are linked and mediated through coping responses, and that the stress of food insecurity may be the mediating factor influencing mental and physical health (Weaver 2009). Stress and depression may lead to overeating, disordered eating, and intake of "comfort foods" to reduce stress (Dallman *et al.* 2003).

National income level appears to be an important explanatory variable for patterning of the relationship between food insecurity and nutritional well-being. Among children in low-income settings, food insecurity is consistently associated with undernutrition. In high-income settings, while less expensive foods tend to be energy dense and of poorer nutritional quality (Drewnowski 2004), food insecurity is not consistently associated with overnutrition as proponents of the food insecurity–overweight paradox have hypothesized (Hadley and Crooks 2012). While food insecurity, poverty, and low socioeconomic status are often associated, exceptions do occur and examination of such variation may help us understand the context-dependent drivers of the link between food insecurity and health outcomes.

Gender-differentiated effects of food insecurity may be mediated through gendered relationships with mothers, who are often primarily responsible for food procurement and provisioning. Women often report sacrificing their own nutrition to ensure the nutrition of their children. Food insecurity influences maternal mental health, and this may be a key modulating variable influencing the effects of food insecurity on children, through maternal parenting and feeding practices (DeCaro *et al.* 2013).

Sustainable Solutions

> All the world's problems can be solved in a garden.
>
> Geoff Lawton, speaking at the Permaculture Research Institute, 2014

The myriad linkages between contemporary agricultural practices and environmental and human health effects argue for a paradigm shift from merely producing food to generating food by employing fertile soil and supporting biodiversity within agricultural and human ecosystems and ensuring equitable access to reduce health disparities. Sub-Saharan Africa is the only region in the world where food production per capita has not increased in the past half century, primarily due to depletion of soil fertility (Sanchez 2004). Improving soil fertility can not only reduce hunger, but also have far-reaching effects on population health. One solution is embodied in the term "EcoHealth," coined by the International Development Research Center, which is short for "ecosystem approaches to human health," and recognizes that many of the problems facing humanity are inherently connected to the environment. An interdisciplinary collaboration between Malawian community nurses and Canadian soil science students that sought to address the high rates of childhood malnutrition in Ekwendeni, Malawi (Charron 2012) provides an exemplary case study showcasing the linkages between improving the soil, ecosystem health, and human health.

Interviews were conducted in 1997 with families whose children were admitted to the Nutrition Rehabilitation Centre at Ekwendeni Hospital. Many families could not afford the rising price of commercial fertilizers, without which crop yields of their staple maize were declining drastically. This food shortage translated into poor children's health and caused stress within families. Women reported that the men had alcohol dependency problems that often resulted in violence. Social stratification was increasing, with associated economic vulnerability and food insecurity for many (Kerr 2005).

Soils, Food, and Healthy Communities (SFHC), a participatory agriculture program, was initiated to educate the community about the relationships between agriculture, human, and environmental health (Kerr 2005; Charron 2012). Their focus was to improve child nutrition through land management. These communities had become accustomed to agricultural extension programs telling them how to farm and public health groups telling them how to feed their children, but when the SFHC group began talking about agriculture at the nutrition hospital, they were surprised. The main change they advocated for was intercropping of legumes within the maize fields. Legumes fix nitrogen in the soil, acting as a natural fertilizer while adding an additional protein and nutrient-rich food source (Shelton 2000). The legumes also cover the area surrounding the maize, so there is less need for weeding or herbicides. The villages were taught to incorporate the residue from the plants into the field after harvest, covering the fields in nutrient-rich compost for the following season.

This multidisciplinary approach included education programs teaching citizens how to link these agricultural methods to nutrition, especially regarding childhood feeding practices. Many mothers and grandmothers fed children maize porridge at a very young age. About 65 percent of children were given food in the first month of life and only 4 percent of children were exclusively breastfed for the first 6 months of life (Kerr, Berti, and Chirwa 2007). In response, SFHC advocated for longer exclusive breastfeeding and advised mothers to include legumes when they introduced porridge.

By 2005, over 4000 farmers had joined the program. An initial focus on improving soil health led to improvements in many measures of health. By facilitating natural systems of fertilization, the communities were producing food without the added cost of fertilizers. This food was made available to children, decreasing the rates of malnutrition. The introduction of new crops diversified their diets and increased their food security.

The research team found that the yields of maize were significantly higher for farmers who participated in the project (Charron 2012). The control households produced an average of 4.4 crops while the intervention groups produced an average of 6.16 crops (Bonatsos, Bezner Kerr, and Shumba 2009). Intervention groups were also found to be about 18 percent less food insecure. Using weight as an indicator of childhood health and nutritional status, children whose families had longer and more active participation in SFHC tended to be an average of 1 kg heavier at the age of 1 and 1.5 kg heavier at the age of 3 (Bezner Kerr, Berti, and Shumba 2011). In this EcoHealth approach, the health of the soil was rejuvenated, in turn benefiting child health, social equity, diet diversity, and community relationships. Years after the SFHC project began and researchers departed, farmers formed the Ekwendeni Farmers Association, demonstrating sustainability of the project. Such interdisciplinary EcoHealth projects are key to a greener revolution in Africa (Snapp *et al.* 2010), and perhaps throughout the world.

Conclusions and Opportunities for Anthropology

This chapter's framework and examples are presented as a *call for action* to anthropologists to conduct broader interdisciplinary research and lay the foundations for more systemic change in environmental and human health by examining agriculture and nutrition (see Figure 2.1). Studying agricultural intensification's unplanned consequences and failures may shed light on human history (Thurston and Fisher 2007b) and contemporary environmental and human health. We must view past and present people as social agents making decisions about subsistence/agricultural strategies within sociopolitical and economic contexts, influenced by factors such as age, gender, and social class. This must be done on multiple levels, and comparatively, as agricultural changes that appear similar may have different underlying causal processes (Thurston and Fisher 2007b). With their long historical and broad comparative perspectives, anthropologists are well positioned to examine why certain innovations or intensification practices are adopted or not, when, and by whom, and to evaluate their intended effects and unintended consequences, and how these in turn affect adoption or rejection of novel methods and strategies. Differential health and mortality by age, sex (usually worse for females), and region in many historical populations (Cohen and Crane-Kramer 2007) serve to caution us against making generalizations about agriculture and diet and their effects on health.

The predominant public health framework of the "Nutrition Transition" argues that most societies progress from states of "undernutrition" to "receding famine" to "nutrition-related non-communicable diseases," and eventually to "medical and policy interventions that lead to behavioral change" (Popkin 2002). This provides a heuristic model of the relationships between food use patterns and nutrition-related disease, but may oversimplify our hunter-gatherer past of omnivory, ecological flexibility, and dietary variability (Dufour and Bender 2012). Most importantly, the model obscures within-population variability, the "specialty" of anthropologists. We need more anthropological data on how macro-level phenomena involved with agriculture and food production systems lead to micro-level changes in individual populations, and vice versa. Paleoanthropologists studying agriculture's effects on health need to distinguish between predominantly genetic variables and more developmentally plastic variables such as stature and tooth size (Cohen and Crane-Kramer 2007). The latter are likely influenced by maternal, fetal, and early childhood nutrition, which provides a link to biological anthropology work being done among contemporary populations on developmental origins of health and disease.

The case study of EcoHealth from Malawi highlights the integration of agriculture, child feeding practices, and human and environmental health. Promoting soil health and diversity is as important as promoting gut health and biodiversity in humans. Our bodies and our gut microflora have evolved to eat a varied diet, and lack of diversity in agriculture and our resulting diet has implications for environmental and human health. Myriad opportunities for biological anthropologists exist to investigate cultural influences on gut microflora, and health and disease. The importance of birth and infant feeding practices which promote colonies of health-supporting gut microflora and later life influences of dietary, environment, and cultural practices may explain some of the observed biological variation and health disparities. Biological variation in ability to access nutrients from the environment is exemplified by *Bacteroides plebeius* strains found in Japanese (but not North American) microbiomes, that have acquired a gene from marine bacteria enabling them to degrade porphyran in edible seaweed (Hehemann *et al.* 2010). Thus nutritional anthropologists interested in the effects of diet on health must expand their focus to include an ecological approach examining microniches of the human gut (Turner and Thompson 2013).

Anthropologists, with their multilevel and evolutionary and ecological approaches, study biocultural factors that influence the foods people eat and their physiological effects. Factors such as human genetic variation, lifestyle differences, infant feeding practices, hygiene, dietary diversity and content, food processing and preparation, and household size and environment, in addition to structural and socioeconomic inequalities, play important roles, and studies must take an explicit ecological approach, considering environmental ecosystems as well as the human-gut microbiome, and place those in a larger sociocultural and political-economic context. For example, soy intake has been correlated with various positive health outcomes such as reduced reproductive cancers, cholesterol, and menopausal symptoms. Yet gut bacteria determine which metabolites are produced and absorbed in the intestines. A higher proportion of the Japanese population appears to have gut bacteria that can convert the isoflavone daizein into the metabolite equol, which has been shown to have increased bioactivity, and may explain some of the observed population differences in epidemiological studies of the relationship between soy and health measures (Setchell, Brown, and Lydeking-Olsen 2002; Setchell and Cole 2006; Melby and Lampl 2011). Our symbiotic gut bacteria appear to be important intermediaries, influencing how food is processed internally, and in turn influencing vulnerability and resilience with respect to infectious and chronic disease.

While some anthropologists focus on the internal human ecosystems, others focus on the external. Farming is a mineral extractive industry: many nutrients and minerals are required to grow plants, yet most industrial farming systems return only three chemical nutrients to the soil, leading to decreasing fertility over time. The insights gained from the study of historical and indigenous practices such as those involved with *terra preta* that supported continued soil fertility can be applied to contemporary problems and projects such as the "City to Soil" project in Australia that aims to overcome the urban–rural disconnect by routing waste destined for landfills into compost for agriculture (Gillespie 2009). Further anthropological study of agricultural practices that support and enhance soil health may provide alternative models to the modern industrial practices that have been documented to decrease soil health. Anthropologists can also examine how agricultural activities (e.g., indigenous Amazonian vs. industrial agricultural practices) affect carbon cycles, and how they impact soil health, and thus affect food security and nutritional quality of foods produced. Furthermore, anthropologists can study traditional agro-ecology practices, as well as study wildlife/pollinator promotion efforts in urban gardening, and examine barriers to and support for ecological diversity.

Dowdall and Klotz's (2014) extensive study of pesticides and global health provides an exemplary model of how to conduct ecological medical anthropology situated in a broader political economic context. They examine the "agricultural treadmill" that affects farmers as they adopt new technologies such as agrochemicals to increase the outputs of the crops they grow, and then must continue buying the newest farm inputs in order to stay ahead of declining market prices. The latter is influenced by the commodification of food (Phillips 2006) and the globalization of agriculture, food production and distribution systems. These influence food choice and nutritional health in complex ways (Himmelgreen, Daza, and Noble 2011), and comparative multilevel anthropological studies may provide understandings and alternatives enabling farmers to get off the treadmill and reverse the unintended consequences of industrial agriculture. One possibility is to explore how citizens and states can start paying farmers to maintain and support ecosystem services that will reduce our costs for clean water and air, reduce antibiotic resistance, and ensure healthy, stable sources of food. Opportunities for anthropologists to study factors influencing agriculture's effects on environmental and human health span the continuum from micro (microbiome) to macro (political economy) levels and encompass themes of ecosystem diversity and variation and unintended consequences for sustainability.

REFERENCES

Aizen, M.A. and Harder, L.D. 2009. "The Global Stock of Domesticated Honey Bees is Growing Slower than Agricultural Demand for Pollination." *Current Biology*, 19(11): 915–918.

Anten, N. 2013. "Ecological Knowledge Offers Perspectives for Sustainable Agriculture." https://www.wageningenur.nl/en/show/Ecological-knowledge-offers-perspectives-for-sustainable-agriculture.htm (accessed November 25, 2015).

Appleby, M.C., Cutler, N., Gazzard, J., Goddard, P., Milne, J.A., Morgan, C., and Redfern, A. 2003. "What Price Cheap Food?" *Journal of Agricultural & Environmental Ethics*, 16(4): 395–408.

Backhed, F. Ley, R.E., Sonnenburg, J.L., Peterson, D.A., and Gordon, J.I. 2005. "Host-Bacterial Mutualism in the Human Intestine." *Science*, 307(5717): 1915–1920.

Badgley, C., Moghtader, J., Quintero, E., Zakem, E., Chappell, M.J., Aviles-Vazquez, K., Samulon, A., and Perfecto, I. 2007. "Organic Agriculture and the Global Food Supply." *Renewable Agriculture and Food Systems*, 22(2): 86–108.

Barker, D.J. 2004. "The Developmental Origins of Adult Disease." *Journal of the American College of Nutrition*, 23(6 Suppl): 588S–595S.

Becher, M.A., Osborne, J.L., Thorbek, P., Kennedy, P.J., and Grimm, V. 2013. "Towards a Systems Approach for Understanding Honeybee Decline: A Stocktaking and Synthesis of Existing Models." *The Journal of Applied Ecology*, 50(4): 868–880.

Berry, W. 1977. *The Unsettling of America: Culture & Agriculture*. San Francisco, CA: Sierra Club Books.

Bezner Kerr, R., Berti, P.R., and Shumba, L. 2011. "Effects of a Participatory Agriculture and Nutrition Education Project on Child Growth in Northern Malawi." *Public Health Nutrition*, 14(8): 1466–1472.

Black, R.E., Allen, L.H., Bhutta, Z.A., Caulfield, L.E., de Onis, M., Ezzati, M., Mathers, C., and Rivera, J. 2008. "Maternal and Child Undernutrition: Global and Regional Exposures and Health Consequences." *The Lancet*, 371(9608): 243–260.

Blaser, M. 2011. "Antibiotic Overuse: Stop the Killing of Beneficial Bacteria." *Nature*, 476(7361): 393–394.

Bonatsos, C., Bezner Kerr, R., and Shumba, L. 2009. "SFHC Food Security Status, Crop Diversity and Dietary Diversity: 2007, 2008 and 2009 Results." In *SFHC Project*. Ekwendeni Hospital, Ekwendeni, Malawi.

Boserup, E. 1965. *The Conditions of Agricultural Growth: The Economics of Agrarian Change Under Population Pressure*. Chicago, IL: Aldine.

Brandt, K. and Mølgaard. J.P. 2001. "Organic Agriculture: Does It Enhance or Reduce the Nutritional Value of Plant Foods?" *Journal of the Science of Food and Agriculture*, 81(9): 924–931.

Brush, S.B. 2007. "Farmers' Rights and Protection of Traditional Agricultural Knowledge." *World Development*, 35(9): 1499–1514.

Burkle, L.A., Knight, T.M., and Marlin, J.C. 2013. "Plant–Pollinator Interactions Over 120 Years: Loss of Species, Co-Occurrence, and Function." *Science*, 340(6127): 1611–1615.

Carolan, M. 2011. *The Real Cost of Cheap Food*. New York: Earthscan.

Charron, D.F. 2012. *Ecohealth Research in Practice*, ed. D.F. Charron. Vol. 1. New York: Springer.

Cohen, M.N. and Armelagos, G.J. (Eds.) 1984. *Paleopathology at the Origins of Agriculture*. Orlando, FL: Academic Press.

Cohen, M.N. and Crane-Kramer, G.M.M. 2007. "Editor's Summation." In *Ancient Health: Skeletal Indicators of Agricultural and Economic Intensification* (pp. 320–343). Gainesville: University Press of Florida.

Curtis, T.P., Sloan, W.T., and Scannell, J.W. 2002. "Estimating Prokaryotic Diversity and its Limits." *Proceedings of the National Academy of Sciences of the United States of America*, 99(16): 10494–10499.

Dallman, M.F., Pecoraro, N., Akana, S.F., La Fleur, S.E., Gomez, F., Houshyar, H., Bell, M.E., Bhatnagar, S., Laugero, K.D., and Manalo, S. 2003. "Chronic Stress and Obesity: A New View of 'Comfort Food'." *Proceedings of the National Academy of Sciences of the USA*, 100(20): 11696–11701.

De Filippo, C., Cavalieri, D., Di Paola, M., Ramazzotti, M., Poullet, J.B., Massart, S., Collini, S., Pieraccini, G., and Lionetti, P. 2010. "Impact of Diet in Shaping Gut Microbiota Revealed by a Comparative Study in Children from Europe and Rural Africa." *Proceedings of the National Academy of Sciences of the USA*, 107(33): 14691–14696.

DeCaro, J.A., Wilson, W., Manyama, M., and Hallgrimsson, B. 2013. "Pathways Toward Differential Maternal and Child Well-being Amidst Food Insecurity in Tanzanian Households: The Role of Child Age and Maternal Affect." *American Journal of Human Biology*, 25: 255–256.

Desowitz, R.S. 1991. "Mal'Aria-the Bad News Airs." In *The Malaria Capers: Tales of Parasites and People* (pp. 143–152). New York: Norton.

Dethlefsen, L., McFall-Ngai, M., and Relman, D.A. 2007. "An Ecological and Evolutionary Perspective on Human-Microbe Mutualism and Disease." *Nature*, 449(7164): 811–818.

Diamond, J. 1987. "The Worst Mistake in the History of the Human Race." *Discover*, 8(5): 64–66.

Dowdall, C.M. and Klotz, R.J. 2014. *Pesticides and Global Health: Understanding Agrochemical Dependence and Investing in Sustainable Solutions*. Walnut Creek, CA: Left Coast Press.

Drewnowski, A. 2004. "Obesity and the Food Environment: Dietary Energy Density and Diet Costs." *American Journal of Preventive Medicine*, 27(3 Suppl): 154–162.

Dufour, D.L. and Bender, R.L. 2012. "Nutrition Transitions: A View from Anthropology." In D.L. Dufour, A.H. Goodman, and G.H. Pelto (Eds.), *Nutritional Anthropology: Biocultural Perspectives on Food and Nutrition*, 2nd ed. (pp. 372–382). Oxford: Oxford University Press.

Dunn, R.R., Fierer, N., Henley, J.B., Leff, J.W., and Menninger, H.L. 2013. "Home Life: Factors Structuring the Bacterial Diversity found within and between Homes." *Plos One*, 8(5): e64133. doi: 10.1371/journal.pone.0064133.

Duram, L.A. 2005. *Good Growing: Why Organic Farming Works.* Lincoln: University of Nebraska Press.

Eaton, S.B. and Konner, M. 1985. "Paleolithic Nutrition. A Consideration of its Nature and Current Implications." *New England Journal of Medicine*, 312(5): 283–289.

Ege, M.J., Mayer, M., Normand, A.-C., Genuneit, J., Cookson, W.O.C.M., Braun-Fahrlaender, C., Heederik, D., Piarroux, R., von Mutius, E., and GABRIELA Transregio 22 Study Group. 2011. "Exposure to Environmental Microorganisms and Childhood Asthma." *New England Journal of Medicine*, 364(8): 701–709.

Ellison, P.T. 2005. "Evolutionary Perspectives on the Fetal Origins Hypothesis." *American Journal of Human Biology*, 17(1): 113–118.

EPA (Environmental Protection Agency). 2014. "About Pesticides." http://www.epa.gov/pesticides/about/ (accessed November 25, 2015).

FAO (Food and Agriculture Organization). 2008. An Introduction to the Basic Concepts of Food Security. http://www.fao.org/docrep/013/al936e/al936e00.pdf (accessed November 25, 2015).

FAO (Food and Agriculture Organization). 2013. *The State of Food Insecurity in the World 2013.* Rome: FAO. http://www.fao.org/docrep/018/i3434e/i3434e00.htm (accessed November 25, 2015).

FAO (Food and Agriculture Organization). 2014. Prevention and Disposal of Obsolete Pesticides. http://www.fao.org/agriculture/crops/obsolete-pesticides/prevention-and-disposal-of-obsolete-pesticides/en/ (accessed November 25, 2015).

Farmer, P., Robin, S. St Luc Ramilus, St.L., and Kim., J.Y. 1991. "Tuberculosis, Poverty, and 'Compliance': Lessons from Rural Haiti." *Seminars in Respiratory Infections*, 6(4): 254–260.

Funkhouser, L.J. and Bordenstein, S.R. 2013. "Mom Knows Best: The Universality of Maternal Microbial Transmission." *PLoS Biology*, 11(8): e1001631.

Garibaldi, L.A., Steffan-Dewenter, I., Winfree, R., Aizen, M.A., Bommarco, R., Cunningham, S.A., Kremen, C. *et al.* 2013. "Wild Pollinators Enhance Fruit Set of Crops Regardless of Honey Bee Abundance." *Science*, 339(6127): 1608–1611.

Garrett, H., Ferguson, J., and Amaranthus, M.P. 2012. *Organic Management for the Professional: The Natural Way for Landscape Architects and Contractors, Commercial Growers, Golf Course Managers, Park Administrators, Turf Managers, and Other Stewards of the Land.* Austin: University of Texas Press.

Gilden, R.C., Huffling, K., and Sattler, B. 2010. "Pesticides and Health Risks." *Journal of Obstetric, Gynecologic, & Neonatal Nursing*, 39(1): 103–110.

Gillespie, G. 2009. "City to Soil: Returning Organics to Agriculture – A Circle of Sustainability." In W.I. Woods, W.G. Teixeira, J. Lehmann, C. Steiner, A. WinklerPrins, and L. Rebellato (Eds.), *Amazonian Dark Earths: Wim Sombroek's Vision* (pp. 465–472). New York: Springer.

Glaser, B. and Birk, J.J. 2012. "State of the Scientific Knowledge on Properties and Genesis of Anthropogenic Dark Earths in Central Amazonia (Terra Preta De Índio)." *Geochimica Et Cosmochimica Acta*, 82(0): 39–51.

Gronlund, M.-M., Lehtonen, O.-P., Eerola, E., and Kero, P. 1999. "Fecal Microflora in Healthy Infants Born by Different Methods of Delivery: Permanent Changes in Intestinal Flora After Cesarean Delivery." *Journal of Pediatric Gastroenterology and Nutrition*, 28(1): 19–25.

Hadley, C. and Crooks, D.L. 2012. "Coping and the Biosocial Consequences of Food Insecurity in the 21st Century." *Yearbook of Physical Anthropology*, 55: 72–94.

Heaton, S. 2013. *Organic Farming, Food Quality and, Human Health: A Review of the Evidence.* http://www.soilassociation.org/LinkClick.aspx?fileticket=cY8kfP3Q%2BgA%3D&%3Btabid=388 (accessed November 25, 2015).

Hehemann, J.-H., Correc, G., Barbeyron, T., Helbert, W., Czjzek, M., and Michel, G. 2010. "Transfer of Carbohydrate-Active Enzymes from Marine Bacteria to Japanese Gut Microbiota." *Nature*, 464(7290): 908–U123.

Himmelgreen, D.A., Daza, N.R, and Noble, C.A. 2011. "Nutrition and Health." In M. Singer and P.I. Erickson (Eds.), *A Companion to Medical Anthropology* (pp. 305–322). Singapore: Blackwell Publishing.

Horrigan, L., Lawrence, R.S., and Walker, P. 2002. "How Sustainable Agriculture can Address the Environmental and Human Health Harms of Industrial Agriculture." *Environmental Health Perspectives*, 110(5): 445–456.

Jabolonka, E. and Lamb, M.J. 2005. *Evolution in Four Dimensions: Genetic, Epigenetic, Behavioral, and Symbolic Variation in the History of Life.* Cambridge, MA: MIT Press.

Jeyaratnam, J. 1990. "Acute Pesticide Poisoning: A Major Global Health Problem." *World Health Stat Q*, 43(3): 139–14.

Jones, K.C. and de Voogt, P. 1999. "Persistent Organic Pollutants (POPs): State of the Science." *Environmental Pollution*, 100(1–3): 209–221.

Kamel, F. and Hoppin, J.A. 2004. "Association of Pesticide Exposure with Neurologic Dysfunction and Disease." *Environmental Health Perspectives*, 112(9): 950–958.

Kerr, R.B. 2005. "Informal Labor and Social Relations in Northern Malawi: The Theoretical Challenges and Implications of Ganyu Labor for Food Security." *Rural Sociology*, 70(2).

Kerr, R.B., Berti, P.R., and Chirwa, M. 2007. "Breastfeeding and Mixed Feeding Practices in Malawi: Timing, Reasons, Decision Makers, and Child Health Consequences." *Food and Nutrition Bulletin*, 28(1): 90–99.

Klein, A.-M., Vaissiere, B.E., Cane, J.H., Steffan-Dewenter, I., Cunningham, S.A., Kremen, C., and Tscharntke, T. 2007. "Importance of Pollinators in Changing Landscapes for World Crops." *Proceedings of the Royal Society B: Biological Sciences*, 274(1608): 303–313.

Kremen, C., Williams, N.M., and Thorp, R.W. 2002. "Crop Pollination from Native Bees at Risk from Agricultural Intensification." *Proceedings of the National Academy of Sciences*, 99(26): 16812–16816.

Kuzawa, C.W. 1998. "Adipose Tissue in Human Infancy and Childhood: An Evolutionary Perspective." *American Journal of Physical Anthropology*, Suppl 27: 177–209.

Lal, R. 2004. "Soil Carbon Sequestration Impacts on Global Climate Change and Food Security." *Science*, 304(5677): 1623–1627.

Larsen, C.S. 1995. "Biological Changes in Human Populations with Agriculture." *Annual Review of Anthropology*, 24(1): 185–213.

Lawton, G. 2014. "The Permaculture Research Institute." http://permaculturenews.org/2008/08/30/ (accessed November 25, 2015).

Lederberg, J. 2000. "Infectious History." *Science*, 288(5464): 287–293.

Leopold, A. 1966. *A Sand County Almanac with Other Essays on Conservation from Round River.* New York: Oxford University Press.

Ley, R.E., Peterson, D.A., and Gordon, J.I. 2006. "Ecological and Evolutionary Forces Shaping Microbial Diversity in the Human Intestine." *Cell*, 124(4): 837–848.

Ley, R.E., Turnbaugh, P.J., Klein, S., and Gordon, J.I. 2006. "Microbial Ecology – Human Gut Microbes Associated with Obesity." *Nature*, 444(7122): 1022–1023.

Linz, B., Balloux, F., Moodley, Y., Manica, A., Liu, H., Roumagnac, P., Falush, D., *et al.* 2007. "An African Origin for the Intimate Association between Humans and Helicobacter Pylori." *Nature*, 445(7130): 915–918.

McMichael, A.J., Powles, J.W., Butler, C.D., and Uauy, R. 2007. "Food, Livestock Production, Energy, Climate Change, and Health." *Lancet*, 370(9594): 1253–1263.

Melby, M.K. and Lampl, M. 2011. "Menopause, A Biocultural Perspective." *Annual Review of Anthropology*, 40(1): 53–70.

Montgomery, D.R. 2007. *Dirt: The Erosion of Civilizations*. Berkeley: University of California Press.

Murray, D., Wesseling, C., Keifer, M., Corriols, M., and Henao, S. 2002. "Surveillance of Pesticide-Related Illness in the Developing World: Putting the Data to Work." *International Journal of Occupational and Environmental Health*, 8(3): 243–248.

Nestle, M. 2002. *Food Politics: How the Food Industry Influences Nutrition and Health*. Berkeley: University of California Press.

Neves, E.G., Petersen, J.B., Bartone, R.N., and Da Silva, CA. 2003. "Historical and Socio-Cultural Origins of Amazonian Dark Earths." In J. Lehmann, D.C. Kern, B. Glaser, and W.I. Woods (Eds.), *Amazonian Dark Earths: Origin, Properties, Management* (pp. 29–50). Dordrecht: Kluwer.

Norton, G.W. 2005. "Ending Hunger in our Lifetime: Food Security and Globalization." *AGEC Agricultural Economics*, 32(3): 329–330.

O'Donnell, A.G., Seasman, M., Macrae, A., Waite, I., and Davies, J.T. 2001. "Plants and Fertilisers as Drivers of Change in Microbial Community Structure and Function in Soils." *Plant and Soil*, 232(1–2): 135–145.

Pennisi, E. 2011. "Microbiology. Girth and the Gut (Bacteria)." *Science*, 332(6025): 32–33.

Pflughoeft, K.J. and Versalovic, J. 2012. "Human Microbiome in Health and Disease." *Annual Review of Pathology*, 7: 99–122.

Phillips, L. 2006. "Food and Globalization." *Annual Review of Anthropology*, 35(1): 37–57.

Pimentel, D. 1974. *Energy use in World Food Production*. Rome: FAO, UN.

Pimentel, D. 2006. "Soil Erosion: A Food and Environmental Threat." *Environment, Development and Sustainability*, 8(1): 119–137.

Pimentel, D. and Pimentel. M. 2003. "Sustainability of Meat-Based and Plant-Based Diets and the Environment." *The American Journal of Clinical Nutrition*, 78(3): 660S–663S.

Pinstrup-Andersen, P., Pandya-Lorch, R., and Rosegrant, M.W. 1999. *World Food Prospects: Critical Issues for the Early Twenty-First Century*. Washington DC: International Food Policy Research Institute.

Pollan, M. 2002. "Power Steer." New York Times, March 31. http://michaelpollan.com/articles-archive/power-steer/ (accessed November 25, 2015).

Popkin, B.M. 2002. "An Overview on the Nutrition Transition and Its Health Implications: The Bellagio Meeting." *Public Health Nutrition*, 5(1A): 93–103.

Price, T. D. 1995. "Social Inequality at the Origins of Agriculture." In T.D. Price and G.M. Feinman (Eds.), *Foundations of Social Inequality* (pp. 129–151). New York: Plenum Press.

Rabinowitz, P. and Conti, L. 2013. "Links among Human Health, Animal Health, and Ecosystem Health." *Annual Review of Public Health*, 34(1): 189–204.

Ramamoorthy, V., Viswanathan, R., Raguchander, T., Prakasam, V., and Samiyappan, R. 2001. "Induction of Systemic Resistance by Plant Growth Promoting Rhizobacteria in Crop Plants Against Pests and Diseases." *Crop Protection*, 20(1): 1–11.

Sanchez, P.A. 2004. "Reducing Hunger by Improving Soil Fertility: An African Success Story." In C.G. Scanes and J.A. Miranowski (Eds.), *Perspectives in World Food and Agriculture* (pp. 75–85). Ames, IA: Iowa State Press.

Searchinger, T., Hanson, C., Ranganathan, J., Lipinski, B., Waite, R., Winterbottom, R., Dinshaw, A., and Heimlich, R. 2013. *Creating a Sustainable Food Future: A Menu of*

Solutions to Sustainably Feed More than 9 Billion People by 2050: World Resources Institute.

Setchell, K.D., Brown, N.M., and Lydeking-Olsen, E. 2002. "The Clinical Importance of the Metabolite Equol – A Clue to the Effectiveness of Soy and Its Isoflavones." *Journal of Nutrition*, 132(12): 3577–3584.

Setchell, K.D. and Cole, S.J. 2006. "Method of Defining Equol-Producer Status and Its Frequency among Vegetarians." *Journal of Nutrition*, 136(8): 2188–2193.

Shelton, H.M. 2000. "Tropical Forage Tree Legumes in Agroforestry Systems." *Unasylva*, 51(200): 25–32.

Singer, M. 2011. "Toward a Critical Biosocial Model of Ecohealth in Southern Africa: The HIV/AIDS and Nutrition Insecurity Syndemic." *Annals of Anthropological Practice*, 35(1): 8–27.

Smith, C., Kerr, K., and Sadripour, A. 2008. "Pesticide Exports from U.S. Ports, 2001–2003." *International Journal of Occupational and Environmental Health*, 14(3): 176–186.

Smith, S.E., Read, D.J., and Harley, J.L. 1997. *Mycorrhizal Symbiosis*. San Diego, CA: Academic Press.

Snapp, S.S., Blackie, M.J., Gilbert, R.A., Kerr, R.B., and Kanyama-Phiri, G.Y. 2010. "Biodiversity Can Support a Greener Revolution in Africa." *Proceedings of the National Academy of Sciences of the United States of America*, 107(48): 20840–20845.

Spivak, M., Mader, E., Vaughan, M., and Euliss, N.H. 2011. "The Plight of the Bees." *Environmental Science & Technology*, 45(1): 34–38.

Stonich, S.C. 1993. *"I Am Destroying the Land!": The Political Ecology of Poverty and Environmental Destruction in Honduras*. Boulder, CO: Westview.

Strachan, D.P. 1989. "Hay Fever, Hygiene, and Household Size." *British Medical Journal*, 299(6710): 1259–1260.

Tanumihardjo, S.A., Anderson, C., Kaufer-Horwitz, M., Bode, L., Emenaker, N.J. Haqq, A.M., Satia, J.A., Silver, H.J., and Stadler, D.D. 2007. "Poverty, Obesity, and Malnutrition: An International Perspective Recognizing the Paradox." *Journal of the American Dietetic Association*, 107(11): 1966–1972.

Thurston, T.L. and Fisher, C.T. 2007a. "Intensification, Innovation, and Change: New Perspectives and Future Directions." In T.L. Thurston and C.T. Fisher (Eds.), *Seeking a Richer Harvest: The Archaeology of Subsistence Intensification, Innovation, and Change* (pp. 249–259). New York: Springer.

Thurston, T.L. and Fisher, C.T. 2007b. "Seeking a Richer Harvest: An Introduction to the Archaeology of Subsistence Intensification, Innovation and Change." In T.L. Thurston and C.T. Fisher (Eds.), *Seeking a Richer Harvest: The Archaeology of Subsistence Intensification, Innovation, and Change* (pp. 1–21). New York: Springer.

Torsvik, V. 2002. "Prokaryotic Diversity – Magnitude, Dynamics, and Controlling Factors." *Science*, 296(5570): 1064–1066.

Tsai, S.M., O'Neill, B.E., Cannavan, F.S., Saito, D., Falcao, N.P.S., Kern, D.C., Grossman, J.M., and Thies, J.E. 2009. "The Microbial World of Terra Preta." In W.I. Woods, W.G. Teixeira, J. Lehmann, C. Steiner, A. WinklerPrins, and L. Rebellato (Eds.), *Amazonian Dark Earths: Wim Sombroek's Vision* (pp. 299–308). New York: Springer.

Turnbaugh, P.J., Ley, R.E., Mahowald, M.A., Magrini, V., Mardis, E.R., and Gordon, J.I. 2006. "An Obesity-Associated Gut Microbiome with Increased Capacity for Energy Harvest." *Nature*, 444(7122): 1027–1031.

Turner, B.L. and Thompson, A.L. 2013. "Beyond the Paleolithic Prescription: Incorporating Diversity and Flexibility in the Study of Human Diet Evolution." *Nutrition Reviews*, 71(8): 501–510.

UN (United Nations). 2013. "Secretary-General's Message on World Food Day." http://www.un.org/sg/statements/?nid=7206 (accessed November 25, 2015).

UNEP (United Nations Environment Programme). 2005. "Ridding the World of POPS: A Guide to the Stockholm Convention on Persistent Organic Pollutants." http://www.unep.org/delc/Portals/119/popseng.pdf (accessed November 25, 2015).

van der Heijden, M.G.A., Bardgett, R.D., and van Straalen, N.M. 2008. "The Unseen Majority: Soil Microbes as Drivers of Plant Diversity and Productivity in Terrestrial Ecosystems." *Ecology Letters*, 11(3): 296–310.

Victora, C.G., Adair, L., Fall, C., Hallal, P.C., Martorell, R., Richter, L., and Sachdev, H.S. 2008. "Maternal and Child Undernutrition: Consequences for Adult Health and Human Capital." *The Lancet*, 371(9609): 340–357.

Villarejo, D. 2003. "The Health of U.S. Hired Farm Workers." *Annual Review of Public Health*, 24(1): 175–193.

Wahlqvist, M. 2013. "Future Directions for Clinical Nutrition in the Asia Pacific Region." Tokyo, Japan, June 11, 2013.

Walter, J. and Ley. R. 2011. "The Human Gut Microbiome: Ecology and Recent Evolutionary Changes." *Annual Review of Microbiology*, 65: 411–429.

Weaver, L.J. 2009. "Moving Beyond Hunger and Nutrition: A Systematic Review of the Evidence Linking Food Insecurity and Mental Health in Developing Countries." *Ecology of Food and Nutrition*, 48(4): 263–284.

Weigel, M.M., Armijos, R.X., Hall, H.P., Ramirez, Y., and Orozco, R. 2007. "The Household Food Insecurity and Health Outcomes of U.S.–Mexico Border Migrant and Seasonal Farmworkers." *Journal of Immigrant and Minority Health*, 9(3): 157–169.

Weiser, S.D., Young, S.L., Cohen, C.R., Kushel, M.B., Tsai, A.C., Tien, P.C., Hatcher, A.M., Frongillo, E.A., and Bangsberg, D.R. 2011. "Conceptual Framework for Understanding the Bidirectional Links between Food Insecurity and HIV/AIDS." *American Journal of Clinical Nutrition*, 94(6): 1729S–1739S.

WHO (World Health Organization). 1948. Preamble to the Constitution of the World Health Organization. http://www.who.int/about/definition/en/print.html (accessed November 25, 2015).

WHO (World Health Organization). 2004. "The Impact of Pesticides on Health." http://www.who.int/mental_health/prevention/suicide/en/PesticidesHealth2.pdf (accessed November 25, 2015).

WHO (World Health Organization). 2011. "Noncommunicable Diseases Country Profiles." http://www.who.int/nmh/publications/ncd_profiles2011/en/ (accessed November 25, 2015).

Wiley, A.S. 2008. "Cow's Milk Consumption and Health: An Evolutionary Perspective." In W. Trevathan, E.O. Smith, and J.J. McKenna (Eds.), *Evolutionary Medicine and Health: New Perspectives* (pp. 116–133). New York: Oxford University Press.

Wilson, E.O. 1992. *The Diversity of Life*. Cambridge, MA: Harvard University Press.

Woods, W.I. and Denevan, W.M. 2009. "Amazonian Dark Earths: The First Century of Reports." In W.I. Woods, W.G. Teixeira, J. Lehmann, C. Steiner, A. WinklerPrins, and L. Rebellato (Eds.), *Amazonian Dark Earths: Wim Sombroek's Vision* (pp. 1–14. New York: Springer.

World Resources Institute. 2002. "People and Ecosystems: The Fraying Web of Life." *Peace Research Abstracts*, 39(1): 3–152.

Worthington, V. 2001. "Nutritional Quality of Organic Versus Conventional Fruits, Vegetables, and Grains." *Journal of Alternative and Complementary Medicine*, 7(2): 161–173.

Wratten, S.D., Gillespie, M., Decourtye, A., Mader, E., and Desneux, N. 2012. "Pollinator Habitat Enhancement: Benefits to Other Ecosystem Services." *Agriculture, Ecosystems and Environment*, 159: 112–122.

Young, J.E., Zhao, X., Carey, E.E., Welti, R., Yang, S.-S., and Wang, W. 2005. "Phytochemical Phenolics in Organically Grown Vegetables." *Molecular Nutrition & Food Research*, 49(12): 1136–1142.

Zivkovic, A.M., German, J.B., Lebrilla, C.B., and Mills, D.A. 2010. "Human Milk Glycobiome and Its Impact on the Infant Gastrointestinal Microbiota." *Proceedings of the National Academy of Sciences*, 108(1): 4653–4658.

CHAPTER 3

Toward "One Health" Promotion

Melanie Rock and Chris Degeling

Introduction

As a field, medical anthropology has contributed robust critiques of biomedical science as well as thoughtful explorations of embodiment at multiple scales (Lock 1993; Nguyen and Peschard 2004; Inhorn 2007; Brotherton and Nguyen 2013). Medical anthropology has certainly sought to raise questions about environmental health, yet contributors have not consistently incorporated anthropological explorations of science, technology, or embodiment (Petryna 2013 [2003]), nor anthropological engagements with the realities of multispecies existence (Mullin 2002; Lestel 2006; Kohn 2007; Kirksey and Helmreich 2010; Blue and Rock 2011; Descola 2013 [2005]). Meanwhile, anthropological theories of space have been advanced (e.g., Jimínez 2003; Low 2009; Ingold 2012), yet thus far, the discipline of geography (e.g., Braun 2005; Hinchliffe and Whatmore 2006; Buller 2014) appears to have received and incorporated this potential line of inquiry more readily than has the field of medical anthropology. In sum, other disciplines and other fields within anthropology are actively engaging with the embodiment and emplacement of more-than-human collectives to an extent that medical anthropology has not. It is possible that foundational terminology in medical anthropology could, in fact, present a discursive boundary to active and reflexive engagement with environmental health – for example, through classifying studies as being *of* illness, *of* sickness, or *in* medicine (Young 1982).

A Companion to the Anthropology of Environmental Health, First Edition. Edited by Merrill Singer.

In response to the virtual absence of engagement with contemporary theorizing about more-than-human collectives in anthropological studies of environmental health, we might ask: are efforts to improve living conditions, and thereby health, necessarily medical or medicalizing in orientation? No, is our answer. To respond more fulsomely, this chapter builds on the recent work of an environmental anthropologist, Tim Ingold. More specifically, we build on his conceptualization of meshwork, which revisits questions of how bodies and environments are fashioned and experienced, while also underscoring the permeability and perishability of both human *and* nonhuman bodies. For Ingold (2011: 68), meshwork denotes "being alive" as a process of "continuous birth" (following Scott 1989). Meshwork, in fact, entails incessant exchange between bodies (human and nonhuman) with their surroundings as the basis for sentience, perception, and emotions. Ingold explicitly rails against the concept of actor networks from science and technology studies (STS), in which the question of whether or not entities are alive is moot or bracketed for the purpose of analysis. While he critiques the work of Bruno Latour under the rubric of actor-network theory, Ingold does not broach recent work aligned to STS that engages with multispecies existence, including that of Donna Haraway, John Law, Annemarie Mol, Sarah Whatmore, or Steve Hinchliffe. Further, Ingold does not explicitly concern himself with health, even as his discussion of "being alive" within and through meshwork resonates with some Indigenous and Western ideas about "being alive well" or "well-being" (Adelson 2000; Rock, Degeling, and Blue 2013).

Following these leads, therefore, we seek to integrate Ingold's meshwork concept with the "One Health" concept, which has gained currency in veterinary medicine and public health (Zinsstag *et al.* 2011), and which is beginning to attract critical attention from social scientists (e.g., Rock *et al.* 2009; Singer *et al.* 2011; Green 2012; Degeling and Kerridge 2013; French and Mykhalovskiy 2013; Hinchliffe *et al.* 2013; Leach and Scoones 2013). "One Health" refers to intricate connections between the health of humans, nonhuman animals, and entire ecosystems, and proponents are beginning to acknowledge the extent to which social organization and social inequality within human populations impact upon outcomes for people, other animals, and environmental integrity (Rock *et al.* 2009; Zinsstag *et al.* 2011). We find Haraway's (2008) discussion of multispecies flourishing, and its politics (following Cuomo 1998), helpful in operationalizing the One Health concept in ways that acknowledge inherent contradictions and pernicious selectivity implied by interventions in any living system for the advantage of human or nonhuman individuals, populations, or their shared ecosystems. Furthermore, in attending to how human life entwines with nonhuman life, we regard Haraway's conceptualization of multispecies flourishing as compatible with Ingold's conceptualization of meshwork. Haraway's discussion of multispecies flourishing, however, emphasizes how scientific knowledge and technology impact upon both human and nonhuman lives.

Ultimately, drawing principally on Ingold and Haraway, we argue for greater attention to nonhuman animals and environments in medical anthropology. In so doing, we call upon anthropologists to engage with a field of public health known as health promotion. To help ground our discussion, policy statements endorsed by the World Health Organization (WHO) are contrasted with policy statements endorsed by the World Animal Health Organization (l'Office international des épizooties, or OIE). We focus particularly on the prescriptions provided by the OIE for the social lives of domestic dogs because, at least in the lived experience and imaginaries of Western societies, dogs exemplify how nonhumans can bridge the divisions between otherness, liminality, and full-fledged kinship.

Welfare, Well-being, and One Health

In veterinary medicine, the term "welfare" is more commonly used in relation to nonhuman animals than is "well-being." Even as animal health professionals increasingly subscribe to what is being described as the "ethological turn," and thereby affective, animal-centered, and positive conceptions of welfare (Bock and Buller 2013), the term "well-being" does not apply to nonhuman animals in common usage, but rather to "a state of being or doing well in life" embodied subjectively by "a person or a community" (OED 2013b). "Welfare" also refers to a "state or condition of doing well," yet this term routinely is used to describe a "person, a community, or a *thing*" (OED 2013a, emphasis added). In part reflecting its origins in economic theory, "welfare," therefore, is a term that is often used to describe nonhumans, whether alive or devoid of life, whereas the term "well-being" is conventionally reserved for human lives.

Crucially, "welfare states" and other kinds of governmental organizations are considered to be things, even as they imbricate with human life (Foucault 1991 [1978]), as well as with nonhuman life (Wadiwel 2009). More generally, anthropologists and other contributors to the interdisciplinary field of science and technology studies have repeatedly shown that the person–thing distinction frequently dissolves in practice, including within Western science and biomedicine (Mol 2002). Moreover, the person–thing distinction is hardly universal (Kopytoff 1982; Kopytoff 1986; Pottage and Mundy 2004; Descola 2013 [2005]).

Accordingly, "welfare" and "well-being" may be fully synonymous in daily life, and we, and others (Nordenfelt 2011), feel fully justified in extending the term "well-being" to nonhuman animals. Nevertheless, distinctions between and amongst humans and nonhuman animals imbue how lives are classified and evaluated, and how bodies are treated and experienced (Blue and Rock 2011). An overview of policies endorsed by the OIE and the WHO provides some insight into the extent to which animal health and welfare have been defined symmetrically with human health and well-being. This exercise illustrates the importance of analyzing contingencies in discursive renderings of human and nonhuman existence, while also pointing to material differences and resemblances. Both discourse and materiality are important in fashioning environments so as to enable well-being for humans and nonhuman species, which is what we mean by One Health promotion.

OIE and WHO Definitions of "Health," "Welfare," and "Well-being"

The OIE was founded in 1924, but it was not until the early 2000s that the welfare of nonhuman animals became a strategic priority for the organization (OIE 2013a). In "[r]ecognizing the essential link between animal health and animal welfare" (OIE 2002), the preamble of the *Animal Welfare Mandate of the OIE* went so far as to state what might appear to be obvious. By implication, during the first 75 years of its existence, the OIE operationalized an understanding of animal health that did not explicitly concern whether nonhuman animals themselves were faring well. As an expression of this new mandate, in 2004 the OIE convened an inaugural Global Conference on Animal Welfare, and a set of "guiding principles on animal welfare" were included within the OIE's *Terrestrial Animal Code* for the first time (OIE 2013a).

The first guiding principle on animal welfare within the OIE Code deliberately echoes the preamble by affirming: "there is a critical relationship between animal health and animal welfare" (OIE 2013b: article 7.1). Both building on and reinforcing the emerging policy importance of animal welfare, the second principle states that the "internationally recognised 'five freedoms'... provide valuable guidance in animal welfare" (OIE 2013b: article 7.1). They are: "freedom from hunger, thirst and malnutrition; freedom from fear and distress; freedom from physical and thermal discomfort; freedom from *pain, injury* and *disease*; and freedom to express normal patterns of behaviour" (OIE 2013b: article 7.2, emphasis added).

Whereas what constitutes "health" in animals is not explicitly defined in the OIE Code, not even in the glossary, "health" is used throughout the document to denote the absence of disease, infection or injury in nonhuman animals and populations (for example, OIE 2013b: article 1.4.3). By contrast, the WHO does not regard human health as synonymous with the absence of disease, injury, or illness. "Health," according to the WHO's (1948) Constitution, "is a state of complete physical, mental and social well-being and not merely the absence of disease or infirmity." Furthermore, another "guiding principle for animal welfare" in the OIE Code recalls the WHO's (1948) definition of human well-being, but not animal welfare, as consisting of something more than "the absence of disease or infirmity." According to this principle, "the use of animals in agriculture, education, and research, and for companionship, recreation and entertainment, makes a major contribution to the *well-being* of people" (OIE 2013b, emphasis added). Yet whether such uses of nonhuman animals protect or enhance *their own* well-being is, to say the least, contested in academe and among advocates for nonhuman animals (Broom 2011). Nevertheless, animal welfare scientists are said to be increasingly adopting complex notions of well-being, vitality, dignity, and integrity that align with multispecies flourishing (Bock and Buller 2013; Harfeld 2013).

From "Health for All" toward Multispecies Flourishing

Whereas the *Terrestrial Animal Health Code* defines animal welfare and provides page after page of specific recommendations for practice (OIE 2013b), the WHO's (1948) Constitution is not nearly as prescriptive when it comes to how to foster or protect health, that is, a "complete state of physical, mental and social well-being" in human populations. The WHO's (1948) definition of human health has not been amended since its adoption in the wake of World War II, yet it has long been criticized for vagueness (e.g., Powers and Faden 2006: 17). Against this backdrop, the *Ottawa Charter* outlined how to achieve the 1948 definition of human health. The stated intent of the Charter was to guide "action to achieve Health for All by the year 2000 and beyond" (WHO 1986). More than 30 years after its adoption, however, the *Ottawa Charter* is little known beyond health promotion as the subfield of public health.

The *Ottawa Charter* operationalized the WHO's (1948) definition of health, as follows: "To reach a state of complete physical, mental and social well-being, *an individual or group must be able to identify and to realize aspirations, to satisfy needs, and to change or cope with the environment*" (WHO 1986, emphasis added). The *Ottawa Charter* never once mentioned nonhuman animals. Needless to say, the "All" in "Health for All" was therefore understood to be limited to humans. In fact, the *Ottawa Charter* defined health promotion as "the process of enabling *people* to increase control over, and to improve, their health" (WHO 1986, emphasis added). Insofar as the *Ottawa Charter* identifies "a stable ecosystem" and "sustainable resources" as among the "fundamental conditions and resources for health," nonhuman animals and environments were construed implicitly as things over which people can and should exert mastery for the sake of human health (WHO 1986).

In our estimation, however, the *Ottawa Charter* could be reinterpreted in support of multispecies flourishing (following Haraway 2008). An especially crucial passage reads:

> Health is created and lived by people within the settings of their everyday life; where they learn, work, play and love. Health is created by caring for oneself and others, by being able to take decisions and have control over one's life circumstances, and by ensuring that the society one lives in creates conditions that allow the attainment of health by all its members. (WHO 1986)

We agree that health can be "created and lived" in the context of everyday life, and would add that nonhuman animals contribute materially to the generation and experience of well-being for people. We also maintain that a collectivity is never purely human, and that nonhuman animals play crucial roles in constituting social life. In fact, the recognized members of many collectivities include nonhuman beings (Descola 2013 [2005]).

Furthermore, in keeping with the OIE's recognition of "five freedoms" as a starting place for operationalizing animal welfare (OIE 2013b: article 7.7.2), we also recognize that "being able to take decisions and have control over one's life circumstances" (WHO 1986) is important for most if not all nonhuman animals, as well as for humans. Even so, terms such as "decision" and "control" may need to be rethought to align with realities and actual practice, which could be helpful to understand the full range of agency exerted by human beings, too. We are thinking, for example, of people with disabilities, as well as of the limited extent to which people exercise control or decide for themselves without social, economic, or cultural influences. Furthermore, we recognize that access to the resources that enable mastery and decision-making capacity are unevenly distributed, to the point of inequity.

The *Ottawa Charter* also foregrounds "[c]aring, holism and ecology" (WHO 1986), which is essential to any extension of the *Ottawa Charter* toward One Health promotion. Even though caring for both human and nonhuman beings can certainly be controlling (Haraway 2008; Law and Mol 2008; Mol 2008 [2006]), implementing the *Ottawa Charter* in ways that acknowledge subjectivity and responsibility for nonhuman animals as well as for human beings could be compatible with multispecies flourishing (Haraway 2008) and with the essence of meshwork (Ingold 2011). In immediate and practical terms, applying the tenets of health promotion as outlined in the *Ottawa Charter* to more-than-human collectivities would reinforce the emergence of new animal-centered and effective animal welfare policies and practices, as well as the adoption of environmental policies and practices that explicitly concern the vitality of both human and nonhuman lives.

One Health Promotion and the Social Lives of Dogs

Dogs are poignant and recurring figures for Haraway (2008) in working out her arguments regarding multispecies flourishing. For the purposes of illustration and theorization, Haraway analyzes her own lived involvement in dog care, which, to name a few examples, includes visits to veterinary clinics; competitive participation in the human–dog sport of agility; visits to nearby beaches so that her dogs can be unleashed to run around and socialize, while owners also socialize; and dog walking in a nature preserve near her home and the university where she is employed, sometimes accompanied by friends and colleagues.

Haraway (2008: 134–135) regards dog care as an ethical imperative; but at the same time, she acknowledges that dog care is riven with contradictions, trade-offs, and ontological multiplicity to an extent that the existing body of health promotion research on dog ownership is not (McNicholas *et al.* 2005; Cutt *et al.* 2007; Toohey and Rock 2011; Christian *et al.* 2013). She notes: "Dogs in capitalist technoculture have acquired the 'right of health,' and the economic (as well as legal) implications are legion" (Haraway 2008: 48). Indeed, dog ownership is increasingly associated with physical activity and social life in some non-Western countries too, including China and Japan (Headey, Fu Na, and Zheng 2007; Oka and Shibata 2009; Shibata *et al.* 2012; Hansen 2013). Practically speaking, to the extent that dogs have become vested with a "right of health," some dogs – along with their human companions – enjoy privileged access to shelter, food, space, biomedical expertise, and protection from predation. Not least on account of shared privilege, "dog–human coflourishing … requires the ongoing work of examined lives" for all the people involved (Haraway 2008: 115).

Responsible Dog Ownership and One Health Promotion

Haraway's (2008) examination of human–canine companionship, as a way of working through the meaning of and the limits inherent to multispecies flourishing, provides fresh insight on the OIE (2013b) Code's subsection on "Stray Dog Population Control." This subsection, as one might expect, addresses concerns surrounding feral dogs. Yet it goes further than that, in at least two notable ways. First, through this policy document, the OIE (2013b: article 7.7.1) endorses "responsible dog ownership" as an ideal, for all dogs. Second, the OIE (2013b: article 7.7.2) recognizes that dog welfare can only be realized within political and ecological systems. Thus, while it might first appear to be just about feral dogs, the OIE Code applies broadly to all dogs and, indeed, to all collectivities within which dogs coexist with people. OIE policy on stray dogs is just as much, if not more, about governing people as it is about controlling dogs.

We are hoping to help shift health promotion as a field toward greater awareness of and attention to nonhuman animals, on ethical grounds and as influences on human well-being. Thus, it is worth noting that many scholars and activists disagree profoundly on moral grounds with defining any nonhuman animal as property, or else favor strict limits on how people can treat nonhuman animals defined as property (Francione and Garner 2010). Our own position is that the legality of dog ownership can be an asset in One Health promotion (Rock and Degeling 2013), but this position invites thorough interrogation of the notion of "responsible pet ownership." In contemporary policy and everyday practice, "responsible pet ownership" combines consideration for the well-being of humans and nonhuman animals (Rock 2013). Examples include leashing dogs in public places and providing pets with veterinary services, both of which can systematically promote health for individual owners, individual pets, other people, and other nonhuman animals (Degeling and Rock 2013; Rock and Degeling 2013; Rock *et al.* 2014). Nevertheless, this emphasis on responsible behavior on the part of pet owners can also individualize culpability and exacerbate social stigma (Graham and Glover 2014).

Following on from recommending the promotion of responsible ownership for all dogs, the OIE (2013b: article 7.7.2) acknowledges that "dog ecology is linked to human activities," such that "control of dog populations has to be accompanied by changes in human behaviour to be effective." Changes are defined as effective if they are consistent with and conducive to responsible dog ownership. Put another way, the OIE links together well-being and control as multispecies endeavors. Furthermore, practical interventions in relation to human–dog companionship could make a difference in the extent to which multispecies flourishing is realized, and to the benefit of whom (Haraway 2008). In these ways, OIE policy statements on dog well-being and dog control broadly cohere with a veterinary conceptualization of One Health as emerging from and depending upon complexity in socioecological systems (Zinsstag *et al.* 2011).

In addition, when interpreting OIE policy statements on dogs in relation to the ideal of multispecies flourishing (Haraway 2008), "recombinant ecologies" could be relevant to promoting health through environmental health justice

(Masuda, Poland, and Baxter 2010). In geography, recombinant ecologies refer to the "dense comings and goings of urban life, rather than the discrete and undisturbed relations between particular species and habitats that are the staple of conservation biology" (Hinchliffe and Whatmore 2006: 123). Even so, given the extent to which humans have influenced multispecies coexistence everywhere, there is no longer any such thing as a pristine habitat or ecosystem. Meanwhile, as geographers, Masuda and colleagues (2010) acknowledge inequity in the distribution and quality of places, and they call upon health promotion researchers to collaborate with disadvantaged collectivities. We simply underline that human beings are not the only species impacted by recombinant ecologies or by environmental health injustice. Dogs, for instance, vary in their access to space and in the quality of their experience while in private or public space, largely as a function of whether they have been claimed as belonging to someone, and, if claimed, of their owners' circumstances and status (Haraway 2008; Tissot 2011; Srinivasan 2013).

Indeed, not all dogs are valued highly, or even tolerated. Sterilization surgery is a prominent application of veterinary expertise, in both higher income and lower income countries (Dalla Villa *et al.* 2010; Scarlett and Johnston 2012; Srinivasan 2013), as a means of preventing the existence of unwanted dogs, and thereby influencing the nature of interactions that people have with dogs. Euthanasia is another prominent application of veterinary expertise, to curtail the size of dog populations and to address threats and nuisances posed by dogs (Dalla Villa *et al.* 2010; Srinivasan 2013). Moreover, not all instances of dog kills could be qualified as "good deaths," in the sense of euthanasia (Dalla Villa *et al.* 2010). Thus, instantiations of multispecies flourishing for people and pet dogs can come at the expense of dogs excluded from a "right of health" (Haraway 2008) and even mere existence. Furthermore, unwanted dogs' bodies comprise a form of waste that can be politically contentious (Instone and Sweeney 2014), as can waste in the form of "dog poo" (Derges *et al.* 2012; Instone and Sweeney 2014). In these ways, canine bodies meld with environmental problems and environmental health injustices.

One Health Promotion through Policies on Pets

In keeping with the notion that dog welfare and human well-being are closely connected, our group recently published a conceptual framework for promoting One Health through policies on dogs and other pet animals. Extrapolating from a "model city" for policies on pets (Rock 2013) and from the social sciences and health promotion, we identified five spheres of activity over which local councils or municipal governments may exert influence in ways that promote well-being for both people and pets: (1) preventing threats and nuisances from pets; (2) meeting pets' emotional and physical needs; (3) procuring pets ethically; (4) providing pets with veterinary services; and (5) licensing and identifying pets (Rock *et al.* 2014). Inspired by the iconic diagram associated with the *Ottawa Charter* (WHO 1986), Figure 3.1 displays how these five spheres fit with health promotion. Indeed, these spheres of activity or influence can reinforce each

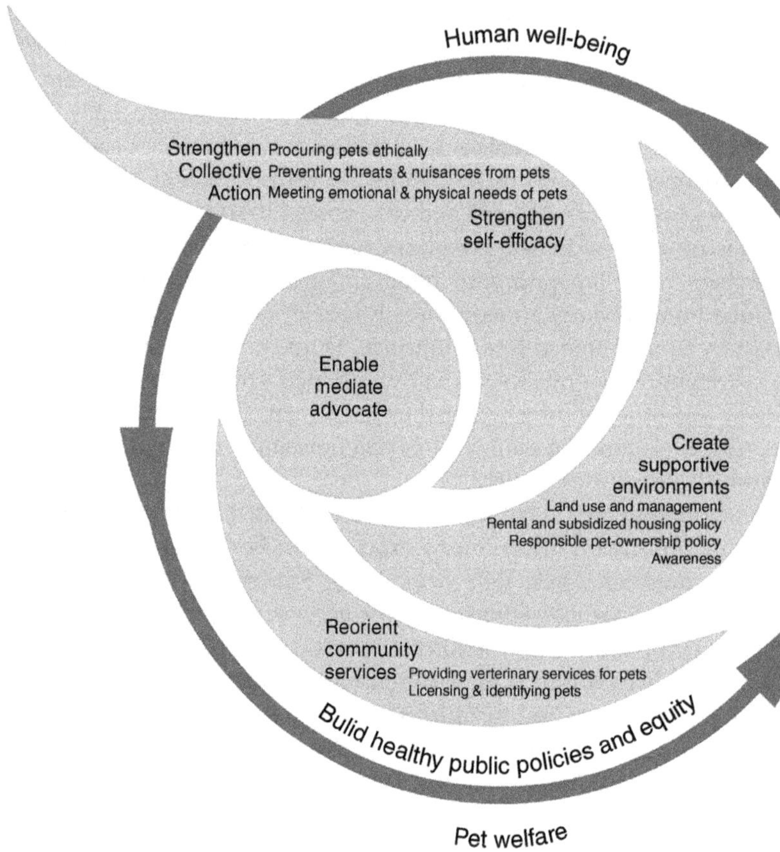

Figure 3.1 Conceptualizing "One Health" promotion through pet-related policies.

other, positively or negatively, depending on the degree of hierarchy within and between human populations as well as the capacity for public engagement and intersectoral cooperation (Rock 2012). Further, any one of these spheres may serve as a point of entry for engaged research and collective action. The potential for positive impacts extends beyond individual pet owners and pets, to the extent of encompassing families, people without pets of their own, entire communities, and even wildlife.

Our conceptual framework for promoting well-being for people and pets within communities and urban areas draws on the concept of "living cities" (Hinchliffe and Whatmore 2006). Whereas Hinchliffe and Whatmore emphasize how wild animals and plants, and the places where these species might be found, contribute to civic associations and galvanize collective action, we emphasize that pet animals participate in community solidarity and social conflict. As stated by Hinchliffe and Whatmore (2006: 124), "This focus on the 'doing' of urban ecologies, on their co-fabrication, implies a shift in the terms on which scientists (including social scientists) engage with the world." Along with Hinchliffe and Whatmore (2006: 124), among many others (e.g., Jasanoff

2004; Wedel *et al.* 2005; Marres and Lezaun 2011; Valverde 2011), we are part of a "turn" in STS and anthropology toward engagement with policy studies.

This turn marks a departure from research in STS on laboratory science and its extensions that sought to side-step any semblance of political allegiance and that shied away from critical reflexivity (Jasanoff 1996), as well as a departure from critiques, inspired mainly by Michel Foucault, of discourses on "healthy cities" and "health promotion" (Petersen and Lupton 1996). Opportunities are thus opening up for vigorous dialogue, within anthropology and beyond, amongst scholars concerned with science, technology, environmental studies, and health studies. Such a dialogue, we suggest, could earnestly embrace health promotion's tenets, while remaining critically attuned to its implications and applications, but not to the extent of disengagement or inaction. In fact, disengagement regarding multispecies entanglements and environments could be considered unethical in social science and health promotion (Masuda, Poland, and Baxter 2010; Rock and Degeling 2015).

Immersion and participation, in fact, are generative of understanding and may require a sense of affinity and common cause (Hinchliffe and Whatmore 2006; Masuda, Poland, and Baxter 2010; Rock and Degeling 2015). Further, engaged social science in health promotion could be enhanced through Ingold's (2011) concept of meshwork. Environmental health research, when viewed as meshwork, necessarily involves bodily experience but also efforts to qualify and transcend the researcher's own experience. Ethnographic research in anthropology that is oriented toward environmental health and multispecies flourishing may thus entail a variant of meshwork, as bodily techniques (following Mauss 2007 [1934]) for appreciating the extent to which well-being is actualized in human and nonhuman lives.

Concluding Remarks

Anthropological theory and related scholarship in STS offers numerous conceptual resources for theorizing and practicing One Health. In this commentary we have emphasized a few exemplars that are especially germane to redrawing the parameters of health promotion, so as to account more explicitly for lived connections between people, other animals, and ecosystems. Ingold's (2011) conceptualization of meshwork and Haraway's (2008) discussion of multispecies flourishing, in our view, are especially important for moving the field of medical anthropology toward engagement with One Health promotion.

Being alive, argues Ingold (2011), requires relationships. And relationships of any depth surpass discrete entities "joined up" heuristically, in the sense of networks. Relationships are not exclusive to human beings or to the human species, according to Ingold (2011), and relationships require space and change over time. To come to terms with multispecies existence, Ingold's concept of meshwork is indebted intellectually to phenemenology. This orientation leads him to stress that human and nonhuman consciousness is rooted in material bodies, yet extends beyond the palpable body into the surrounding environment.

Ingold (2011) recognizes that nonhuman animals are sentient, exert agency, and may reason. According to Ingold (2011: 93), however, human beings are unique as a species in the extent of our "cognitive ability to work things out in advance, in the head, prior to implementation in the world." Nevertheless, as Ingold (2011: 94) also observes, "a creature that could do nothing that had not been fully thought out in advance could never, in practice, do anything at all." Yet we would acknowledge that human beings are unique in the extent to which social life revolves around the use of technologies to predict, control, and participate. Moreover, this assertion echoes earlier contributions (e.g., Callon and Latour 1981) to STS, in which primatology figured centrally (for discussion, see Ingold 2012), and which led to the concept of actor networks that Ingold (2011) would later critique.

Overall, we accept Ingold's assertion that anthropology is founded on "inquiry into conditions and possibilities for human life in the world." Yet we follow Ingold's (2011, 1988) own lead and that of Haraway's (2008) in underscoring that human beings do not exist separate and apart from nonhuman species in this world. It follows that human health, understood as "physical, mental, and social well-being" (WHO 1948, 1986), cannot exist or undergo improvement without reference to nonhuman animals and shared environments. In fact, the material environment sometimes qualifies as a veritable being (Ingold 2000; Ingold 2012).

Given the importance of nonhuman animals and environments for how health is generated and for how inequity is perpetuated in daily life, we maintain that research, ethics, and interventions in health promotion would all be enhanced through engagements with the concept of One Health. Thus, we urge medical anthropologists and environmental anthropologists to engage in discussions about One Health to the extent of actually practicing One Health promotion. We also urge health promotion researchers and medical anthropologists to give more thought to the material difference that nonhuman animals make to social life. This chapter, we hope, will assist with such rapprochement and with improving the lives of nonhuman animals and human beings alike.

REFERENCES

Adelson, N. 2000. *"Being Alive Well": Health and the Politics of Cree Well-Being*. Toronto: University of Toronto Press.

Blue, G. and Rock, M.J. 2011. "Trans-Biopolitics: Complexity in Interspecies Relations." *Health: an Interdisciplinary Journal for the Social Study of Health, Illness & Medicine*, 15: 353–368.

Bock, B. and Buller, H. 2013. "Healthy, Happy and Humane: Evidence in Farm Animal Welfare Policy." *Sociologia Ruralis*, 53: 390–411.

Braun, B. 2005. "Environmental Issues: Writing a More-Than-Human Geography." *Progress in Human Geography*, 29: 635–650.

Broom, D.M. 2011. "A History of Animal Welfare Science." *Acta Biotheoretica*, 59: 121–137.

Brotherton, P.S. and Nguyen, V.-K. 2013. "Revisiting Local Biology in the Era of Global Health." *Medical Anthropology*, 32: 287–290.

Buller, H. 2014. "Animal Geographies I." *Progress in Human Geography*, 38: 308–318.

Callon, M. and Latour, B. 1981. "Unscrewing the Big Leviathan: How Actors Macrostructure Reality and How Sociologists Help Them Do So." In K.D. Knorr Cetina and A.V. Cicourel (Eds.), *Advances in Social Theory and Methodology: Toward an Integration of Micro and Macro-Sociologies* (pp. 227–303). Boston, MA: Routledge.

Christian, H.E., Westgarth, C., Bauman, A., Richards, E.A., Rhodes, R., and Evenson, K.R. 2013. "Dog Ownership and Physical Activity: A Review of the Evidence." *Journal of Physical Activity & Health*, 10: 750–759.

Cuomo, C. 1998. *Feminism and Ecological Communities: An Ethic of Flourishing.* Boston, MA: Routledge.

Cutt, H.E., Giles-Corti, B., Knuiman, M., and Burke, V. 2007. "Dog Ownership, Health and Physical Activity: A Critical Review of the Literature." *Health & Place*, 13: 261–272.

Dalla Villa, P., Kahn, S., Stuardo, L., Iannetti, L., Di Nardo, A., and Serpell, J.A. 2010. "Free-Roaming Dog Control among OIE-Member Countries." *Preventive Veterinary Medicine*, 97: 58–63.

Degeling, C. and Kerridge, I. 2013. "Hendra in the News: Public Policy Meets Public Morality in Times of Zoonotic Uncertainty." *Social Science & Medicine*, 82: 156–163.

Degeling, C. and Rock, M. 2013. "'It Was Not Just a Walking Experience': Reflections on the Role of Care in Dog-Walking." *Health Promotion International*, 28: 397–406.

Derges, J., Lynch, R., Clow, A., Petticrew, M., and Draper, A. 2012. "Complaints about Dog Faeces as a Symbolic Representation of Incivility in London, UK: A Qualitative Study." *Critical Public Health*, 22: 419–425.

Descola, P. 2013 [2005]. *Beyond Nature and Culture.* Chicago: Chicago University Press.

Foucault, M. 1991 [1978]. "Governmentality." In G. Burchell, C. Gordon, and P. Miller (Eds.), *The Foucault Effect: Studies in Governmentality with Two Lectures by and an Interview with Michel Foucault* (pp. 87–104). Chicago: University of Chicago Press.

Francione, G.L. and Garner, R. 2010. *The Animal Rights Debate: Abolition or Regulation?* New York: Columbia University Press.

French, M. and Mykhalovskiy, E. 2013. "Public Health Intelligence and the Detection of Potential Pandemics." *Sociology of Health & Illness*, 35: 174–187.

Graham, T.M. and Glover, T.D. 2014. "On the Fence: Dog Parks in the (Un)Leashing of Community and Social Capital." *Leisure Sciences*, 36: doi: 10.1080/01490400.01492014.01888020.

Green, J. 2012. "One Health, One Medicine, and Critical Public Health." *Critical Public Health*, 22: 377–381.

Hansen, P. 2013. "Urban Japan's 'Fuzzy' New Families: Affect and Embodiment in Dog–Human Relationships." *Asian Anthropology*, 12: 83–103.

Haraway, D. 2008. *When Species Meet.* Minneapolis: University of Minnesota Press.

Harfeld, J.L. 2013. "Telos and the Ethics of Animal Farming." *Journal of Agricultural and Environmental Ethics*, 26: 691–709.

Headey, B., Fu Na, and Zheng, R. 2007. "Pet Dogs Benefit Owners' Health: A 'Natural Experiment' in China." *Social Indicators Research*, 87: 481–493.

Hinchliffe, S., Allen, J. Lavau, S., Bingham, N., and Carter, S. 2013. "Biosecurity and the Topologies of Infected Life: From Borderlines to Borderlands." *Transactions of the Institute of British Geographers*, 38: 531–543.

Hinchliffe, S. and Whatmore, S. 2006. "Living Cities: Towards a Politics of Conviviality." *Science as Culture*, 15: 123–138.

Ingold, T. 1988. "Introduction." In *What Is an Animal?* (pp. 1–16). Unwin Hyman.

Ingold, T. 2000. *The Perception of the Environment: Essays on Livelihood, Dwelling and Skill.* New York: Psychology Press.

Ingold, T. 2011. *Being Alive: Essays on Movement, Knowledge and Description.* London: Routledge.

Ingold T. 2012. "Toward an Ecology of Materials." *Annual Review of Anthropology*, 41: 427–442.

Inhorn, M.C. 2007. "Medical Anthropology at the Intersections." *Medical Anthropology Quarterly*, 21: 249–255.

Instone, L. and Sweeney, J. 2014. "Dog Waste, Wasted Dogs: The Contribution of Human–Dog Relations to the Political Ecology of Australian Urban Space." *Geographical Research*, 52(4): 355–364: doi: 10.1111/1745-5871.12059.

Jasanoff, S. 1996. "Beyond Epistemology: Relativism and Engagement in the Politics of Science." *Social Studies of Science*, 26: 393–418.

Jasanoff, S. 2004. *States of Knowledge: The Co-Production of Science and the Social Order.* London: Routledge.

Jimínez, A.C. 2003. "On Space as Capacity." *Journal of the Royal Anthropological Institute*, 9: 137–153.

Kirksey, S.E. and Helmreich, S. 2010. "The Emergence of Multispecies Ethnography." *Cultural Anthropology*, 25: 545–576.

Kohn, E. 2007. "How Dogs Dream: Amazonian Natures and the Politics of Transspecies Engagement." *American Ethnologist*, 34: 3–24.

Kopytoff, I. 1982. "Slavery." *Annual Review of Anthropology*, 11: 207–230.

Kopytoff, I. 1986. "The Cultural Biography of Things: Commoditization as Process." In A. Appadurai (Ed.), *The Social Life of Things: Commodities in Cultural Perspective* (pp. 64–91). Cambridge: Cambridge University Press.

Law, J. and Mol, A. 2008. "The Actor-Enacted: Cumbrian Sheep in 2001." In L. Malafouris and C. Knappett (Eds.), *Material Agency towards a Non-Anthropocentric Approach* (pp. 57–78). New York: Springer.

Leach, M. and Scoones, I. 2013. "The Social and Political Lives of Zoonotic Disease Models: Narratives, Science and Policy." *Social Science & Medicine*, 88: 10–17.

Lestel, D. 2006. "Ethology and Ethnology: The Coming Synthesis." *Social Science Information*, 45: 147–153.

Lock, M. 1993. "Cultivating the Body: Anthropologies and Epistemologies of Bodily Practice and Knowledge." *Annual Review of Anthropology*, 22: 133–155.

Low, S.M. 2009. "Towards an Anthropological Theory of Space and Place." *Semiotica*, 2009: 21–37.

Marres, N. and Lezaun, J. 2011. "Materials and Devices of the Public: An Introduction." *Economy and Society*, 40: 489–509.

Masuda, J.R., Poland, B., and Baxter, J. 2010. "Reaching for Environmental Health Justice: Canadian Experiences for a Comprehensive Research, Policy and Advocacy Agenda in Health Promotion." *Health Promotion International*, 25: 453–463.

Mauss, M. 2007 [1934]. "Techniques of the Body." In M. Lock and J. Farquhar (Eds.), *Beyond the Body Proper.* Durham, NC: Duke University Press.

McNicholas, J., Gilbey, A., Rennie, A., Ahmedzai, S., Dono, J.A., and Ormerod, E. 2005. "Pet Ownership and Human Health: A Brief Review of Evidence and Issues." *BMJ (British Medical Journal)*, 331: 1252–1254.

Mol, A. 2002. *The Body Multiple: Ontology in Medical Practice.* Durham, NC: Duke University Press.

Mol, A. 2008 [2006]. *The Logic of Care: Health and the Problem of Patient Choice.* London: Routledge.

Mullin, M. 2002. "Animals and Anthropology." *Society & Animals*, 10: 387–394.

Nguyen, V.-K. and Peschard, K. 2004. "Anthropology, Inequality, and Disease: A Review." *Annual Review of Anthropology*, 32: 447–474.

Nordenfelt, L. 2011. "Health and Welfare in Animals and Humans." *Acta Biotheoretica*, 59: 139–152.

OED (Oxford English Dictionary). 2013a. "Welfare." http://dictionary.oed.com.

OED (Oxford English Dictionary). 2013b. "Well-Being." http://dictionary.oed.com.

OIE (l'Office international des epizooties). 2002. *New Mandates*. Resolution No. XIV, Adopted by the International Committee of the OIE on May 29, 2002: Animal Welfare Mandate of the OIE. http://www.oie.int/en/about-us/key-texts/basic-texts/new-mandates/ (accessed November 27, 2015).

OIE (l'Office international des epizooties). 2013a. *OIE's Achievements in Animal Welfare*. http://www.oie.int/animal-welfare/animal-welfare-key-themes/ (accessed November 27, 2015).

OIE (l'Office international des epizooties). 2013b. *Terrestrial Animal Code*. http://www.oie.int/index.php?id=169&L=0&htmfile=chapitre_1.7.1.htm (accessed November 27, 2015).

Oka, K. and Shibata, A. 2009. "Dog Ownership and Health-Related Physical Activity among Japanese Adults." *Journal of Physical Activity & Health*, 6: 412–418.

Petersen, A.R. and Lupton, D. 1996. *The New Public Health: Health and Self in the Age of Risk*. Los Angeles, CA: Sage.

Petryna, A. 2013 [2003]. *Life Exposed: Biological Citizens after Chernobyl*. Princeton, NJ: Princeton University Press.

Pottage, A. and Mundy, M. 2004. *Law, Anthropology and the Constitution of the Social*. Cambridge Studies in Law and Society. Cambridge: Cambridge University Press.

Powers, M. and Faden, R. 2006. *Social Justice: The Moral Foundations of Public Health and Health Policy*. Oxford: Oxford University Press.

Rock, M. 2012. "Connecting Lives: Reflections on a Syndemic Approach to Prevention Involving Research on How People Relate to Pets." *Annals of Anthropological Practice*, 36: 312–327.

Rock, M.J. 2013. "Pet Bylaws and Posthumanist Health Promotion: A Case Study of Urban Policy." *Critical Public Health*, 23: 201–212.

Rock, M.J., Adams, C.L., Degeling, C., Massolo, A., and McCormack, G.R. 2014. "Policies on Pets for Healthy Cities: A Conceptual Framework." *Health Promotion International*. doi: 10.1093/heapro/dau1017.

Rock, M.J., Buntain, B., Hatfield, J., and Hallgrímsson, B. 2009. "Animal–Human Connections, 'One Health,' and the Syndemic Approach to Prevention." *Social Science & Medicine*, 68: 991–995.

Rock, M.J. and Degeling, C. 2013. "Public Health Ethics and a Status for Pets as Person-Things: Revisiting the Place of Animals in Urbanized Societies." *Journal of Bioethical Inquiry*, 10: 485–495.

Rock, M. and Degeling, C. 2015. "Public Health Ethics and More-Than-Human Solidarity." *Social Science & Medicine*, 129: 61–67.

Rock, M.J., Degeling, C., and Blue, G. 2013. "Toward Stronger Theory in Critical Public Health: Insights from Debates Surrounding Posthumanism." *Critical Public Health*. doi: 10.1080/09581596.09582013.09827325.

Scarlett, J. and Johnston, N. 2012. "Impact of a Subsidized Spay Neuter Clinic on Impoundments and Euthanasia in a Community Shelter and on Service and Complaint Calls to Animal Control." *Journal of Applied Animal Welfare Science*, 15: 53–69.

Scott, C. 1989. "Knowledge Construction among the Cree Hunters: Metaphors and Literal Understanding." *Journal de la Société des Américanistes*, 75: 193–208.

Shibata, A., Oka, K., Inoue, S., Christian, H., Kitabatake, Y., and Shimomitsu, T. 2012. "Physical Activity of Japanese Older Adults Who Own and Walk Dogs." *American Journal of Preventive Medicine*, 43: 429–433.

Singer, M.C., Herring, A., Livingston, J. and Rock, M. 2011. "Syndemics in Global Health." In M. Singer and P.I. Erickson (Eds.), *Companion to Medical Anthropology* (pp. 159–180). Oxford: Blackwell.

Srinivasan, K. 2013. "The Biopolitics of Animal Being and Welfare: Dog Control and Care in the UK and India." *Transactions of the Institute of British Geographers*, 38: 106–119.

Tissot, S. 2011. "Of Dogs and Men: The Making of Spatial Boundaries in a Gentrifying Neighborhood." *City & Community*, 10: 265–284.

Toohey, A.M. and Rock, M.J. 2011. "Unleashing Their Potential: A Critical Realist Scoping Review of the Influence of Dogs on Physical Activity for Dog-Owners and Non-Owners." *International Journal of Behavioral Nutrition and Physical Activity*, 8: 46. doi: 10.1186/1479-5868-1188-1146.

Valverde, M. 2011. "Seeing Like a City: The Dialectic of Modern and Premodern Ways of Seeing in Urban Governance." *Law & Society Review*, 45: 277–312.

Wadiwel, D.J. 2009. "The War against Animals: Domination, Law and Sovereignty." *Griffith Law Review*, 18: 283–297.

Wedel, J.R., Shore, C., Feldman, G., and Lathrop, S. 2005. "Toward an Anthropology of Public Policy." *The Annals of the American Academy of Political and Social Science*, 600: 30–51.

WHO (World Health Organization). 1948. *Preamble to the Constitution of the World Health Organization as Adopted by the International Health Conference, New York, June 19–22, 1946.* Signed on 22 July 1946 by the Representatives of 61 States (Official Records of the World Health Organization, No. 2, p. 100) and Entered into Force on 7 April 1948. http://www.who.int.

WHO (World Health Organization). 1986. *Ottawa Charter for Health Promotion.* http://www.phac-aspc.gc.ca.

Young, A. 1982. "The Anthropologies of Illness and Sickness." *Annual Review of Anthropology*, 11: 257–285.

Zinsstag, J., Schelling, E., Waltner-Toews, D., and Tanner, M. 2011. "From 'One Medicine' to 'One Health' and Systemic Approaches to Health and Well-Being." *Preventive Veterinary Medicine*, 101: 148–156.

PART II

Ecobiosocial Interactions and Health

CHAPTER 4

Conceptualizing Ecobiosocial Interactions: Lessons from Obesity

Stanley Ulijaszek, Amy McLennan, and Hannah Graff

Introduction

In 1997, the World Health Organization (WHO) recognized obesity as an emerging global public health concern (WHO, Division of Noncommunicable Diseases 1998). It convened an expert consultation on obesity with the aim of reviewing epidemiological data and making recommendations for future research, treatment, and prevention. The report from the meeting reiterated the existing clinical perspective: that obesity is fundamentally a result of sedentary lifestyles and the consumption of high-fat, energy-dense diets. It also pointed to new research attention being paid to the role of environments in population-level weight gain (WHO 1998). The report suggested that exposure to unfavorable environments may accelerate obesity, but acknowledged that identifying and studying environmental factors that contribute to weight gain was extremely challenging.

By the time of the WHO's recognition that environments may play a role in obesity emergence, researchers had already begun to argue for a shift in thinking about obesity. In 1997, Egger and Swinburn proposed an ecological framework

A Companion to the Anthropology of Environmental Health, First Edition. Edited by Merrill Singer.

for understanding obesogenesis which took into account biological, behavioral, and environmental factors. They described examples of "micro" and "macro" environmental factors (for example, food in the home and food industry policies respectively) and argued that a "paradigm shift to understanding obesity as 'normal physiology within a pathological environment' signposts the directions for a wider public health approach to the obesity pandemic" (Egger and Swinburn 1997: 480). Similarly, following the publication of the WHO report, Hill and Peters argued that "to stop and ultimately reverse the obesity epidemic, we must 'cure' this environment" (1998: 1373). Swinburn and colleagues continued to develop their argument and published a framework describing the "obesogenic environment" in 1999 (Swinburn, Egger, and Raza 1999). This is one of two frameworks further elaborated in this chapter.

More recent reviews focusing on obesogenic aspects of the environment illustrate the extent to which these and other calls for a shift in thinking about obesity resulted in a proliferation of ecological approaches to obesity in the years that followed. For example, literature on the built environment and obesity has largely been published since 2002 (Papas *et al.* 2007). Food environments, initially through the analytical category of the "food desert" – an area characterized by limited access to healthy, affordable food – began to be associated with obesity in 1995 (Lang and Caraher 1998). Literature on retail planning and geographical implications for obesogenesis is recent (White 2007). In 2009, Harris and colleagues reviewed existing data and called for new approaches to studying the implications of the media and marketing environments for childhood obesity (Harris *et al.* 2009). A review of the relationships between physical activity and obesity highlighted the need for policy makers to consider not just recreation facilities, but also broader features of location, including socioeconomic context, neighborhood, workplaces, and land use (Fox and Hillsdon 2007). Various pathways have been hypothesized to link the environment to obesity; these continue to be investigated but are increasingly framed as complex and multifactorial. Genetics, epigenetics, social change, and cultural change may all play a role.

The proliferation of research relating to obesity and the environment has resulted in the description of a series of discrete yet intersecting environments and environmental factors which have been linked to obesogenesis through evidence from a wide range of disciplines. Environments at once shape our diets and are shaped (often degraded) by large-scale food production (Leatherman and Goodman 2005). Industrial agriculture, for example, is linked in numerous ways to environmental and public health outcomes (Horrigan, Lawrence, and Walker 2002). Built environments, and our interaction with them, impact on activity levels and access to food (Papas *et al.* 2007). Activity levels, for instance, may be linked to the walkability of streets or access to green space, while food access may depend on the relative proximity of retailers of fast or fresh food (Beaulac, Kristjansson, and Cummins 2009). Local food environments are shaped by social determinants and political-economic and commercial factors (Drewnowski 2004), while prenatal or fetal environments can shape future body fatness through metabolic, genetic, and epigenetic mechanisms (Whitaker and Dietz 1998).

The resultant "cacophony" of obesogenic environmental factors, ecological analyses, and policy solutions (Lang and Rayner 2007) added to the complexity of the obesity-related policy challenge. In an effort to overcome this challenge, the UK government, through the Foresight think tank process, used systems science to link diverse forms of evidence. The resultant "obesity system," graphically represented as the Foresight Obesity System Map (FOSM) (Butland *et al.* 2007; Vandenbroeck, Goossens, and Clemens 2007), remains one of the most complex political ecological models of obesity today. This is the second framework further elaborated in this chapter.

In this chapter, we use the *obesogenic environment* (as framed by Swinburn, Egger, and Raza 1999) and the *obesity system* (as described by Butland *et al.* 2007) frameworks as the basis for exploring the potential for ecobiosocial conceptualizations of obesity. In the following section we discuss the two frameworks in more detail, describing the context of their development and the way in which they conceptualize environmental impacts on health. We then examine each of them to identify the ways in which environmental, biological, and social factors are synthesized. Application of anthropological data to the two frameworks points to several places where ethnographic data detailing lived experience do not fit well into these frameworks. Social relations and historical processes are particularly absent. We conclude by suggesting that an ecobiosocial framing of obesity has the potential to contribute a greater understanding of this global health concern. A focus on processes (and not simply factors), which is rooted in ethnographic inquiry, may be a useful way to develop such a framework.

Frameworks for Conceptualizing Obesity

The Obesogenic Environment

The concept of the obesogenic environment, and the analytical framework with which it was described, was developed by researchers in the field of public health in the late 1990s. It was developed in response to an identified need for methods that would allow the environment – which was increasingly being acknowledged as a contributor to population-level obesity – to be rigorously and systematically studied.

The ANGELO (Analysis Grid for Environments Linked to Obesity) framework, which Swinburn *et al.* (1999) proposed as a tool to systematically describe and analyze the obesogenic environment, was an extension of their ecological framework for understanding obesity (Egger & Swinburn 1997). It permitted them to progress obesity theory from acknowledging the environment's contribution to obesity in broad terms, to identifying individual factors and features of the environment that could be studied, measured, and potentially modified. The framework was refined and tested in collaboration with communities in Australia and the Pacific islands, and it continues to be used for the purposes of policy making, intervention design, and priority setting.

The ANGELO framework is a grid that divides the environment into one of two sizes and one of four types; each environmental factor can be placed

Table 4.1 The ANGELO framework developed by Swinburn *et al.* (1999). All environmental factors are classified into one of eight grid cells.

Size \ Type	*Physical*		*Economic*		*Political*		*Sociocultural*	
Micro (settings)	Food	Physical activity	Food	Physical activity	Food	Physical activity	Food	Physical activity
Macro (sectors)	Food	Physical activity	Food	Physical activity	Food	Physical activity	Food	Physical activity

Source: Modified from Swinburn *et al.* (1999: 565).

somewhere in this eight-cell grid (Table 4.1). In terms of size, the environment is classified as either micro (local settings with which individuals interact, which are to some degree modifiable by the individual) or macro (broader sectors which are generally beyond the control of an individual). Examples of each are given by the authors: micro settings include festivities, neighborhoods, schools, homes, churches, and markets; macro settings include transport and the health regulatory system. Within each of these settings there are different types of environments. Swinburn *et al.* (1999) categorize these as being physical, economic, political, or sociocultural. Food and physical activity are subcategories within each of the eight grid cells.

Factors may be identified by researchers, policy makers, or local community representatives; the framework is a tool which facilitates communication between different stakeholders. They are then sorted into one of the grid squares. In the small Pacific island of Nauru, for example, one significant barrier to physical activity is the ferocious feral dog population which roams the streets. These dogs limit the extent to which people walk, especially in the mornings and evenings. This community opinion was formalized in the World Health Organization STEPS survey, where 58 percent of respondents reported that the presence of dogs in their area was a barrier to walking (Government of Nauru & World Health Organization 2007). Such a factor would be considered in the ANGELO framework to be micro level (and so somewhat modifiable at the individual and local level) and part of the physical environment. Other factors, such as international trade agreements that facilitate the import of some foods and drinks and are barriers to others, would be classified as macro level (not modifiable at the local level) and part of the political environment.

The ANGELO grid is not only a tool for researchers to classify aspects of the environment. It can also be used by community health workers and nutritionists to systematically think about the ways in which the environment may impact health in their local communities, as well as to systematically list factors alongside each other so that their relative importance and feasibility of intervention can be discussed and assessed. It could be used, for example, to discuss, debate and compare factors as diverse as feral dogs and trade policy: which could be feasibly addressed, by whom, in which timescales, and to what ends? Swinburn *et al.* (1999) tested their framework amongst nutritionists from across the Pacific islands. After initially populating the grid through brainstorming, participants could then use the tool to prioritize interventions and future research. Each factor was ranked according to three key criteria: validity (based on existing research evidence for its influence on diet and physical activity), relevance (to the community in question), and changeability (or its potential as a target for intervention). Scores for these areas could be aggregated to prioritize interventions. This framework continues to be useful for prioritizing research attention and intervention design in particular locales.

Through the application of the ANGELO framework, it becomes clear that certain environmental factors are more significant than others in different places, and to different people. For governments, for example, addressing feral dogs and individual physical activity levels is a much more feasible target for intervention than engaging in renegotiation of trade policies. This is especially the case in small island nations, which have comparatively little power in global trade policy negotiations, including those concerning poor-quality cuts of meat or industrially processed foods like two-minute noodles (e.g., Gewertz and Errington 2010; Errington, Fujikura, and Gewertz 2012; Snowdon and Thow 2013). Matters such as global economic power and inequality, colonial histories of exploitation, and changing local social relations are not considered by the model, which deals more with the factors resulting from these complex processes.

The description of the obesogenic environment using the ANGELO framework progressed the conceptualization of the environment because it permitted systematic analysis of what had previously been a somewhat nebulous concept. This research succeeded in breaking the environment down into analytically manageable units or factors. Early application of the framework highlighted the complexity of factors in the environment that contribute to obesity and health more broadly, as well as the powerlessness of individuals and communities to address many of these factors. This remains somewhat discordant with the clinical and health promotion approaches to obesity which largely continue to focus on the individual as the key locus of change.

Application of the framework also highlighted the balance of attention that had already been paid to different aspects of the environment. While a great deal of research had already been carried out regarding economic factors, for example, the authors pointed to the ongoing difficulties in measuring sociocultural aspects of the environment. Over the subsequent years, increasing numbers of social, technological, economic, behavioral, political, biological, and psychological factors were identified as contributing to the obesogenicity of the environment.

The Obesity System

The obesity system, graphically represented as the FOSM (Butland *et al.* 2007; Vandenbroeck *et al.* 2007), was developed almost a decade after the obesogenic environment construct of Swinburn *et al.* (1999). It was the result of a policy-making initiative, and the outcome of an identified need to bring many forms of evidence about the obesogenicity of environmental factors together along with biological ones, for the purposes of long-term policy planning.

The obesity system characterized by the FOSM is arguably the most complex political ecological framing of obesity to date. It was constructed over a period of two years in consultation with over 200 experts from a broad range of non-governmental organizations and academic, commercial, and governmental sectors, and captured both evidence-based research findings and expert opinion. The FOSM features 108 "nodes," each representing a factor thought by experts to contribute to obesity etiology. Nodes are grouped in four major areas: human physiology, physical activity patterns, psychology, and the food environment (Vandenbroeck *et al.* 2007). These areas are, in turn, divided into seven thematic clusters, also described as subsystems or themes, on the system map (Butland *et al.* 2007: 82–85): physiology (which is interchangeably labeled as "biology" in some parts of the report), individual physical activity and physical activity environment, individual psychology and social psychology (which is interchangeably labeled as "societal influences" in some parts of the report), and food consumption and food production.

Each thematic cluster, and each node therein, feeds into a central loop of energy imbalance. Nodes are linked according to the systems designers' observations of the experts' discussions of how the factors associated with obesity are connected. While the nodes themselves are of equal size, the weighting of linkages between them (indicated by the weight of the lines drawn between nodes) varies depending on the extent to which a particular factor has been shown (or hypothesized) to impact the factor to which it is connected. The map is intended to be dynamic, with countless feedback loops of positive and negative reinforcement between nodes.

The *walkability of the living environment*, which may include factors such as feral dogs, as seen on Nauru, is one of the nodes on the FOSM. The node is located in the physical activity cluster, and is iteratively connected to the node representing the *dominance of motorized transport*, through which it contributes to *overall level of transport activity* and hence *overall physical activity levels.* The *walkability of the living environment* is also directly connected to *perceived lack of time*, a node in the social psychology cluster which is closely connected – via *stress* – to *psychological ambivalence.*[1] In this way, the matter of feral dogs in Nauru may be understood through the framework as being associated with obesity via at least two major pathways: dogs reduce physical activity because walking is (often correctly) perceived to be dangerous, they increase stress, and they contribute to psychological ambivalence as people struggle to follow health guidelines. The FOSM depicts all of these factors feeding into generating positive energy balance in individual bodies. While this depiction is complex, comparison with ethnographic data shows that it does not capture the interwoven social, economic, political, and historical underpinnings of the factor. Understanding how factors (or nodes) on the map have contributed to obesity – itself a phenomenon which has emerged over time – is complicated insofar as factors on the map remain asocial and ahistorical.

In the obesity system, many different factors are brought together in a map that connects them conceptually. Importantly, this highlights the complexity of obesity and the interdependence of environmental factors which contribute to it. At the time, it also demonstrated the discordance between environmental factors as they interact in practice, academic categorizations of them, and governmental sectors in whose jurisdictions they fell. The FOSM has continued to inform UK government action and further international research on the drivers and prevention of obesity (Morgan and Dent 2010; Department of Health for England 2011). It is one of a number of approaches that aim to incorporate increasingly sophisticated systems modeling techniques (including agent-based modeling, data modeling, and mathematical modeling) into conceptualizing global concerns such as obesity or climate change.

The obesity system added two new dimensions to framing obesogenic environments. First, it attempted to unite data from different academic disciplines and to overcome the delineations between the factors they elaborated (Foresight 2005). Second, it attempted to capture, using systems mapping and concepts such as feedback loops, the iterative interactions between different factors. This is particularly important for understanding the broader impacts of intervening at any one point in the system; it is also useful for understanding the cross-sector and cross-departmental collaboration likely to be required to effect population-wide change.

Disentangling the Environmental, Biological, and Social Factors in Each Framework

The ANGELO framework and FOSM were developed for different reasons, at different times, and based on different bodies of evidence. In the obesogenic environment, environment is framed as all encompassing. The purpose of the ANGELO framework is to describe elements of this environment in systematic detail. A range of factors, including the four types explicitly listed in the framework (physical, economic, political, and sociocultural), are conceptualized as falling within a person's environment. Environment is also framed as multilayered: factors may be either micro-environmental or macro-environmental. The micro environment is framed as being local (and potentially amenable to local change) while the macro environment is defined by larger structures that cannot be altered by local action or local actors. Micro-environmental settings are described as places, people, and groups who gather for physical activity and/or food; examples include homes, schools, neighborhoods, gyms, churches, or supermarkets. These are embedded in, and shaped by, geographically diffuse macro-environmental sectors such as industry, media, food production, and transport systems.

The obesogenic environment defined using the ANGELO framework is described as being linked to obesity in the way that it impacts an individual's eating and physical activity behavior; this, in turn, acts through biological metabolic systems to effect weight change. For example, poor access – physically and financially – to fresh food and comparatively close proximity of processed food vendors to schools and places of work may result in increased calorie intake and obesity (Mitchell, Cowburn, and Foster 2010). An illustrative example of this is described in Warin's (2011) ethnographic analysis of obesity in Rotherham, a northern English town at the center of a reality TV show highlighting poor health and nutrition. Alternatively, a neighborhood equipped with well-maintained footpaths, accessible sporting facilities and safely lit streets may encourage people to walk, cycle, and spend more time outdoors, which would directly impact on their physical activity levels.

The ANGELO conceptualization aligns well with epidemiological data which indicate that obesity emergence has, for example, coincided with changing physical activity behaviors in a variety of domains. At the micro level are transportation, everyday (or incidental) activity, work, and play (Wareham 2007). These are shaped at the macro level by changes to the natural environment, loss of outdoor green space, and urbanization. Urban environments vary in their physical infrastructure, access to services, and availability of food and green space. However, the population-level change that comes with the nutrition and behavior transition of urbanization has been linked to shifts in body composition and higher levels of obesity in diverse settings (see Popkin 1999, 2004). This resultant built environment has been associated with increased levels of physical inactivity and obesity emergence (Fox and Hillsdon 2007).

In the obesity system characterized by the FOSM, the environment is framed as one part of a broad range of factors contributing to obesity. Environmental factors are concentrated in four of the seven thematic clusters: "food production" and "food consumption" (which together constitute the food environment), "individual activity," and "activity environment." Food production structures possible food consumption patterns, while the activity environment structures possible individual physical activity patterns. Both food consumption and individual physical activity are framed as acting through energy imbalance to produce obesity. The food supply chain – as part of a food environment – and the multinational corporations and government stakeholders that control it, impacts on the prices and fiscal accessibility of food (e.g., Hawkes 2006). In this way, transportation, everyday activity, built environment, space for recreation, food production and consumption, for example, are all depicted as exerting iteratively interacting forces in the overall system.

The framework of the obesogenic environment proposed by Swinburn *et al.* (1999) mentions biology in several places. All environmental factors act through metabolic systems to effect weight change. This reflects the classic biomedical framing of obesity as an imbalance between energy intake (eating) and energy expenditure (exercise). This means that any obesogenic environmental factor is seen as ultimately either increasing people's calorie consumption or decreasing physical activity levels. Biology is also depicted as something that ultimately drives behavior; all aspects of behavior which cannot be attributed directly to biological causes are depicted as arising from environmental impacts. The biological has two places in the FOSM as well. Biological drivers feature prominently as mediators at the center of the model, as all factors on the model are depicted as ultimately influencing energy balance in an individual. But within the model there is also a separate thematic domain, one of seven in total, for "physiology" (it is also referred to as "biology" in some parts of the report which accompanies the systems map). This includes nodes for resting metabolic rate, predisposition to activity, quality and quantity of breastfeeding, and genetic or epigenetic predisposition.

In Swinburn *et al.*'s (1999) framework, the "sociocultural environment" is one of four different parts of the overall environment, the others being political, physical, and economic components. Social factors as depicted in the model include local attitudes, beliefs, and values explicitly related to physical activity or food, such as the cultural importance of high-fat foods. In the obesity system, the label of "social psychology"/"societal influences" is given to one of seven thematic clusters. Factors that fall within this cluster include media consumption, peer pressure, education, acculturation, and conceptualization of obesity as a disease.

For anthropologists, a number of factors that fall outside of this thematic cluster also have social dimensions. Food and its use, for example, are inherently social. Food environments are not simply physical settings; rather, people are involved in food preparation, production, distribution, and consumption. Political and economic factors can significantly alter this setting through policies, subsidies, import restrictions, marketing regulation, and taxes. Taxes or duties are not simply fiscal measures but have deeply rooted social links based on political, economic, and historical context (Timpson, Lavin, and Hughes 2013). Timpson *et al.* (2013), for example, describe how attitudes and beliefs about taxes differ based on socioeconomic status and geographic location of individuals and communities. A number of taxation models have been developed to suggest the health benefits of taxes placed on specific ingredients (for example, certain amounts of salt, sugar, or saturated fat) or on specific types of food (for example, cookies or soft drinks), the thinking being that people will change their buying and then their consumption behaviors if the price of food changes drastically (Landon & Graff 2012; Mytton, Clarke, and Rayner 2012; Barquera, Campos, and Rivera 2013). Longstanding tobacco excise taxes have proven to be a powerful environment-changing tool for reducing tobacco use globally by shifting consumption patterns through cost (Chaloupka, Yurekli, and Fong 2012). However, even models of taxation schemes are fraught with political debate, conflicting stakeholder interests, local dissention, and passionate arguments both for and against them (Landon and Graff 2012) and are just one part of an individual's environment. Such matters are inherently social, but are largely considered in both models to fall within political or economic domains.

Both ANGELO and FOSM integrate the environmental, biological, and social into one model, but they do so in very different ways. ANGELO frames environment (of which the social is one discrete part) as all-encompassing, biology being the mediator between environment and health outcomes. ANGELO does not take into account the mediating role culture and social factors play between environment and health. In FOSM, environmental factors, biological factors, and social factors are each separate and are depicted as iteratively intersecting. Metabolic systems are the mediator between all of these factors and health outcomes. Comparison with anthropological examples highlights the assumptions implicit in both frameworks. Environments and the foods produced in them, for example, are shaped by complex social, cultural, and economic forces. This was demonstrated well by Mintz in his classic anthropological research documenting the rise of sugar consumption in Britain (Mintz 1985).

Ecobiosocial models have previously been developed for studying infectious diseases such as dengue fever, as a way to bring together environmental, biological, and social data about disease patterns (Arunachalam *et al.* 2010). Insofar as both of the obesity models discussed here illustrate the extent to which obesity is the product of the interaction of environmental, biological, and social factors, both illustrate that obesity may be considered to be an ecobiosocial phenomenon. Reframing obesity from a biomedical to an ecobiosocial phenomenon invites attention from nonmedical fields of research and links it to other complex global phenomena such as climate change.

What Is Missing from These Ecobiosocial Frameworks?

The processes behind the development of both ANGELO and FOSM moved the obesity research agenda forward in striking ways. However, despite the conceptual links between obesity and the environment that have been firmly established over the past decades, interventions largely continue to target individuals and their eating and physical activity behaviors, habits, and choices (Swinburn *et al.* 2011). This is in part because population-wide measures to impact food and physical activity environments are often politically difficult to implement and may not be allowed the lifespan needed to see long-term change in a population. Examples of this can be seen in various attempts to impose taxes and other fiscal measures on fats, sugars, and alcohol across Europe (Landon and Graff 2012). There is a contradiction between the ecobiosocial framing of obesity and the individualist intervention strategies for it.

Other factors also contribute to this evidence/practice contradiction. Both frameworks reviewed here are based on implicit biomedical assumptions about obesity, health, and the body; they ultimately still depict individual diet and exercise to be the locus of health and therefore of change. Interventions which target individuals can be delivered through existing clinical services, are more cost-effective, and are less politically charged. Ecobiosocial interactions do not conform to a cause-and-effect model and so it is difficult to gather sufficient longitudinal evidence to politically justify ecobiosocial intervention. In addition, environmental determinants are often linked to large industrial organizations or institutions, which have comparatively more power to resist change than individuals. At the same time, obesity remains a significant global public health concern, and the stigmatization of obese individuals is perpetuated on an increasingly global scale (Brewis *et al.* 2011). Underlying social values may unknowingly bias research and intervention design and implementation. This can be partly attributed to challenges – such as those outlined by Swinburn *et al.* (2011) – faced in creating and evaluating policies based simultaneously on environmental, biological, and social principles.

Our examination of the two models, and attempts to fit ethnographic data into them for the purposes of illustrating how they might be applied, highlight additional points of contradiction between the frameworks and lived experience which may contribute to the mismatch between ecobiosocial framings of obesity and the interventions that arise from them. Stray dogs were not a problem on Nauru in the 1960s, but they are today. Likewise, obesity has emerged in Nauru between the 1960s and today; for this reason, a historical perspective may be informative. In the 1960s, dogs had to be registered with the government (nonregistration was punishable by fines), most were de-sexed by local veterinarians, and stray dogs were impounded by environmental health officers. Over time, and with increasing national liberalization, registration was less strictly enforced and fines no longer administered. Environmental health budgets were redirected as a result of increasing concerns about communicable and noncommunicable diseases (which were, at the time, largely attributed to individual diet and exercise). Rapid political changes meant that longer term policies were difficult to adopt and enact. An economic downturn had several impacts: for instance, veterinary and environmental health services were further reduced, and changing social relations meant that personal security became an increasing concern and increasing numbers of households invested in ferocious guard dogs which they could not always afford to feed. While people continue to call on the government to address the issue, government spending priorities lie elsewhere. For example, the Department of Transport struggles to maintain roads and sewerage systems, and the Department of Health struggles to provide adequate acute care; both of these are of greater concern to local people, and to international aid donors, than stray dogs. The classification of stray dogs as part of the micro-level physical environment does not acknowledge that the walkability of the environment is as much political, economic, and social as it is physical. Likewise, it is as much a macro-environmental matter as it is micro-environmental. Issues of class, power, race, and (global) inequality are also omitted. Such points of contradiction between lived experience and the existing ecobiosocial models may form additional barriers to the design and implementation of interventions based on the two frameworks.

Neither ANGELO nor FOSM explicitly considered how environmental, biological, and social factors come together and are negotiated and experienced in everyday life over time and cross-culturally. Anthropologists have recently defined the term "ecobiosocial" as referring to interacting "economic, ecological, biological and social relational forces that impact human health" (Singer and Erickson 2011: 517). This is distinct from the epidemiological application of ecobiosocial modeling discussed in the previous section insofar as it emphasizes the importance of "social relational forces" or processes, and not simply "social factors," for understanding human interactions with the environment.

While social factors are incorporated as individual research nodes in both frameworks of obesity considered here, social relations infuse all environmental factors the frameworks contain. In the ANGELO framework, physical, economic, and political environments (and not simply those in the sociocultural category) are inherently relational. Physical environments are constructed, designed, shaped (intentionally and unintentionally), and lived in by people. Economic and political factors, such as farm subsidies, agribusiness, socioeconomic status, or household spending are linked to relations of power, gender, and ethnicity. The FOSM captures some of the interaction between different factors and its conceptualization of the relational is more sophisticated.

Practices that anthropologists have studied as being inherently social do not necessarily fall within the social portion of the FOSM. Quality and quantity of breastfeeding, for example, is listed as a "biological" factor in the obesity system, but has been anthropologically linked to historical, political, gender-related, and economic factors (Wall 2001). Even ambient temperature, a node that appears in the physical activity environment portion of the FOSM, is relational. Buildings or vehicles may be climate-controlled, and hours spent working or traveling are related to patterns of employment, socioeconomic status, political power (or lack thereof), kinship, exchange practices, and so on. The outdoor ambient temperature is equally relational, being linked to urban design, the balance of built and natural environments, and complex issues such as global climate change, risk, and vulnerability (Baer and Singer 2009; Baer and Singer 2014).

Another reason for the contrasts between ANGELO and FOSM and their operationalization into policy and practice emerges when comparing them to the phenomenon of obesity they seek to describe. While obesity emergence has occurred over the past 60 years, which in itself should suggest focusing on changes in social and political processes, both frameworks consider only the contemporary environment. This contrasts with evidence suggesting that insecurity linked to neoliberal political systems emergent in the past 30 years or so contributes to obesity (Offer, Pechey, and Ulijaszek 2012). This is important, because the environment and our interaction with it are rooted in historical and political economic processes (e.g., Mintz 1985; Steel 2009). The purpose of ANGELO is to describe and analyze the contemporary environment; it makes no claim to study historical processes, and these would not be expected to be captured in the model. The FOSM aims to capture processes of change and interaction between nodes of influence. However, while inter-nodal relationships are depicted as having the potential for dynamicity, the structure of the overall environment (or the nodes depicted in the system) remains fixed. Thus the nodes represent factors at a specific point in time and they are dynamic only in their relationships to each other, not through time.

Obesity has emerged gradually as a population-level phenomenon in the latter half of the twentieth century. Some authors have shown that trends in increasing BMI (body mass index) can be identified in even earlier time periods (Komlos and Brabec 2010). However, neither framework considered here has a time-depth that matches, or exceeds, the historical emergence of obesity over time, and neither refers to historical data in its construction. The environment, as well as the iterative human–environment interactions that shape our relationships with and within it, has changed markedly over the past century. This historical dynamicity is yet to be captured in the modeling of obesity. While obesity could be considered an outcome of ecobiosocial interactions over time, social relational interactions and time remain less well elaborated in the frameworks we have discussed.

CONCLUSION

In this chapter we argue that obesity is an outcome of ecobiosocial interactions, but that frameworks representing these interactions remain to be developed. Anthropological understandings of ways in which the environment can make and unmake health may be useful in developing ecobiosocial frameworks of obesity. In practice, social relations and historical processes are central to shaping environments and human interactions within them, which rebound in diverse ways on individual health, and these are likely to be important in the case of obesity.

A reason that the relational is important is because it permits abstract models to connect with everyday lives. While the ANGELO framework was practical in policy-making terms, as illustrated by its successful trial with stakeholders from island communities, it did not take into account the complex and iterative interactions between different factors that could, for instance, undermine interventions put in place (Finegood, Merth, and Rutter 2010). The FOSM took these interactions into account where possible, but in doing so it became a complex tool for policy development and design and became removed from everyday realities. A focus on social relations in addition to social factors may permit future frameworks, including ecobiosocial ones, to move more readily from theory to practice. While it is difficult to capture the fluid nature of human relationality, some efforts have been made to situate the production of obesity within social relations. For example, social relations and their links to population-level obesity emergence have already begun to be elucidated in research focusing on social networks (Christakis and Fowler 2007), social capital (Ulijaszek 2012), socioeconomic status (Offer *et al.* 2012), and cultural consensus modeling (Ulijaszek 2007).

Time, and change over time, is also important. A comparison of the frameworks described illustrates the progress from systematic description of a static environment to beginning to conceptualize relations of feedback and reinforcement within it. However, both models depict the environment as a fixed framework. For the purposes of policy design, models are used to project and predict future outcomes at a hypothetical level. Historical analysis, and an understanding of the processes through which a certain environment has taken shape, may contribute to developing interventions based not on hypothetical projections but on evidence. In order to capture historical processes, however, frameworks must somehow depict the environment as a dynamic relational field rather than a fixed framework of factors.

Obesity is a good example of where human interaction with the environment can make and unmake health in many societies. The two frameworks examined here conceptualize the links between obesity and our environment. In doing so, they also illustrate how obesity can be understood as an ecobiosocial phenomenon, resulting from complex and intersecting environmental, biological, and social factors. Close examination of these frameworks in the context of ethnographic data, however, points to places where they – as well as the concept of ecobiosociality more broadly – might be further refined in the future.

Anthropologists have recently highlighted the importance of social relations and processes, and not simply social factors, in developing such models. Social relations weave environmental and biological factors together. They encompass a multitude of important aspects of everyday life which contribute to health outcomes, including ethnicity, power, politics, and exchange relations, as well as habits, social values, and historical changes in all of these. Through the example of obesity, it is possible to see that "ecobiosocial" is not simply the sum of environmental, biological, and social *factors*. These domains could also be seen as dynamic relational *processes*, iteratively interrelated over time, and negotiated by people in their everyday lives. Ecobiosocial frameworks informed by anthropological inquiry and focusing on processes rather than factors may be useful in describing obesity emergence in future.

NOTE

1 See an interactive version of the FOSM at: http://www.shiftn.com/obesity/FullMap.html.

REFERENCES

Arunachalam, N., *et al.* 2010. "Eco-bio-social Determinants of Dengue Vector Breeding: A Multicountry Study in Urban and Periurban Asia." *Bulletin of the World Health Organization*, 88(3): 173–184.

Baer, H.A. and Singer, M. 2009. *Global Warming and the Political Ecology of Health: Emerging Crises and Systemic Solutions.* Walnut Creek, CA: Left Coast Press.

Baer, H.A. and Singer, M. 2014. *The Anthropology of Climate Change: An Integrated Critical Perspective.* London: Routledge, Earthscan.

Barquera, S., Campos, I., and Rivera, J.A. 2013. "Mexico Attempts to Tackle Obesity: The Process, Results, Push Backs and Future Challenges." *Obesity Reviews*, 14(S2): 69–78.

Beaulac, J., Kristjansson, E., and Cummins, S. 2009. "A Systematic Review of Food Deserts, 1966–2007." *Preventing Chronic Disease*, 6(3): 1–10.

Brewis, A.A., Wutich, A., Falletta-Cowden, A., and Rodriguez-Soto, I. 2011. "Body Norms and Fat Stigma in Global Perspective." *Current Anthropology*, 52(2): 269–276.

Butland, B., *et al.* 2007. *FORESIGHT. Tackling Obesities: Future Choices – Project Report*, 2nd ed. London: UK Government Office for Science.

Chaloupka, F.J., Yurekli, A., and Fong, G.T. 2012. "Tobacco Taxes as a Tobacco Control Strategy." *Tobacco Control*, 21(2): 172–180.

Christakis, N.A. and Fowler, J.H. 2007. "The spread of Obesity in a Large Social Network over 32 Years." *The New England Journal of Medicine*, 357(4): 370–379.

Department of Health for England. 2011. *Healthy Lives, Healthy People: A Call to Action On Obesity in England.* London: Department of Health.

Drewnowski, A. 2004. "Obesity and the food Environment: Dietary Energy Density and Diet Costs." *American Journal of Preventive Medicine*, 27(3 Suppl): 154–162.

Egger, G. and Swinburn, B.A. 1997. "An 'Ecological' Approach to the Obesity Pandemic." *BMJ*, 315(7106): 477–480.

Errington, F., Fujikura, T., and Gewertz, D. 2012. "Instant Noodles as an Antifriction Device: Making the BOP with PPP in PNG." *American Anthropologist*, 114(1): 19–31.

Finegood, D.T., Merth, T.D.N., and Rutter, H. 2010. "Implications of the Foresight Obesity System Map for Solutions to Childhood Obesity." *Obesity*, 18(Suppl.1): S13–16.

Foresight, 2005. *Trends and Drivers of Obesity: A Literature Review for the Foresight Project on Obesity*. London.

Fox, K.R. and Hillsdon, M. 2007. "Physical Activity and Obesity." *Obesity Reviews*, 8(Suppl. 1): 115–121.

Gewertz, D. and Errington, F. 2010. *Flap Food Nations in the Pacific Islands*. Berkeley: University of California Press.

Government of Nauru and World Health Organization. 2007. *Nauru NCD Risk Factors STEPS Report*. Suva: World Health Organization Western Pacific Region (WHOWPR).

Harris, J.L., Pomeranz, J.L., Lobstein, T., and Brownell, K.D. 2009. "A crisis in the Marketplace: How Food Marketing Contributes to Childhood Obesity and What Can Be Done." *Annual Review of Public Health*, 30: 211–225.

Hawkes, C. 2006. "Uneven Dietary Development: Linking the Policies and Processes of Globalization with the Nutrition Transition, Obesity and Diet-Related Chronic Diseases." *Globalization and health*, 2(1): 4.

Hill, J.O. and Peters, J.C. 1998. "Environmental contributions to the obesity epidemic." *Science*, 280(5368): 1371–1374.

Horrigan, L., Lawrence, R.S., and Walker, P. 2002. "How Sustainable Agricultre Can Address the Environmental and Human Health Harms of Industrial Agriculture." *Environmental Health Perspectives*, 110(5): 445–456.

Komlos, J. and Brabec, M. 2010. "The Trend of Mean BMI Values of US Adults, Birth Cohorts 1882–1986 Indicates that the Obesity Epidemic Began Earlier than Hitherto Thought." *American Journal of Human Biology*, 22(5): 631–638.

Landon, J. and Graff, H. 2012. *What Is the role of Health-Related Food Duties?* London: National Heart Forum (now UK Health Forum).

Lang, T. and Caraher, M. 1998. "Access to Healthy Foods: Part II. Food Poverty and Shopping Deserts: What Are the Implications for Health Promotion Policy and Practice?" *Health Education Journal*, 57(3): 202–211.

Lang, T. and Rayner, G. 2007. "Overcoming Policy Cacophony on Obesity: An Ecological Public Health Framework for Policymakers." *Obesity Reviews*, 8(S1): 165–181.

Leatherman, T.L. and Goodman, A. 2005. "Coca-colonization of Diets in the Yucatan." *Social Science & Medicine*, 61(4): 833–846.

Mintz, S.W. 1985. *Sweetness and Power: The Place of Sugar in Modern History*. New York: Penguin.

Mitchell, C., Cowburn, G., and Foster, C. 2010. *Assessing the Options to Use the Regulatory Environment to Promote Local Physical Activity and Healthy Eating*. London: National Heart Forum.

Morgan, L. and Dent, M. 2010. *The Economic Burden of Obesity*. Oxford: National Obesity Observatory.

Mytton, O., Clarke, D., and Rayner, M. 2012. "Taxing Unhealthy Food and Drinks to Improve Health." *British Medical Journal*, 344: 2931.

Offer, A., Pechey, R., and Ulijaszek, S.J. (Eds.) 2012. *Insecurity, Inequality and Obesity in Affluent Societies*. Oxford: Oxford University Press.

Papas, M.A., Alberg, A.J., Ewing, R., Helzlsouer, K.J., Gary, T.L., and Klassen, A.C. 2007. "The Built Environment and Obesity." *Epidemiologic Reviews*, 29(27): 129–143.

Popkin, B.M. 1999. "Urbanization, Lifestyle Changes and the Nutrition Transition." *World Development*, 27(11): 1905–1916.

Popkin, B.M. 2004. "The Nutrition Transition: An Overview of World Patterns of Change." *Nutrition Reviews*, 62(7): S140–S143.

Singer, M. and Erickson, P.I. 2011. "Introduction." In M. Singer and P. I. Erickson (Eds.), *A Companion to Medical Anthropology* (pp. 1–6). Chichester, UK: Wiley-Blackwell.

Snowdon, W. and Thow, A.M. 2013. "Trade Policy and Obesity Prevention: Challenges and Innovation in the Pacific Islands." *Obesity Reviews*, 14(S2): 150–158.

Steel, C. 2009. *Hungry City: How Food Shapes Our Lives.* London: Vintage.

Swinburn, B.A., *et al.* 2011. "The Global Obesity Pandemic: Shaped by Global Drivers and Local Environments." *The Lancet*, 378(9793): 804–814.

Swinburn, B.A., Egger, G., and Raza, F. 1999. "Dissecting Obesogenic Environments: The Development and Application of a Framework for Identifying and Prioritizing Environmental Interventions for Obesity." *Preventive Medicine*, 29: 563–570.

Timpson, H., Lavin, R., and Hughes, L. 2013. *Exploring the Acceptability of a Tax on Sugar-Sweetened Beverages: Insight Work.* Liverpool, UK: John Moores University.

Ulijaszek, S.J. 2007. "Frameworks of Population Obesity and the Use of Cultural Consensus Modeling in the Study of Environments Contributing to Obesity." *Economics and Human Biology*, 5(3): 443–457.

Ulijaszek, S.J. 2012. "Socio-economic Status, Forms of Capital and Obesity." *Journal of Gastrointestinal Cancer*, 43(1): 3–7.

Vandenbroeck, P., Goossens, J., and Clemens, M. 2007. *Tackling Obesities: Future Choices – Building the Obesity System Map.* London: Foresight – Government Office for Science.

Wall, G. 2001."Moral Constructions of Motherhood in Breastfeeding Discourse." *Gender and Society*, 15(4): 592–610.

Wareham, N. 2007. "Physical Activity and Obesity Prevention." *Obesity Reviews*, 8(Suppl. 1): 109–114.

Warin, M. 2011. "Foucault's Progeny: Jamie Oliver and the Art of Governing Obesity." *Social Theory & Health*, 9(1): 24–40.

Whitaker, R.C. and Dietz, W.H. 1998. "Role of the Prenatal Environment in the Development of Obesity." *The Journal of Pediatrics*, 132(5): 768–776.

White, M. 2007. "Food Access and Obesity." *Obesity Reviews*, 8(Suppl. 1): 99–107.

WHO (World Health Organization), Division of Noncommunicable Diseases. 1998. *Obesity. Preventing and Managing the Global Epidemic. Report of a WHO Consultation on Obesity (Geneva, 3–5 June 1997).* Geneva: World Health Organization.

CHAPTER 5

Environmental Racism and Community Health

Melissa Checker

Beryl Thurman, president of the North Shore Waterfront Conservancy (NSWC) of Staten Island, New York liked to joke that her neighborhood looked like an industrial "Girls Gone Wild Video." This 5.2-acre stretch of waterfront on Staten Island's north shore contained approximately 21 contaminated properties including two private waste transfer stations, a Department of Sanitation garage, a Con Edison plant, a sewer treatment plant, several bus depots, a former lead paint factory, and a radioactive site that was part of the Manhattan Project. Four properties were on the federal Superfund list, and another seven appeared on New York State's priority cleanup list. Just 70 feet away from these sites, the North Shore's dense residential neighborhoods housed the city's fastest growing populations of Hispanics, African Americans, and low-income families (Checker 2009). Unsurprisingly, the North Shore also reported the borough's highest asthma rates, and children on the North Shore exhibited lead levels that were up to 15 percent higher than New York City averages (NYC DOHMH 2010, 2006). Long before Hurricane Sandy, residents here raised alarms about the risks they faced from contamination as well as increased flooding caused by rising sea levels and storm surges. They constantly lobbied city, state, and federal officials to mitigate both contaminants and flooding, and to permit new development with these issues in mind (Checker 2012).

Several hundred miles to the south, in the mid-sized city of Augusta, Georgia, low-income residents of the Hyde Park neighborhood also coped with extensive and long-term contamination. This neighborhood was originally set aside for

A Companion to the Anthropology of Environmental Health, First Edition. Edited by Merrill Singer.

African Americans in the 1940s, giving former sharecroppers the opportunity to purchase and build their own homes. Moreover, the area was bordered by two factories and a brickyard, which offered the kinds of jobs available to African Americans under Jim Crow. Eventually, seven polluting facilities, as well two sets of railroad tracks and a local highway, enclosed the neighborhood in a "toxic donut." In the late 1980s, the Environmental Protection Agency (EPA) discovered that one of those industries had leaked high levels of arsenic, chromium, PCBs (polychlorinated biphenyls), lead, and dioxins. When those chemicals were also found in Hyde Park's soil, residents began to link them to high rates of asthma, certain cancers, and reproductive problems. But subsequent risk assessments yielded contradictory and inconclusive reports about the degree to which residents' health problems were connected to chemical contaminants. In addition, because the neighborhood was surrounded by several waste-producing facilities, and, until 1970, it did not contain running water, sewer, or gas lines, residents had been exposed to contaminants through multiple pathways; thus, they were unable to definitively pinpoint one source of the pollution. Too poor to move on their own, these residents thus remained stuck in their contaminated neighborhood (Checker 2005).

Unfortunately, neither of these two cases is unique. Across the United States and around the world, countless studies show that communities of color and low-income areas host a disproportionate number of toxic waste-producing facilities, and they bear the brunt of environmental degradation, natural disasters, toxic waste, and climate change. In the late 1980s, the US environmental justice movement was galvanized to address environmental disparities in policy, practice, and enforcement. Today, over two decades later, environmental justice activists have made some significant progress in convincing public agencies to incorporate guidelines and procedures that address environmental inequality. Several recent studies (including two by the EPA's own Office of Inspector General), however, reveal that the disproportionate siting of hazardous waste facilities in communities of color has grown worse over the last two decades (see EPA Office of Inspector General 2004, 2006; Bullard *et. al.* 2007).

In this chapter, I use an anthropological approach to explore some of the roadblocks that inhibit the success of the environmental justice movement. Specifically, I focus on risk uncertainties, and how environmental risk assessments obscure the links between chemical contaminants and illness. Recent ethnographic research on risk ambiguities reveals how corporate polluters take advantage of uncertainty and offer partial accommodations, thereby co-opting local opposition and reshaping people's understandings of risk. I contribute to this work by presenting three examples from my own research that demonstrate a similar dynamic between state agencies and local communities. In these cases, state actors agreed to remediate contaminated sites, but they tied that remediation to redevelopment incentives. I argue that, in so doing, the state linked contamination to its redevelopment agenda and thus delinked it from public health concerns. In each of these cases, residents challenged the ascendance of economic interests and continually reasserted their own priorities, affirming the importance of including community perceptions and actions in assessing structural factors in environmental health.

After briefly introducing some of the issues driving the US environmental justice movement, as well as its major impacts, I focus on obstacles that continue to impede progress toward achieving a more environmentally just and healthy society. In particular, I investigate why the environmental risk assessment process tends to produce inconclusive reports that fail to legitimate environmental justice communities' claims that poor health is linked to environmental toxins. While in some cases, inconclusive risk assessments disable or mitigate collective action, in my own research I find that it inspired activists to find alternative mechanisms for remediating toxic contamination while circumventing the risk assessment process. The final three sections use case examples from my own research to explore one such mechanism – brownfield redevelopment. This program offers incentives to private developers to clean up and redevelop contaminated sites in low-income areas. Yet, I argue that brownfields crystallized neoliberal ideals which cast economic development as a cure-all for urban ills, including issues of contamination. As a result of this philosophy, economic concerns drove the entire cleanup process, from site assessment and selection, to remediation, to redevelopment. However, in the case studies presented, I show how residents continually reasserted their own priorities and worked to reconnect contamination to public health concerns.

Environmental Siting and Health Disparities in the United States

Since 1987, when the United Church of Christ (UCC) released a landmark report on environmental disparities in the United States, study after study has found that race, not income, is the most potent variable in predicting the location of hazardous waste facilities in the United States – more powerful than income, land values, and home ownership rates (Commission for Racial Justice 1987; see also US GAO 1983; Bullard 2000; Pace 2005). According to the UCC report, people of color made up approximately two-thirds of residents in areas that host multiple hazardous-waste facilities, and blacks were more than twice as likely as whites to live in neighborhoods where industrial pollution was suspected of being the greatest health danger (Commission for Racial Justice 1987). Such findings fueled the rise of the US environmental justice movement, as well as a robust body of social science research that continues to document the degree to which environmental burdens disproportionately fall on the shoulders of low-income communities of color (see Bryant 1995; Bullard 2000; Bullard *et al.* 2007).

Activists and scholars point out that environmental racism is embedded in historic and contemporary policies, practices, and institutions. Due to this historic and contemporary discrimination, residents of environmental justice communities lack access to a host of resources (adequate health care, transportation, education, employment, housing, etc.) that could help improve their circumstances.

For example, because local zoning and planning boards have historically been composed primarily of white people, people of color had little say in factory or incinerator siting decisions. To this day, minority neighborhoods are more likely than white neighborhoods to be rezoned (again, often by predominantly white planning boards) from residential to commercial or light industrial uses (Mantaay 2002). In addition, despite the Fair Housing Act and other civil rights reforms, fair housing evaluations routinely show that realtors continue to steer African Americans toward existing "ghettos," and minorities with the same resources and credit cards as whites are denied mortgages twice as often as whites (Massey and Denton 1993; Hannah-Jones 2012). All of these factors lead to constraints in the residential choices of people of color (Brown *et al.* 2005). Segregated housing markets then lead to inequality in schools, which combines with more overt racism to limit employment opportunities (Cole and Foster 2001; see also Bullard 2000). The health effects of living amidst contamination perpetuate this vicious cycle. For instance, growing up with lead, dioxin, or mercury poisoning makes children miss or perform more poorly in school, further curtailing their educational and job opportunities (see Pulido 1996; Faber 1998; Harper 2004; Brown 2007). Unequal access to opportunity also makes communities of color vulnerable to "job blackmail," or trading environmental quality for promises of jobs and economic opportunities (Bullard 2000; see also Checker 2005).

Exacerbating such inequalities, clean-air and water legislation in the 1970s imposed stiffer environmental regulations that enabled local residents to oppose hazardous-waste-generating facilities in their neighborhoods. As middle-class white communities began to protest, "Not in my backyard" (NIMBY), garbage dumps, incinerators, and landfills routinely ended up in poor, communities of color, which lacked the time, education, and social networks necessary to oppose them. As sociologist Robert Bullard observes, public officials and private industries "responded to the NIMBY phenomenon using the place-in-blacks'-backyards (PIBBY) principle" (Bullard 2000: 4). All of these cumulative and recursive issues contribute to the conditions and factors that attract polluting industries to people of color neighborhoods and make it difficult for people of color to move out of contaminated neighborhoods.

To address the multiple inequities that produce environmental injustice, activists initially defined the environment as "where we live, work, and play." In other words, the environment included their air, water, and soil *as well as* housing, schools, employment, and other resources subject to discrimination (Novotny 1995b; Harvey 1996; Checker 2005). Movement leaders sought to diversify mainstream environmental organizations, create more equitable environmental policies and procedures, and to protect communities from present and future contamination (Bullard 2000). In 1994, President Clinton issued Executive Order 12898, which called for federal agencies to incorporate environmental justice into their missions. Many states and municipalities followed suit. Among other things, this meant that the environmental justice impacts of proposed publicly funded projects came under new scrutiny, as did the degree to which environmental justice communities had the opportunity to participate in environmental decision making. The Order also called for "improved methodologies for assessing and mitigating impacts, health effects from multiple and cumulative exposure" (Bullard *et al.* 2007), an issue I address in the following section.

Despite the adoption of environmental justice guidelines and procedures by federal, state, and local agencies, environmental disparities persist across the United States. A 2005 study conducted by the Associated Press reported that "blacks were 79 percent more likely than whites to live in neighborhoods where industrial pollution is suspected of posing the greatest health danger" (Pace 2005). In 2007, a comprehensive national survey conducted to mark the 20th anniversary of the UCC report showed that people of color were *more* concentrated in areas with commercial hazardous sites than they were in 1987 (Bullard *et al.* 2007). In the following section, I show how an anthropological perspective informs our understandings of the discourses, practices, and entrenched biases that perpetuate uneven environmental geographies and environmental health disparities.

Assessing Environmental Health Risks

To determine the chance that a particular facility will produce harmful effects on human health or ecological systems, and to define the nature and magnitude of health risks to humans (e.g., residents, workers, recreational visitors) from chemical contaminants,[1] regulatory agencies require an environmental risk assessment. In turn, these assessments provide key evidence in siting decisions, lawsuits, remediations, and relocations. However, over the past two decades, a growing body of critical scholarship has revealed a number of biases and assumptions that underlie the environmental risk assessment process and exclude the experiences of people of color. In particular, the risk assessment process prevents environmental justice communities from definitively linking local contaminants to their health problems (see Wigley and Schrader-Frechette 1996; see also Bryant 1995; Novotny 1995b; Kriebel *et al.* 2001). The Hyde Park case provides a vivid illustration of the problems associated with the risk assessment process.

Three years after Hyde Park residents learned that their neighborhood was contaminated, and after they had waged a concerted campaign for relocation, the EPA agreed to conduct a comprehensive environmental risk assessment. The first step in the assessment was to study the level of individual chemicals in the neighborhood's soil, air, and groundwater. However, EPA scientists did not consult with residents about how deeply to bore into the soil. As one man said, "They sent out some people to do that testing out here and they scooped little bit of dirt with spoons on the ground. Hey, I done put dirt on top of dirt trying to get rid of the floods and things we been having out here for years" (Checker 2005). In other words, samplers failed to recognize that many residents had covered their yards with imported topsoil, and to adjust their boring depths accordingly. The next phase of the process included dose-response assessment. Here, the Agency for Toxic Disease Registry (ATSDR) provided data about the dose levels at which contaminants poses a risk to humans (Wigley and Shrader-Frechette 1996; Tesh 2000; Kriebel *et al.* 2001). For obvious reasons, chemicals are not tested on humans, so scientists extrapolate from animal research. Yet, lab rodents are bred to be genetically similar, whereas people are genetically and geographically diverse (Kriebel *et al.* 2001; see also Douglas and Wildavsky 1983; Nachman *et al.* 2011). In addition, to extrapolate risk levels from animals to humans, scientists use a hypothetical adult (known as "Reference Man"). As defined by the EPA, Reference Man is a "Caucasian male …154 pounds, five feet seven inches tall, and "Western European or North American in habitat and custom" (Shipak 2007: 7; see also Kuehn 1997: 259–276). In other words, standard comparison techniques fail to provide information on the range of ways in which women, children, elderly, or already sick people – far more susceptible groups of people – might react to a chemical (Fitchen 1988; Shrader Frechette 2010). In addition, dose response studies only examine whether certain chemical exposures cause particular illnesses, not whether such exposures increase susceptibility to certain illnesses. For example, a recent study published by the American Diabetes Association found strong correlations between concentrations of persistent organic pollutants and the prevalence of diabetes (Lee *et al.* 2006). Not only can certain toxic agents provoke Type I diabetes, but having diabetes also creates metabolic impairments, which can make a person susceptible to toxic-related illness (Hubbard and Wald 1993: 78). In the third phase, risk assessors estimate the extent of human exposure to various contaminants – that is, who may have been exposed, for how long or how frequently, and how much.[2] Here again, methods of assessment do not necessarily take the specific experiences of a community into account. For instance, the EPA studied contaminant levels in fish that lived in a popular local fishing spot. The ATSDR then compared those findings to its standards for safe fish consumption among nonrecreational and nonsubsistence fish consumers and determined that fish consumption posed no threat to Hyde Park residents (ATSDR 1994). Yet, Hyde Park residents claimed that the ATSDR underestimated their fish consumption. Had the agency actually interviewed the residents, they would have found that many of them actually had subsistence fished in the past, and some continued that practice in the present.

Perhaps the most controversial aspect of the entire process is risk characterization, or the development of conclusions about the nature and extent of residents' risks, based on their exposure to harmful chemicals. Hyde Park's assessment, for instance, characterized residents' risks for each individual chemical found in its soil (arsenic, lead, cadmium, chromium, etc.). Like most environmental justice communities, however, residents were exposed to dozens of different chemicals over time, both within their neighborhood and through their jobs as factory workers, mechanics, domestics, and so on. (Checker 2005). But environmental scientists know little about the additive, compound, and synergistic effects of toxins (Dietrich 2013). While the Clinton Executive Order and the EPA have emphasized the need to develop methodologies for studying multiple and cumulative risks (see EPA 2006), these methods are still nascent and not widely used. As medical anthropologist Alexa Dietrich states, "[the methods] are costly to develop, and they create new realms of uncertainty for government agencies with interest in approving projects, as well as for industries looking to cover their legal bases at the least cost" (2013: 61–62).

The issues described above have led to a prevalence of inconclusive risk assessments and determinations (see Fitchen 1988; Novotny 1998b; Dietrich 2013). As a result, all kinds of environmental justice remedies – including legal settlements, government-sponsored relocations, ongoing health care and monitoring, or the closing or modifying of operations at polluting facilities – become impossible. The social implications of inconclusive risk assessments are also far reaching. In the next section, I highlight some recent anthropological work that studies how inconclusive risk assessments influence social perceptions of risk and environmental justice activism.

The Aftermath of Uncertainty

Building on anthropology's long disciplinary history of exploring the cultural contingency of risk perceptions, some anthropologists have begun to explore the social construction of risk uncertainty (Douglas and Wildavsky 1983; Gunter and Kroll-Smith 2006; Petryna 2013; Button 2010; Cepek 2013; Little 2014). In particular, this research examines how institutional frameworks along with experiences and identities based on gender, class, religion, ethnicity, race, and/or age, shape how people understand and act upon risk. For example, Kelly Alley finds that, according to Hindu beliefs, the highly polluted Ganga River was a goddess, able to purify herself of toxins. Viewing the river as polluted would thus violate strongly held convictions, so people were reluctant to organize for its protection (2002). More recent anthropological work on risk perception focuses on prolonged and indeterminate cases, asking how individuals and collectivities cope with ambiguity over extended periods of time (Aureyo and Swistun 2008; Button 2010; Cepek 2013; Dietrich 2013). In their landmark study of a community living near an oil refinery in Flammable, Argentina, for instance, Aureyo and Swistun (2009) argue that inconsistent messages put forward by scientists, the petrochemical company, the state, and the medical establishment inflected residents with doubts about the severity and source of their health problems, dissuading them from taking any kind of sustained collective action. Anthropologist Merrill Singer (2011) builds on these findings in his research with a Louisiana community living near chemical manufacturing plants and agribusinesses. Comparing his findings to those of Aureyo and Swistun, Singer finds that residents in the community he studied were fairly certain that local companies were to blame for their poor health but they believed that they were powerless to do anything "given their socioeconomic status and the unresponsiveness of the local or state government" (2011: 158). As a result, Singer concludes that community members lived in a state of prolonged "toxic frustration."

Gwen Ottinger's (2013) research with a Louisiana community near an oil refinery also explores the impact of corporate accommodations on environmental justice activism. In this case, the oil refinery offered residents who chose to stay in their homes cash payments, home improvement monies, and multiple opportunities for community–industry dialogue. The concessions, which many residents accepted, downplayed the dangers of contamination and appealed to their visions of themselves as educated homeowners capable of making informed choices that balanced concerns about risk with concerns for quality of life. Meanwhile, the company was able to incorporate neoliberal values of transparency, social responsibility and cooperation into its public image and to continue to control (and downplay) conversations about risk. Alexa Dietrich (2013) also examines how companies deter collective opposition in her study of a Puerto Rican neighborhood surrounded by pharmaceutical factories. Although few local residents were employed in the factories, their parent companies established a kind of patronage by participating in local rituals, funding social programs, and including community and NGO representatives on their boards and other bodies. Residents were then disinclined to jeopardize these relationships by speaking out against the companies. Finally, Peter Little (2014) researched how residents in upstate New York coped with long-term contamination from vapor intrusion. Here the polluting industry (owned by IBM) agreed to mitigate contamination through partial remediations. In this case, residents did not accept IBM's accommodations, and they insisted that partial remediations did not go far enough in reducing their health risks. Little traces sustained local opposition to residents' experiences with deindustrialization and economic uncertainty, as well as to local power dynamics.

Importantly, all of these cases illustrate how, in a deindustrializing economy where manufacturing and other blue-collar jobs are few and far between, new kinds of corporate patronage replaced traditional forms of "job blackmail." In the remainder of this essay, I expand on that notion by examining how government bodies also worked to persuade environmental justice communities to accept risk in exchange for neighborhood revitalization. While such programs provided a way to clean up contamination without undergoing problematic environmental assessments, by linking remediation to economic development, and promises of economic prosperity, they threatened to dilute environmental justice goals and elide concerns about health and safety.

BOA Constrictions

On a damp Thursday night in January, 2012, I joined about 20 North Shore residents in the basement of the Reformed Church of Staten Island, an historic landmark dating back to the late 1600s. Around the church, gabled Victorian homes (some from the 1800s) lined narrow streets that ambled toward the waterfront. These picturesque scenes, however, were frequently interrupted by vacant businesses, dilapidated homes, empty lots, and waterfront industries. Indeed, in addition to being one of Staten Island's oldest districts, Port Richmond was also one of its poorest. The average income for a family of three in Port Richmond was approximately $19,000,[3] according to a local community group, and unemployment among adults aged 20–24 was as high as 25 percent

(United States Census Bureau 2011). Those who were employed, especially the area's large number of undocumented immigrants, often worked for exploitative wages. These conditions led the New York State Department of Environmental Conservation to name Port Richmond to its Brownfield Opportunity Area (BOA) program in 2005.

The BOA program was rooted in a federal initiative known as the Brownfield Program. Launched by the EPA under the Clinton administration in 1995, one year after the Executive Order on environmental justice, brownfields were defined as "propert[ies], the expansion, redevelopment, or reuse of which may be complicated by the presence *or potential presence* of a hazardous substance, pollutant, or contaminant."[4] Brownfield grants provided seed moneys to municipalities as an incentive to private investors to purchase, assess, clean, and redevelop these sites. In some ways, the program marked a victory for environmental justice groups as it did not require an environmental risk assessment to prove that a site qualified for remediation. Rather, if a perception of contamination prevented a site's redevelopment, it was considered a brownfield. Because the program prioritized low-income neighborhoods, it appealed to all kinds of environmental justice and community-based activists, as well as real estate professionals, businesses, and local governments. Within a decade, all 50 states had created their own brownfield incentive programs.

By incentivizing private investors to clean up and redevelop contaminated sites, these brownfield programs crystallized neoliberal ideas which held that free of government "interference", market-based economies will efficiently and optimally allocate public resources (Robbins 2014: 100). Neoliberal policies thus encouraged the privatization of public services and prioritized economic growth, largely through urban redevelopment which was touted as the way to cure nearly all of the problems plaguing the postindustrial city (including environmental pollution) (Logan and Molotch 2007; Eisinger 1988; see also Zukin 1993). For proponents of neoliberalism, Brownfield programs presented a "win–win" scenario – by providing seed money to municipalities to incentivize private investment, they simultaneously encouraged revitalization and the cleanup of toxic properties.

In recent years, however, brownfield programs have begun to face criticism from environmental justice activists and scholars who question the degree to which these incentives advantage large developers and property owners and facilitate neighborhood gentrification and displacement (Essoka 2010). For instance, Gamper-Rabindran and Timmins (2011) correlate the cleanup of hazardous sites with changes in neighborhood income levels, finding that gentrifying neighborhoods are more likely to receive cleanups than those whose income levels are stable or declining (Harvey 1996; Ageyman, Bullard, and Evans 2003; Pellow and Brulle; 2005; Checker 2011). BOA initiatives sought to address some of these criticisms by demarcating zones where revitalization was hindered by the presence of multiple contaminated sites. BOA funding also targeted local development organizations (rather than municipalities or private entities) by offering grants to create comprehensive, community-based plans for redevelopment and revitalization.[5] In 2012, Staten Island's Northfield Community Local Development Corporation (NCLDC) received a grant to develop such a plan.

The meeting at the Reformed Church was the first in a series of public sessions to solicit input into the BOA planning process. NCLDC leaders began the meeting by announcing that they had decided to hire New York City's Department of City Planning (DCP) to create the BOA plan. The agency had already "done the legwork," they explained, in the course of producing a number of previous planning documents that suggested ways to revitalize Port Richmond. DCP planners then took the microphone and narrated a PowerPoint presentation that introduced their approach to the BOA. They began by defining its purpose: "[to] identify potential strategic brownfield sites, analyze economic and market trends and work with the community to identify potential redevelopment strategies."[6] These strategies included "supporting new retail services and jobs, strengthening the working waterfront, and providing needed amenities including open space and waterfront access."[7] Local residents were familiar with this language – it appeared in several previous (and highly contested) DCP plans for the North Shore. It also described the Bloomberg administration's approach to neighborhood redevelopment throughout the city, especially on former industrial waterfronts.

Under Bloomberg, one-third of the city was rezoned, mostly to lift height restrictions and to allow for taller buildings and the creation of residential and commercial developments in areas formerly restricted to manufacturing zones.[8] Almost all of this development served Bloomberg's agenda to rebrand New York as a "luxury city," which included transforming low-income and industrial neighborhoods into loft and commerce-filled zones designed to attract tourists and upwardly mobile professionals (Brash 2011). According to this ideology, revenue from high-end development would increase the city's tax base and eventually "trickle down" to benefit all kinds of public services. In the meantime, some of those services, such as the cleaning of toxic sites, could be privatized and incorporated into the city's overarching redevelopment agenda (Angotti 2008). Yet, for North Shore residents, revitalization was not the answer to their environmental problems. Not only could it price them out of their neighborhood, but they also believed that the gentrification of waterfronts in Brooklyn, Queens, and Manhattan had displaced waste-producing industries from those places, and relocated them to the North Shore. As Victoria Gillen, leader of the Elm Park Civic Association and the North Shore Community Coalition for Environmental Justice, commented, "Creating all the wonderful new playgrounds and high-value waterfront residential areas pushes HEAVY industrial use, into parts of Queens and Staten Island."

Back at the BOA meeting, residents were not shy about challenging the DCP's plan. First, they insisted on the need to identify "strategic brownfield sites" according to the threat the site posed to the community, not "economic and market trends." As one man said, "We need more enforcement and cleanup before we need more development." Second, residents pointed out that the BOA did not address already overburdened environmental infrastructure. Area sewers, for instance, overflowed with each heavy rain and discharged into the Kill Van Kull. Similarly, for years they had been asking the city to repair and augment flood protections along the waterfronts. Moreover, Port Richmond

Avenue, the neighborhood's main traffic artery, was already clogged with cars, trucks, and buses. "How dare you talk about drawing in new populations?" the local president of the NAACP (National Association for the Advancement of Colored People) demanded.

DCP and NLDC leaders responded to such questions by assuring residents that all of their concerns would be solved by an influx of residential and commercial developments, which would trigger infrastructure improvements, school expansions, further cleanups, and so on. But most meeting-goers did not agree. In fact, for them, the intrusion of a market-based agenda into brownfield cleanup was a crushing blow. As Gillen said at the end of the meeting, "I heard about this and thought, oh Brownfield, yeah great. We need that. But now I'm stunned." The next section provides a second example from the North Shore that highlights the implications of brownfield remediation for community health concerns.

Storage Wars[9]

In the spring of 2012, Joelle Morrison and her husband moved their belongings to Devon Storage, a 2-year-old facility on Staten Island's North Shore. The Morrisons had just sold their house and were finishing renovations on a new one. In the interim, they were staying in an apartment. Then Hurricane Sandy hit. The storage facility, which sat on a former wetland, filled with water that covered its entire first floor. "About 20 percent [of our belongings] are left," Morrison told me a few weeks after the storm, "and it all has to be cleaned ... It smells terrible." Not only was Devon located near a sewage treatment plant that had discharged during the storm, but it also sat on the North Shore's heavily contaminated waterfront, and just a few yards from the equally toxic Kill Van Kull.

What the Morrisons did not know was that Devon Self Storage, a former shipbuilding and maintenance yard, had recently signed on to New York City's new Brownfield Cleanup Program (BCP). Initiated in 2010, the BCP was the first municipally run brownfield program in the country. It targeted sites with low to moderate contamination, thus complementing state and federal programs' tendencies to focus on larger sites. Once enrolled, the city offered developers (and their lenders) protection from future liability and allowed them to deduct cleanup costs from federal taxes.[10] In addition, developers needed only to apply to one agency, the Office of Environmental Remediation (OER). Thus, they avoided seeking cumbersome City Council or Community Board approvals, or even more onerous public reviews. This streamlined process answered those neoliberal critics who blamed slow and heavy-handed regulatory bureaucracies for impeding economic redevelopment. The time from application to the start of remediation for private developers usually took less than a year (Checker 2011).

Devon's owners applied to the BCP soon after its launch. Three years earlier, they had discovered soil vapors containing high levels of PCEs (perchloroethylenes) and TCEs (trichloroethylenes) during construction of the facility. Both compounds are used as industrial solvents, and long-term exposure to them is associated with disorders of the central nervous system and several types of cancers in humans, especially of the kidney, liver, cervix, and lymphatic system. While levels were low enough to allow storage operations to go forward, they were high enough to impede the future reuse of the site for residential or certain commercial purposes. The BCP enabled Devon's owners to clean the site, and expanded their options for redeveloping it in the future.

Once accepted into the BCP, Devon's owners were required to post their remediation work plan on the OER web site, making it available for public comment for 6 weeks. Although such documents are highly technical, over the years, North Shore environmental justice activists had become fluent in the specialized language of environmental consultants and engineers. Both Victoria Gillen and Beryl Thurman submitted comments on the work plan, challenging its proposal to partially remediate the site by capping the contamination and covering it with a hard surface.

Gillen's comment pointed out that the site's proximity to a residential area made a partial remediation risky: "Noting the presence of residential property within several hundred feet of the cleanup site, and being exquisitely aware of the preponderant historic disregard for residential interests on Staten Island's North Shore, we hereby request, as is our right, an assessment of proposed remedies by a professional in the environmental remediation field." Thurman took a different tack, arguing that because the waterfront property was built on landfill, increasing storm surges could displace the containment:

> This property like many of the waterfront properties on Staten Island's North Shore is vulnerable to sea level rising, storm surges and flooding from the Kill Van Kull. In such an event it is highly likely that even paved, or black topped properties would be damaged causing any contaminants that were below the hard surface to become exposed during a storm and then swept towards the residential communities and then back into the nearby waterways such as in the case with New Orleans' Ninth Ward and Hurricane Katrina in 2005.

This reference to New Orleans was well taken. Research conducted in the aftermath of Hurricane Katrina demonstrates that floodwater dislodged and distributed heavy metals (Rotkin-Ellman *et al.* 2010; Zahran *et al.* 2010). Other research shows that storm surges have breached retaining walls and other barriers meant to seal in toxic contaminants (Valhouli 2012). Partial remediations seem especially risky in waterfront neighborhoods with multiple toxic sites. Rising sea levels and storm surges generate more frequent and intense flooding that endangers the stability of contaminant structures. Once dislodged, floodwater can disseminate these contaminants and mix them with other chemicals in the area. Although the OER's director took notice of Thurman and Gillen's comments, and met with each of them separately to discuss their concerns,[11] the final version of the work plan remained almost identical to the original.

The Devon case reflects national trends in the cleanup of toxic urban sites. A study by geographer Deb Ranjan Sinha (2011) finds that across the country the partial remediation of brownfield sites is becoming increasingly common, as is the privatization of the entire cleanup process. Not only do private consultant firms conduct site assessments (often offered on spec), but they also tend to be the same firms that coordinate site cleanups. Thus, assessments are akin to bids, aimed at securing cleanup contracts. Accordingly, they stress cost-saving measures that emphasize the minimum, rather than the maximum, necessary and technically possible environmental solutions (Sinha 2011; see also Downs *et al.* 2009). Privatization of brownfields cleanups also entails less transparency and meaningful public input (Chess and Purcell 1999; Downs *et al.* 2009). For instance, by timing opportunities for public comments to occur after project approval, the BCP process rendered public participation futile. Like the case of the Port Richmond BOA, economic interests, rather than health risks, ultimately drove remediation (Checker 2012). In the next section, I return to Hyde Park to show how local residents also challenged the brownfield process and, ultimately, succeeded in resisting the very idea of redevelopment and remediation.

"Sore Eye"

"[Brownfields] sounded like our best lead so far," said Charles Utley, President of HAPIC (Hyde and Aragon Park Improvement Committee), recalling his reaction to learning about the federal Brownfield program in 1997. Seven years earlier, he and his neighbors had filed a lawsuit charging the wood-preserving factory that had leaked contaminants into their neighborhood with endangerment and neglect. Yet, they could not prove that the wood-preserving factory was the sole source of their contamination. Moreover, after the EPA's risk assessment failed to link the contaminants to local health problems, neither the lawsuit nor a government-sponsored relocation looked promising. As HAPIC leaders continued to seek alternatives, they discovered the EPA's Brownfield Pilot Grants. At the time, only municipalities could apply for the funds, so HAPIC leaders convinced Augusta's mayor to submit an application.[12] After two tries, Augusta became one of the first cities in the nation to receive a Brownfield pilot grant in 1999.

Importantly, early brownfield grants focused exclusively on assessing and redeveloping commercial or industrial sites, not residential properties. Accordingly, Hyde Park's grant centered on a 10.8 acre scrap metal yard that, over the years, had overtaken part of a street and sprawled into the backyards of nearby residents (see Figure 5.1). Towers of tires and scrap metal rose high above the roofs of the neighborhood, and during heavy rains, foul-smelling water flowed from the site and flooded the yards of nearby residents. An assessment of onsite contamination at the scrap yard revealed the presence of heavy metals, primarily lead, and PCBs in soils, low concentrations of metals in groundwater, and small pockets of petroleum throughout the site (Gannett Fleming 2004). Cleanup costs were estimated at $10 million. Because this sum was more than a private developer could be expected to spend, the EPA joined with the Georgia EPD to remove 20,000 tons of surface waste that included 12,000 tons of hazardous lead-contaminated soil and 181 tons of mercury-contaminated

(a)

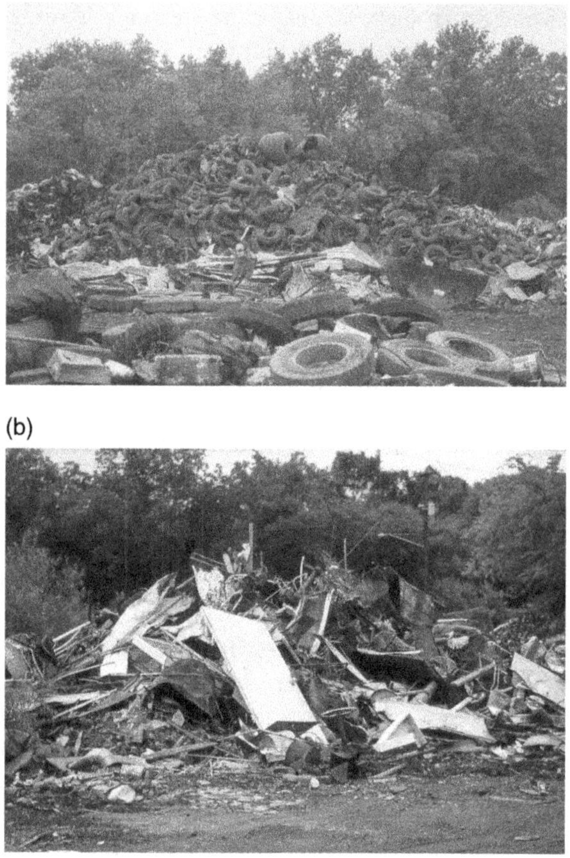

(b)

Figure 5.1 Goldberg Brothers scrap metal yard – Hyde Park, Augusta, Georgia circa 1999.

debris (Checker 2005). Once the site was cleaned, city leaders began searching for a developer to purchase and repurpose it.

Residents had mixed reactions to the Brownfield Pilot grant. On one hand, they were unanimously relieved that the junkyard, so long a "sore eye" (*sic*), was clean of debris and contaminants. On the other hand, because the brownfield program excluded residential properties, it was unclear whether and how this process would address contamination in people's yards. In other words, residents resisted the brownfield program's "trickle down" strategy, where redevelopment of the scrap yard would spur wider neighborhood revitalization and eventually accrue benefits to individual households and enable them to move if they desired. Moreover, most residents believed that the neighborhood was not remediable. "You can't clean this up," one woman said. "We need to move everyone out and make the whole neighborhood an industrial park." Residents thus continued to lobby for relocation, even as city leaders continued to pursue brownfield redevelopment.

In 2003, a second federal brownfield grant expanded the scope of the first to include an adjacent metal recycling center. This grant took advantage of the fact that the EPA now allowed some assessment of contaminants in residential properties surrounding brownfield sites and included funds to study properties within a certain radius of both scrap yards.[13] The ensuing study, released in 2006, showed pockets of cadmium, copper, lead, mercury, zinc, and PCBs that exceeded regulatory standards across the study area. It concluded, "Pockets of contaminated soil exceeding the Georgia Environmental Protection Division (EPD) Type 1 (residential) Risk Reduction Standard (RRS) are located throughout the study area, including the residential Hyde Park community" (Gannett Fleming 2006: 32). Study engineers surmised that these metals had come from the scrap yards and were being circulated by storm runoff and flooding (Gannett Flemming 2006). Importantly, this assessment was not meant to evaluate health risks, but to measure contaminant levels and recommend methods for remediating them to acceptable standards for commercial development. It included only a brief statement about human health risks, pointing out the potential for human exposure "to site contaminants through ingestion, dermal contact, or inhalation" (Gannett Flemming 2006: 22). Later, however, the study engineer publicly stated that he believed relocation to be the best course of action (Checker 2012).

For Hyde Park residents, of course, the health implications of the assessment were primary (see Checker 2012). Their insistence on relocation now grew stronger and louder, and they appeared in local media outlets calling on city leaders to "do something." Meanwhile, the city stayed its course with the brownfield program, continuing to work on redeveloping the former scrap yards. To that end, a city-sponsored community visioning workshop in the fall of 2008 brought in brownfield consultants from Atlanta to lead a design "charrette"[14] meant to elicit community members' visions for neighborhood revitalization. When the consultants distributed boxes of crayons and paper to residents, their opposition to redevelopment came to a head. "Crayons?!" they exclaimed later. "Peoples out here are dying and they brought us crayons?!" For them, crayons symbolized years of being patronized and having their needs dismissed. They refused to spend an afternoon envisioning redevelopment. Passing the crayons and paper on to their children, they insisted on bypassing the visioning session and skipping to the question and answer period. Now, they asked questions about their property taxes, community center maintenance problems, and other issues of immediate concern.

Hyde Park residents continued to pursue relocation, rather than redevelopment, for the next few years. In 2010, their city councilor announced a plan to relocate Hyde Park residents and turn the entire neighborhood into a 20-acre storm water detention pond to alleviate flooding throughout the city.[15] The relocation would adhere to the Uniform Relocation Act, which stipulates that people displaced in connection with federally funded projects are "made whole."[16] In this case, homeowners would receive enough compensation to buy a property comparable to their current home, and their moving expenses would be paid. Neighborhood support for the proposal was unanimous, and after several delays, the City Council approved it. In the summer of 2013, David and Thomasine Jackson, who had lived on the edge of the scrap yard and experienced the worst flooding in the neighborhood, became the first family to undergo relocation. About 6 months later, I sat with the Jacksons in the living room of their new home, atop the highest hill in their subdivision. "Now when it rains," said David, holding his palms up to the sky, "I just say let it come."

While Hyde Park was one of just a few environmental justice communities in the United States to win a relocation (Bullard *et al.* 2007), theirs was not an unmitigated victory. Because the relocation was impelled by an infrastructure project, not contamination or health risks, residents had to continue to fight for a way to address their health problems. As Charles Utley told me, "We're still asking them for a program to monitor people's health." At the time of publication, that particular fight continues. Thus, while residents successfully resisted redevelopment and the "trickle down" strategy for environmental justice that it represented, they were unsuccessful in persuading government agencies to address their health concerns.

Conclusions

Over 20 years into the environmental justice movement, and despite some legislative gains, uneven siting practices continue. That means people of color are still consigned to live in polluted and contaminated neighborhoods, and practical victories are few and far between. The perniciousness of environmental disparities is linked to historically and cumulatively embedded forms of discrimination. For instance, close examination of environmental risk assessments reveal the many ways in which they exclude the multiple exposures and vulnerabilities of poor people and people of color and obscure the links between toxic chemicals and local health problems. In turn, indeterminate risk assessments have far-reaching consequences for local communities. Recent anthropological work finds that, in an environment of risk uncertainty, corporate polluters use partial accommodations and practices of "corporate responsibility" to downplay local health risks and discourage local opposition, in part by appealing to neoliberal values of homeownership and financial independence. I suggest that these practices reconfigure traditional forms of "job blackmail" for a postindustrial era of job scarcity. In other words, rather than asking communities to accept hazardous facilities for the sake of the jobs they might supply, today's corporations provide support to local social programs, minimal payouts to homeowners, and risk mitigation measures in exchange for community quiescence and acceptance (see also Ottinger 2013).

My own research extends these findings by exploring how government bodies similarly exploit situations of risk uncertainty in order to advance neoliberal redevelopment agendas. I focus on public programs that incentivize private investors to clean and redevelop contaminated properties. In linking remediation to redevelopment and private investment, such programs prioritize economic interests and emphasize cost-saving measures such as partial remediation, while eliding public health concerns. Thus, rather than jobs, government entities offered environmental justice communities promises of neighborhood revitalization and eventual economic mobility as an exchange for risk acceptance. But local communities resisted these promises and challenged the notion that neoliberal forms of redevelopment provide a cure-all for urban ills. Instead, residents continued to assert their own environmental health and justice priorities.

NOTES

1 http://epa.gov/riskassessment/basicinformation.htm#arisk.
2 http://www.cdc.gov/nceh/ehs/Publications/Guidance_Flooding.htm#Figure_1.
3 Make the Road, a local immigrant rights organization, reported this figure on its web site: http://www.maketheroad.org/whoweare_aboutourcommunity.php.
4 http://www.epa.gov/brownfields/basic_info.htm; italics mine.
5 http://www.dec.ny.gov/chemical/8650.html.
6 http://www.nyc.gov/html/dcp/html/portrichmondboa/index.shtml.
7 http://www.nyc.gov/html/dcp/html/portrichmondboa/index.shtml.
8 http://www.nytimes.com/newsgraphics/2013/08/18/reshaping-new-york/.
9 Portions of this section, including its subtitle, were previously published in Checker (2015).
10 Quotes in this paragraph can be found at http://www.nyc.gov/html/planyc2030/html/theplan/brownfields.shtml.
11 I was not privy to those conversations.
12 See Checker (2012) for a fuller description of this process, in which the mayor allowed HAPIC leaders (with help from a pro bono consultant and me) to draft the grant proposal.
13 A city engineer initiated this grant proposal and I assisted him with it.
14 See http://www.ced.uga.edu/pdfs/outreach/charrettes/final-hydepark-report.pdf (accessed December 6, 2015).
15 Detention ponds reduce flood damage by gathering storm water and slowly releasing it, while retention ponds retain water on a more permanent basis.
16 http://portal.hud.gov/hudportal/HUD?src=/program_offices/comm_planning/affordablehousing/training/web/relocation/overview.

REFERENCES

Agyeman, J., Bullard, R.D., and Evans, B. 2003. *Just Sustainabilities: Development in an Unequal World.* Cambridge, MA: MIT Press.

Alley, K.D. 2002. *On the Banks of the Gaṅgā: When Wastewater Meets a Sacred River.* Ann Arbor: University of Michigan Press.

Angotti, T. 2008. *New York For Sale: Community Planning Confronts Global Real Estate.* Boston, MA: MIT Press.

ATSDR (Agency for Toxic Substances and Disease Registry) 1994. "Petitioned Public Health Assessment Addendum, Southern Wood Piedmont Augusta, Richmond County, Georgia, Appendix 3 – March 1994 Health Consultation." Atlanta, GA.

Auyero, J. and Swistun, D. 2008. "The Social Production of Toxic Uncertainty." *American Sociological Review*, 73(3): 357–379.

Auyero, J. and Swistun, D. 2009. *Flammable: Environmental Suffering in an Argentine Shantytown*. Oxford: Oxford University Press.

Brash, J. 2011. *Bloomberg's New York: Class and Governance in the Luxury City*. Athens, GA: University of Georgia Press.

Brown, M.K., Carnoy, M., Currie, E., Duster, T.D., Oppenheimer, D.B., Schultz, M.M., and Wellman, D. 2005. *Whitewashing Race: The Myth of a Color-Blind Society*. Princeton, NJ: University of California Press.

Brown, P. 2007. *Toxic Exposures: Contested Illnesses and the Environmental Health Movement*. New York: Columbia University Press.

Bryant, B.I. 1995. *Environmental Justice: Issues, Policies, and Solutions*. Washington, DC: Island Press.

Bullard, R.D. 2000. *Dumping in Dixie: Race, Class, and Environmental Quality*, 3rd ed. Boulder, CO: Westview.

Bullard, R.D, Mohai, P., Saha, R., and Wright, B. 2007. "Toxic Wastes and Race at Twenty, 1987–2007: A Report Prepared for the United Church of Christ Justice & Witness Ministries." Cleveland, OH: United Church of Christ.

Button, G. 2010. *Disaster Culture: Knowledge and Uncertainty in the Wake of Human and Environmental Catastrophe*. Walnut Creek, CA: Left Coast Press.

Cepek, M.L. 2013. "Indigenous Difference: Rethinking Particularity in the Anthropology of Amazonia." *The Journal of Latin American and Caribbean Anthropology*, 18(2): 359–370. doi: 10.1111/jlca.12034.

Checker, M. 2005. *Polluted Promises: Environmental Racism and the Search for Justice in a Southern Town*. New York: New York University Press.

Checker, M. 2009. "Staten Island's Toxic Stew." *Gotham Gazette*. http://old.gothamgazette.com/article/environment/20090526/7/2923 (accessed December 16, 2015).

Checker, M. 2011. "Wiped Out by the 'Greenwave': Environmental Gentrification and the Paradoxical Politics of Urban Sustainability." *City & Society*, 23: 210–229.

Checker, M. 2012. "Chicken Little, a Ferris Wheel and Disorderly Development on Staten Island's North Shore." *Gotham Gazette*. http://www.gothamgazette.com/index.php/development/2133-chicken-little-a-ferris-wheel-and-disorderly-development-on-staten-islands-north-shore (accessed December 16, 2015).

Chess, C. and Purcell, K. 1999. "Public Participation and the Environment: Do We Know What Works?" *Environmental Science & Technology*, 33(16): 2685–2692. doi: 10.1021/es980500g.

Commission for Racial Justice. 1987. *Toxic Wastes and Race in the United States: A National Report on the Racial and Socioeconomic Characteristics of Communities with Hazardous Waste Sites*. New York: United Church of Christ.

Cole, L. and Foster, S. 2001. *From the Ground Up: Environmental Racism and the Rise of the Environmental Justice Movement*. New York: New York University Press.

Dietrich, A.S. 2013. *The Drug Company Next Door: Pollution, Jobs, and Community Health in Puerto Rico*. New York: New York University Press.

Douglas, M. and Wildavsky, A. 1983. *Risk and Culture: An Essay on the Selection of Technological and Environmental Dangers*. Berkeley, CA: University of California Press.

Downs, T., Ross, L., Patton, S., and Rulnick, S., *et al.* 2009. "Complexities of Holistic Community-based Participatory Research for a Low Income, Multi-ethnic Population Exposed to Multiple Built-environment Stressors in Worcester, Massachusetts." *Environmental Research*, 109: 1028–1040.

Eisinger, P.K. 1988. *The Rise of the Entrepreneurial State: State and Local Economic Development Policy in the United States*. Madison: University of Wisconsin Press.

EPA Office of Inspector General. 2004. "EPA Needs to Consistently Implement the Intent of the Executive Order on Environmental Justice." Evaluation Report 2004-P-00007.Washington,DC.http://www.epa.gov/oig/reports/2004/20040301-2004-P-00007.pdf.

EPA Office of Inspector General. 2006. "EPA Needs to Conduct Environmental Justice Reviews of Its Programs, Policies, and Activities." Evaluation Report 2006-P-00034.Washington,DC.http://www.epa.gov/oig/reports/2006/20060918-2006-P-00034.pdf.

Essoka, J. 2010. "The Gentrifying Effects of Brownfields Redevelopment." *The Western Journal of Black Studies*, 34(3): 299–316.

Faber, D. 1998. *The Struggle for Ecological Democracy: Environmental Justice Movements in the United States.* New York: Guilford.

Fitchen, J. 1988. "Anthropology and Environmental Problems in the US: The Case of Groundwater Contamination." *Practicing Anthropology*, 10(3–4): 5.

Gannett Fleming 2006. "Phase II Environmental Site Assessment and Site Reuse Feasibility Study, Augusta Brownfields Study Area, Augusta, Georgia." Augusta, Georgia. On File with Author.

Gunter, V. and Kroll-Smith, S. 2006. *Volatile Places: A Sociology of Communities and Environmental Controversies.* Sage.

Hannah-Jones, N. 2014. "Living Apart: How the Government Betrayed a Landmark Civil Rights Law." *ProPublica.* http://www.propublica.org/article/living-apart-how-the-government-betrayed-a-landmark-civil-rights-law (accessed March 15, 2014).

Harper, J. 2004. "Breathless in Houston: A Political Ecology of Health Approach to Understanding Environmental Health Concerns." *Medical Anthropology*, 23: 295–326. doi: 10.1080/01459740490513521.

Harvey, D. 1996. *Justice, Nature and the Geography of Difference.* Oxford: Blackwell.

Hubbard, R. and Wald, E. 1993. *Exploding the Gene Myth: How Genetic Information Is Produced and Manipulated by Scientists, Physicians, Employers, Insurance Companies, Educators, and Law Enforcers.* Boston, MA: Beacon Press.

Kriebel, D., Tickner, J., Epstein, P., Lemons, J., Levins, R., Loechler, E.L., Quinn, M., … Stoto, M. 2001. "The Precautionary Principle in Environmental Science." *Environmental Health Perspectives* 109 (9): 871–876.

Kuehn, R.R. 1997. "An Analysis of the Compatibility of Quantitative Risk Assessment with the Principles of Environmental Justice in the United States." *Risk Decision and Policy*, 2(3): 259–276.

Lee, D., Lee, I., Song, K., Steffes, M. Toscano, W., Baker, B., and Jacobs, D.R. 2006. "A Strong Dose-Response Relation between Serum Concentrations of Persistent Organic Pollutants and Diabetes: Results from the National Health and Examination Survey 1999–2002." *Diabetes Care*, 29(7): 1638–1644.

Little, P.D. 2014. *Toxic Town IBM, Pollution, and Industrial Risks.* New York: NYU Press.

Logan, J.R. and Molotch, H.L. 2007. *Urban Fortunes: The Political Economy of Place.* Berkeley, CA: University of California Press.

Maantay, J. 2002. "Industrial Zoning Changes in New York City: A Case Study of 'Expulsive Zoning.'" *Projections*, 3: 63–108.

Massey, D.S. and Denton, N.A. 1993. *American Apartheid: Segregation and the Making of the Underclass.* Cambridge, MA: Harvard University Press.

Nachman, K.E., Fox, M.A., Sheehan, M.C., Burke, T.A., Rodricks, J.V., and Woodruff, T.J. 2011. "Leveraging Epidemiology to Improve Risk Assessment." *Open Epidemiology Journal*, 4: 3–29.

Novotny, P. 1995a. "Popular Epidemiology and the Struggle for Community Health in the Environmental Justice Movement." In *The Struggle for Ecological Democracy: Environmental Justice Movements in the United States* (pp. 137–138). New York: Guilford.

Novotny, P. 1995b. "Where We Live, Work and Play: Reframing the Cultural Landscape of Environmentalism in the Environmental Justice Movement." *New Political Science*, 23.

NYC DOHMH (NYC Department of Health and Mental Hygiene). 2006. "Community Health Profile: Port Richmond." http://www. nyc.gov/html/doh/downloads/pdf/data/2006chp-501.pdf.

NYC DOHMH (NYC Department of Health and Mental Hygiene). 2010. "Lead Poisoning in New York City: 2009 Annual Data Report." http://www.nyc.gov/html/doh/downloads/pdf/lead/lead-2009report.pdf.

Ottinger, G. 2013. *Refining Expertise: How Responsible Engineers Subvert Environmental Justice Challenges.* New York: New York University Press.

Pace, D. 2005. "'More Blacks Live with Pollution.'" *Associated Press*, December 13. hosted.ap.org/specials/interactives/archive/pollution/part1.html.

Pellow, D.N. and Brulle, R.J. 2005. *Power, Justice, and the Environment: A Critical Appraisal of the Environmental Justice Movement.* Cambridge, MA: MIT Press.

Petryna, A. 2013. *Life Exposed: Biological Citizens after Chernobyl.* Princeton, NJ: Princeton University Press.

Pulido, L. 1996. *Environmentalism and Economic Justice: Two Chicano Struggles in the Southwest.* Tucson: University of Arizona Press.

Robbins, R.H. 2014. *Global Problems and the Culture of Capitalism.* Boston, MA: Allyn & Bacon.

Shipak, M. 2007. "*Listening to Environmental Justice Communities: A Model for Government Agencies Identifying Environmental Health Problems and Solutions.*" Washington, D.C.

Shrader-Frechette, K. 2010. "Analyzing Public Participation in Risk Analysis: How the Wolves of Environmental Injustice Hide in the Sheep's Clothing of Science." *Environmental Justice*, 3(4): 119–123.

Singer, M. 2011. "Down Cancer Alley: The Lived Experience of Health and Environmental Suffering in Louisiana's Chemical Corridor." *Medical Anthropological Quarterly*, 25(2): 141–163.

Sinha, D. 2011. "The Environmental Kuznets Curve Hypothesis and Legacy Pollution: A Geohistorical Analysis of the Environmental Consequences of Industrialization in Worcester, Massachusetts." *The Industrial Geographer*, 7(2): 1–18.

Tesh, S.N. 2000. *Uncertain Hazards: Environmental Activists and Scientific Proof.* Ithaca, NY: Cornell University Press.

US GAO (General Accounting Office). 1983. *Siting of Hazardous Waste Landfills and Their Correlation with Racial and Economic Status of Surrounding Communities.* Washington, DC: US GAO.

United States Census Bureau. 2011. 2007–2011 *American Community Survey 5-Year Estimates.*

Wigley, D. and Shrader-Frechette, K. 1996. "Environmental Racism and Biased Methods of Risk Assessment." *Risk: Health, Safety and Environment*, 7, 55–58.

Valhouli, C. 2012. "Mold News: Sandy Leaves Toxic Trouble." *New York Observer*, November 7. http://observer.com/2012/11/youre-soaking-in-it-sandy-leaves-toxic-trouble/.

Zahran, S., Mielke, H.W., Gonzales, C.R., Powell, E.T., and Weiler, S. 2010. "New Orleans before and after Hurricanes Katrina/Rita: A Quasi-Experiment of the Association between Soil Lead and Children's Blood Lead." *Environmental Science & Technology*, 44(12): 4433–4440.

Zukin, S. 1993. *Landscapes of Power: From Detroit to Disney World.* Berkeley, CA: University of California Press.

CHAPTER 6

Medicine, Alternative Medicine, and Political Ecologies of the Body

Joseph S. Alter

Introduction

Taking a hardline position, many advocates for "Nature Cure" claim that treatment with water, earth, sunlight, air, and diet can cure many if not all diseases. Given what is known about pathology, etiology, and the social determinants of health and disease, most scholars, policy makers, and health care professionals would regard these claims to reflect cruel, perverse, misguided quackery. But what is being said about public health by making seemingly outrageous medical claims about efficacy?

Nature Cure, along with other forms of alternative medicine, is often criticized for essentializing and valorizing cultural beliefs, shifting medical responsibility to the individual, and generally ignoring problems of social inequality and power (Baer 2001, 2004). Sympathetic anthropologists, taking a relativist stance, might argue that Nature Cure should be understood in terms of the logic of culture, cultural history, and the politics of cultural identity (see Nissen and Manderson 2013). And naturopaths have recently argued that the incipient "holism" of their approach is broadly compatible with anthropological holism, and that this can be taken advantage of to engineer a rapprochement of critical medical anthropology and complementary and alternative medicine (Flesch 2012; Tippens, Oberg, and Bradley 2012). However, there are important

A Companion to the Anthropology of Environmental Health, First Edition. Edited by Merrill Singer.

epistemological problems involved in reconciling critical medical anthropology and constructionist perspectives on culture (see Baer 1997). Furthermore relativism and holism would seem to come up short on the ultimate question of evidentiary efficacy, particularly since Nature Cure has a long history of being reductively deterministic in authoritatively claiming the power of nature as a definitive cure-all. The practice of Nature Cure constantly begs the hard question: Does it work?

This chapter provides an answer in order to further question the relevance of culture to the practice of medicine, as medicine – in all of its various ethno-manifestations – lays claim to the domain of health in terms of remedial, individualistic healing. Thus a more radical claim is made for Nature Cure in terms of a political ecology of public health than is made by practitioners and proponents intent on demonstrating efficacy and/or holistic complementarity. In doing so this chapter provides a broad theoretical perspective on a "political ecology of the body," as this perspective provides a way to think past or problematize discourses of efficacy (see Craig 2012) to understand multiple levels of consciousness and awareness about the relationship among social distinctions, health, biology, and the environment.

Using material from a study of Nature Cure in India, the argument presented here is that culture and the logic of cultural analysis unto itself is not very helpful in understanding what is significant about a rich, textured, and elaborate "cultural" system of medicine. It will be argued that culture makes "nonsense" of the sense that is reflected in a political ecology of the body and the biosocial configuration of the body's ecological health. This political ecology is fundamentally epidemiological and transcends domains of cultural difference and distinction, even as local cultural practices seek to bracket the meaning of the body, and its therapeutic manipulation, in particular ways.

By contrasting the "sense" of biosocial ecology with the "nonsense" of culture, what I mean is that the idea of using water to cure people of infectious diseases is nonsensical in light of what is known about pathology and the efficacy of pharmaceutical interventions. Hydrotherapy and other Nature Cure modalities of treatment, can, nevertheless, be understood as aspects of an ecologically grounded, materialist response to the impress of power, and experiences of health risk and alienation as shaped by power relations in society. These experiences and the cultural responses to them make sense in terms of two centuries of increasingly powerful and pervasive social determinants of health, namely, population density and urbanization, poor sanitation, mobility, compromised nutrition, work- and labor-related risk, and, most specifically, epidemic-scale iatrogenesis in the context of biomedical institutionalization at the turn of the nineteenth century. Relative poverty and wealth structure risk in this environment, but it is particularly among the rapidly growing, and inherently precarious, middle class – resolutely modern, entrepreneurial, and upwardly mobile, but conscious of increased risk and vulnerability – that we can see the articulation of a political ecology of the body over the past 150 years.

Analysis is based on the results of research that involved intensive participant observation in half a dozen Nature Cure hospitals in six different cities of India, as well as ethnohistorical archival research that provided insight on the globalization of Nature Cure theory and practice. Invented in nineteenth-century south central Europe (Kirchfeld and Boyle 1994), the global history of Nature Cure parallels, overlaps with, and reflects historical developments in biomedicine, thus shaping a broad history of public health at the interstices of two radically different approaches to the problem of disease. Significantly, it is this global history, and theories and practices shaped by this history, that defines a political ecology of the body in contemporary practice.

A Political Ecology of the Body

In many ways and on many levels scientific understandings of physiology, pathology, and epidemiology have come to define humans and other organisms in very specific ways. In conjunction with this, environments are often conceptualized in terms of a hierarchy of organisms and their problematic interaction, with humans in a more or less discrete, unique, and superior position, able to manipulate interaction to their advantage based on increasingly specialized knowledge. The discovery of germs and the development of virology in the late nineteenth century dramatically reflect this and highlight the way in which the body itself has increasingly come to be understood in terms of eco-pathology, infection, immunization, and the isolation and control of disease vectors.

The value of this conceptualization of the body is obvious and can hardly be exaggerated. But it has also produced a peculiar attitude toward health and disease (see Rose 2007; Cohen 2009). In many respects this attitude is simply an extension and "hardening" of an attitude that correlates with culture most broadly as a boundary marker based on the exceptionalism of shared knowledge that is learned and communicated by a single species.

Research on the human diet in relation to health and diseases is a striking case that illustrates the contradictions and paradoxes of exceptionalism in terms of evolutionary adaptation, cultural change, and social inequality (Cordain *et al* 2005). But, arguably, revolutionary innovations in medicine over the past 150 years have produced a profound sense of alienation as our bodies are managed, delineated, and bounded in increasingly comprehensive and complex ways, ranging from vaccination to genetic engineering. In this regard, it is useful to keep in mind that critical theoretical insights on biosociality, new biotechnologies (Lock *et al.* 2000; Landecker 2007), global pharmaceutical regimes (Petryna, Lakoff, and Klienman 2006; Singer 2008; Dumit 2012), and biocapitalist medical research and development (Petryna 2009; Sunder Rajan 2012) provide a refined and nuanced understanding of biosocial processes that began to take shape in the late nineteenth century.

Over roughly the same period of time, since the 1860s, three interdependent major changes have had a significant impact on health and, therefore, on our bodies. Dramatic population growth, urban development, and a demographic shift in the configuration of social hierarchy, first in Europe and then elsewhere, corresponded directly to the industrialization of food production and processing, and changes in nutrition based on new patterns of consumption (Cordain *et al.* 2005; Barrett and Armeligos 2013: 15–48). By the turn of the century, revolutions in medicine (Waller 2002; Lindeman 2010), industry, and food production – as well as the deterioration of urban public health (see Barrett and Armeligos 2013: 49–78) – contributed to extreme articulations of class distinction, privilege, and inequality (Rees 2001; Grell, Cunningham, and Roeck 2005) that were clearly manifest in the emergence and reemergence of infectious diseases during this epidemiological transition (Barrett *et al.* 1998). Given the close correlation at this time between burgeoning structural inequalities, revolutions in medicine and medical technology, and the growth and development of industrial capitalism, the insights of critical medical anthropology might be as productively applied to the analytical "provincialization" (see Chakrabarty 2009) of European medical history as they have been to international and global health (see Singer and Baer 1995; Baer, Singer, and Susser 2003; Farmer 2003, 2013; Nichter 2008; Pfeiffer and Nichter 2008).

Precisely because of the growing structure of national public health interventions and the development of new medical technologies at the *fin de siècle*, and despite inequities and exploitation, the urban poor, the expanding working class, the rapidly growing middle class, and the industrial corporate elite were all increasingly subject to the same structure of alienation (see Cohen 2009) whereby their bodies and their health became more and more atomized, isolated, and objectified, and yet, ironically, more and more dependent on layers of technology that produced as much risk and suffering as they did promise of universal health, wealth, and happiness (Berg and Cocks 2002; Waddington 2011).

It is important to keep in mind that a political ecology of the body is a very broad analytical framework that helps to clarify the underlying structure of a more specific political economy of health focused on problems of clean drinking water, sanitation, nutrition, affordable health care, and immunization, as these things impinge on people's health (see Navarro 1978). In analyses that focus on the political ecology of the body, "politics" has to do with who controls the nature of nature, the internal and external bio-ecology of the body. This is a different kind of politics from the politics of activism in the arena of global health (McMichael and Beaglehole 2003; see Janes and Corbett 2010 for an excellent review), but it is a micro politics of the body-as-and-in-the-environment that is compatible with critical interventions concerning environmental health and the larger scale of global political ecology (Baer 1996; Little 2013; Leatherman 2005; Singer 2008; Singer and Baer 2009).

Hierarchical, organismic atomization is, therefore, a historically constructed "power-full" perspective on the environment and ecology, as this perspective became extremely hardened and dramatically embodied around the turn of the nineteenth century. Although intimately linked to the methods and insights of science, hierarchical, organismic atomization is by no means an intrinsically objective or inherently accurate representation of nature. A radically different perspective, historically constructed as an alternative political ecology, can be characterized in terms of three broadly similar theoretical postulates: systematics

(Bateson1987), bio-semiotics (Barbieri 2008; Hoffmeyer 2010; see also Alter forthcoming) and actor-network theory (Latour 2004, 2005). In its purest form these postulates provide a way to focus on ecological health as defined in terms of systemic networks and organic reciprocity rather than by defensive isolation and/or offensive domination.

In this formulation, health is an embodied, interactive attribute of ecological adaptation rather than an intrinsic state of being. As such, this alternative conceptualization of health produces a radically different political ecology of the body. It takes the question of efficacy, which is charged with intense self-interest and heavily marked with the politics of culture, and turns it on its head. Medical projects that focus on remedial health can and do provide important insights on fundamental problems of public health, but often precisely because of the way in which measures of efficacy at the level of the individual do not add up to good public health, and beg important questions about environmental health as well as the health of the environment. A person who is cured or immunized most likely continues to live in an unhealthy environment, and this "estrangement" can be understood in terms of alienation (see Alter forthcoming). Political ecologies of the body engage with this problem, either directly or indirectly, in terms of the development of forms of embodied consciousness that resist atomization and seek to establish various forms of organic reciprocity.

The definitive impact of biological factors in human and nonhuman experience, and the organic facticity of such things as death, disease, pain, and debility, cyclically reproduce social facts in human experience that correlate with, but are less open to creative manipulation than, ideas about what has cultural value or significance with respect to health and healing in general. Nature Cure is a system of medicine defined by a history of critical engagement with the structural, political, and economic problems that relate to the social facticity of health in the context of modernity – especially as reflected in the culture of biomedicine – even though what is proposed as a solution by practitioners might be called utopian fantasy rather than rational utilitarian pragmatism. In any case, to make sense of Nature Cure in terms of cultural meaning is to make sense of "nonsense" rather than see what is at stake with respect to various manifestations of power at the intersection of the body and the environment.

One way to understand what is at stake is this: Over the course of several decades the burden of disease in India has shifted dramatically from communicable to noncommunicable diseases (Shah and Mathur 2010; Deepa *et al.* 2011), with cardiovascular disease (CVD) now the leading cause of death in a country that still carries the burden of many other diseases as well as the burden of vast inequities (WHO NCD Country Profiles 2011). Half of all CVD deaths occur among those between the ages of 30 and 69, which is, on average, 10 years younger than in other so-called established market economies (Gupta *et al.* 2014). As an index of human biology reacting to an environment shaped by dramatic changes in lifestyle and patterns of consumption – that is, by a compressed history of wealth, class disparity, and nutritional health (see Pandey *et al.* 2013; Singh *et al.* 2013) – India's "silent epidemic" of cardiovascular heart disease is diagnostic of a political ecology of the body in terms of concrete risk factors, but also in the broadest sense of the term (see Umamahesh 2014).

However, a critical perspective on this ecology only comes to light by contrasting-in-context the leading cause of death with the second most common cause, diarrheal disease. The vast majority of diarrheal deaths are among infants born into environments where drinking water is contaminated with human waste (Manna *et al.* 2013). The significance of the etiological difference between acute CVD and diarrheal disease (*pace* Ghosh 2012) is what highlights the absurdity of cultural distinctions in the practice of different "systems" of medicine. There are, I think, moral, ethical, and political problems in proposing the same range of alternative options to a 35-year-old man with arteriosclerosis and his dehydrated 2-year-old daughter.

The contrast also defines a cultural ecology of modernity and a political economy of compounded structural inequality on the level of intra-village health where an intimately local epidemiological transition from CVD to diarrheal disease would seem farcical if it were not tragically true (Kumar *et al.* 2012). This political ecology is profoundly at odds with public health in general on any level, but especially as manifested in India (Gwatkin, Guillot, and Heuveline 1999; Ramraj and Alpert 2008). On this scale of consciousness both CVD and diarrhea are symptomatic of the same overarching biocultural problem: the problem of living hierarchically in an environment that does not accommodate hierarchical, organismic atomization, except in terms of exploitation, injustice, and violence – being able to eat too much of too many unhealthy things as a consequence of biosocial privilege or being in a position where water is unhealthy as a consequence of biosocial factors such as structural poverty. At the nexus of this ecology are men, women, children, and infants who collectively embody the symptoms of civilization and its discontents, albeit it in radically different ways; for the history of culture is a history of progressive conceptual alienation from the environment of our animal origins and from other organisms, human and nonhuman.

As we shall see, people articulate the possibility of an alternative ecology of health in terms of the "nonsense" of cultural systems of medicine that contribute to the alienation of particularism and the inequality that is inherent to questions of efficacy. Culture as a system of meaning is, fundamentally, the problem. On one level, Nature Cure reflects this quite clearly and dramatically. But in its radical elemental simplicity, and its insistence on dealing with CVD and diarrhea as symptoms of a deeper, more entrenched problem of bio-ecology and human exceptionalism, Nature Cure also presents a revolutionary alternative conceptualization of embodied health.

The Nature of Culture: Ecology, Modernity, and the Body

Nature Cure is institutionalized and professionalized in terms that are remarkably standardized throughout India. For reasons explained below, what developed in south central Europe as a modern form of hydrotherapy in the second half of the nineteenth century is now supported by the government of India as one of six recognized systems of medicine (see Wujastyk and Smith 2008). Practitioners with certified degrees from over a dozen training colleges around the country provide treatment to patients with a range of chronic diseases, mostly CVD, hypertension, arthritis, diabetes, a spectrum of symptoms associated with menopause, and a number of neurological conditions. Most patients are overweight and are, on average, over 50 years old. Although there is some variation in the cost and quality of services at different institutions, all patients are middle class, and roughly half are men and half women. Treatment is specifically designed for each person, and typically involves 10 to 20 days of inpatient care. Treatment always includes a dietary regimen of simple, minimally processed vegetarian food, enemas, hydrotherapy, massage, and a combination of mud and sun baths. Based exclusively on the use of so-called natural elements – earth, air, sunlight, water, and ether – treatment involves the use of technology in the form of tubs, tubes, showers, cloth wraps, steam closets, helio-therapeutic colored glass chambers, and special kinds of soil, among other things.

The institutionalization of Nature Cure reflects several interrelated features of cultural history (see Alter 2000, 2004). First, its popularity is linked to extreme disaffection with and antipathy toward biomedicine, as this attitude took shape as a well-articulated critique in Europe at the turn of the nineteenth century. Nature Cure in India is explicitly based on this critique, but also draws directly on philosophical, ideological, and technological innovations associated with the American health reform movement of the early twentieth century (Whorton 1982, 2002). Second, the popularity of Nature Cure is directly linked to Mohandas K. Gandhi's advocacy of a program of anticolonial agitation and embodied nonviolence based on diet reform, hydrotherapy, enemas, and mud baths, among other things (Alter 2000). Third, yoga was incorporated into the practice of Nature Cure early in the twentieth century, and since *asana* and *pranayama* were being subject to intensive study at this time – both clinical and purely experimental – a powerful discourse of scientific veracity developed to support arguments for a bio-ecological and bio-moral link between the body and two key yogic elements, air and ether (Alter 2004).

The institutionalization of Nature Cure in India throughout the twentieth century reflects a synthesis of diverse trajectories of cultural knowledge, German, English, American, and Indian (Sporn and Baer 2009). Although it is possible to find logical coherence in this synthesis, one is still left with a sense that in terms of cultural meaning Nature Cure is an ad hoc pastiche of influences. In relation to this it is no wonder that Gandhi – influenced by Henry Salt, Leo Tolstoy, Louis Kuhne, Adolf Just, and the Bhagavad Gita – was often referred to as a health faddist and an eccentric quack. At least part of the problem is that the cultural logic of Nature Cure is inherently idiosyncratic, arcane, quixotic, and exotic, thus undermining the nature of its political purpose.

Ecology and biosocial political activism come together in the experiences of individuals who experimented with Nature Cure and, subsequently, in the way in which health and disease were reconceptualized by these individuals in terms of a radical understanding of physiology and pathology. This reflected – and in turn generated – a discourse of public health, explicated below, that critically identified environmental problems in relation to patterns of risk and risk behavior in the context of the class distinctions and inequities that characterized modern urban life. Here Nature Cure's "invention" in the second half of the nineteenth century, and the history of its subsequent development, reveals a remarkably consistent, rational, and pragmatic approach to health.

Nature Cure is a distinctly modern innovation, albeit with roots in premodern Hippocratic humoralism, the monastic fetishization of mineral springs, and European bathing practices (Anderson and Tabb 2002; Bradley 2012). Four interrelated points will make this clear.

First, the invention of "the water cure" to treat all symptoms of distress is attributed to Vincent Pressnitz, an early nineteenth-century Silesian peasant who cured himself, began to treat others in his community, and became well known throughout Europe by mid-century. Pressnitz was inspired to experiment with the healing properties of water after watching a wounded deer wallow in a mountain stream. What Pressnitz did was to use cold water as a form of modern medicine for the treatment of diseases that were being conceptualized as modern ailments. He provided treatment for notables and the aristocracy of south central Europe as well the growing industrial middle class in the Danube valley (Claridge 1842). In conjunction with the fact that he was a successful healer, Pressnitz's fame grew because of how inexpensive print media attracted patients from all over the continent as well as from England and the United States. Beyond promotion as such, it is important to appreciate the extent to which the publication and distribution of print media produced a culture of popular health promotion based on middle-class anxiety and frustration (Porter 1992, 2001).

Second, although Pressnitz developed simple methods for the administration of treatment, other early innovators, such as Father Sabastian Kneipp, focused on the "technoscience" of hydrotherapy, developing precise ways to manipulate the temperature, force, and composition of water as steam, liquid, and solid. He designed tubs, built showers, and adapted watering cans for use in hydrotherapy (Kirchfeld and Boyle 1994). In the second half of the nineteenth century some advocates of Nature Cure prescribed bathing in streams, rivers, and lakes. But jumping into the frigid waters of the Danube and walking barefoot in the snow – as Kneipp was wont to do when first experimenting on himself – did not fit well with the scientific and technological ambitions and perquisites of modern Nature Cure as a commercialized "biocapitalist" enterprise. Building on this, an entrepreneur industrialist from Leipzig named Louis Kuhne turned Kneipp's biomechanical innovations into high-tech "industrial strength" forms of urban indoor treatment. Based on a materialist and pragmatic conception of physiology and pathology he devised a factory mode of "natural" health production (Singh 1980).

Third, Nature Cure in the nineteenth century was closely linked to broad epidemiological patterns in the prevalence of infectious diseases, as well as to revolutionary innovations in biomedical theory and practice. It also developed in response to the professionalization of medicine within the changing political structure of Europe. Thus, from its inception Nature Cure was defined by an explicit form of activism against the "toxicity" of modern life and the way in which biomedicine and doctors were implicated in the production of a toxic, unhealthy environment. Many doctors were, in turn, highly critical of hydrotherapy, fasting, mud baths, and heliotherapy. As biomedicine was increasingly shaped by scientific experimentation and regulation of various kinds, Nature Cure came to be regarded by physicians as anachronistic, irrational. Quackery pure and simple.

But acrimony, prejudice, and rank self-interest aside, activism by the likes of Pressnitz, Kneipp, and Adolf Just can better be understood with reference to the abominable state of public health in nineteenth-century Europe, including the portentous problem of iatrogenesis which persisted even after the discovery of germs and the implementation of sanitation protocols in hospitals. In conjunction with rapid social change, urbanization, and industrialization, dramatic disparities in wealth and exploitative labor practices also profoundly shaped public health at this time (Barrett and Armeligos 2013).

As the distinction between the country and the city took shape in both epidemics and endemic diseases, Nature Cure may be understood as a political ecology of health that provided an embodied response to the alienation, distress, and dystopia of class disparities and industrial-strength pollution, both inside and outside the body.

To some extent this response was out of synch with revolutionary developments in bacteriology that led to the control of diseases and lower death rates, but only to some extent (see Rosen 1993: 168–312; for an understanding of the persistence of miasmatic reasoning and the paradox of why germ theory "did not matter" in the context of sanitary reform, see Barrett and Armeligos 2013: 49–53). Advocates of Nature Cure at the *fin de siècle* were, to some extent, fighting an old battle that was clearly being won in a different way on a different front. From their perspective, however, this was simply symptomatic of a long-standing problem: using drugs to cure diseases without addressing more fundamental problems of health. To adapt and extend an old adage, if the battle seemed to have been lost, it simply meant that the struggle moved both more deeply into the body and more explicitly into the domain of professionalized medicine. From the standpoint of Nature Cure, powerful and potent drugs masked a more fundamental problem: the more effective commercialized drugs became, the more profound and insidious the disparity between "real" public health and the "illusion" of having solved a problem by eliminating diseases such as smallpox and yellow fever.

A fourth feature that distinguished Nature Cure was its conceptualization as a distinct system of medicine, allegedly based on rational procedures, rather than an ad hoc set of anachronistic, mystical, or folk remedies involving the four basic elements of earth, water, sunlight, and air. Fundamentally, it was organic and natural, but also new and innovative rather than "traditional." Practitioners justified the treatment they prescribed in terms of empirical observation, experimentation, and – above all – the proof of recorded cases and word-of-mouth recommendation. As such, Nature Cure took shape as an increasingly codified and systematized form of medicine grounded in a distinct theory of physiology, health, and disease. Thus it may be understood as a discrete tangent of medical history on a curving trajectory of development that is different from – but as logically consistent as – the one that is thought to connect Hippocrates and Galen to Pasteur and Koch via Vesalius, Leeuwenhoek, and Nicholas Andry in terms of microbiology. As can be seen in a seminal book published by Louis Kuhne (1893), Nature Cure was, in some respects, industrialized post-humoralism, with several important modifications that define its political structure in relation to physiology, public health, and ecology.

Louis Kuhne's *The New Science of Healing* (1893) is a fascinating book for many reasons. Among other things it seems to have hit a nerve in colonial India where translations became very popular (Venkat Rao 1979; Singh 1980). Besides providing instructions on how to use water, earth, sunlight, and air in self-treatment, Kuhne simplified and clearly expressed a basic theory of physiology and pathology. In some important respects his theory was also a philosophy of medicine and a politics of public health. Given the extent to which alternative medicine has come to be defined as complementary – that is, structurally "complementing" biomedicine – it is important to highlight the extent to which Kuhne, Gandhi, and other advocates of Nature Cure were reactionary radicals rather than passive proponents of alternative medicine. They were interested in revolutionary change not holistic, balanced New Age reconciliation.

The new science of healing is based on three interrelated principles:

1 As a natural organism, the body heals itself.
2 All diseases are caused by accumulated foreign matter that produces toxicity in the body. All diseases are symptoms of this basic bio-ecological problem.
3 Symptoms, however traumatic, are not discrete problems. They are signs that the body is healing itself. Consequently, distress, however uncomfortable, is a positive sign of recovery.

Natural elements are used to produce a pristine bio-ecology – and a kind of internalized return-to-nature environmentalism – that facilitates this process of natural healing. Drugs of any kind, even herbs, leaves, flowers, or the pure extract of plants, must never be used as medicine. By only treating the symptoms of specific diseases – including viral infections, tumors, and gangrene – pharmaceutical medicine undermines an organic healing process that is facilitated by a seamless interface between the ecology of the body and the elements of the natural environment. Diet is very important, but must be purely "natural." Food should be unprocessed, including nuts, fruits, vegetables, and sprouted grains. This reduces the buildup of toxicity. Fasting is integral to the whole process and is one of the most effective ways to purge toxins and purify the body.

As articulated by Kuhne, the new science of healing became a means by which to embody a political position against biomedicine. However, his theory also provided a broad understanding of how urban life and modern patterns of consumption were unhealthy in terms of nature and ecology, as this encompassed the more specific problem of epidemics, sepsis, and infection. In other words, and reflecting a common theme in populist health advocacy at the *fin de siècle* (see Whorton 1982, 2002; Cayleff 2010; Zweiniger-Bargielowska 2010), modern life made people sick, even if they did not understand the nature of the problem in relation to their symptoms. Or even that they were suffering from symptoms at all. The toxic nature of modernity changed the shape of their bodies, quite literally. It was on this basis that Kuhne developed his theory of "facial diagnosis," a protocol that extended well beyond the etiological significance of appearance – a kind of diagnostic eyes, ears, nose, and throat specialization – to an interpretation of how the insidious accumulation of foreign matter produced physiological deformities and anatomical anomalies all over the body. As microbiology began to diagnostically focus on the scientific evidence for pestilent organisms, invisible to the naked eye, Nature Cure emphasized a "macrobiology" of pollution, posture, and protuberances that seemed to be hiding in plain sight, right on the naked surface of the diseased and distorted body of everyman. Adolf Just gave clear expression to the larger bio-ecological project in his book *Return to Nature!* (1903), a strident manifesto that shows how Nature Cure fit with popular forms of late nineteenth-century German romanticism, most especially the rugged nudism of the *Wandervogel* movement.

Nature Cure in India

Adolf Just's and Louis Kuhne's books hit a nerve in modern India precisely because they were not metaphysical or spiritual. Although obviously cultural in the generic sense that everything is, the appeal of the books is in their presentation of hydrotherapy and mud baths as intrinsically and intuitively naturalistic and rational. *The New Science of Healing* appeared to transcend cultural distinctions by appealing to personal experience and the logic of elemental materialism. Based on the purported truth of natural laws, common sense is presented in Kuhne's argument as a critique of culture and cultural reason. Culture is taken to reflect a fundamental problem with the structure of modernity, especially the aspects of artificiality, superficiality, and the misplaced priorities of taste and distinction.

Kuhne locates these problems of abstract value precisely in the bowels of everyman. In light of this, the fact that Nature Cure probably does, in fact, reflect a key aspect of German culture is completely beside the point, given that enemas fit into the logic of detoxification and internal elemental purification quite literally, regardless of what they might signify about Teutonic fecal fetishism. The same is true for South Asia, where yoga and various articulations of Ayurveda involve purgation, emetics, and gastrointestinal hydration, but have nothing to do with procedures such as colon hydration within the rubric of modern, rational Nature Cure (see Alter 2015). *The New Science of Healing*'s appeal in *fin de siècle* South Asia seems to have had very little to do either with intracultural or cross-cultural continuity, beyond very broad and ultimately superficial similarities between the *arche* of elements in Greek medical theory – as vaguely reflected in the structure of Nature Cure – and the five *maha bhuta* elements of nature in *samkhya* philosophy. On this point my earlier analyses (Alter 1997, 2000) are, if not wrong, at least symmetrically superficial by virtue of focusing exclusively on culture and cultural constructions of meaning that produce an illusion of coherence.

Nature Cure is popular in India because people feel that it works. That much is obvious. But the work that it does is more broadly political, as reflected in stories of dramatic cure and recovery at the interface of colonialism, modernity, and disease ecology. Personal accounts of recovery and advocacy for Nature Cure based on these experiences become pointed critiques of public health at this particular point of interface.

Kuhne's theory was not only practical and functional; it was also presented as an argument that could be extended from the embodied experience of personal recovery to a bio-ecological critique of public health. And although Kuhne made this argument based on his experience in Germany, his argument fed into a more general sense of middle-class anxiety and alienation in many parts of the world. In India this "sense" of disequilibrium and disaffection with modernity was profoundly embodied, but Kuhne's theory provided a way to act on these concerns – especially the disjuncture of rural and urban lifestyles – in terms of middle-class consciousness independent of nationalism or the derivative cultural perquisites and formulations of colonialism. In a very important sense, it is necessary to recognize that Nature Cure innovators in India were acting in terms of their class status within a social history of global public health. Their interlocutors were German, French, British, American, Russian, and South African (Singh 1980). Mohandas Gandhi, K. Lakshmana Sharma, Vittaldas Modi, and others spoke as critics of public health in the context of global modernity even though academic disciplines born in the shadow lands of colonialism understand them to *simply* be nationalists or *just* advocates for things Indian – which ultimately comes to the same thing.

Without question epidemics produced a profound disease burden in the nineteenth century that has shaped the history of modern medicine in many ways. As in other areas of the world, the structure of this burden in colonial India was linked to urbanization, patterns of trade, and sanitation. Throughout the century tuberculosis, cholera, plague, and other infectious diseases produced patterns of risk that defined health in the public sphere – and, therefore public health policies – but also created a kind of broad collective consciousness about the nature of illness and disease in society at large, as well as within the inwardly concentric domains of region, community, neighborhood, family, and self. Clearly epidemics with high and sudden mortality rates – as in the case of cholera (see Barrett and Armeligos 2013) – dramatically reshaped this consciousness in specific locations, especially once their etiology was understood But relatively slow-moving epidemics such as tuberculosis produced what might be called a pervasive habitus of morbidity in large areas of Europe, Asia, and the Americas. While this fit into the entrenched logic of miasmic reasoning, it also supported the claims of Nature Cure advocates that persistent diseases like consumption were diagnostic of widespread bio-ecological toxicity, and that this established an environment for the growth and spread of epidemics.

More generally, however, it is useful to draw a broad correlation between developments in the burden of disease over specific periods of time, the history of epidemic cycles, and public health policies and development projects that institutionalize and reinforce social disparities based on class, gender, and race. In relation to these factors, in many parts of the world – but certainly in India – health consciousness changed dramatically over the course of three generations from approximately 1850 to 1925. In broad terms this included an increased sense of personal risk, a corresponding sense of individual responsibility for reducing that risk (by finding the right doctor and having the necessary money to spend), and a sense that one's own lifestyle as an older adult did not correspond to one's parents' habitus of health and one's own memories – positive or negative – of childhood within that habitus. Add to this a rapid rural-to-urban demographic shift and corresponding increases in urban class disparity, and what you have is a foundation for dramatic biosocial change.

Between 1896 and 1899 an epidemic of bubonic plague devastated many parts of India, especially Bombay, killing over 2 million people by 1903. Harsh measures by the colonial administration to impose sanitation protocols and quarantine caused widespread protests and riots (Pati and Harrison 2008; Kumar 2010). By the middle of the century cholera had spread from Bengal to many parts of the world with major outbreaks in formerly unaffected cities. Following a major, widespread epidemic in 1868 the colonial government identified pilgrimage, religious festivals, and the movement of troops as contributing to the spread of the disease, and imposed restrictions on each of these in different ways and with radically different sets of priorities. Following the construction of railway lines and large-scale irrigation systems throughout the subcontinent in the early part of the century, malarial fever came to be the leading cause of death, with areas of intensive development often becoming associated with high risk. Charles Bentley's 1911 report for the Malaria Investigation Committee showed that as much as 75 percent of all fevers in the city of Bombay were caused by malaria, resulting not just in high mortality but an economic loss equivalent to the value of more than 1.2 million rupees (Mushtaq 2009). Tuberculosis, a particularly insidious disease commonly associated with poverty, increased in prevalence in India throughout the nineteenth century, although never to the level of some European cities where it caused as much as 40 percent of all deaths among the working class. And then, of course there was the global influenza pandemic of 1918 which, in South Asia, caused the death of at least 17 million people or 5 percent of population. Unlike other epidemics, mortality was remarkably high among otherwise healthy young adults, because more senior individuals may have had a degree of immune protection from previous exposure to relatives of the implicated influenza virus.

Response to all of this – and especially to the sense of risk produced by the conjunction of an intensified disease burden, class-based social and economic anxiety and the pressure and alienation of a rapidly and constantly changing urban environment – was embodied in various ways. This does not mean that first-, second-, and third-generation individuals living at this time were necessarily aware of epidemiological and demographic factors in terms of statistical values. What they were aware of, and what is important, is the fact that premature death, disability, and disfigurement – Kuhne's protuberances – were increasingly and alarmingly common, and that symptoms of disease on this scale – fever, diarrhea, pustules, vomiting, and pneumonia – indexed modernity as a chronic condition, if not a disease unto itself. Literacy and media certainly played a major role in raising people's awareness of the scale and scope of the problem, although the intricacies and importance of this factor in the development of a new consciousness of public health can only be alluded to here (see Briggs 2011).

Without question Mohandas Gandhi (1869–1948) was the most well known public figure to advocate the exclusive use of Nature Cure to prevent and cure all diseases. As I have argued elsewhere (Alter 2000), Gandhi's visionary politics of public health encompassed his nationalism and defined his political position on all issues in terms of a kind of bio-moral materialism. It is wrong – analytically, philosophically, and historically – to try and disentangle Gandhi's position on the moral principles of political nonviolence from his struggle to embody the morality of vegetarianism. They are one and the same.

Gandhi's interest in Nature Cure came out of his experiences in England and South Africa. The experiments he conducted on himself, in terms of fasting, diet, hydrotherapy, and celibacy, continued to take shape through elaboration after he returned to India in 1915. And there is much to be learned about bio-ecology by way of Gandhi's writings (Gandhi 1967, 2000). But Gandhi was by no means alone, nor the first. Following the translation of Kuhne's *The New Science of Healing* into Telagu in 1894 and then into Hindi and Urdu in 1904, Nature Cure became increasingly popular, especially in Calcutta, Bombay, Madras, and smaller cities in Andhra. In 1928, Dr. S. J. Singh published a book called *Practical Naturopathy* – adopting the terminology of Benedict Lust, a German-American exponent of Kneipp's water-cure method and founder of naturopathy in the United States. Lust, whose own books also became integral to training programs in India, helped popularize and professionalize Nature Cure in the United States after being treated by Kneipp in Germany and then allegedly using hydrotherapy to cure himself of tuberculosis in the late 1890s. Between 1930 and 1960, Dr. S. J. Singh played a leading role in the professionalization of Nature Cure in India, especially as this process was manifested in the founding of the All Indian Nature Cure Federation in 1956 and the establishment of Bharatiya Prakritic Chikitsa Vidyapeet, a training college for Naturopaths in Calcutta in 1963. An Indian Nature Cure Practitioners Association was founded in 1973, followed, in 1978, by the formalization of government support through the Central Council for Research on Yoga and Naturopathy under the Ministry of Health and Family Welfare (Singh 1980).

Since Krishna Swaroop Shrotriya's translation of *The New Science of Healing* in 1904 and his construction of a sanatorium in Bijnor on the model of the much larger one built by Kuhne in Leipzig, Nature Cure facilities in India have changed very little over the course of the past century. What has changed dramatically is the nature of public health, which is now characterized by the very heavy burden of the diseases of advanced capitalist societies – atherosclerosis, diabetes, obesity, and COPD (chronic obstructive pulmonary disease) – much more so than infectious diseases, although malaria, dengue, tuberculosis, and HIV/AIDS are still significant problems. Regardless of whether treatment is for asthma, pneumonia, hypertension, malarial fever, or diabetes, Nature Cure treatment continues to define a political ecology of the body set against the impress of risk in the very structure of civilization. This is why it has not changed very much. The bio-ecological solution it provides for the culturally constructed disjuncture of body from environment is fundamentally the same, even though the "symptoms" of the disjuncture have become more insidiously chronic and less virulently contagious – or, in the case of India, the worst of both epidemiological worlds.

As evidenced through participant observation in six facilities in different parts of the country as well as a basic survey of infrastructure and administration at 20 clinics and hospitals, technologies, procedures, and protocols are standardized for Nature Cure by the Central Council for Research on Yoga and Naturopathy (www.ccryn.org). Treatment is always based on diagnostic assessment, most often with patients providing biomedical records, clinical test results, and a list of medications they are taking. They are always told to continue taking medications until advised not to. Based on diagnosis, using biomedical disease categories, patients are then prescribed a regimen of treatment that may last for anywhere from 6 or 7 to 30 days or more.

The ideal scenario is for a patient to adopt Nature Cure as a lifestyle and to continue treatment as a way of life in order to prevent disease and promote health. Thus a person who comes to a facility to be treated for chronic hypertension should become a person whose body is thereafter shaped by a regimen of water and mud baths, enemas, *pranayama* (breathing exercises) and *asana* (postures), and the consumption of raw, unprocessed foods.

Although there is significant variation in the regimens prescribed to patients with different kinds of problems – and variation in prescriptions between facilities – almost all regimens involve warm- and cold-water baths, steam baths, mud baths, enemas, and massage. In this sense, Nature Cure clinics are training centers where patients learn how to reconnect their bodies to the elements of the environment as constructed within the system's ideology. This is completely different in almost every way from the development of an ethos of mystical communion with nature based on the principles of outdoor adventure and ecological environmentalism. Trees to hug, animals to save, and biodiversity to promote for the greater good are simply not part of this picture, which is equal parts physiological, elemental, and technological in a late Victorian mode. To be sure, Nature Cure is viscerally affective, as I have argued elsewhere (Alter 2015). But the visceral point of connection is through the grounded materialism of elements that bring a physical sense of nature into contact with urban bodies.

Bringing the elements of nature into contact with the body is only part of the picture. What Nature Cure therapy does, most fundamentally, is purge the toxins of modern life. Fasting, enemas, and baths combine with raw food – fruits, vegetables, nuts, and some grains – to restore the body to what is thought to be its natural state or organic balance. Alcohol, tobacco, and caffeinated drinks are never consumed. Coincidentally – but very significantly in relation to lifestyle diseases – such a restricted diet reduces the intake of sodium, removes meat and most dairy products, and promotes weight loss. Whether this is, in any sense, a "natural" diet for our species is, needless to say, an open question, if a question at all, given that nature and diet are cultural constructs. But for most middle-class people it is a healthy alternative to what they eat most of the time, and certainly a radical alternative to what they most desire to eat and commonly consume. Many people who adopt a Nature Cure lifestyle adapt their diet to include adequate nutrition, but the emphasis is always on less rather than more, and on simple rather than complex and unprocessed food, rather than food that has been prepared for taste on the basis of refined recipes.

In many respects, this diet is designed to counteract the negative effects of a long history of food fetishization in civilization, beginning with the domestication of animals and crops, and the taste that our species has developed for sugar (see Mintz 1985) and refined and polished grains of relatively marginal nutritional value such as wheat, rice, and corn. But food and consumption is not simply taken to be symptomatic of civilization as such. The refinement of taste is directly correlated with distinctions of class status, as status is a function of wealth and patterns of consumption. Thus there is a close correlation between the impress of upward mobility and nutritional health as well as structural poverty and the manifold health problems associated with hunger and malnutrition. Diet reform, as most dramatically advocated by Mohandas K. Gandhi, seeks to provide a single answer to these apparently very different problems. A simple, natural diet serves to redistribute resources in society at large, purging the toxicity of excess in those who eat too much and restoring balance in the bodies of those whose poverty prohibits them from eating enough.

Conclusion: Biosocial Ecology

To the extent that Nature Cure generalizes the logic of Gandhian diet reform, it could be dismissed as paternalistic idealism. It is certainly utopian from the standpoint of public health. But to draw these conclusions is to understand Nature Cure as a cultural system of healing that has to work like medicine if it is to be considered useful. The deterministic question of efficacy – on the level of an individual or the sum total of individuals in a society – obscures a biosocial history of the political ecology of the body structured in relation to problems of environmental health, class distinction, and the hierarchical, organismic atomism of medicine. When practitioners insist that Nature Cure is "completely effective," they are making a much more radical, revolutionary, and ultimately defensible claim than those who insist that it "really works" for the treatment of a particular disease.

The case of Nature Cure in India is presented here as a particular example of how other forms of alternative and complementary medicine might be analyzed and understood in terms of distinct political ecologies of the body, as these political ecologies share common features, but also reflect the particularities of each case. Thus, an analytical examination of homeopathy might be structured around the problem of a political economy of scale and ecology as articulated in Heinemann's theory of dilution and the principle that like cures like. This would lead away from questions of efficacy and cultural history – and, perhaps more problematically, away from engaged agency and claims of legitimacy based on experience – to a consideration of how homeopathy articulates a broad and deep critique of ontological assumptions about health, physiology, and nature in the practice of biology, ecology, and other forms of medicine. One possibility would be to understand homeopathy in terms of a political ecology of the body structured in terms of a semiotics of scaled correspondence, compatibility, and similarity as against hierarchical domination structured by violence, destruction, and elimination.

Similarly, a political ecology of the body would be analytically useful in understanding the distinctions between osteopathy and chiropractic in relation to principles of functional anatomy, physiology, and pathology in the context of changing patterns of office work and workplace motility, Fordist factory regimentation, and corseting at the *fin de siècle*. In this context, both chiropractic and osteopathy articulate subtle differences in a populist sense of body/mind/spirit integration that locates the healing power of a "universal intelligence" in the body itself. The bio-ecological embodiment of innate intelligence serves as a vital antidote to the way in which work, lifestyle, and fashion manifest themselves in the maladjustment of the spine and its symptomatic articulations. In this context the strong anti-intellectual bent of both chiropractic and osteopathy can be understood in relation to a kind of moral materialism that links body, environment, and spirit. The fact that contemporary chiropractic and osteopathy have become more and more biomedicalized, professionalized, and "intellectualized" has overdetermined the problem of efficacy, on the one hand, and criticisms of pseudoscience and quackery, on the other, relative to historically contextualized critical political ecologies of embodied health.

In more general terms, the conclusion to be drawn from this argument is to not let the impress of cultural meaning and individual predilections of taste define the significance of alternative medicine, thereby exaggerating the importance of the problem of efficacy in relation to the sociological relevance of biology, ecology, and power to a history of the present (Mintz 1985).

REFERENCES

Alter, J.S. 1997. "A Therapy to Live By: Public Health, the Self, and Nationalism in the Practice of a North Indian Yoga Society." *Medical Anthropology*, 17: 309–335.

Alter, J.S. 2000. *Gandhi's Body: Sex, Diet, and the Politics of Nationalism*. Philadelphia: University of Pennsylvania Press.

Alter, J.S. 2004. *Yoga in Modern India: The Body between Science and Philosophy.* Princeton, NJ: Princeton University Press.
Alter, J.S. forthcoming. Gattungswesen: The Ecology Of Species Being: Alienation, Biosemiotics and Social Theory. Anthropos.
Alter, J.S. 2015. "Nature Cure and Ayurveda: Nationalism, Viscerality, and Bio-ecology in India." *Body and Society*, 21(1): 3–28.
Anderson, S.C. and Tabb, B.H. 2002. *Water, Leisure and Culture: European Historical Perspectives.* Oxford: Berg.
Baer, H.A. 1996. "Bringing Political Ecology into Critical Medical Anthropology: A Challenge to Biocultural Approaches." *Medical Anthropology*, 17: 129–141.
Baer, H.A. 1997. "The Misconstruction of Critical Medical Anthropology: A Response to a Cultural Constructivist Critique." *Social Science & Medicine*, 44: 1565–1573.
Baer, H.A. 2001. *Biomedicine and Alternative Healing Systems in America: Issues of Class, Race, Ethnicity, and Gender.* Madison: University of Wisconsin Press.
Baer, H.A. 2004. *Toward an Integrative Medicine: Merging Alternative Therapies with Biomedicine.* Walnut Creek, CA: AltaMira Press.
Baer, H.A. and Singer, M. 2009. *Global Warming and the Political Ecology of Health: Emerging Crises and Systemic Solutions.* Walnut Creek, CA: Left Coast Press.
Baer, H.A., Singer, M., and Susser, I. 2003. *Medical Anthropology and the World System.* Westport, CT: Praeger.
Barbieri, M. 2008. *Introduction to Biosemiotics: The New Biological Synthesis.* Dordrecht: Springer.
Barrett, R. and Armeligos, G. 2013. *An Unnatural History of Emerging Infections.* Oxford: Oxford University Press.
Barrett, R., Kuzawa, C., McDade, T., and Armelagos, G. 1998. "Emerging Infectious Diseases and the Third Epidemiological Transition." *Annual Review of Anthropology*, 27: 247–271.
Bateson, G. 1987. *Steps to an Ecology of Mind: Collected Essays in Anthropology, Psychiatry, Evolution, and Epistemology.* Northvale, NJ: Aronson.
Berg, M. and Cocks, G. 2002. *Medicine and Modernity: Public Health and Medical Care in the Nineteenth- and Twentieth-Century Germany.* Cambridge: Cambridge University Press.
Bradley, I.C. 2012. *Water: A Spiritual History.* London: Bloomsbury.
Briggs, C.L. 2011. "'All Cubans are doctors!' News coverage of health and bioexceptionalism in Cuba." *Social Science & Medicine*, 73: 1037–1044.
Cayleff, S. 2010. *Wash and Be Healed: The Water Cure Movement and Women's Health.* Philadelphia: Temple University Press.
Chakrabarty, D. 2009. *Provincializing Europe: Postcolonial Thought and Historical Difference.* Princeton, NJ: Princeton University Press.
Claridge, R.T. 1842. *Hydropathy; or, the cold water cure, as practised by Vincent Priessnitz, at Graefenberg, Silesia, Austria.* London: J. Madden.
Cohen, E. 2009. *A Body Worth Defending: Immunity, Biopolitics, and the Apotheosis of the Modern Body.* Durham, NC: Duke University Press.
Cordain, L., *et al.* 2005. "Origins and Evolution of the Western Diet: Health Implications for the 21st Century." *American Journal of Clinical Nutrition*, 81: 341–354.
Craig, S. 2012. *Healing Elements: Efficacy and the Social Ecology of Tibetan Medicine.* Berkeley: University of California Press.
Deepa, M., *et al.* 2011. "Non-communicable Diseases Risk Factor Surveillance: Experience and Challenge from India." *Indian Journal of Community Medicine Supplement*, 1: s50–56.
Dumit, J. 2012. *Drugs for Life: How Pharmaceutical Companies Define Our Health.* Durham, NC: Duke University Press.

Farmer, P. 2003. *Pathologies of Power: Health, Human Rights, and the New War on the Poor.* Berkeley: University of California Press.

Farmer, P. 2013. *Reimagining Global Health: An Introduction.* Berkeley: University of California Press.

Flesch, H. 2012. Comments on Baer and colleagues' "A Dialogue between Naturopathy and Critical Medical Anthropology: What Constitutes Holistic Health?" *Medical Anthropology Quarterly*, 26: 287–291.

Gandhi, M.K. 1967. *Key to Health.* Ahmadabad: Navajivan.

Gandhi, M.K. 2000. *Gandhi's Health Guide.* Freedom, CA: Crossing Press.

Ghosh, R. 2012. "Child Mortality in India: A Complex Situation." *World Journal of Pediatrics*, 8: 11–18.

Grell, O.P., Cunningham, A., and Roeck, B. 2005. *Health Care and Poor Relief in 18th and 19th Century Southern Europe.* Burlington, VA: Ashgate.

Gupta, S., *et al.* 2014. "Emerging Risk Factors for Cardiovascular Diseases: Indian Context." *Indian Journal of Endocrinology and Metabolism*, 17: 806–814.

Gwatkin, D.R., Guillot, M., and Heuveline, P. 1999. "The Burden of Disease among the Global Poor." *Lancet*, 354: 586–589.

Hoffmeyer, J. 2010. *A Legacy for Living Systems.* Dordrecht: Springer.

Janes, C.R. and Corbett, K.K. 2010. "Anthropology and Global Health." In B.J. Good, M.M.J. Fischer, S.S. Willen, and M.-J. DelVecchio Good (Eds.), *A Reader in Medical Anthropology: Theoretical Trajectories, Emergent Realities* (pp. 405–421). Chichester, UK: Wiley-Blackwell.

Just, A. [1903] 1898. *Return to Nature!: The Natural Method of Healing and Living and the True Salvation of the Soul. Paradise Regained.* New York: Lust Publications.

Kirchfeld, F. and Boyle, W. 1994. *Nature Doctors: Pioneers in Naturopathic Medicine.* East Palestine, OH: Buckeye Naturopathic Press.

Kuhne, L. [1893] 1891. *The new science of healing; or, the doctrine of the oneness of all diseases forming the basis of a uniform method of cure, without medicines and without operations. An instructor and adviser for the healthy and the sick.* New York: Lust Publications.

Kumar, D. 2010. "Probing History of Medicine and Public Health in India." *Indian Historical Review*, 37: 259–273.

Kumar, R., *et al.* 2012. "Epidemiological Transition in a Rural Community of Northern India: 18-Year Mortality Surveillance Using Verbal Autopsy." *Journal of Epidemiology and Community Health*, 66: 890–893.

Landecker, H. 2007. *Culturing Life: How Cells Became Technologies. Cambridge.* MA: Harvard University Press.

Latour, B. 2004. *Politics of Nature: How to Bring the Sciences into Democracy.* Cambridge, MA: Harvard University Press.

Latour, B. 2005. *Reassembling the Social: An Introduction to Actor-Network Theory.* Oxford: Oxford University Press.

Leatherman, T. 2005. "A Space of Vulnerability in Poverty and Health: Political-Ecology and Biocultural Analysis." *Ethos*, 33: 46–70.

Lindemann, M. 2010. *Medicine and Society in Early Modern Europe.* Cambridge: Cambridge University Press.

Little, P.C. 2013. "Vapor Intrusion: The Political Ecology of an Emerging Environmental Health Concern." *Human Organization*, 72: 121–131.

Lock, M.M., Young, A., and Cambrosio, A. 2000. *Living and Working with the New Medical Technologies: Intersections of Inquiry.* Cambridge: Cambridge University Press.

Manna, B., *et al.* 2013. "Determinants of Health Care Seeking for Diarrheal Illness in Young Children in Urban Slums of Kolkata, India." *American Journal of Tropical Medicine and Hygiene*, 89: 56–61.

McMichael, T. and R. Beaglehole, 2003. "The Global Context for Public Health." In R. Beaglehole (Ed.), *Global Public Health: A New Era* (pp. 1–23). Oxford: Oxford University Press.

Mintz, S.W. 1985. *Sweetness and Power: The Place of Sugar in Modern History.* New York: Viking.

Mushtaq, M.U. 2009. "Public Health in British India: A Brief Account of the History of Medical Services and Disease Prevention in Colonial India." *Indian Journal of Community Medicine*, 34: 6–14.

Navarro, V. 1978. "The Crisis of the Western System of Medicine in Contemporary Capitalism." *International Journal of Health Services*, 8: 179–211.

Nichter, M. 2008. *Global Health: Why Cultural Perceptions, Social Representations, and Biopolitics Matter.* Tucson: University of Arizona Press.

Nissen, N. and Manderson, L. 2013. "Researching Alternative and Complementary Therapies: Mapping the Field – Introduction." *Medical Anthropology*, 32: 1–7.

Pandey, R., *et al.* 2013. "Determinants of Urban Rural Differences in Cardiovascular Risk Factors in Middle-Aged Women in India: A Cross Sectional Study." *International Journal of Cardiology*, 163: 157–162.

Pati, B. and Harrison, M. 2008. *The Social History of Health and Medicine in Colonial India.* New York: Routledge.

Petryna, A. 2009. *When Experiments Travel: Clinical Trials and the Global Search for Human Subjects.* Princeton, NJ: Princeton University Press.

Petryna, A., Lakoff, A., and Kleinman, A. 2006. *Global Pharmaceuticals: Ethics, Markets, Practices.* Durham, NC: Duke University Press.

Pfeiffer, J. and Nichter, M. 2008. "What Can Critical Medical Anthropology Contribute to Global Health?" *Medical Anthropology Quarterly*, 22: 410–415.

Porter, R. 1992. *The Popularization of Medicine, 1650–1850.* New York: Routledge.

Porter, R. 2001. *Bodies Politic: Disease, Death, and Doctors in Britain, 1650–1900.* Ithaca, NY: Cornell University Press.

Ramraj, R., and Alpert, J.S. 2008. "Indian Poverty and Cardiovascular Disease." *American Journal of Cardiology*, 102: 102–106.

Rees, R. 2001. *Poverty and Public Health 1815–1948.* Oxford: Heinemann.

Rose, N. 2007. *The Politics of Life Itself: Biomedicine, Power, and Subjectivity in the 21st Century.* Princeton, NJ: Princeton University Press.

Rosen, G. 1993. *A History of Public Health.* Baltimore, MD: Johns Hopkins University Press.

Shah, B. and Mathur, P. 2010. "Surveillance of Cardiovascular Disease Risk Factors in India: The Need and Scope." *Indian Journal of Medical Research*, 132: 634–642.

Singer, M. 2008. *Drugs and Development: The Global Impact on Sustainable Growth and Human Rights.* Long Grove, IL: Waveland.

Singer, M. 2009. "Reproducing Inequities: Poverty and the Politics of Population in Haiti." *Global Public Health*, 4: 215–217.

Singer, M. and Baer, H.A. 1995. *Critical Medical Anthropology.* Amityville, NY: Baywood Publishing Company.

Singer, M. and Baer, H.A. 2009. *Killer Commodities: Public Health and the Corporate Production of Harm.* Walnut Creek, CA: AltaMira.

Singh, R., *et al.* 2013. "Body Composition Parameters as Correlates of Coronary Artery Disease." *Indian Journal of Medical Research*, 138: 1016–1019.

Singh, S. J. 1980. *History and Philosophy of Naturopathy.* Nature Cure Council of Medical Research.

Sporn, S. and Baer, H.A. 2009. *Naturopathy around the World: Variations and Political Dilemmas of an Eclectic Heterodox Medical System.* Hauppauge, NY: Nova Science Publishers.

Sunder Rajan, K. 2012. *Lively Capital: Biotechnologies, Ethics, and Governance in Global Markets.* Durham, NC: Duke University Press.

Tippens, K.M., Oberg, E., and Bradley, R. 2012. "A Dialogue between Naturopathy and Critical Medical Anthropology: Toward a Broadened Conception of Holistic Health." *Medical Anthropology Quarterly*, 26: 257–270.

Umamahesh, K., *et al.* 2014. "Incidence of Cardiovascular Diseases and Associated Risk Factors among Subjects with Type 2 Diabetes – An 11-Year Follow Up Study." *Indian Heart Journal*, 66: 5–10.

Venkat Rao, B. 1979. "Development of Naturopathy in Andhra Pradesh." *Bulletin of the Indian Institute of History of Medicine (Hyderabad)*, 9: 41–45.

Waddington, K. 2011. *An Introduction to the Social History of Medicine: Europe since 1500.* Basingstoke, UK: Palgrave Macmillan.

Waller, J. 2002. *The Discovery of the Germ: Twenty Years That Transformed the Way We Think about Disease.* New York: Columbia University Press.

WHO (World Health Organization). 2011. India, NCD country profiles, 2011. Washington, DC: WHO.

Whorton, J.C. 1982. *Crusaders for Fitness: The History of American Health Reformers.* Princeton, NJ: Princeton University Press.

Whorton, J.C. 2002. *Nature Cures: The History of Alternative Medicine in America.* Oxford: Oxford University Press.

Wujastyk, D. and Smith, F.M. 2008. *Modern and Global Ayurveda: Pluralism and Paradigms.* Albany, NY: SUNY Press.

Zweiniger-Bargielowska, I. 2010. *Managing the Body: Beauty, Health and Fitness in Britain, 1880–1939.* Oxford: Oxford University Press.

CHAPTER 7

Asthma and Air Pollution: Connecting the Dots

Helen Kopnina

Introduction

This chapter focuses on the relationship between asthma and car-induced increases of particulate matter in the air, on the one hand, and patient awareness of the link between air pollution and respiratory conditions, on the other. It begins with a discussion of the link between air pollution and asthma, subsequently turning to the phenomenon of "car culture" in general and in the Netherlands in particular as it relates to rising rates of air pollution and environmental health.

In the discussion section, I inquire why international health institutions and patient organizations have not put pressure on international environmental organizations, and national environmental ministries, let alone the actual polluters such as automobile industry. My discussion culminates in reflection on the massive corporate support for the ongoing use of motor vehicles, resulting in a situation in which patient organizations composed of pollution-related disease sufferers and their supporters are more focused on mitigation of the symptoms than addressing the ultimate causes of asthma.

In this chapter, I argue that to fully address the issue of respiratory health, international health organizations as well as national health ministries, patient organizations, and the general public must recognize the link between vehicular dependency, air pollution, and asthma. Consequently, I recommend explicitly linking vehicular dependency to the state of poor

A Companion to the Anthropology of Environmental Health, First Edition. Edited by Merrill Singer.

respiratory health, both in the specific case of the Netherlands and globally. More broadly, I argue that raising environmental health awareness among existing and potential asthma patients, by explicitly linking vehicular dependency to the state of poor respiratory health, may help in efforts to lobby the government to raise air quality standards and control polluting industries more effectively.

Asthma and Air Pollution

The respiratory system is a primary body nexus for diverse environmental threats to cluster, intermingle, and multiply their adverse impacts as well as a site for harmful disease interactions sparked by changing environmental conditions (Baer and Singer 2008; Singer 2013). Many conditions have been linked in some way to environmental pollution. Studies also have shown that food contaminants, indoor pollution, and climate change can all affect respiratory health (Astma Fonds; Asthma UK; WHO 2014).

Asthma is a chronic disease characterized by recurrent attacks of breathlessness and wheezing, which vary in severity and frequency from person to person (WHO 2014). The prevalence of asthma has changed in recent decades due to better diagnostic and treatment technologies, on the one hand, and environmental factors, such as pollution or changing lifestyles, on the other (Kopnina and Keune 2010; WHO 2014). There is a growing awareness in the areas of environmental health and in fields as diverse as medical anthropology and toxicology of the negative effects of air pollution on occurrence of asthma (American Lung Association; EPA; NRDC; Helman 2007). As the collected essays in this volume demonstrate, medical anthropology in particular has heightened awareness of the centrality of culture to human experience, and brought about recognition of the importance of social structure and an environmentally mediated political economy on health.

Two key air pollutants affect asthma: ozone, found in smog, and particle (or particulate matter) pollution. Studies show a direct relationship between the number of hospitalizations for asthma and increases of particulate matter in local air, including dust, soot, fly ash, diesel exhaust particles, smoke, and sulfate aerosols (e.g., NRDC; Morris, Sale, and Wakefield 2000; Salam, Islam, and Gilliland 2008; Balmes 2009; Tramuto *et al.* 2011). Increasingly, the Centers for Disease Control and Prevention (CDC) has linked asthma and both indoor and outdoor air pollution. According to the American Lung Association, car exhaust, smoke, and factory emissions make outdoor air dangerous, while tobacco smoke, presence of dust mites, and household chemicals and inadequate ventilation of stoves are just a few of the indoor hazards that can impact respiratory health.

There is now strong evidence associating the development of asthma with residence near roads that have heavy traffic and especially those used by diesel-fueled vehicles, which are the source of most particulate matter pollution (EHHI; Independent 2004; Krivoshto *et al.* 2008; Vidal 2013). An Italian study of urban air pollution and adult emergency room admissions for respiratory symptoms, for example, demonstrates that exposure to ambient levels of air pollution is an important determinant of emergency room (ER) visits for acute respiratory symptoms (Tramuto *et al.* 2011).

Increases in adult asthma are equally true of childhood asthma. Recent studies show a clear relationship between exposure to air pollutants and both the occurrence of the disease and exacerbation of childhood asthma (GINA; Zmirou *et al.* 2004; McConnell *et al.* 2006). There is also growing evidence of asthma symptoms in children who live near congested roadways (Van Vliet *et al.* 1997; Venn *et al.* 2001; Nicolai *et al.* 2003; Jerrett *et al.* 2008). The recent population-based matched case-control study of children by Li *et al.* (2011) examined the relationship between individual exposure to air pollution and severity of asthma symptoms. The study found that asthma events were associated with proximity to primary roads with asthma events becoming less likely the greater the distance between a person's residence and a primary road. Simultaneously, there are also serious health risks associated with the use of asthma medication, particularly the long-acting Beta-agonists in most prescribed non-alternative asthma corticosteroid inhaled medication (e.g., Nieto *et al.* 2007; Ducharme *et al.* 2010; Kopnina 2010; Jacobs, Jones, and Macginnitie 2012).

Environmental Health and Social Justice

The issue of environmental health is related to a larger discussion in the social sciences about environmental justice and studies that show that the poorest people tend to live in the most polluted environments. In the rural areas of the developing world, the poor often have been forced into marginal areas (Sahsuvaroglu *et al.* 2009). First, environmental justice seeks to redress inequitable distribution of environmental burdens to vulnerable groups and economically disadvantaged populations. Second, environmental justice highlights the unequal exposure to environmental risks and benefits in developed and developing countries. Third, temporal environmental justice refers to issues associated with intergenerational justice or concern for future generations of humans. In all three cases, environmental justice entails equitable distribution of burdens and benefits to different nations or social groups. By contrast, ecological justice involves biospheric egalitarianism or justice between species (Kopnina 2014a, 2014b).

Environmental racism, related to the three types of justice listed above, typically involves placement of economically disadvantaged or minority communities in proximity to environmentally degraded environments or, conversely, the placement of polluting industries or practices near disadvantaged communities (Melosi 1995; Singer and Hodge, this volume). Environmental racism includes any policy or practice that negatively affects the living environment of low-income or ethnically marginalized communities to a greater degree than affluent communities (Holifield 2001; Singer and Evans 2013).

Patient Organizations and Asthma

There is considerable literature on how emerging patient organizations attempt to address environmental health issues. In recent years, patient group platforms were established and new legal instruments came into place, including Patients' Rights laws and Charters of the Rights of Patients. Patients' rights groups have also been more active at the European Union (EU) level since the late 1980s. Seen as the extension of human rights generally, the rights of patients is an issue that has become recognized in Europe in the past two decades. The European Consultation on the Rights of Patients, held in Amsterdam in 1994 under the auspices of the World Health Organization's Regional Office for Europe (WHO-EURO), defined principles and strategies for promoting the rights of patients, within the context of the health care reform process in Europe.

However, few nongovernmental organizations or patient organizations, such as the American Lung Association, Asthma UK, and Astma Fonds, embrace an understanding that would enable them to put pressure on air-control, pollution-control, or environmental standards agencies, let alone the actual polluters, such as the fossil fuel and car industries. The social composition of these groups tends to consist of educated, mostly middle-class individuals, as these tend to be more aware of risks as well as more "empowered" to act than the less privileged classes. The pursuit of health has become a prominent lifestyle goal among sections of the upper middle classes but often this is framed in terms of individual decisions and actions.

While changes in air quality and the release of greenhouse gases are tied to practices like the massive corporate support for the ongoing use of motor vehicles (Baer 2009; Singer 2013; Baer, this volume), and increased prominence of "car culture" globally, patient organizations seem more focused on treating the symptoms rather than addressing the ultimate causes of disease. In cases where patients' organizations' interests may clash with industrialist groups, the governments of most neoliberal democracies do not seem prepared to ignore industrial lobbies in favor of population health.

A famous example of the clash between industrialist and patients' groups' interests involves asthma patients' organizations and the tobacco industry. This will be further discussed below in the section entitled "Connecting the Dots." More broadly, the state of public health efforts focused on traffic and asthma seems quite uncertain, to say the least. There are some studies of emic understandings of asthma and environmental risks but they tend to be largely inconclusive (e.g., Brown *et al.* 2002, 2003).

Car Culture and Environmental Health

Anthony Giddens opens his book, *Politics of Climate Change* (2009), with a question about sports utility vehicles (SUVs):

> Why does anyone, anyone at all, for even a single day longer, continue to drive an SUV? Their drivers have to be aware that they are contributing to a crisis of epic

> proportions concerning the world's climate? On the face of things, what could be more disturbing than the possibility that they are helping to undermine the very basis of human civilization?

Treating SUVs as a metaphor, Giddens goes on to provide a number of socio-economic, political, and psychological theories intended to account for the reasons that, despite environmental awareness, "we are all SUV drivers" (Giddens 2009: 2). Less apocalyptically, McShane (1994) and Holtz Kay (1997) express their concerns about widespread car use, linking it to a number of negative social and environmental effects. However, like Giddens, they do not discuss the effect of cars on environmental health.

Yet a number of health-related effects of cars have been discerned (see Baer, this volume). Aside from the links between and inhalation of harmful fumes and incidence of such diseases as asthma and cancer, there is an obvious toll claimed by traffic accidents (the statistics of which are truly frightening). Car driving also has been linked to health because of the lack of movement of the drivers (affecting their muscular and cardiovascular systems, and causing obesity). The very process of car production is polluting, causing immediate toxic pollution and far-reaching effects such as global warming. Threats to respiratory health being ushered in by global warming include ecosyndemics that entail harmful disease interactions sparked by changing environmental conditions (Singer 2013). Another consequence of having over a billion cars in the world is that an increasing area of land is covered by tarmac, allowing less of the green "filtering" that counteracts greenhouse gas buildup (Sperling and Gordon 2009; Kopnina and Keune 2010; Kopnina 2011).

What Drives This Car Dependency?

The automobile industry has long sought to highlight its products' appeal to people based on their desire for control, power, social status, and self-esteem. The idea of the car as a status symbol and the perception of driving as adventurous, thrilling, and pleasurable is now universal. These trends may be linked to the larger question of the apparent universality of a consumer culture appeal being driven by globalism. Kopnina (2013) has noted that despite differences in their religious, cultural, or social values or ideologies, Ukrainian, Zimbabwean, Brazilian, Japanese, Turkish, and Dutch citizens generally do not seem to be prepared to give up their personal possessions and comforts (such as cars) for the sake of (nonmaterialist) religious or ideological ideals. While "new urbanism," "smart growth," and eco-cities are gaining ground in contemporary discourse, hybrid and electric vehicles are increasing their market share, and "green" consumerism is becoming mainstream in many developed countries, none of this activity has made much difference, apart from fostering the illusion of progress (Rees 2009). In order to explain the cross-cultural love affair with cars more generally, we may ponder the widespread desire of human beings to distinguish their status and identity with the markers of material possessions through "conspicuous consumption" (Veblin 1902), and other features of human nature (Rees 2008; Kopnina 2013). However, conspicuous consumption has not always been universal, as illustrated by counter-examples like northwestern potlatch and pacific yam display. Rather, conspicuous consumption could be seen as a reflection of a need generated within a particular historic context and mode of production rather than a universal human trait.

More specifically, car dependency can be linked to various socioeconomic features of advanced industrial societies. These features involve the power hegemony of the industry that produces cars, and the drivers' addiction to cars, fueled by clever marketing strategies and governments' support of this industry. The American car-maker Henry Ford started buying tracks of railroads in order to build highways for cars, turning a car into one of the symbols of being American, progressive, and successful.

James J. Flink (1975: 40–41) accounts for the American car culture in relationship to the government's laissez faire policy in supporting the automobile industry and promoting cheaply produced products for mass consumption as playing on culturally constituted core values of individualism, autonomy, and freedom.

Aside from these affective factors, it is the speed, flexibility, and convenience of cars, and the affective benefits of driving, such as being independent, gaining a sense of personal identity and "enjoyment of driving," that account for the globalizing love of cars (Lefrançois 1998; Stradling, Meadows, and Beatty 1999; Sandqvist and Kriström 2001). Steg (2005) reflects on the research, examining various motives for car use on the basis of a model of the meaning of material possessions, feelings of sensation, power, superiority, and arousal. This is similar to general observations about the social functions of "conspicuous consumption." It is clear that people's psychological attachment to cars, and the automobile industry's calculated grip on the market, are not deterred by concerns about road safety, environmental sustainability, the impact of road kill on local species, and many other negative effects of cars. Despite the guilty feelings of a few individuals, cultural prioritizing of transportation and energy policies places "mobility" and "modernity" as priorities before one of the many "collateral damages" of cars (Desmond 2013).

Ecological modernization proponents and clever car manufacturers argue that electric or hybrid cars are much less harmful. At the same time, car manufacturers and automobile organizations introduce various schemes to encourage "ecological driving," alternative fuels, CO_2 taxation, car-related noise reduction, and so forth. However, opponents point to the "rebound effect" of such technologies, namely (a) an increase in the number of vehicles; (b) an increase in fuel consumption in response to increases in technical efficiency; and (c) an increase in vehicle miles traveled (Greening, Greene, and Difiglio 2000). According to Isenhour (2010), the increasing affordability of energy-efficient vehicles also drives demand for resource extraction for new car production, regardless of the functionality of existing automobiles or the absence of plans for their disposal.

Air Pollution and Transportation in the Netherlands

The Netherlands relies for 92 percent of its energy on fossil sources. Emissions and waste include carbon monoxide (CO), particulate matter (PM10, PM2.5), nitrates (NOx), sulfates (SOx), heavy metals (As, Cd, Cr-VI, Ni, Hg, Pb), volatile organic components (VOCs), and polycyclic aromatic carbohydrates (PACs).

It appears that the Netherlands is one of the most polluted countries in Western Europe, according to the Dutch environmental group Stichting Natuur en Milieu (Foundation Environment and Nature). The organization bases its claim on a survey commissioned by the European Commission (NRC 2008) A number of studies published in the leading medical journal *Lancet* show that poor air quality in the Netherlands correlates with incidences of respiratory illness and death (Brunekreef and Holgate 2002; Hoek *et al.* 2002). With more than seven million passenger vehicles on its roads, the Netherlands is the sixth largest automotive market in Europe (ACEA). Car density in the Netherlands in 2009 was 462 per 1000 inhabitants, up from 371 per 1000 in 1991 (Eurostat 2014). This is remarkable, because the Netherlands is a territorially small country with a highly developed public transportation system and is an alleged leader in ecological modernization (Kopnina 2014a, 2014b). Do not those bicycles used by many Amsterdam residents account for greener transportation trends? Unfortunately not, as owners of the Dutch bicycles own cars as well, and the presence of bike lanes in all major Dutch cities does not stop the continuous expansion of Dutch motorways.

Within the European Union, the Netherlands appears to be one of the worst countries for air pollution in terms of emissions from diesel cars. In October 2011, the government of the Netherlands launched its Sustainability Agenda designed to examine how key sectors can help the country attain green growth, with the goal of having 15,000– 20,000 electric cars on the roads by 2015 (OECD 2011). In an article titled "Dirty Dikes" in the *Economist*, the Netherlands is described as a "sink-hole of pollution" with its water "brimming with nitrates and phosphates, and the air is clogged with particulate matter":

> The Netherlands … scores particularly badly on the quality of its soil, where those phosphates and nitrates linger in large quantities. They seep into surface water, the quality of which is also below EU guidelines. Emissions of nitrogen monoxide and dioxide are triple the EU average. Carbon-dioxide emissions rose by 15% between 1990 and 2010. Only vast purchases of emission rights keep the Netherlands below its Kyoto targets. (Economist 2012)

Despite European Environmental Agency regulations, emissions in the Netherlands had decreased much less than anticipated by the EU standards defined in the past decade, and in fact the number of (nonelectric) car users has increased (Eurostat 2014). Moreover, recent studies of Dutch children's perception of cars indicate that future generations of Dutch citizens are not likely to start using public transport (Kopnina 2011; Kopnina and Williams 2012).

According to national research on Mobility in the Netherlands, Mobiliteitsonderzoek Nederland, there are 7348 million households in the country. Four out of five (79.1%) owns one or more cars. There are very few car-less families (4%), and four in five single-parent families own a car. According to Hans Jeekel (2011), 20 percent of the car-less persons in the country simply cannot afford a car.

Asthma in the Netherlands

According to the Dutch Ministry of Public Health, there are 519,800 (236,800 men and 283,000 women) registered asthma patients in the Netherlands, among whom 115,000 are children (Astma Fonds; RIVM 2014). In a Dutch cross-sectional study (Van Vliet *et al.* 1997) examining whether motor vehicle exhaust from freeways has an effect on the respiratory health of children, 1068 children attending schools situated less than 1000 meters from major freeways carrying between 80,000 and 150,000 vehicles per day in the Province of South Holland were asked to participate. Chronic respiratory symptoms reported in the questionnaire were analyzed using logistic regression. Distance from the freeway and traffic intensity was used as exposure variables. Coughing, wheezing, runny nose, and doctor-diagnosed asthma were significantly more often reported for children living within 1000 meters of the freeway. Those living closer to the freeway and to greater truck traffic exposure tended to be poorer, underprivileged, or members of minority groups. Environmental racism is also related to "transit racism," as minority communities in the United States, for example, have higher morbidity rates (among other factors, due to traffic) than white communities and, as a result, are more readily affected by debates over environmental factors and subsequent public health and government efforts. Considering the international studies presented above, it is not unreasonable to assume that the Dutch data are consistent with general patterns of vehicular-related negative effects on respiratory health.

Remarkably, however, environmental awareness of the adverse effects of personal vehicle pollution and health in Dutch society is very low (Kopnina 2011, 2014a, 2014b). What does this tell us about the potential for linking car dependency with awareness of negative effects of traffic pollution and other health effects associated with cars? To answer this question, I examine more general trends in the health and antitoxin awareness movement.

Health and Antitoxin Awareness Movement

Concerns about the occupational hazards in industrial society have intensified since the turn of the previous century, and a global antitoxics movement has emerged, closely linked to a consumers' movement that arose in the late 1960s. The publication of the book *The Silent Spring* by Rachel Carson in 1962 warned the public about the use of chemical pesticides and their influence on health and environment, and began a process of raising awareness of the dangers of environmental chemicals.

Awareness of environmental health risks was also triggered by the technology-caused disasters that have occurred since the turn of the twentieth century. One of the earlier examples of this occurred at the Love Canal chemical waste dump in Niagara Falls, New York, when the link between human illness and the dumping of chemicals in the water was discovered in the 1970s. Another example was the so-called toxic fog in London, UK, in 1952, which involved a combination of air pollution and extreme weather conditions; by some estimates this led to hundreds of lives being lost in less than a year, and thousands of cases of respiratory diseases (e.g., Bell, Davis, and Fletcher 2004).

Such disasters have caused heightened public awareness of environmental health risks and widespread public protests in Western countries. Zavestovsky (2010) traces the global antitoxics movement to 1971 when David Weir, who was working for the US Peace Corps in Afghanistan, noticed that a packet of Kool-Aid he had bought listed cyclamates among its ingredients. This sweetener had been recently been banned in the United States. This discovery led to Weir's investigation into the problem of US corporations dumping their banned products on overseas markets. Weir (1987) subsequently published a book focusing on the dumping of pesticides, illustrating how chemical companies were protecting profits by selling, or dumping, products that had been banned in their country of production in countries without such stringent regulatory infrastructure.

One of the worst accidents of the previous century, the Bhopal disaster in India in 1984, was caused by a gas leak from Union Carbide India Ltd. which killed at least 4000 local residents instantly and caused health problems in perhaps 500,000 others, people who still suffer from chronic disease consequential to gas exposure (Morehouse and Sarangi 2005). Following this, there was the Chernobyl accident, oil spills in the Gulf of Mexico, and, more recently, the Fukushima nuclear disaster.

What is worrying is not the sudden and intense occurrence of industrial disasters so much as the common everyday pollution, such as the particulate matter emitted by cars, or the massive amounts of plastic found in the oceans, seas, lakes, rivers, and city parks. According to Zavestovsky (2010), just as the consumer movement identified multinational corporations as the primary source of new risks related to the global spread of harmful consumer products, so too did the nascent global antitoxics movement come to see multinational corporations as the driving force behind new toxic risks. In fact, many environmental health threats are the result of the by-products of the manufacturing of consumer goods, or the processing of the raw materials to make those goods. Yet, focusing strictly on the risks related to the goods themselves, as the consumers' movement does, is insufficient. For example, through drift and absorption into groundwater, the chemicals used in agriculture and elsewhere are having a much broader impact. So too are the indirect consequences of car ownership, through the building of roads, parking lots, garages, and so on, which has caused a decline in natural areas, and a lowering of the quality of air.

Connecting the Dots

Social scientists need to continue to draw connections between particular environmental problems (e.g., global warming, toxic dumping, pollution) and human health problems, such as asthma (Baralt 2010; Kopnina and Keune 2010). Whitelegg (1993) provides a critical environmental analysis of European transportation, asserting that the conceptual basis of current transportation policy must be changed to ensure future sustainability. Congestion in cities, pollution, the health-damaging effects of traffic, privatization of transport infrastructure, and the social distribution of mobility are discussed in the context of European modernity. Through such contextual examination of European modernity, Whitelegg also gains insights into affective motives that perpetuate car culture. Thus, we need to look more closely at similar studies demonstrating that symbolic and affective motives are linked to cars and thus to psychological resistance to abandoning cars in favor of public transport use (Van Vugt, Meertens, and Van Lange 1995; Tertoolen, Van Kreveld, and Verstraten 1998; Abrahamse *et al.* 2009), as well as studies linking corporate pressure from the automobile industry on both consumers (through marketing) and government (through public lobbying and financial contributions) (Baer 2009). We need to ask the following questions: Are weak government policies targeted at reducing car use likely to affect drivers' choices? Given the relative balance of power of patients' and consumers' groups, on the one hand, and polluting industries, on the other, is government failure to protect the weaker party and allow the powerful industrial lobbies to have their way likely to continue?

Other actions, such as government support for polluting industries (e.g., in the United States the Obama administration's bailout of the auto industry), clearly indicate that political preference is strongly biased toward industry, rather than public health. Public attitudes toward policy measures for reducing private car use testify to complex and not always rational (in terms of price or effort reduction) but often social and effective considerations for car use (Loukopoulos *et al.* 2005). Such studies of car use suggest that policy makers should not exclusively focus on instrumental motives, but should also consider the many social and affective motives involved. Thus, on the one hand, if international health organizations such as WHO, as well as national health ministries, patient organizations, and general publics, were to recognize the direct link between vehicular dependency and asthma, the case for addressing car culture could be made stronger. Strategic policy efforts then should explicitly link the present pattern of mobility to public health. But also – and quite significantly – researchers could help the public to realize that governments may never do enough to address health issues in the status quo because they have vested interests in industries, including polluting industries, that have large financial and political leverage.

Due to rapid culture change, children are more likely to depart from the attitudes and habits of their parents, including with regard to transportation (Kopnina and Williams 2012). Thus, it may be of paramount importance to address existing – and changing – attitudes of children, who may yet find new ways for sustainable transportation. Research on parent–child transition of values may provide a clue to the formation of views of future transportation users. Because of the increasing tendency of parents to take children by car to various activities, children's attitudes might be partially influenced by the habits their parents develop for them (Lindén and Carlsson Kanyama 1999; Nillson and Küller 2000). Considering the proverbial wisdom and empirical reality that parents worry about their children's health, we may postulate that rising environmental health awareness in connection to cars among parents might have a greater effect not only on their own choice of transportation, but on that of the future generations. Thus, another strategic policy move would involve targeting both parents and children for increasing recognition of the negative effects of cars on children's health.

To sum up, a number of recommendations can be drawn. It appears that psychological attachment to cars and the automobile industry's calculated grip upon the market is not deterred by concerns about road safety, environmental sustainability, and many other negative effects of cars. Adult asthma patients and parents of children with asthma need to be made more aware of the direct connection between private transport use and the occurrence of asthma. It is also of paramount importance to address existing attitudes of children to transportation. Making this additional health concern more explicit will assist in making progress in consciously reducing car dependency.

In order to enable this change a number of stakeholders need to consider certain actions. Researchers need to inform the public about the connection between cars and respiratory health. Ideally, concerted efforts by the public could inform governments' strategic policy making, which could reinforce the positive loop of awareness and action. Strategic policy needs to target both parents and children in recognizing the negative health effects of cars, particularly in regard to transportation. The greatest challenge of this strategic policy will be to control the perpetrators, the powerful fossil fuel energy corporations and the car industry. Last but not least, it could help if we, the researchers, looked more often in the mirror to see how our own "mobility" and adaptation to modern comforts can contribute to making clear the linkages that will enable improvement in environmental health on a global scale.

REFERENCES

Abrahamse, W., Steg, L., Gifford, R., and Vlek, C. 2009. "Factors Influencing Car Use for Commuting and the Intention to Reduce It: A Question of Self-Interest or Morality?" *Transportation Research-F: Psychology and Behaviour*, 12(4): 317–324.

ACEA (European Automobile Manufacturers' Association). ACEA "Country Profiles." http://www.acea.be/index.php/country_profiles/detail/netherlands#text (accessed February 8, 2014).

American Lung Association. Making the Connection – Asthma and Air Quality. http://www.lung.org/about-us/media/top-stories/making-the-connection-asthma-and-air-quality.html (accessed December 1, 2015).

Astma Fonds. http://www.longforum.nl/ (accessed December 1, 2015).

Asthma UK. Air Pollutants. http://www.asthma.org.uk/knowledge-bank-pollutants.

Baer, H. 2009. "Environmental and Health Consequences of Motor Vehicles: A Case Study in Capitalist Technological Hegemony and Grassroots Responses to It." In M. Singer and H. Baer (Eds.), *Killer Commodities: Public Health and the Corporate Production of Harm* (pp. 95–118). Landham, MD: AltaMira.

Baer, H. and Singer, M. 2008. *Global Warming and the Political Ecology of Health: Emerging Crises and Systemic Solutions.* Walnut Creek, CA: Left Coast Press.

Balmes, J.R. 2009. "Can Traffic-Related Air Pollution Cause Asthma?" *Thorax*, 64: 646–647.

Baralt, L. 2010. "Biomedical and Environmental Health Perspectives: The Example of Confronting Breast Cancer." In H. Kopnina and H. Keune (Eds.), *Health and Environment: Social Science Perspectives.* New York: Nova Science Publishers.

Bell, M., Davis, D., and Fletcher, T. 2004. "A Retrospective Assessment of Mortality from the London Smog Episode of 1952: The Role of Influenza and Pollution." *Environmental Health Perspectives*, 112(1): 6–8.

Brown, P. Zavestoski, S. Luebke, T., Mandelbaum, J., McCormick, S., and Mayer, B. 2003. "The Health Politics of Asthma: Environmental Justice and Collective Illness Experience in the United States." *Social Science and Medicine*, 57: 453–464.

Brown, P., Zavestoski, S., Mayer, B., McCormick, S., and Webster, W. 2002. "Policy Issues in Environmental Health Disputes." *Annals of the American Academy of Political and Social Science*, 584: 175–202.

Brunekreef, B. and Holgate, S.T. 2002. "Air Pollution and Health." *The Lancet*, 360(9341): 1233–1242.

Carson, R. 1962. *The Silent Spring.* Boston, MA: Houghton Mifflin.

CDC Centers for Disease Control and Prevention. Air Pollution & Respiratory Health. http://www.cdc.gov/nceh/airpollution/.

Desmond, J. 2013. "Requiem for Roadkill: Death and Denial on America's Roads." In H. Kopnina and E. Shoreman-Ouimet (Eds.), *Environmental Anthropology: Future Trends* (pp. 46–58). New York: Routledge.

Ducharme, F.M., Ni Chroinin, M., Greenstone, I., and Lasserson, T.J. 2010. "Addition of Long-acting Beta2-Agonists to Inhaled Steroids versus Higher Dose Inhaled Steroids in Adults and Children with Persistent Asthma." *Cochrane Database Syst Rev.* 14(4): CD005533.

The Economist. 2012. "Pollution in the Netherlands: Dirty Dikes." http://www.economist.com/printedition/2012-02-04.

EPA (European Environmental Agency). 2010. "The Netherlands. Air Pollution." http://www.eea.europa.eu/soer/countries/nl/soertopic_view?topic=air%20pollution.

Eurostat. 2014. "Motorization Rate Cars per 1.000 Inhabitants." http://epp.eurostat.ec.europa.eu/statistics_explained/index.php/The_EU_in_the_world_-_transport.

EHHI (Environment and Human Health, Inc.). "The Harmful Effects of Vehicle Exhaust." http://www.ehhi.org/reports/exhaust/summary.shtml (accessed December 1, 2015).

EPA. 2012 US Environmental Protection Agency. "Heavy-Duty Highway Diesel Program." http://www.epa.gov/oms/highway-diesel/.

Flink, J.J. 1975. *The Car Culture.* Cambridge, MA: MIT Press.

Giddens, A. 2009. *Global Politics and Climate Change.* Oxford: Polity.

GINA (Global Initiative for Asthma). http://www.ginasthma.org/.

Greening, L.A., Greene, D.L., and Difiglio, C. 2000. "Energy Efficiency and Consumption – The Rebound Effect – A Survey." *Energy Policy*, 28(6/7): 389–401.

Helman, C.G. 2007. *Culture, Health and Illness.* London: Hodder Arnold.

Hoek, G., Brunekreef, B., Goldbohm, S., Fisher, P., and van den Brandt, P. 2002. "Association between Mortality and Indicators of Traffic-Related Air Pollution in the Netherlands: A Cohort Study." *The Lancet*, 360(9341): 1203–1209.

Holifield, R. 2001. "Defining Environmental Justice and Environmental Racism." *Urban Geography*, 22(1): 78–90.

Holtz Kay, J. 1997. *Asphalt Nation: How the Automobile Took Over America and How We Can Take It Back*. Los Angeles, CA: University of California Press.

Independent. 2004. "Focus: New link between Asthma and Diesel Fumes Shows the Campaign Must Go On." http://www.independent.co.uk/life-style/health-and-families/health-news/focus-new-link-between-asthma-and-diesel-fumes-shows-the-campaign-must-go-on-6171275.html.

Isenhour, C. 2010. "On Conflicted Swedish Consumers, the Effort to Stop Shopping and Neo-Liberal Environmental Governance." *Journal of Consumer Behavior*, 9: 454–469.

Jacobs, T.S, Jones, B.L, and Macginnitie, A.J. 2012. "Long-acting Beta-agonists and the Risk of Intensive Care Unit Admission in Children." *Journal of Asthma*, 49(5): 450–455.

Jeekel, H. 2011. "The Car-Dependent Society" (De autoafhankelijke samenleving) Eboron, The Netherlands. http://www.eburon.nl/de_autoafhankelijke_samenleving?language_code=nl.

Jerrett, M., Shankardass, K., Berhane, K., *et al.* 2008. "Traffic-related Air Pollution and Asthma Onset in Children: A Prospective Cohort Study with Individual Exposure Measurement." *Environmental Health Perspectives*, 116: 1433–1438.

Kopnina, H. 2010. "Contesting Asthma Medication: Patients' View of Alternatives." *Journal of Asthma*, 47(6): 687–694.

Kopnina, H. 2011. "Kids and Cars: Environmental Attitudes in Children." *Transport Policy*, 18: 573–578.

Kopnina, H. 2013. "The Grand Old Theory of Human Nature and Environmental Problems." *Journal of Ecological Anthropology*, 16(1): 61–68.

Kopnina, H. 2014a. "Christmas tale of (Un)Sustainability: Reflecting on Consumption and Environmental Awareness on the Streets of Amsterdam." *Sustainable Cities and Society*, 10: 65–71.

Kopnina, H. 2014b. "Environmental Justice and Biospheric Egalitarianism: Reflecting on a Normative-Philosophical View of Human–Nature Relationship." *Earth Perspectives*, 1: 8.

Kopnina, H. and Keune, H. (Eds.) 2010. *Health and Environment: Social Science Perspectives*. New York: Nova Science Publishers.

Kopnina, H. and Williams, M. 2012. "Car Attitudes in Children from Different Socio-Economic Backgrounds in the Netherlands." *Transport Policy*, 24: 118–125.

Krivoshto, I.N. Richards, J.R., Albertson, T.E., and Derlet, R.W. 2008. "The Toxicity of Diesel Exhaust: Implications for Primary Care." *Journal of the American Board of Family Medicine*, 21(1): 55–62.

Lefrançois, R. 1998. "Mobility Patterns and Attitudes Toward Driving a Car among the Elderly Living in Small Towns and Rural Areas." *Rural Society*, 1(1): 17–27.

Li, S., Batterman, S., Wasilevich, E., Elasaad, H., Wahl, R., and Mukherjee, B. 2011. "Asthma Exacerbation and Proximity of Residence to Major Roads: A Population-Based Matched Case-Control Study among the Paediatric Medicaid Population in Detroit, Michigan." *Environmental Health*, 10: 34.

Lindén, A.L. and Carlsson Kanyama, A. 1999. "Differences in Resource Consumption and Lifestyles – What Are the Implications for Sustainability?" *Ecological Economics Bulletin*.

Loukopoulos, P., Jakobsson, C., Gärling, T., Schneider, C.M., and Fujii, S. 2005. "Public Attitudes towards Policy Measures for Reducing Private Car Use: Evidence from a Study in Sweden." *Environmental Science and Policy*, 8(1): 57–66.

McConnell, R., Berhane, K., Yao, L., *et al.* 2006. "Traffic, Susceptibility, and Childhood Asthma." *Environmental Health Perspectives*, 114: 766–772.

McShane, C. 1994. *Down the Asphalt Path*. New York: Columbia University Press.

Melosi, M. 1995. "Equity, Eco-racism and Environmental History." *Environmental History Review*, 19(3): 1–16.

Morehouse, H.B.W. and Sarangi, S. (Eds.) 2005. *The Bhopal Reader. Remembering Twenty Years of the World's Worst Industrial Disaster*. Apex Press.

Morris, S.E., Sale, R.C., and Wakefield, J.C. 2000. "Hospital Admissions for Asthma and Chronic Obstructive Airways Disease in East London Hospitals and Proximity of Residence to Main Roads." *Journal of Epidemiology and Community Health*, 54: 7.

Nicolai, T., Carr, D., Weiland, S.K., *et al.* 2003. "Urban Traffic and Pollutant Exposure Related to Respiratory Outcomes and Atopy in a Large Sample of Children." *European Respiratory Journal*, 21: 956–963.

Nieto, A., Mazon, A., Pamies R., Linana, J.J., Lanuza, A., Jiménez, F.O., Medina-Hernandez, Nieto, F.J. 2007. "Adverse Effects of Inhaled Corticosteroids in Funded and Nonfunded Studies." *Archives of Internal Medicine*, 167(19): 2047–2053.

Nillson, M. and Küller, R. 2000. "Travel Behavior and Environmental Concern." *Transportation Research Part D: Transport and Environment*, 5(3): 211–234.

NRC. 2008. *Dutch Air Pollution among Worst in Europe*. http://vorige.nrc.nl/international/article2069254.ece/Dutch_air_pollution_among_worst_in_Europe.

NRDC (Natural Resources Defense Council). "Asthma and Air Pollution." http://www.nrdc.org/health/effects/fasthma.asp.

OECD 2011. *Green Growth in Action: The Netherlands*. http://www.oecd.org/greengrowth/greengrowthinactionthenetherlands.htm.

Rees, W. 2008. "Human Nature, Eco-footprints and Environmental Injustice." *Local Environment*, 13(8): 685–701.

Rees, W. 2009. "The Ecological Crisis and Self-Delusion: Implications for the Building Sector." *Building Research and Information*, 37(3): 300–311.

RIVM. 2014. Nationaal Kompas Volksgezondheid, Dutch Ministry of Public Health http://www.nationaalkompas.nl/gezondheid-en-ziekte/ziekten-en-aandoeningen/ademhalingswegen/astma/astma-samengevat/.

Roberts, K. 1999. *Leisure in Contemporary Society*. New York: CABI Publishing.

Sahsuvaroglu, T., Jerrett, M., Sears, M., *et al.* 2009. "Spatial Analysis of Air Pollution and Childhood Asthma in Hamilton: Canada: Comparing Exposure Methods in Sensitive Subgroups." *Environmental Health*, 8(14): 1–13.

Salam, M.T, Islam, T., and Gilliland, F.D. 2008. "Recent Evidence for Adverse Effects of Residential Proximity to Traffic Sources on Asthma." *Current Opinion in Pulmonary Medicine*, 14(1): 3–8.

Sandqvist, K. and Kriström, S. 2001. "Getting along Without a Family Car. The Role of Automobiles in Adolescents' Experience and Attitudes. Part I." *Inner City Stockholm*. Institutionen för Individ, Omvärld och Lärande, Stockholm, Sweden.

Singer, M. 2013. "Respiratory Health and Ecosyndemics in the Time of Global Warming." *Health Sociology Review*, 22(1): 98–111.

Singer, M. and Evans, J.M. 2013. "Water Wary: Understandings and Concerns about Water and Health among the Rural Poor of Louisiana." In H. Kopnina and E. Shoreman-Ouimet (Eds.), *Environmental Anthropology: Future Trends* (pp. 172–187). New York: Routledge.

Sperling, D. and Gordon, D. 2009. *Two Billion Cars: Driving Toward Sustainability*. New York: Oxford University Press.

Steg, L. 2005. "Car Use: Lustand Must. Instrumental, Symbolic and Affective Motives for Car Use." *Transportation Research Part A: Policy and Practice*, 39(2–3): 147–162.

Stradling, S.G., Meadows, M.L., and Beatty, S. 1999. *Factors Affecting Car Use Choices*. Transport Research Institute, Napier University, Edinburgh, UK.

Tertoolen, G., Van Kreveld, D., and Verstraten, B. 1998. "Psychological Resistance against Attempts to Reduce Private Car Use." *Transportation Research A*, 32: 171–181.

Tramuto, F., Cusimano, R., Cerame, G., Vultaggio, M., Calamusa, G., Carmelo, M.M., and Vitale, F. 2011. "Urban Air Pollution and Emergency Room Admissions for Respiratory Symptoms: A Case-Crossover Study in Palermo, Italy." *Environmental Health*, 10: 34.

Van Vliet, P., Knape, M., de Hartog, J., *et al.* 1997. "Motor Vehicle Exhaust and Chronic Respiratory Symptoms in Children Living Near Freeways." *Environmental Research*, 74: 122–132.

Van Vugt, M., Meertens, R.M., and Van Lange, P.A.M. 1995. "Car versus Public Transportation? The Role of Social Value Orientations in a Real-Life Social Dilemma." *Journal of Applied Social Psychology*, 25: 258–278.

Veblin, T. 1902. *The Theory of the Leisure Class: An Economic Study of Institution.* New York: Macmillan.

Venn, A.J, Lewis, S.A., Cooper, M., *et al.* 2001. "Living near a Main Road and the Risk of Wheezing Illness in Children." *American Journal of Respiratory Critical Care Medicine*, 164: 2177–2180.

Vidal, J. 2013. "Diesel Fumes More Damaging to Health than Petrol Engines." *Guardian*, January 27. http://www.theguardian.com/uk/2013/jan/27/diesel-engine-fumes-worse-petrol.

Weir, D. 1987. *The Bhopal Syndrome: Pesticides, Environment and Health.* San Francisco, CA: Sierra Club Books.

Whitelegg, J. 1993. *Transport for a Sustainable Future: The Case for Europe.* London: Belhaven Press.

WHO (World Health Organization). 2014. Asthma.

Zavestoski, S. 2010. "Environmental Health Organizing in a Globalizing World: The Emergence of a Global Anti-Toxics Movement and its Political, Legal and Economic Challenges." In H. Kopnina and H. Keune (Eds.), *Health and Environment: Social Science perspectives.* New York: Nova Science Publishers.

Zmirou, D., Gauvin, S., Pin, I., *et al.* 2004. "Traffic Related Air Pollution and Incidence of Childhood Asthma: Results of the Vesta Case-Control Study." *Journal of the Epidemiological Community Health*, 58: 18–23.

CHAPTER 8

Washing Away Ebola: Environmental Stress, Rumor, and Ethnomedical Response in a Deadly Epidemic

Ivo Ngade, Merrill Singer, Olivia Marcus, and José E. Hasemann Lara

Introduction

Emerging infectious diseases are a critical issue in contemporary global environmental health. Ebola outbreaks, which have occurred over the last 40 years, signal the growing threat to human health of infectious zoonotic diseases that originate in animals and have the ability to cross over into human populations. Notably, the 2014/15 Ebola epidemic in West Africa become the largest, most widespread outbreak of this viral disease to date. Among its various impacts, the epidemic triggered a proliferation of rumors about possible emergent ethnomedical cultural responses. Rumor, an enduring feature of human social environments, can be a significant force in cultural change in times of social upheaval. Spreading across the complex topography of face-to-face and electronic social networks, rumor can quickly cause panic in a society, especially

A Companion to the Anthropology of Environmental Health, First Edition. Edited by Merrill Singer.

during disasters, wars, epidemics, and other environmental disruptions (Noji 2005; Nekovee *et al.* 2007).

The power of rumors lies in their ability to "attract attention, evoke emotion, incite involvement, [and] affect attitudes and actions" (DiFonzo and Bordia 2007: 12). The 2011 Fukushima-Daiichi nuclear disaster in Japan, for example, triggered a rumor-driven salt-buying frenzy in China, impacting both social behavior and the price of this commodity (Zhao and Wang 2013). In the context of the HIV/AIDS epidemic, two harmful rumors—that the virus was developed in a laboratory in a Western country and that a public health team inoculated tens of thousands of Africans with an untested vaccine that caused the pandemic—became widespread in Africa and beyond (Laccino 2014). As these examples suggest, rumor is a factor in environmental health, a feature of how societies monitor and respond to changing environmental conditions.

Specifically, both of these examples demonstrate that rumors emerge when a social group is struggling to make sense of ambiguous, uncertain, or confusing situations, especially environmental contexts that are perceived as both threatening and immediate. Research suggests that people have a core psychosocial need to understand the world around them and to act effectively in it; therefore ambiguity in a threatening situation is often highly discomforting (Fiske 2004). Prevailing cultural constructions normally satisfy this need by providing symbolic webs of meaning and significance that help reinforce confidence in prevailing worldviews during times of change (Geertz 1973). Culture "impose[s] system on an inherently untidy experience" (Douglas 1966: 4). When events cannot be meaningfully understood in terms of existing cultural frameworks, however, novel ideas emerge and are shared among peers, may be changed and adapted through processes of group communication, and sometimes are adopted as a basis for subsequent action in the world. This process, which Williams (2009: 137) labeled "emergent culture," is a pathway along which "new meanings and values, new practices, new relationships and kinds of relationships are continually being created." Shibutani (1966) has proposed that when formal information is weak or absent—as certainly has been the case during the 2014/15 Ebola outbreak in West Africa—people compensate by informally interpreting what is going on around them, giving rise to snowballing rumors. Rumors, in short, can serve as a mechanism of group sense making when existing cultural models of environmental reality no longer seem to make sense to people (Rosnow 1988). Yet this is not a well-understood aspect of environmental health. As Mitman, Murphy, and Sellers (2004: 12) observe, "[m]uch history of environment and health is about what we don't, or don't quite, know," and the role of rumor in human–environment relations is certainly a part of what we need to know much better if we are to respond effectively in times of health crises (Grein *et al.* 2000).

Based on qualitative interviews conducted in two cities in Cameroon, we examine the rise and spread of Ebola rumors, most notably popular ideas about the protective value of bathing in and/or drinking salt water. These rumors are significant for various reasons, but most notably because of the new health risks they introduced in the midst of the Ebola epidemic. Our concern in this chapter is with examining the special contribution anthropology can make to assessing and effectively responding to adverse rumors that magnify environmental health risks during epidemics. With the continual emergence of new infectious diseases in disrupted environments – such as anthropogenic deforestation and the rise of Ebola as a human disease – the stakes have increased and the specific ways communities respond to emergent environmental threats are now critical to understand.

Ebola and Rumor in Cameroon

The recent Ebola epidemic in West Africa highlights the ways that rumors, by influencing how decisions are made in an emergency-disrupted environment, can have lasting effects in society (Zhang and Zhang 2009). Allport and Postman (1947: ix) define rumor as "a specific proposition for belief, passed along from person to person, usually by word of mouth, without secure standards of evidence being present." In the contemporary world of instantaneous communication, this definition must be broadened to include electronic venues of interconnection, including text messages, e-mail, and mobile phone calls. Various theories of rumor have been developed by social psychologists, folklorists, communications researchers, and anthropologists. Generally, this body of work views rumor as a form of individual and collective information seeking when gaps and uncertainty of important information exist in formal channels of communication, such as public health recommendations during an epidemic (Rosnow and Fine 1976). This gap may be the result of incomplete authoritative information or be a product of popular mistrust of official sources of information. Thus, it is necessary to pay close attention to "the special role of confusion and uncertainty" in the generation and spread of rumor (Stewart and Strathern 2004: xii).

It has been observed that this experience of ambiguity and uncertainty emerges when deviation occurs from a supposedly steady state (Ferreira, Boholm, and Lofstedt 2001). Mary Douglas (1966: 40) recognized that "any given culture must confront events which seem to defy its assumptions." Frequent in experience in the modern world, argue Ferreira and coworkers (2001), are imagistic transgressions of familiar contexts, such as the terrifying print and electronic media images of dead and dying Ebola victims and of unearthly-looking public health workers shrouded head to foot in personal protective garments. These kinds of depictions, to paraphrase Douglas's (1966: 36) definition of dirt (i.e., "matter out of place"), can be thought of as "images out of place" from a cultural perspective. Research on how people remember events indicates that (a) understanding is enhanced when news stories are visually engaging; and (b) highly visual and dramatic events tend to promote high recall levels, although people often exaggerate the content of such events (Bell 1991; Flynn *et al* 2001). Moreover, Zinn (2008: 191) has stressed that "[t]he violation of cultural boundaries [created by disruptive images] ... can ... contribute to the establishment of new meaning."

In this process of disruption and meaning construction rumor may be especially critical. As anthropological studies of rumor have emphasized, rumor is noteworthy because it is comprised of texts that have a wide circulation and serves to embed meanings that go beyond the interests of any one small group (meanings for smaller in-groups being referred to as gossip) (Lienhardt 1975; Kapferer 1990; Stewart and Strathern 2004; Paz 2008). Rumors not only reflect issues of broad heightened concern, they travel widely and often quickly.

Rumor is critical as well because, quite literally, it can be deadly (Feldman-Savelsberg, Ndonko, and Schmidt-Ehry 2000; Stewart and Strathern 2004). This power, in part, rests in the fact that "rumours can spread astoundingly fast through social networks" and impact the understandings and behaviors of many people who have an emotional connection with the content of a rumor (Nkpa 1975; Kostka, Oswald, and Wattenhofer 2008). This was apparent at a certain moment in the Ebola epidemic when rumors about the prophylactic value of saltwater bathing and drinking went viral in Cameroon in social media venues as well as on the street, and in other social spaces (e.g., church and community functions). Although it is not precisely clear how this rumor spread to Cameroon—a country that has not recorded a single case of this viral disease—it appears likely that it emerged when the Ebola outbreak was reported in Nigeria. Shortly after reports surfaced of the first cases in Nigeria, a country with a porous border with Cameroon, rumors swiftly spread that the virus had been detected at the government hospital in Douala, Cameroon (Kindzeka 2014). Moreover, just as the idea that salt bathing and/or drinking as an Ebola preventive was being disseminated in Cameroon, the Nigerian government began trying to dissuade its own citizens from engaging in these same behaviors being promoted by popular messages. This Nigerian government response was provoked by reports of the deaths of 20 people who excessively drank (and bathed in) salt water in Abuja, Nigeria. Ultimately it appears that two people, both being sufferers from high blood pressure, did die of drinking excessive amounts of salt water and at least 20 more were hospitalized (Neporent 2014).

Rumor in a Time of Social Media and Mobile Communication

Symplur, a company that tracks health information trends based on Twitter posts, reported that Nigerians first began sending tweets using the words "Ebola," "salt water," and "drinking" on August 4, 2014. Four days later, social network traffic concerning these issues reached a daily peak of approximately 450 tweets (Neporent 2014). In Cameroon, the hope that salt water would shield people from the deadly Ebola virus also soon gained popular credence as people began receiving text messages from friends and relatives and otherwise hearing about this simple, inexpensive strategy to spare them from a disease that seemed at the time to be sweeping through all of West Africa.

It is clear that the adoption of mobile phones into local lives among Cameroonians facilitated the rapid and wide circulation of various alleged preventive approaches. Our data indicate that Internet forums also have been an important source of information, evinced by participants' reports of searching the Internet for Ebola remedies. Beyond the use of salt water, other scientifically unsubstantiated, yet readily available, remedies were rumored to be effective, including eating several large onions, drinking a mixture of coffee and cocoa powder, using Vaseline, eating bitter kola nut, and avoiding the consumption of bushmeat (Basu 2014). While these other popular preventive strategies probably did not introduce new health risks, the drinking of large quantities of salt water appears to have had severe negative effects in some cases, which signals the importance of better understanding the emergence and spread of rumors about protective behaviors that people, lacking other options and struggling with uncertainty, quickly adopt in the midst of a frightening epidemic.

Ethnomedical Responses to Stress and Danger

Anthropology, given its methodological focus on ethnographic engagement with the on-the-ground processes and relationships of everyday life, may be particularly suited for discovering and decoding rumor and other forms of popular communication (Pietilä 2007; Besnier 2009). It has been noted that anthropologists steeped in daily affairs can systematically observe, report on, interpret, and explain local perspectives on the Ebola epidemic response in community settings (Hewlett and Hewlett 2008). Understanding such responses and interpreting them within a particular social or cultural framework is one way anthropologists can differentiate emerging health risks from the encompassing social "noise" generated by an Ebola outbreak (Abramowitz 2014). Because of their methodological toolkit and participation as socially embedded researchers, anthropologists are well equipped to discriminate rumor from tradition and to help guide health and public health professionals toward greater efficacy in improving the environmental health of communities.

The term "ethnomedicine" has been used in anthropology to describe the cultural subsystem that responds to health threats and troubling health conditions (Erickson 2008). Ethnomedical systems – local, regional, and national approaches for understanding disease and mobilizing meaningful action – can be viewed as "sociocultural adaptive strategies" that promote well-being and respond to health threats by drawing broadly on people's symbolic webs of meaning as they have been formed by exposure to traditional, emergent, and biomedical approaches to healing (Foster and Anderson 1978: 33). Reflecting this kind of openness to new situations, the salt water preventive emerged in West Africa within prevailing frameworks of regional ethnomedical beliefs and practice that, while not protective from the actual virus, did offer psychosocial relief from the pressing and burdensome fear of deadly contagion. The salt water rumor, in other words, presented a reassuring idea about a way to ward off an anticipated environmental danger, and, in so doing, helped people to cope with their fears of the epidemic.

From a health perspective, fear itself is dangerous. As Ropeik (2004: S56) stresses,

> some of the decisions we make when we are fearful … and because of the ways our bodies react to chronically elevated levels of stress, the hazards of [fear] … may be more significant than any of the individual risks about which we fret … A … comprehensive risk analysis approach must recognize that … fears pose an actual danger that needs to be understood, accounted for … and reduced every bit as much as the threat from any physical hazard.

An enduring sense of looming danger is known to produce identifiable psychosocial reactions, including disruption of appetite, lifestyle routines, social relationships, sleep, and job performance. Chronic worry and emotional stress also can produce a host of physical reactions triggered by the release of stress hormones like cortisol. These hormones can elevate blood sugar and triglycerides, substances that the body uses for fuel. But the continued release of these hormones under conditions of prolonged stress can also cause physical reactions like difficulty swallowing, dizziness, fast heartbeat, fatigue, headaches, irritability, muscle aches, and nausea. These symptoms, if persistent, not only lead people to feel "stressed out," but produce "wear and tear" on the body and exacerbate pathophysiology (McEwen 1998a, 1998b; Dressler 2011). In such situations, people often seek relief, sometimes through the adoption of harmful but short-term, stress-reducing behaviors like overeating, smoking, and the use of alcohol and other drugs (Singer 2006; Krieger 2011). Other behavior changes may also occur as people seek to lower their physical and emotional sense of distress, including, in the case under discussion, the adoption of various alleged preventive behaviors like salt water bathing and/or drinking in a time of Ebola.

Why salt? Salt, a vital environmental resource, has long been seen as having healing power for a range of health problems, and therefore is an ingredient used in many ethnomedical treatments in West Africa. However, more broadly, one can observe the use of salt in health remedies the world over: for example, gargling warm salt water is often used to soothe a sore throat (Cirillo *et al.* 1994). Research in Port Harcourt, Nigeria has shown that salt is used to prepare leaves from a shrub of the asertacease family (*Vernonia amygdalina*) into a juice that is consumed three times a day for stomach ache (Nwauzoma and Dappa 2013). Similarly, in their survey of ethnobotanical and ethnomedical practice in Oyo State, Nigeria, Borokini and colleagues (Borotini *et al.* 2013) report the use of salt in several healing preparations employed to treat various illness conditions. Use of salt in ethnomedical treatment also has been described in both the Nkongsamba Region (south region) and in the Lebialem highlands (southwest region) of Cameroon (Noumi 2009, Focho, Ndam and Fonge 2009). Shortly after the Ebola outbreak began in 2014, the titular head of the Igala Kingdom (also called the Kingdom of Idah) in north-central Nigeria, Idakwo Michael Ameh Oboni, specifically prescribed salt water bathing as an ethnomedical vaccine against Ebola (Ogala, Ibeh, and Audu 2015). According to local reports, the Igala monarch claimed that to bathe in a solution comprised of a pinch of salt in 15 liters of water would be sufficient to prevent infection. The prescription, which originally was intended only for people of the Igala Kingdom, was quickly disseminated to friends and family via word of mouth, social media, and the Internet, and soon reached people far beyond the kingdom.

Many people who heard about the bath were eager to take any action possible that might prevent Ebola, and soon began exchanging telephone calls and text messages with members of their social network, advising them to use saltwater solution. In addition, news about this strategy began circulating in web-based forums, such as the popular Nigerian message board, Nairaland, and among news sources as well. Reports of a salt-buying frenzy in Maiduguri (in the north of Nigeria) began surfacing after locals from this community received text messages about the salt bath and/or drink remedy (Ogala *et al.* 2015). This ethnomedical prophylaxis was further reinforced when Ejike Mbaka, a popular and politically outspoken Catholic priest in Enugu, Nigeria, was rumored to have suggested that his parishioners drink salt water (Ogala *et al.* 2015). In fact, he publically condemned this practice in a sermon delivered in his church in August of 2014 (Nairaland Forum 2014).

Based on Buckner's (1965) analysis of the theory of rumor transmission, which explains that rumor often is spread by people who cannot accurately assess the veracity of a statement or situation, it is likely that in both Nigeria and Cameroon people who received and texted messages about the salt bath/drinking treatment were not motivated by an experiential knowledge of the effectiveness of these strategies. Nonetheless, as the prescription began to reach many people in Cameroon, the rumor was amplified by new components, including the idea that people needed to brush their teeth with salt in the morning, rub their bodies with Vaseline, and that they needed to drink a cup of salt water (Mughe 2014). Commenting on the epidemic and the motivations for the adoption of these behaviors, the *Guardian Post* newspaper (2014) reported: "The fear of death has never been manifested so much in Cameroon as that evoked by the Ebola virus" (Mughe 2014).

Methods

Data for this paper were collected during two qualitative studies conducted in two cities in Cameroon, Yaoundé and Limbe. Between the two studies, 90 interviews were conducted among adult residents to assess:

1 Local knowledge, local action: popular ethnomedical response to the Ebola threat in Yaounde, Cameroon; and
2 Local attitudes toward bushmeat consumption at the time of Ebola in Limbe, Cameroon.

Papers on the primary topics of these studies are under review. The investigators did not specifically ask participants about salt bathing as an Ebola preventive, yet found that this topic was raised frequently by participants.

In study 1, conducted in a large public market in the capital city of Yaoundé, data on salt bathing and/or drinking were retrieved from responses to the following questions:

- *Do you worry about Ebola coming into Cameroon?*
- *What is your biggest worry about Ebola?* or *How much do you worry about this?*
- *Did this message prompt you to seek further information?*
- *Do you do anything to protect yourself from Ebola? What?*

In study 2, conducted using a door or interview format in the border city of Limbe, answers to the following questions elicited responses on salt bathing:

- *Do you think about Ebola very much?*
- *Are you worried about getting Ebola? How worried?*

For this paper, responses to these questions were analyzed for information about attitudes, beliefs, and behaviors involving salt bath and/or salt water drinking as well as other purported protective strategies.

We also conducted online searches for mentions of the salt bath and/or drink preventive for Ebola, examining electronic news items and online blogs with references to the use of saltwater bath solution in Nigeria and Cameroon. Blogs and forums—frequently modified web pages with dated entries—have become increasingly analyzed venues for tracking changes and trends in new knowledge, popular ideas, and attitudes (Jones and Alony 2008). With the emergence of social media in developing countries, blogging has become a popular source for rapidly sharing new knowledge, engaging in community discussion, and reflecting on current events (e.g., Bortree 2005). Also of particular interest for our study were prominent news sources such as the *Guardian Post* (Cameroon), *Premium Times* (Nigeria), and the forum Nairaland (Nigeria), among others.

Results

Relevant findings from the two studies are organized into the following themes: fears about Ebola spreading to Cameroon; sources of information about salt bathing (and/or drinking); message-sharing practices about salt bathing and/or drinking; and using salt bath and/or drinking to avoid Ebola infection.

Fears about Ebola Spreading to Cameroon

Participants' fears about Ebola spreading into Cameroon were expressed in two ways: (a) feelings of vulnerability in the face of a deadly disease; and (b) as a source of worry in their lives.

First, asked if they were concerned about Ebola entering Cameroon, almost all 90 participants across the two studies expressed considerable anxiety. Participants' statements expressing this apprehension included: "In short,

I panic," "I feel traumatized when I imagine how Ebola can attack my family," "I just feel sad," and "I feel frightened." Typical was the statement of a 31-year-old male master's student and teaching assistant at Yaoundé University, who said: "I worry a lot because in the months of December 2014 and January 2015 whenever I watched news on Afrique Media I got frightened with the number of deaths. If it comes to Cameroon, the death situation will be the same [here]." Another participant, a 25-year-old female student, said: "[I am afraid] to the extent that I cry when I watch TV about cases in Liberia."

As these comments indicate, the sudden appearance and swift spread of Ebola in West Africa left people in Cameroon feeling in harm's way, fearing that they might be the next to feel the devastating impact of a disease they little understood but one that they knew could bring misery to them and their friends and families. Moreover, they felt helpless and exposed and were anxious to find protection in a time of growing uncertainty and threat.

Second, participants' fears of Ebola also were elicited when asked about what was their biggest worry. In this regard, participants said they felt desperate because "[Ebola] is very contagious" (student in Yaoundé, age 28), "deadly" (unemployed male, age 29), "has no cure" (female BA graduate, age 22), and "kills rapidly" (male student, age 21). Additionally, one participant told us her fear of Ebola grew out of the "fact it kills rapidly and America hasn't discovered any vaccine yet as we hear" (female bitter kola vendor in the market, age 50). Similarly, another stated, "My biggest worry is that a cure be found" (female student, age 25).

An interesting theme among some participants was the comparison of Ebola with endemic diseases, namely malaria and HIV/AIDS. For example, one participant told us that Ebola "is a very unusual disease because at first we thought AIDS was the worst, but now Ebola is the biggest enemy disease" (female, unemployed, age 24). A 25-year-old male student even expressed a preference: "Yes I prefer malaria or typhoid as these can be cured but Ebola threatens even first class medical doctors." As these comments reflect, participants had once believed that AIDS was the greatest infectious disease threat in their lives, but AIDS was now a treatable condition while Ebola lacked a cure or vaccine. Consequently, participants felt the need to take some action to avoid the plague they dreaded was swiftly coming their way.

Sources of Information about Salt Bathing (and/or Salt Drinking)

Participants reported several sources of information about Ebola and about possible preventive measures. These sources included television, radio, church, markets, bars, schools, hospitals, community meetings, newspapers, Internet, street conversations, workplaces, funeral ceremonies, at home, neighbors, phone calls, and text messages. Between the two studies, 43 participants (48%) (37 from study 1 and 6 from study 2) mentioned text messages as a source of information about Ebola and of ways to prevent infection. Ten of these reported receiving text messages about bathing and/or drinking salt water as prophylaxes.

The discrepancy between the studies may be explained by the fact that participants were directly asked about their texting behavior in study 2, whereas it was discussed without prompting in study 1.

About one-fourth of the participants in study 2 (12 of 50) reported that they sought more information after receiving texts, either by calling their sources directly or searching the Internet for confirmation or more knowledge. A 23-year-old job seeker, for example, said: "*Yes at my free times I will read on internet about Ebola.*" Another responded: "Yes it made me to go to cyber cafes each time to read on internet about the latest of Ebola, how it can be prevented and how it can spread" (female student, age 23). Others commented: "Yes it motivated me to seek further information especially through social media … I exchanged a lot of ideas on ebola through Facebook and other social networking sites" (female student, age 27); "Yes I always logged on internet to read about remedies" (male student, age 23); "Yes I used internet to seek further information to explain to my parents and sisters" (male student, age 25).

Sources of information are important to individuals when considering trust in the information provided, the gravity of the information, and motivation to seek further information. It is evident from our interviews that hearing news from a face-to-face, electronic, or other source marked the beginning, for some participants, of learning about Ebola, its nature and potential threat; it was the start of their efforts to assess their risk and to lower it by taking measures that they learned about. It was also the beginning of their attempt to warn and educate others in their social networks.

Message-sharing Practices about Salt Bath and/or Salt Water Drinking

Ten participants acknowledged receiving and/or sending text messages about salt bathing or drinking among three groups of social network members: friends, relatives, and colleagues. Discussing the messages he had received, for example, one participant reported a list of preventive strategies: "Don't eat bushmeat because it causes Ebola, wash your hands with medicated soap, bath with salt water and eat bitter kola" (male, in the military, age 32). Another stated he received text messages that informed him: "Ebola is real and deadly thus several measures have to be taken: 1) avoid bushmeat; 2) wash hands; and 3) bath in salt water and 4) eat bitter kola as it prevents ebola" (male trader, age 35).

Others report being sent or sending messages saying: "Ebola and the need to prevent it by avoiding bushmeat and also eating bitter kola and bathing in salt water" (female student, age 24); "That there is a dangerous disease called Ebola that is spreading and can be transmitted by eating bushmeat … that eating bitter kola and bathing in salt water can prevent it" (female, businesswoman, age 35); "That Ebola kills fast and can be prevented in the following ways; washing hands, avoiding contact, avoiding bushmeat, bathing in salt water and eating bitter kola" (female student, age 19).

As seen from these statements, text messaging and mobile phones have enhanced the sharing of information through social networks in the midst of an epidemic. Another likely form of information sharing about salt bathing and/or salt water drinking was through Facebook. For example, a 27-year-old female student said, "I exchanged a lot of ideas on Ebola through Facebook and other social networking sites." Today Facebook is deeply integrated into the lives of many Cameroonians (especially youth), as are other channels of electronic communication.

Salt Bathing and/or Drinking in Relation to Changes in Behavior to Avoid Ebola

Behavior change is a salient topic in understanding disease spread because what people do determines their level of risk. Information, and the cultural meanings and emotions embedded therein, can impact social attitudes and behaviors in both negative and positive ways relative to risk exposure. In a context of perceived threat and uncertainty, receptivity—the openness and willingness of people to take in new ideas and enact behavioral change as a result—may be significantly accentuated. The greater a group's "receptivity to new information from the environment, the more influential is the new information" (Walker and Schafer 2011: 233). Behavior change in the case of salt bathing/drinking information is precipitated by conditions of uncertainty and social panic. Because of these conditions of perceived peril, people become increasingly prepared to do whatever it takes, sometimes "just in case" – as long as it fits with their preexisting understanding – to reduce their risk. Thus, at the height of the Ebola epidemic in Sierra Leone, Ofeibea Quist-Arcton, a journalist covering the epidemic, reported during an interview:

> It was on Saturday, very early in the morning. There was this buzz. Everybody was talking. Mothers were calling their grown children up at 1, 2, 3 o'clock in the morning to pray over salt water and then bathe in it. Some were told to drink a little. People were being woken out of a deep sleep to perform this ritual literally in the middle of the night. We were told there were instances of town criers going up and down the streets instructing people to bathe with hot salt water. And it was Christians and Muslims. It may be an indicator of how much Ebola is taking hold of people's consciousness. It just swept everybody away. It was certainly widespread and not just in the capital. The calls and texts and Whatsapp [text] messages were spinning around the country. (Silver 2014)

Online sources (blogs) and media sources reported that a student started the salt water bathing rumor as a joke (Radford 2014). It has been reported that the originator of the idea designed a text message advising Nigerians to start salt water bathing and drinking as much salt water as possible as soon as they received the message. Reportedly, many people who were recipients of the message hurried immediately into bathrooms to take a salt bath and later drank water with salt (Radford 2014). The student in question later apologized online for the hoax. Nevertheless, this "joke" reveals how mobile phones and the Internet, both of which now are ubiquitous in Cameroon's communication landscape, have the potential to quickly reach many people with unsubstantiated rumors or even intentionally fabricated falsehoods of supposedly effective courses of action in times of peril.

Ten of our participants in Cameroon indicated they bathed in and/or drank salt water to protect themselves from Ebola. Comments on this behavior are as follows: "I started bathing with salt water and then ate bitter kola that I wasn't eating previously" (female businesswoman, age 30); "That Ebola is a dangerous disease and could be avoided through several measures: ... [Now] I bath in salt water a few times" (female businesswoman, age 28); "[I] wash my hands, bath in salt water and eat bitter kola" (female tailor, age 19).

Another participant (male NGO volunteer, age 25) stated: "Yes! I bath with salt water which they told us in church is another option. They also told us in church that putting a moderate amount of salt in water to drink also prevents Ebola, so I do this. Often, I also wash my hands with medicated soup on a running tap. This was another option we were told to follow. Another thing I did to protect myself from Ebola is that I stopped playing volleyball, my hobby, ... I think a lot of people also stopped their hobbies especially those that require interaction with others."

Conclusion and Recommendation

Based on her study of rumor and gossip in African social history, White (1994) maintained that the study of rumor is a window into community response to global, national, and environmental events. The analysis of rumor, consequently, is a means of understanding the local in light of its relationship to, and assessment of, both the global and of the contextual (Turner 1993). In contexts of perceived environmental risk and cultural ambiguity, "the mobilization of public opinion is an important catalyst, and in this process rumor and gossip ... are crucially effective" (Stewart and Strathern 2004: xiii). Hence, it is important to keep a close eye on patterns of rumor formation and dissemination – including, in particular, channels of rumor communication – during periods of environmental health threat.

Anthropological research affirms that the control of Ebola requires understanding local views and responses to an outbreak (Hewlett and Amola 2003). Examining emergent ethnomedical belief and practice is one way to engage local views because ethnomedicine is often a flexible system that is sensitive to changing material conditions. It is, in other words, an adaptive mechanism used by people in times of uncertainty and fear (Singer and Baer 2011). Understanding patterns of local action during an epidemic can help in the development of reality-based health promotion strategies that recognize that people are not passive in the face of disease-triggered fear but, instead, use existing cultural models, adjust available models in light of new conditions, adopt new models, and blend ideas from multiple sources. The development of electronic communication significantly enhances the capacity for cultural change, allowing the rapid exchange of ideas and the spread of new cultural behaviors at an accelerated pace. Affirming the insights of Sharon Abramowitz (2014) about the potential contribution of anthropologists in an epidemic, our study shows that Ebola not only provokes considerable fear and panic, but it also motivates people to seek new cultural forms and strategies to prevent infection. Awareness of the changing cultural landscape in contemporary crisis situations, and the role of rumor and social media in processes of change, is vital in terms of expanding environmental health knowledge and in developing useful public health interventions rather than poorly designed ones that assume culture is a fixed system of tradition-bound ideas and practices. Consequently, we argue, formal public health communication in a health crisis will be strengthened by anthropological studies of rumor development and transmission in response to uncertainty, fear, and perceived urgency. Further, we maintain that in viewing environmental health as comprising all of the health-related factors external to people that shape their well-being (WHO 2015), it is important to analyze rumor as a mechanism that prepares communities for change in the face of environmental threats and disruptions.

REFERENCES

Abramowitz, S. 2014. "Ten Things That Anthropologists Can Do to Fight the West African Ebola Epidemic." Somatosphere. http://somatosphere.net/2014/09/ten-things-that-anthropologists-can-do-to-fight-the-west-african-ebola-epidemic.html (accessed December 2, 2015).

Allport, G. and Postman, L. 1947. *The Psychology of Rumor.* New York: Henry Holt.

Bell, A. 1991. *The Language of News Media.* Oxford: Blackwell.

Basu, I. 2014. "The Superstition That Is Dramatically Escalating the Ebola Outbreak." *The Week Magazine.* http://theweek.com/articles/444857/superstition-that-dramatically-escalating-ebola-outbreak (accessed December 5, 2015).

Besnier, N. 2009. *Gossip and the Everyday Production of Politics.* Honolulu, Hawaii: University of Hawaii Press.

Borokini, T., Ighere, D.A., Clement, M., Ajiboye, T.O., and Alowonle, A. 2013. "Ethnobiological Survey of Traditional Medicine Practice for Women's Health in Oyo State." *Journal of Medicinal Plants Studies*, 1(5): 17–29.

Bortree, D. 2005. "Presentation of Self on the Web: An Ethnographic Study of Teenage Girls' Weblogs." *Education, Communication & Information*, 5(1): 25–39.

Buckner, H.T. 1965. "A Theory of Rumor Transmission." *Public Opinion Quarterly*, 29: 54–70.

Cirillo, M., Capasso, G., Leo, V.A.D., and Santo, M.G.D. 1994. "A History of Salt." *American Journal of Nephrology*, 14(4–6): 426–431.

DiFonzo, N. and Bordia, P. 2007. *Rumor Psychology: Social and Organizational Approaches.* Washington, DC: American Psychological Association.

Douglas, M. 1966. *Purity and Danger: An Analysis of Concepts of Pollution and Taboo.* New York: Praeger.

Dressler, W. 2011. "Culture and the Stress Process." In M. Singer and P. Erickson (Eds.), *A Companion to Medical Anthropology* (pp. 119–134). San Francisco: Blackwell.

Erickson, P. 2008. *Ethnomedicine.* Long Grove, IL: Illinois Waveland Press.

Feldman-Savelsberg, P., Ndonko, F., and Schmidt-Ehry, B. 2000. "Sterilizing Vaccines or the Politics of the Womb: Retrospective Study of a Rumor in Cameroon." *Medical Anthropology Quarterly*, 14(2): 159–179.

Ferreira, C., Boholm, A., and Lofstedt, R. 2001. "From Vision to Catastrophe: A Risk Event Search of Images." In J. Flynn, P. Slovic, and H. Kunreuther (Eds.),

Risk, Media and Stigma: Understanding Public Challenges to Modern Science and Technology (pp. 301–308). Abingdon, UK: Earthscan.

Fiske, S. 2004. *Social Beings: A Core Motives Approach to Social Psychology*. New York: Wiley.

Flynn, J., Peters, E., Mertz, C., and Slovic, P. 2001. "Risk, Media, and Stigma at Rocky Flats." In J. Flynn, P. Slovic, and H. Kunreuther (Eds.), *Risk, Media and Stigma: Understanding Public Challenges to Modern Science and Technology* (pp. 309–329). Abingdon UK: Earthscan.

Focho, D., Ndam, W., and Fonge, B. 2009. "Medicinal Plants of Aguambu Bamumbu in the Lebialem Highlands, Southwest Province of Cameroon." *African Journal of Pharmacy and Pharmacology*, 3(1): 1–13.

Foster, G. and Anderson, B. 1978. *Medical Anthropology*. New York: John Wiley & Sons.

Geertz, C. 1973. *The Interpretation of Cultures*. New York: Basic Books.

Grein, T., Kamara, K., Rodier, G., Plant, A., Bovier, P., Ryan, M., Ohyama, T., and Heymann, D. 2000. "Rumors of Disease in the Global Village: Outbreak Verification." *Emerging Infectious Diseases*, 6(2): 97–102.

Hewlett, S.B. and Amola, P.R. 2003. "Cultural Context of Ebola in Northern Uganda." *Emerging Infectious Diseases*, 9(10): 1242–1248.

Hewlett, B. and Hewlett, B. 2008. *Ebola, Culture and Politics: The Anthropology of an Emerging Disease*. Belmont, CA: Wadsworth.

Jones, M. and Alony, I. 2008. "Blogs the New Source of Data Analysis." *Journal of Issues in Informing Science and Information Technology*, 5: 433–446.

Kapferer, J.-N. 1990. *Rumors: Uses, Interpretations, and Images*, rev. ed. Trans. Bruce Fink, trans. New Brunswick, NJ: Transaction.

Kindzeka, M. 2014. "Cameroon Fears Ebola Spread from Nigeria." Voice of America. http://www.voanews.com/content/cameroon-fears-ebola-spread-from-nigeria/2410738.html (accessed December 2, 2015).

Kostka, J., Oswald, Y., and Wattenhofer, R. 2008. "Word of Mouth: Rumour Dissemination In Social Networks." *Structural Information and Communication Complexity*, 5058: 185–196.

Krieger, N. 2011. *Epidemiology and the People's Health: Theory and Context*. Oxford: Oxford University Press.

Laccino, L. 2014. "Ebola 'Caused by Red Cross' and Other Conspiracy Theories." *International Business Times*. http://www.ibtimes.co.uk/ebola-caused-by-red-cross-other-conspiracy-theories-1469896 (accessed December 2, 2015).

Lienhardt, P. 1975. "The Interpretation of Rumour." In J. Beattie and R.G. Lienhardt (Eds.), *Studies in Social Anthropology: Essays in Memory of E. E. Evans-Pritchard* (pp. 105–131). Oxford: Clarendon Press.

McEwen, B. 1998a. "Protective and Damaging Effects of Stress Mediators: Allostasis and Allostatic Load." *New England Journal of Medicine*, 338: 171–179.

McEwen, B. 1998b. "Stress, Adaptation, and Disease: Allostasis and Allostatic Load." *Annals of the New York Academy of Science*, 840: 33–44.

Mitman, G., Murphy, M., and Sellers, C. 2004. "Introduction: A Cloud over History." In G. Mitman, M. Murphy, and C. Sellers (Eds.), *Landscapes of Exposure: Knowledge and Illness in Modern Environments*. Osiris 19:1 17. Chicago: University of Chicago Press.

Mughe, M. 2014. "Pork, Bush-Meat Vendors Go off Business." *Guardian Post*. http://guardianpostonline.blogspot.com/2014_08_01_archive.html.

Nairaland Forum. 2014. "Measures to Contain Ebola in the Church – Fr. Mbaka." http://www.nairaland.com/1851217/measures-contain-ebola-church-fr#25367308 (accessed December 2, 2015).

Nekovee, M., Moreno, T., Bianconi, G., and Marsili, M. 2007. "Theory of Rumour Spreading in Complex Social Networks." *Physica A*, 374(1): 457–470.

Neporent, L. 2014. "Nigerian Ebola Hoax Results in Two Deaths." ABC News. http://abcnews.go.com/Health/nigerian-ebola-hoax-results-deaths/story?id=25842191 (accessed December 2, 2015).

Nkpa, N. 1975. "Rumors of Mass Poison in Biafra." *Public Opinion Quarterly*, 41(3): 332–346.

Noji, E. 2005. "Public Health Issues in Disasters." *Critical Care Medicine*, 33(1): 29–33.

Noumi, E. 2009. "Treating Asthma with Medicinal Plants. An Ethnomedicinal Case Study from Baré-Bakem, Nkongsamba Region, Cameroon." *Syllabus Review*, 1: 10–15.

Nwauzoma. A.B. and Dappa, M.S. 2013. "Ethnobotanical Studies of Port Harcourt Metropolis, Nigeria." *ISRN Botany*. doi: 10.1155/2013/829424.

Ogala, E., Ibeh, N., and Audu, O. 2015. "Ebola Sparks Panic across Nigeria as Citizens Scramble for Salt-Water Bath 'Remedy.'" *Premium Times*. http://www.premiumtimesng.com/news/166257-ebola-sparks-panic-across-nigeria-as-citizens-scramble-for-salt-water-bath-remedy.html (accessed December 2, 2015).

Paz, A. 2008. "The Circulation of Chisme and Rumor: Gossip, Evidentiality, and Authority in the Perspective of Latino Labor Migrants in Israel." *Journal of Linguistic Anthropology*, 19(1): 117–143.

Pietilä, T. 2007. *Gossip, Markets, and Gender: How Dialogue Constructs Moral Value in Post-Socialist Kilimanjaro*. Madison: University of Wisconsin.

Radford, B. 2014. "Social Media Ebola Hoax Causes Deaths." *D News*. http://news.discovery.com/human/psychology/social-media-ebola-hoax-causes-deaths-14100.htm (accessed December 2, 2015).

Ropeik, D. 2004. "The Consequences of Fear." *EMBO Reports*, 5 (Suppl. 1): S56–S60.

Rosnow, R. 1988. "Rumor as Communication: A Contextualist Approach." *Journal of Communication*, 38(l): 12–28.

Rosnow, R. and Fine, G. 1976. *Rumor and Gossip: The Social Psychology of Hearsay*. Oxford: Elsevier Rumor.

Shibutani, T. 1966. *Improvised News: A Sociological Study of Rumor*. New York: Bobbs-Merrill.

Silver, M. 2014. "Pray Over Hot Salt Water, Then Bathe In It: An Anti-Ebola Ritual." National Public Radio. http://www.npr.org/sections/goatsandsoda/2014/08/12/339638348/pray-over-hot-salt-water-then-bathe-in-it-an-anti-ebola-ritual (accessed December 2, 2015).

Singer, M. 2006. *Something Dangerous: Emergent and Changing Illicit Drug Use and Community Health*. Prospect Heights, IL: Waveland Press.

Singer, M. and Baer, H. 2011. *Introducing Medical Anthropology: A Discipline in Action*, 2nd ed. Lanham, MA: Altamira.

Stewart, P. and Strathern, A. 2004. *Witchcraft, Sorcery, Rumors and Gossip*. Cambridge: Cambridge University Press.

Turner, P. 1993. *I Heard It Through the Grapevine: Rumor in African-American Culture*. Berkeley: University of California Press.

Walker, S. and Schafer, M. 2011. "Dueling with Dictators: Explaining the Strategic Interaction Patterns of U.S. Presidents and Rogue Leaders." In S. Walker, A. Malici, and M. Schafer (Eds.), *Rethinking Foreign Policy Analysis: States, Leaders and the Microfoundations of Behavioral International Relations* (pp. 223–144). New York: Routedge.

White, L. 1994 "Between Gluckman and Foucault: Historicizing Rumour and Gossip." *Social Dynamics* 20(1): 75–92.

WHO (World Health Organization). 2015. "Environmental Health." Online at http://www.who.int/topics/environmental_health/en/.

Williams, R. 2009. "Base and Super Structure in Marxist Cultural Theory." In M.G. Durham and D.M. Kellner (Eds.), *Media and Cultural Studies: Keyworks* (pp. 130–143). Malden, MA: Wiley-Blackwell.

Zhang, Z.-L. and Zhang, Z.-Q. 2009. "An Interplay Model for Rumour Spreading and Emergency Development." *Physica A*, 388(19): 4159–4166.

Zhao, X. and Jianzhong, W. 2013. "Dynamical Model about Rumor Spreading with Medium." *National Discrete Dynamics in Nature and Society*. doi: 10.1155/2013/586867.

Zinn, J. 2008. "A Comparison of Sociological Theories on Risk and Uncertainty." In J. Zinn (Ed.), *Social Theories of Risk and Uncertainty: An Introduction* (pp. 168–200). Malden, MA: Blackwell.

CHAPTER 9 Paradise Poisoned: Nature, Environmental Risk, and the Practice of Lyme Disease Prevention in the United States

Abigail Dumes

Susan is an artist who lives with her husband and son in a farmhouse in western Connecticut.[1] Her studio is located in a barn that is adjacent to the house. From the windows of both buildings, the windswept fields and surrounding woods create verdant tableaus that are her art's inspiration. When I interviewed Susan at her home in 2010, she had been undergoing treatment for Lyme disease since 1994, when she discovered a "bull's eye" rash on the back of her neck.[2] In addition to the toll that 16 years of ill health had taken on her, Susan described being haunted by the fact that she continues to live in an area where she and her family are at risk for getting more tick bites. She explained,

> A part of me would like to just get the hell out of here; part of me would like to move where there are no ticks. That's just the worst thing about being here. It's awful, it's like a scourge. It has definitely changed how I understand nature. I love the country so much, but I'm not going to walk out in those fields. I only walk on mowed lawn. There's no careless running through the forest anymore.

A Companion to the Anthropology of Environmental Health, First Edition. Edited by Merrill Singer.

This chapter, which draws upon 18 months of ethnographic fieldwork among Lyme patients, physicians, and scientists in the northeastern United States, explores the complicated relationship between how individuals in Lyme endemic areas understand their natural environment and the ways in which they understand and act upon their health.[3] Unlike other infectious diseases, the viability of Lyme disease depends upon a natural ecology suitable to the habitat preferences of the blacklegged tick, small rodents, and deer. And because the transmission of Lyme disease to humans requires exposure to this landscape, Lyme and other tick-borne diseases draw unique analytic attention to contemporary ideas about – and practical engagements with – nature. The first section of this chapter provides a broad historical context for the production of an aesthetic of nature in the United States. Here, I suggest that because an American aesthetic of nature encompasses the affective spectrum between attraction and repulsion – nature is beautiful, in part, *because* it is frightening – the contours of Lyme disease can be better understood through what I call an *epidemiology of affect*. That is, who gets Lyme disease and why is more than just a matter of demographic and geographic correlations of risk; it is also about how Americans in Lyme endemic areas understand and act upon their competing feelings toward their natural environment.

The second section examines the underbelly of an aesthetic of nature in the United States: environmental risk. The task here is to identify what constitutes "the environment" and what part of that environment individuals in Lyme endemic areas find risky. I suggest that, for some Lyme disease patients, Lyme disease is just one risk in a constellation of environmental risks that can be broadly described as a toxic environment. That this is so points to a reality in which the environment is not confined to the "outside" and where individuals perceive environmental risk to exist on an almost indistinguishable continuum between the inside and the outside.

The third and final section ends with an exploration of the practical consequences – in this case, prevention practices – produced by the tension between an attraction to nature and an awareness of environmental risk in Lyme endemic areas. Drawing from Saba Mahmood's Aristotelian-inspired work on "exteriority as a means to interiority," I explore a range of emerging "bodily practices" related to tick bite prevention and how they shape ideas about nature and environmental risk (Mahmood 2005: 134; Lock 1993). Here, I argue that, in the lives of the people who enact them, the *effects* of tick bite prevention practices – what they incidentally happen to produce across relations – become more important than their efficacy, and these practices constitute the active building of new individualized environments, or what biologist Jacob von Uexkull terms "environment-worlds" (Agamben 2004: 40).

An American Aesthetic of Nature

It is not a coincidence that, during his 2012 presidential campaign, candidate Mitt Romney often quoted lines from "America the Beautiful," a song that celebrates "spacious skies" and "purple mountain majesties above the fruited plain": in the United States, nature has become inextricably linked with ideas of beauty *and* with what it means to be an American. Environmental historian Roderick Nash observes in his now classic text, *Wilderness and the American Mind*, that as "the basic ingredient of American culture," nature has, since the late nineteenth century, been understood as "beautiful, friendly, and capable of elevating and delighting the beholder" (Nash 2001: 4). But this was not always the case. Prior to the 1800s and the emergence of Romanticism in Europe, nature was considered to be unsightly, without moral merit, and a threat to "civilizing" tendencies. One of the most compelling examples that Nash provides is that of the mountain. Now emblematic of natural splendor – reaching the peak of which is, for many, the true test of a nature-compatible constitution – mountains in the seventeeth century were, as Nash describes, "generally regarded as warts, pimples, blisters and other ugly deformities on the earth's surface" and were, fittingly, given such names as "Devil's Point" (Nash 2001: 45). However, under the Romantics' eyes, the boundless unruliness of forests, crevasses, and mountainscapes became a means to transcendence. More critically, philosopher Kate Soper, in *What is Nature?*, argues that although nature had been represented as a duality between terror and serenity since the days of Homer, the Romantics' representations differed in that, for them, the "chaos" of nature became "endowed with its own aesthetic appeal" (Soper 1995: 222).

Nash describes how, like their European counterparts, American pioneers and frontiersmen also perceived nature to be "cursed" and "ungodly." As journals and other narratives attest, living in proximity to the wilderness was not perceived to be a source of pleasure or inspiration but rather a forced necessity. However, as Nash also describes, the ideological momentum generated by the Romantic movement in Europe gradually translated to changing understandings of nature in America. And, for a former colony like America, nature and the unique features of the American landscape quickly became a means by which to distinguish itself from Europe. This was especially true for Henry David Thoreau, who saw in American wildness a clean slate for national moral growth. In *Thoreau's Nature: Ethics, Politics, and the Wild*, political theorist Jane Bennett observes that, from Thoreau's perspective, "the milk of (American) Wildness flows freely, and this is, as we know, crucial to recrafting the self. The Wildness of the American wilderness is the condition of possibility of a new man, a 'new Adam'" (Bennett 1994: 114). In the eyes of Thoreau, what America once had too much of, it now had in enviable quantity and in kind conducive to moral advantage.

While at the beginning of the nineteenth century many Americans distinguished themselves through the unique wilderness of their national landscape, environmental historian Daniel J. Philippon (2005) argues that, toward the century's end, the suburban garden came to assume an equally important place as a natural refuge. Just as the Romantics saw the wilderness as a site for moral instruction, early suburban architects saw in the proximity of suburbs to nature the possibility of social uplift. Of these architects and planners, Philippon suggests that Andrew Jackson Downing was among the most influential. Through texts like *Treatise on the Theory and Practice of Landscape Gardening* (1841) and

Architecture of Country Houses (1850), Downing argued that daily exposure to natural beauty would strengthen individual integrity and reinforce family values. In a piece entitled *Rural Essays*, he wrote: "in the United States, nature and domestic life are better than society and the manners of towns … hence, all sensible men gladly escape, earlier or later, and partially or wholly from the turmoil of cities" (Philippon 2005: 77).

Finally, over the last three decades, nature and one's exposure to it have not only become about a better life, but also about a healthier one. Of course, ideas about the health benefits of nature are longstanding. In the late nineteenth century, physicians began to advocate for pure mountain air as a treatment for tuberculosis and other lung diseases. And by the mid-nineteenth century, the abovementioned suburban architect, Andrew Jackson Downing, edited a gardening book targeted at white, middle-class women in the hopes that it "would increase, among our own fair country women, the taste for these delightful occupations in the open air, which are so conducive to their own health, and to the beauty and interest of our homes" (Philippon 2005: 77). But contemporary understandings about the health benefits of nature – whether that nature is located in the wilderness of Alaska or in the suburbs of Fairfield County, Connecticut – are myriad and range from obesity prevention to the abatement of neurological conditions to the reduction of childhood behavioral disorders. As a result, a movement has coalesced around concerns that individuals – and children in particular – are suffering from nature deprivation. One of the most vocal advocates for this movement is Richard Louv, who coined the term "nature deficit disorder." In his book, *Last Child in the Woods: Saving our Children from Nature-Deficit Disorder*, Louv (2005) argues that increasing diagnoses of childhood behavioral disorders, such as attention deficit disorder, are not a result of increasing pathology but of the absence of the biophysical benefits of nature in individuals' lives. To support his argument, he cites a range of studies that show that children who live and play closer to nature are better able to concentrate and are less obese (Louv 2005: 39–54).

In the case of Lyme disease, however, Louv's means to health (nature) is also a threat to it. Indeed, due to the natural ecology of Lyme disease, individuals who tend to contract Lyme are either those who prefer to live near the woods or those who like to spend time in the woods. This fact lies at the heart of my argument for why tick-borne disease, and Lyme disease in particular, can only fully be understood through an *epidemiology of affect*. As a cornerstone of public health, epidemiology can be defined as "the study of how often diseases occur in different groups of people and why."[4] Traditionally, epidemiological explanations for disease incidence among particular populations are based on statistical analysis of demographic and socioeconomic factors including age, racial and ethnic background, and income status. However, Lyme disease makes a strong case for the role of affect in the incidence and distribution of tick-borne disease. Understanding how people navigate the tension between their competing feelings of affection for *and* aversion to nature helps to shed light on who gets Lyme disease and why; it also helps to explain why Lyme disease prevention proves to be so challenging, as the primary "risk" for acquiring Lyme disease – exposure to "nature" – is simultaneously and collectively valued as a personal and cultural "benefit." Following an epidemiology of affect, then, an aesthetic of nature tends to be particularly strong among patients who *end up* having Lyme disease.[5] Although there are many Lyme patients and physicians who have a dramatically estranged relationship with nature after their experience with Lyme disease, there are as many for whom the aesthetic, moral, and health benefits outweigh its risks.

Take, for example, Regina and Mary, two women who founded and lead a Lyme disease support group that I attended almost every month for 18 months. Both Regina and Mary describe enduring long struggles with Lyme disease. They, as well as their children, have been treated for Lyme disease over the years, and, although they report that they have recovered, they explained to me that their children continue to struggle with symptoms, a reality that often triggered tearful conversations during support group meetings. For Regina and Mary, however, the importance of living near the outdoors continues to be paramount – so much so that Regina moved her family from Texas back to Connecticut when her three children were young so that they could "grow up near Nature." "I wanted them to have what I had," she explained. "Horseback riding and fields to run in. If only I knew that moving here is what would make my children sick." During our interview together, Mary echoed the same sentiments: "We were always big outdoors people. We loved to camp and stuff. And I struggle with, I just can't live in a house. I need to be outdoors, you know, so I just can't live in a vacuum and I think my kids are the same way. I wouldn't let them go running in a field, but ..." her voice trailed off. It was clear from Mary's expression that, as much hardship as her family had gone through *because of* nature, the thought of living *without it* was impossible to imagine.

For individuals like Regina and Mary, the importance they ascribe to nature influences how they choose to navigate environmental risk. In the case of Lyme disease, the salience of nature's aesthetic, moral, and health dimensions makes possible the idea of *risks worth taking* and transforms what in other contexts would be perceived as irresponsible and reckless behavior into noble and courageous action. This tension is nicely captured in the blog entry of one Lyme disease patient, who writes:

> I hope that you may take heart and continue to explore wild, wooded places free from concern about menacing, infectious ticks and vector-borne illnesses. Just rock the pants-tucked-into-socks look and have an OCD friend check you for unwanted guests afterward. No illness, or threat thereof, should keep you from enjoying the breathtaking beauty and majesty of nature.

Another revealing example is that of Dr. Childs, a mainstream Lyme physician whose practice I observed on several occasions. Dr. Childs is a self-identified nature enthusiast who wakes up early before work to row on the Connecticut River and spends weekends bird watching with his wife. He loves to hike, and, during the time I spent with him, he was often busy planning his next outdoor adventure in a country that he had never visited. One of the few photos in his office is of him and his children triumphantly astride the peak of a mountain range. Dr. Childs found it hard not to share his enthusiasm for the outdoors when he discovered that his patient was also an outdoors enthusiast; and he seemed particularly pleased when a patient was determined to continue their outdoor activities. One patient described how much he loved hiking in the woods and how he was excited to get back in the woods when his knee got better. "That's the spirit!" Dr. Childs chimed in. Another patient exclaimed, "I've hunted and fished all my life. And nothing, not even Lyme disease, is going to keep me from hunting and fishing!" Dr. Childs nodded approvingly in agreement.

Even those who continue to admire nature, however, often recognize that they no long feel comfortable *in* it, a recognition that is met with a certain degree of sadness and nostalgia. A physician I interviewed named Dr. Reed explained:

> I like the outdoors, always have. I love to camp. I'm also an assistant scout leader. I used to feel safe, but now I don't. I'm constantly worried that a bug will bite me. Now when I go into the woods, I have gaiters that I put on. I lay them down and spray them with permethrin. And then I put DEET on my skin … and I STILL don't like to go into the woods. My family looks at me like I'm nuts, but so far, knock on wood, we haven't found a tick on any of our family members.

The regime of bodily practices that Dr. Reed engages just so that he can feel safe enough to enjoy the woods that he still loves will be discussed in the final section of this chapter. What is important here, and what I have explored in this section, is the difficulty that individuals like Dr. Reed face in navigating the gap between their love for and fear of nature. In 2009, the *New Yorker* published a cartoon depicting Adam and Eve in the Garden of Eden. As Adam inspects a lifted leg, Eve says, "It's Eden. You don't have to keep checking for ticks." For Thoreau, American nature was a prospect more hopeful than the actual Garden of Eden because "it remains to be seen" how the "backwoodsman in America" – the "Adam in the wilderness" – turns out (Bennett 1994: 114). Thoreau, it seems, could not have anticipated that, for some, the rise of Lyme disease would be a fall from nature as disillusioning as that which followed the original eaten apple.

Environmental Risk Outside In

As the previous section made clear, ideas of nature are intimately linked to perceptions of environmental risk. Sociologists Alan Petersen and Deborah Lupton observe that the limitation of "nature discourse," or what I describe as an American aesthetic of nature, is that nature is also "responsible for death, destruction, (and) disease" (Petersen and Lupton 1999: 106). However, identifying what actually *constitutes* environmental risk is no easy task (Beck 1992; Douglas 1992; Harthorn and Oaks 2003; Pidgeon, Simmons, and Henwood 2006). In the case of Lyme disease, ticks and the pathogens they carry might appear to be the most obvious environmental risk for Lyme patients. But as I came to learn, in Lyme patients' everyday lives, Lyme disease is just one part of a larger constellation of environmental risks that can be described as "toxins" and, in general, individuals' concerns tend to be more broadly centered around environmental *toxicity*, whether man-made (e.g., pesticides) or natural (e.g., tick-borne pathogens). In this way, environmental risk is located less in the wildness of nature and more in the diffuse and ubiquitous quality of a toxic environment. In light of this, I suggest that the practices and ideas surrounding Lyme disease help to shed light on a broader emerging relationship between the body and the environment, in which the risk of the environment is not a matter of the "outside" but of an immanent environment that we engage with – and in – irrespective of whether we are inside or outside.

For example, during one of my many conversations with a mainstream Lyme physician named Dr. Elway, she asked, "Did I tell you what I find so interesting about chronic Lyme patients? In general, they tend to be really concerned about toxins – about the potential harm of what they're putting in their bodies – and yet they seem to be perfectly fine with exposing their bodies to years of antibiotics." While it is true that chronic Lyme patients are often concerned about exposure to toxins, their concerns are not unique. In the last couple of decades, many Americans have come to perceive toxins – both inside and outside the home – as an increasing menace to health and wellness. Among the most effective vehicles for the construction and operationalization of the body as a site of toxicity have been biomonitoring studies. The first, conducted by the Centers for Disease Control and Prevention and published in 2001, confirmed the presence of 27 chemicals in American bodies.[6] The most recent report in this series was published in 2009 and expanded the list of chemicals to 212, many of these known carcinogens.[7] No longer theoretical, the traffic between the outside and inside of the body is now variously visualized and responded to in everyday practice. As one woman observed at a Lyme disease support group meeting, "The skin is the largest organ on the body. (Why wouldn't I be) afraid of chemicals getting inside of me?"

In *Shopping Our Way to Safety*, sociologist Andrew Szasz (2007) describes individuals' response to what they perceive as an increasing toxic threat – and the porousness of the boundaries between toxins and their bodies – as the "inverted quarantine." The inverted quarantine describes a shift from a popular understanding of the "classic" quarantine, in which the underlying assumption is that "the overall collective environment is basically healthy," to one in which the "whole environment is toxic, illness-inducing" (2007: 5). Practices that proceed from this shift include a range of behaviors centered around isolating the body from "disease-inducing surroundings," including installing water and air filtration systems, purchasing organic produce, wearing organic clothing, using toxin-free cosmetics and cleaning supplies, and ensuring that building materials adhere to the strictest regulations for toxicity (2007: 5). In a move that mirrors trends in public health toward a greater emphasis on individual responsibility, the inverted quarantine operates under the assumption that individuals can circumvent failures in mass regulation by protecting themselves and the ones they love. Szasz argues that there is not only no way to shop our way to safety, but that the illusion of doing so translates to further neglect of mass regulation.

I would push Szasz's argument one step further and suggest that even as many individuals create barriers to toxin exposure, many also recognize the limitations of these barriers. That is, they recognize that there is only so much they can do. The result of this understanding is an emerging and focused attention on toxin *removal*. Accordingly, while the consequence of a diminishing gap between the inside and the outside is that *no* place is safe anymore, the solution is that, once toxic, the body can often be *detoxified*. This is no more so the case than it is for Lyme patients. When I began to observe Lyme patient support group meetings, I was surprised to discover that a significant part of most meetings was occupied by strategies for eliminating toxins from the body. This reality is rooted in an idea shared by many chronic Lyme patients and Lyme-literate practitioners that Lyme disease is particularly pernicious, not merely in and of itself, but in its synergy with other ailments of the body, most notable among them being toxicity. At support group meetings, seasoned members often tried to communicate to newcomers that addressing Lyme disease is only addressing one piece of the unwellness puzzle. One woman explained, "If you have a toxic swamp in your body, that's what Lyme prefers. You have to get rid of toxic soup." For many Lyme patients, heavy metals are perceived to be a frontrunner of toxicity, but toxins like "xenoestrogens," "yeast," "bacterial die-off," and the antibiotics that many patients credit as critical to their recovery are close behind. When it comes to removal, what has worked and what has not worked for patients spans the spectrum: loofah scrubs, Epsom salt baths, sweating out toxins by sitting in saunas or exercising, colloidal silver, chelation, colonic enemas, diets and fasts, and herbs like milk thistle and dandelion root.[8]

If a toxin can be both biological and chemical and can be found inside and outside, it also happens that one substance can be toxic or beneficial depending on its context. The subtle distinctions that constitute when and where something is or is not a toxin plays out, for example, in the case of mold. As one Lyme patient explained,

> After we detox, I can come home and smell mold. I smell the mold from the ground, which isn't a problem, because it's outside and I don't have a problem. You can't stop living outside; you *can* remedy it in your home. I felt like I've always been sick in my house because I wake up every day and have a dull headache.

Perhaps most striking here is the reason for why outside mold is not a toxic threat, while inside mold is. The issue is not that one type of mold is more toxic than the other; they are perceived to be the same mold. The issue is that the ability to control outside mold is out of one's hands, while inside mold is perceived to be controllable. The extent to which something is perceived to be controllable is a good barometer for how it will be perceived as a toxin. As one patient explained, "I like to focus on the things I can control."

Another good example of the environmental toxin's contextual nature can be found in Lyme patients' use of the Rife machine and the seemingly contradictory actions some take to limit their exposure to other electromagnetic frequencies. The Rife machine, a contraption that emits electromagnetic frequencies, was developed in the 1930s by a researcher named Royal Rife. A subscriber to the school of thought that cancer has a bacterial or viral basis, Rife created a machine that he believed targeted bacteria and viruses at their own unique frequencies and, in doing so, "devitalized" them (Hess 1996: 664). Initially taken seriously by medical institutions, the machine was tested in clinical trials conducted at University of California, San Francisco and University of Southern California, only to become the center of a heated lawsuit and meet the fate of being banned by the California Department of Health (Hess 1996: 664–665). As of this writing, the Rife machine has yet to be approved by the Food and Drug Administration. Patients and alternative practitioners have continued to use the machine for a range of maladies, and they have done so in an underground fashion by purchasing the machine in parts and assembling it on their own. Because the machine costs upward of a couple of thousand dollars, patients often collectively purchase one and share its use.

Among Lyme disease patients, the Rife machine is increasingly used in conjunction with antibiotics or on its own. However, the same patients who use the Rife machine to achieve health benefits are often simultaneously concerned about the risks of their exposure to everyday electromagnetic frequencies. Like concerns about toxins in general, concerns about an electromagnetically toxic environment are not unique to Lyme patients. As questions about the potentially harmful effects of everyday electronic devices, like cell phones and laptops, have become more common in popular media, many Americans have begun to take precautionary action, such as using cell phone headsets to create a perceived safe distance between the phone's output and the ear or placing a lap guard on one's lap for laptop use. But for many Lyme patients, even these efforts taken by some concerned consumers are not sufficient. Several support group meetings I attended were spent strategizing about how to best limit exposure to electromagnetic frequencies. Some members suggested removing all electronic equipment from one's bedroom. Others thought that just turning off the wireless router at night would be sufficient. Still others suggested more aggressive action, recommending that filters or nodes be applied to all electromagnetic devices that a person owns in their home, office, and cars. One patient named Nancy explained, "I have electromagnetic sensitivity. All I do is read. I can't sit in front of the computer or the television." To protect herself from what she understands are the harmful effects of electromagnetic radiation, Nancy has installed technology throughout her home that is purported to interfere with frequencies and "renaturalize" them so that they are no longer harmful. "It's expensive, but it works," she said. "I can feel all my cells open up. It makes me feel more open." Another support group member agreed. "I'm so much less sleepy when I drive," the woman exclaimed. "I can tell immediately when the node is not in place."

The tension in this example turns on the fact that while Nancy and other chronic Lyme patients go to great lengths to accommodate "electromagnetic sensitivity" and to prevent themselves from being exposed to electromagnetic frequencies, many are nevertheless willing to use an electromagnetic frequency machine to target the bacterium that causes Lyme disease. The difference, of course, is that in the case of everyday exposure, the exposure is not on these patients' terms and is outside of their control. In the case of the Rife machine, the exposure is on their terms and within their control. And unlike everyday exposure, the Rife machine has a targeted and expected health effect. In the end, the toxicity of electromagnetic frequency is not necessarily gauged according to dose – on how much or how little is used – but on the intent and outcome of its use.

If Lyme patients often perceive their health predicament as of one of choosing *between* toxic environmental evils (i.e., strategically accommodating one toxin to mitigate the toxic effect of another), it makes sense that, when it comes to pesticides, the environmental toxin par excellence, Lyme patients are often its greatest proponents. During a conversation with a mother of two daughters, all three of whom were being treated for chronic Lyme disease, the mother exclaimed, "We're almost completely organic except that we spray the most horrible toxins on the yard. We also spray ourselves like crazy!"[9] Another woman I interviewed had made it her year's mission to persuade her local drugstore to provide a continuous supply of an insecticide called permethrin to its customers. For these Lyme patients, even in the face of their concern for toxin exposure, there is no such thing as being too careful when it comes to tick eradication. As the woman above explained, "We try to have our lawn sprayed at least six times per year." Another patient admitted, "Of course I spray my lawn! I'm a nut job – I'm very careful. I also take permethrin, spray it on cotton balls, and stuff it in paper tubes. Squirrels and chipmunks nest in there and it kills the ticks. Ever since I began spraying, I haven't found one tick on my property."

For most patients with whom I spoke, the decision to use pesticides was a choice between two personal health risks: the risk of pesticide exposure and the risk of Lyme disease infection. As one patient explained, "When it comes to applying repellants, some people believe that it's dangerous to them. I respect that because that's pretty much where I was coming from, too. But you get neurological Lyme and you have Lyme long term and you start reevaluating your opinions." Some individuals also considered the environmental impact of pesticides when making their decision. For example, one chronic Lyme patient I interviewed, a 25-year-old college student, reasoned, "It might be horrible for the environment, but of course I'm going to spray pesticides. What's the point of having a world if you can't live in it?" Another patient, a middle-aged government employee, exclaimed, "I've always been a really ecological friendly person. But there wasn't hesitation when it came to my health and protecting my family. That outweighed the possibility of the effects of it leaching into the Farmington River. The immediacy of Lyme disease, that made the difference. When it comes to ticks, I don't care what I have to do." In both cases, the risk of Lyme disease was almost always prioritized over the risk of pesticides to human and environmental health.

As the examples in the section have demonstrated, one answer to the question posed by Dr. Elway in the beginning of this section is that the simultaneity of Lyme patients' use and avoidance of substances that they recognize as toxic is not contradictory. Rather, toxin avoidance is merely an attempt to limit further exposure to a toxic environment of which, through their antibiotic and pesticide use, Lyme patients are an inextricable part. From ticks and mold to electromagnetic frequencies and pesticides, the case of Lyme disease makes clear that what constitutes the "environment" in the United States is often much more than just the "outside" and that, for many individuals in Lyme endemic areas, ticks are just one risk in a range of environmental risks that are perceived to be "toxic."

The Practice of Lyme Disease Prevention

While the previous two sections examined *how* individuals in Lyme endemic areas who are concerned about Lyme disease navigate the tension between their attraction to nature and their fear of environmental risk, this section concludes by examining the practical consequences of that tension – more specifically, the emerging bodily practices that individuals increasingly enact to keep ticks off them. Here, I argue that as a way of being in and engaging with an environment whose salience to the self is constantly changing, tick prevention practices become less about whether or not they actually work and more about what they incidentally happen to produce across social relations. As I demonstrate in the example of the tick check, a personal prevention practice that often requires the help of someone else, it is the *effects* of these practices – for example, quality time spent between parents and children, intimate time spent between partners, and a collective feeling of greater safety – that individuals come to value over the efficacy of the practices themselves.

Described by first-century Roman naturalist Pliny the Elder as the "foulest and most vile of creatures," ticks, which attach to a host and draw blood unnoticed for up to three days, have long made humans uneasy (Edlow 2003: 84). In 1749, a Swedish naturalist named Pehr Kalm, documenting his travels through the northeastern United States, wrote of ticks: "To these I must add the wood-lice, with which the forests are so pestered, that it is impossible to pass through a bush without having a whole army of them on your clothes, or to sit down, though the place be ever so pleasant" (Stafford 2007: 1).

The dense annoyance of ticks that Kalm experienced in 1749 changed, however, at the turn of the twentieth century, when forests were cleared for farmland and deer (which are tick carriers) were hunted out of the landscape. Entomologist Kirby Stafford describes how an entomologist in 1872 declared ticks to be nearly extinct along the path that Pehr Kalm had traveled 100 years before (Stafford 2007: 2). It was not until after World War II that the perfect storm of reforestation, deer reintroduction, and the expansion of suburbs into forested areas allowed for the return of the tick. As a result, Americans, often preferring to live close to the woods but not in them, became increasingly familiar with and wary of tick encounters.

In *Cure Unknown: Inside the Lyme Epidemic,* journalist Pamela Weintraub describes how this threat of tick encounters estranged her from the nature she had always loved. She writes:

> Before I realized our environment was making us sick, I viewed the natural beauty around me as a gentle, beneficent luxury, a reward for my success. ... Before Lyme, I threw parties on my forty-foot deck, going out at dusk to barbeque skewers of mushrooms and steak, all the while dazzled by another red sunset beyond the pines. After Lyme, I woke up at dawn and, venturing out on my forty-foot deck, saw twenty deer grazing in my yard. I'd clang my pots loud, making them bolt and run. Before Lyme, I hiked deep into the woods, smelling the cool moist breath of pine needles and moss. After Lyme, I hesitated even stepping on the grass in Chappaqua without high socks and boots, my suburban version of the Hazmat suit. What had once seemed pristine now felt toxic and ruined. (2008: 105)

Like Pamela, many of the individuals I spoke with during the course of my fieldwork moved to or remained in forested suburbs to be "close to nature." But "after Lyme," many described an experience of becoming "prisoners of their own paradise." As one patient exclaimed, "I don't go out. I used to always go out. I love nature and I love animals. Now I don't like grass or walking through the woods. If I see people walking through the woods, I want to say, 'You're going to get sick!'" Another patient explained,

> The deck outside is my world. It's way above the ground. I don't go on the lawn. I don't go to picnics. My life is totally changed. I used to be outside camping, hiking, hiking 80 miles per week. Now I walk on the pavement and come back. That's it. I'm afraid to go on any grasses. Also, I heard that a tick came in on someone's Christmas tree, so I've have been putting up artificial ones for the past couple years.

Yet another patient, a television producer in his early forties who, unlike the other two women, continues to venture outside, explains that he does so with great unease. "Now I'm freaked out," he admits, "even when I take the dog for a walk. And now that it's summer, I see a tick waiting to jump off every leaf. My perception of where ticks are has changed – ticks are totally on my radar screen."

Because the greatest risk for tick exposure occurs in one's backyard, Lyme disease has transformed mundane domestic objects – like lawns, playgrounds, and stone walls – into frightening and difficult-to-decipher menaces. One father I met, whose children were not allowed to walk on the lawn without permission, recounted how his young son, in reaction to a pile of leaves he had raked together, exclaimed, "Look, Dad, a pile of ticks!" Upon later seeing a cartoon depicting children playing in leaves, his son asked, "Why would their parents let them do that?" Another woman described a recent Christmas-shopping-in-July outing where she passed over some deer-themed Christmas cards because the sight alone had made her cringe. In a similar instance, another woman explained, "When I see kids playing in the grass or people walking dogs in the grass, I grimace. We hear stories about Lyme every day. I feel bad, because kids want to go out in the backyard, but my granddaughter will never go in my backyard. It's a shame, I love the woods. All those big rock formations in the back!"

Some families, overwhelmed by the idea of living in such close contact with ticks, have moved to non-Lyme endemic areas (and many have at least contemplated it). But most stay, for a variety of reasons. One woman explained, "I've lived my whole life in Connecticut. My family is here and my husband's whole family is here. So I just can't imagine. I've heard that people have moved to California, though." Other patients I spoke with, like Regina and Mary who lead the support group meeting I described in this chapter's first section, gestured to their constitutional incompatibility with city life. "We could move to New York City and not have grass, and that's not the kind of life I want. I like grass. It's nice." Another woman echoed this sentiment: "I know that there are enough things that you can do to prevent Lyme disease without moving to the concrete jungle. We would never move. But I also don't let my kids go in the woods. Isn't that crazy? I live in a rural area and don't want to go in the woods!"

In making the decision to stay, many turn to what they describe as the only thing at their disposal: prevention. Tick bite prevention includes an ever-expanding range of bodily practices, such as tick checks, repellants, knee-high socks, wearing socks with sandals, tucking pants into socks, light-colored clothing, wearing a hat, avoiding grass, avoiding leaf litter, keeping animals outside (or at least not letting them in bed with you), only having pets with white fur, spraying the yard with pesticides, putting clothes in the dryer after coming inside, and bathing after coming inside. Some individuals and families conscientiously engage in as many of these practices as they can. As Sue, a stay-at-home parent with two daughters, explained,

> When we're in the garden, we wear khaki pants with white socks. We also wear hats and socks on our hands. And, of course, we spray ourselves like crazy. When we come inside, we take our clothes off in the garage and then shower. We also try to find other things we like to do, like bike riding and skiing. And we try to spray six times per year. The other thing is that knee highs have come back in fashion, so it's much easier to get my girls to wear long socks.

In a similar vein, another woman explained,

> I cannot get bitten again. I have to take all the precautions that I can in order not to get bit: tick checks, repellants, pesticides, you name it. We even have a protocol for washing clothes: we take off clothes in garage and then put them in a garbage bag until they go to laundry. They also get twisty tied.

Others find focusing on just one or two prevention practices more manageable. For instance, one woman explained how if she walks through her yard, she wears rubber boots. Another man, who lets his dog sleep on his bed, pulls down the covers every night and looks for ticks. He added, "And I insist on only solid sheets. It's the only way you can see the ticks."

In general, some prevention practices are rarely done. As one patient with whom I spoke rhetorically asked, "Who's going to wear long pants on a hot summer day?" But some, like tick checks and remembering to shower after coming indoors, have, for many, become part of the daily repertoire of bodily hygiene. Eileen, a 43-year-old woman who used to work at an optical lens factory explained, "Am I using permethrin? No. Am I using DEET? No. Just last weekend I was outside just doing a very little bit of yard work and then I was inside taking a shower. My husband's also following me saying, 'Take a shower.' That's one of the most effective things." Echoing Eileen, Judy, a 60-year-old woman who works as a freelance writer, explained, "I have two sons and we all take showers immediately when coming back in. We also use loofahs. It's basic hygiene really. Some people I look at and think, 'Hello, you haven't taken a shower for a week, no wonder you're crawling with ticks!'"

That tick checks and showering after coming indoors have become part of some individuals' "basic hygiene" is notable given that personal hygiene as a means to a disease-free life has, over time, become a less urgent priority for many Americans. Indeed, in the United States, everyday attention to and care for the body, as a functional barrier between the contagion of the outside and the health of the inside, has become the stuff of outdated parental expressions like, "Don't forget to wash behind your ears." Broadly speaking, public health measures, like waste management, municipal drinking water, and vaccines, have dramatically reduced the menace of communicable diseases that produced vigilant inspection of the body's planes and folds up until the middle of the twentieth century. In the *Gospel of Germs: Men, Women, and the Microbe in American Life*, medical historian Nancy Tomes observes how, in the early 1900s, "revelations that skin, hair, and body cavities harbored millions of germs provided abundant material for heightening anxieties about bodily hygiene" (Tomes 1998: 165). For women, germ anxiety took the form of a nationwide campaign to wear shorter dresses and skirts, so that hemlines would not become Petri dishes of contagion. For men, it meant a new aesthetic that valued shorn, beardless faces (Tomes 1998: 159). This broader shift in public health from collective to individual responsibility in the form of personal hygiene behaviors became institutionalized through public education. For example, Suellen Hoy, in *Chasing Dirt: The American Pursuit of Cleanliness*, describes how schoolteachers in the mid-twentieth century conducted toothbrush drills and required daily inspections of hair, hands, ears, and necks (Hoy 1995: 128).

Unlike tooth brushing and hair washing, which, for some, have become habits of an aesthetic nature with little conscious attention to health (let alone life and death), tick checks are bodily practices explicitly enacted in health's pursuit and with a keen attention to risk of disease. But they are also a new breed of bodily practice in that they are acts of personal hygiene that are inherently social (Lock 1993). This is, in large part, because of the habits of ticks themselves. Built for moist environments, ticks leave leaf litter only to, when they happen upon a human, make their way to the floral equivalent of the human body: armpits, the bra line, hairlines, around the anus, and tucked within the creases of male and female genitalia. The irony is that these most intimate places, which most would prefer to inspect in privacy, are not easily inspectable by their bearer and require the help of another set of eyes and hands. It is in this way that the sociality of tick checks is always already linked to questions of intimacy, sexuality, and the obscene.

For example, at a tick-borne disease prevention conference in the spring of 2011, an entomologist stepped up to the microphone during a question and answer session. Frustrated with the gap between concept and practice, and working on a hunch that most people do not do thorough enough tick checks, the entomologist said, "Without someone to check me, a tick guy like me needs a tick guy sized mirror." He proceeded to bend over, so that his rear faced the panel, and then mimed spreading his cheeks open, his head peering around his body as if looking into the imaginary mirror before him. The discomfort in the audience was palpable. One could only imagine that it was a discomfort operating on two levels: discomfort with the idea of checking one's own body in that way and discomfort with the idea of having to check someone else's body in that way. The entomologist's simple mime also reinforced the idea that ticks prefer hard-to-reach intimate places and that ticks checks are better performed by intimates than by the self, even if both practices might, at times, be perceived to be unpleasant.

However, as has been the theme of this chapter, revulsion and attraction are two sides of the same coin. Helped along in no small part by country legend Brad Paisley's song, "Ticks," which cleverly seeks to persuade a woman to walk into the sticks so he can check her for ticks, the term "tick checks" has also become a sexual innuendo with the same clinical valence of something like, "Let's play doctor." The salience of this term was confirmed during an interview with a male Lyme patient. After talking at length about hunting and camping and other outdoor activities, I asked the patient whether he performed tick checks and, transitioning from an up-until-then serious tone to one that was markedly mischievous, he responded, with a knowing smirk, "Only for fun." And in a letter penned in support of a Lyme advocacy group by a famous Hollywood actor who also happens to have been a Lyme patient, the actor wrote, "Tick checks are great foreplay. Enjoy them!" Vector-borne disease health officials had hoped to capitalize on the emerging colloquial traction of the term by coining the prevention message, "Get Naked," but I was told by a health official at another conference in the fall of 2010 that this idea was only too quickly given the kibosh by STD health officials who warned that anything having to do with nudity and sexuality was infringing on their public health marketing territory.

Given all of this, it is easy to see how tick checks can quickly become a sensitive subject between parents and children. As one patient I interviewed explained,

> When my son was a baby, we used to have what we called "tick patrol" and I would bring him in and strip him down every night and we would check every area of his body and I can tell you, I took a tick off his penis. I mean that's … I remember that … but I would check him constantly. But he's 18 now. I'm hoping … well, I tell him he has to check himself.

Like this mother, parents whom I spent time with often complained that once their children reached a certain age, they and their children no longer felt comfortable doing certain types of tick checks with each other. Even though they had taught their children to check themselves, they worried that they would not do them thoroughly enough or, more likely, that they would forego the check completely. As another mother asked, "Can you imagine getting a 12-year-old boy to take a tick check seriously?" On the other hand, limited tick checks (of the hair, back, and shoulders) very much remain within the bounds of family intimacy. One physician explained how his children, now teenagers, still asked to be checked for ticks because they just liked it. "It's one of the things that they grew up doing with me," he explained. In the end, the intimate tick checks that families enjoy and the more sexual tick checks that Brad Paisley croons about are not as thorough as the miming entomologist would like them to be, while the thorough tick checks that he advocates for are not the ones that most people want to do.

In addition to the limitations of when and where tick checks are considered appropriate, tick checks are also plagued by the problem of ticks' small size. The juvenile, or nymphal, stage of the blacklegged tick is the size of a period and is understood to be the primary vector of *Borrelia burgdorferi* to humans (Clover and Lane 1995; Diuk-Wasser *et al.* 2006; Embers *et al.* 2013). As demonstrated by the boy in the example above who conflated leaves with ticks, ticks *are* so small that they could be anywhere and anything, and, for all intents and purposes, they might as well be leaves. As one mother admitted, "We're very religious about checking them for ticks but I'm also, you know, they still roll around in the grass and hike in the woods and I have two boys. They both have long hair. If my older one gets a tick, I'm not going to find it, you know, he's got curly, long hair."

More disconcerting still is when the ambiguous *there* of the outside becomes the ambiguous *here* of the body. For example, several informants described the experience of watching a mole grow, only to discover too late that the mole was, in fact, a tick. By then, the tick had already had a full blood meal and was given plenty of time to transmit infection, its removal no longer an act of prevention but a mere detachment. Central to the experience and practice of tick checks, then, is the idea of *the one you do not find*. Because most Lyme disease cases are the result of a tick that was not found (or found too late), tick checks are haunted by the specter of their own inefficacy. That is, irrespective of how many ticks are found during any given tick check, they are always a reminder of the one tick that might not have been and, therefore, the one tick that might have mattered.

Oddly enough, the inefficacy of tick checks is the very thing that leads to their continuation, to their being performed again and again, for the limitations of realizing that a tick might not have been found is simultaneously the acceptance of the infinite possibility that there is *always* a tick to be found. It is a cycle propelled by absence rather than presence. Failure also inheres in the rest of the things that people do to keep ticks off them. A public health official I interviewed explained that although most tick prevention practices seem to be commonsensical, we "really don't know if most of them work." For example, in the case of the application of pesticides to lawns, this official said that, in the absence of relevant studies, the recommendation to do this merely operates on an assumption that lower tick populations translate to lower Lyme disease infection rates.[10] Among the patients with whom I spent time, however, I was not surprised to hear that, irrespective of outcome, many felt that they would rather do something that *might not work* than *nothing at all.* Indeed, if not everyone likes tick checks or believes that they are effective, then many, at least, have gotten used to doing them and, in doing them, have come to value their effects.

This section built on the previous section by examining how an environment that is increasingly immanent and less and less defined by the divide between inside and outside is *also* produced in and through individuals' practical engagement with it. In 1909, biologist Jacob von Uexkull coined the term *Umwelt*, or "environment-world," to give expression to the idea of a "surrounding world" (Agamben 2004: 40; Buchanan 2008: 147). Uexkull argued that, when it comes to the relationship between organisms and their environment, attention should be paid to "subjective universes," whereby each organism creates its own environment through interaction. As a result, "the environment" becomes "environments," with the potential for there to be as many environments as there are organisms (Buchanan 2008: 22). When it comes to Lyme disease, I have suggested that, in the context of the increasingly affective relationship between humans and their environments, the emerging bodily practices of tick bite prevention constitute the active building of new "environment-worlds." And the environment-world of tick bite prevention practice is one in which protecting the self is also a matter of knowing the other, and where tick checks, whether they work or not and although exacted on the individual body, are increasingly, if not incidentally, made meaningful across human relations.

Conclusion

Together, this chapter's three sections explored why a Lyme patient like Susan, who lives in nature and whose art is inspired by nature's "beauty," is also terrified of nature. As tick-borne diseases like Lyme disease become an increasing threat in the United States, individuals who live in Lyme endemic areas face the difficult task of negotiating the competing demands between their attraction to nature and their concerns over the health risks of a "toxic" environment, an environment that crosses the boundary between "inside" and "outside" and of which Lyme disease is just one small part. In doing so, these individuals must also navigate and make choices about which toxins – from bacterial pathogens to antibiotics to pesticides – are "less risky" than others. Drawing from interviews with and observations of Lyme patients, physicians, and scientists throughout the northeastern United States, I have argued that the experience of having and preventing Lyme disease can be better understood through the construct of an "epidemiology of affect," whereby individuals' feelings about nature inform their engagement with it and produce an emerging range of everyday prevention practices uniquely characterized by affective social relations. More broadly, this study highlights the importance of ethnographic attention to human experiences and practices in better understanding the changing landscape of environmental health.

NOTES

1 To protect the privacy of my informants, all names used in this chapter are pseudonyms.
2 Lyme disease is a tick-borne bacterial infection that was discovered in Lyme, Connecticut in 1982 (see Bulled and Singer, this volume). Since then, there has been heated debate over how to diagnose and treat it. While proponents of the "mainstream" standard of care claim that Lyme disease is easily diagnosed and treated, proponents of the "Lyme-literate" standard of care claim that diagnostic tests are unreliable and that Lyme disease can persist in the form of "chronic Lyme disease," a condition which mainstream proponents do not recognize but which Lyme-literate proponents argue should be treated with extended courses of antibiotics. In this chapter, I use "Lyme patient" to describe any patient who identifies with having or having had Lyme disease, irrespective of their medical history. Although most of the patients whom I interviewed and observed described experiences with Lyme disease marked by chronicity, I do not make a distinction between chronic Lyme disease and Lyme disease when referring to the ideas and experiences of these patients because most patients and Lyme-literate physicians understand chronic Lyme disease to be one point on the timeline of the Lyme disease experience and not a qualitatively different disease state from acute Lyme disease. Moreover, although patients often refer to themselves as chronic Lyme patients, they also perceive the use of this term by mainstream physicians as a means to distinguish them from what mainstream physicians perceive to be "real" Lyme patients. Because I am only interested in the ideas and experiences of my project's participants, the terms I use in this chapter reflect the positionality of the individuals who use them, as well as the social contexts in which they are used.
3 The research methods I used were a familiar anthropological combination of participant observation, unstructured and semi-structured interviews, and popular, academic, and virtual media analysis. As a participant observer, I shadowed physicians on either side of the standard of care divide, and I regularly attended critical sites of discourse and practice in the Lyme disease controversy, including patient support group meetings, scientific laboratory and public health meetings, fundraising events, and scientific conferences. In addition to conducting hundreds of informal interviews at these sites, I also conducted 145 semi-structured interviews with patients, physicians, scientists, health officials, politicians, and patient advocates. Finally, because a significant portion of Lyme disease discourse takes place online, I tracked the daily publication and circulation of relevant articles, blog posts, and listserv e-mails. Together, the data derived from the range of methods I used allowed me to piece together analytical insights into the lived experience of Lyme's controversy.
4 http://www.bmj.com/about-bmj/resources-readers/publications/epidemiology-uninitiated/1-what-epidemiology (accessed December 2, 2015).
5 I emphasize the phrase "end up" to underscore the contingency of the relationship between having Lyme disease and loving nature.
6 http://www.cdc.gov/media/pressrel/r010321.htm (accessed December 2, 2015).
7 http://www.cdc.gov/exposurereport/pdf/fourthreport.pdf (accessed December 2, 2015).
8 Chelation therapy is the ingestion or injection of a chemical compound that binds with metal ions. The result is a chemical complex that is water-soluble; it then enters the bloodstream and is excreted in the urine. While chelation therapy for heavy metal poisoning is used for acute cases in mainstream medicine, its popularity among some complementary, alternative, and integrative medicine practitioners for subclinical cases has been the subject of much scrutiny.

9 For some, the opposite is true. Another woman I interviewed said that she would not spray her yard because she did not want to be exposed to any more chemicals. But when I asked her if the same logic applied to her food, she replied, "No. A little funny, huh? Anything but. You know what, if I had all the money in the world, I'd probably eat organic but, to me, it's too expensive. Every once in a while I try and buy, like, chicken that doesn't have antibiotics or whatever in it. A lot of people say well you have to at least do the organic milk and I don't even do that."

10 To address this evidence gap, the CDC (Centers for Disease Control and Prevention) initiated a study in the spring of 2011 to test the relationship between a single lawn application and Lyme disease infection rates.

REFERENCES

Agamben, G. 2004. *The Open: Man and Animal.* Stanford, CA: Stanford University Press.

Beck, U. 1992. *Risk Society: Towards a New Modernity.* London: Sage.

Bennett, J. 1994. *Thoreau's Nature: Ethics, Politics, and the Wild.* Thousand Oaks, CA: Sage Publications.

Buchanan, B. 2008. *Onto-Ethologies: The Animal Environments of Uexküll, Heidegger, Merleau-Ponty, and Deleuze.* Albany, NY: SUNY Press.

Clover, J.R. and Lane, R.S. 1995. "Evidence Implicating Nymphal *Ixodes pacificus* (Acari: Ixodidae) in the Epidemiology of Lyme Disease in California." *American Journal of Tropical Medical Hygiene*, 53: 237–240.

Diuk-Wasser, M. *et al.* 2006. "Spatiotemporal Patterns of Host-Seeking *Ixodes scapularis* Nymphs (Acari: Ixodidae) in the United States." *Journal of Medical Entomology*, 43: 166–176.

Douglas, M. 1992. *Risk and Blame: Essays in Cultural Theory.* London: Routledge.

Edlow, J.A. 2003. *Bull's Eye: Unraveling the Medical Mystery of Lyme Disease.* New Haven, CT: Yale University Press.

Embers, M., Grasperge, B.J., Jacobs, M.B., and Philipp, M.T. 2013. "Feeding of Ticks on Animals for Transmission and Xenodiagnosis in Lyme Disease Research." *Journal of Visualized Experiments*, 78:1–19.

Harthorn, B.H. and Oaks, L. (Eds.) 2003. *Risk, Culture, and Health Inequality: Shifting Perceptions of Danger and Blame.* Berkeley, CA: University of California Press.

Hess, D.J. 1996. "Technology and Alternative Cancer Therapies: An Analysis of Heterodoxy and Constructivism." *Medical Anthropology Quarterly*, 10: 657–674.

Hoy, S. 1995. *Chasing Dirt: The American Pursuit of Cleanliness.* Oxford: Oxford University Press.

Lock, M. 1993. "Cultivating the Body: Anthropology and Epistemologies of Bodily Practice and Knowledge." *Annual Review of Anthropology*, 22: 133–155.

Louv, R. 2005. *Last Child in the Woods: Saving our Children from Nature-Deficit Disorder.* Chapel Hill, NC: Algonquin Books of Chapel Hill.

Mahmood, S. 2005. *Politics of Piety: The Islamic Revival and the Feminist Subject.* Princeton, NJ: Princeton University Press.

Nash, R. 2001. *Wilderness and the American Mind.* New Haven, CT: Yale University Press.

Petersen, A.R. and Lupton, D. 1999. *The New Public Health: Health and Self in the Age of Risk. St.* Leonards, Australia: Allen & Unwin.

Philippon, D.J. 2005. *Conserving Words: How American Nature Writers Shaped the Environmental Movement.* Athens: University of Georgia Press.

Pidgeon, N., Simmons, P., and Henwood, K. 2006. "Risk, Environment, and Technology." In P. Taylor-Gooby (Ed.), *Risk in Social Science.* Oxford: Oxford University Press.

Soper, K. 1995. *What is Nature?: Culture, Politics and the Non-Human*. Oxford: Blackwell.

Stafford, K. 2007. "Tick Management Handbook: An Integrated Guide for Homeowners, Pest Control Operators, and Public Health Officials for the Prevention of Tick-Associated Disease." Connecticut Agricultural Experiment Station, New Haven, CT.

Szasz, A. 2007. *Shopping Our Way to Safety: How We Changed from Protecting the Environment to Protecting Ourselves*. Minneapolis, MN: University of Minnesota Press.

Tomes, N. 1998. *The Gospel of Germs: Men, Women, and the Microbe in American Life*. Cambridge, MA: Harvard University Press.

Weintraub, P. 2008. *Cure Unknown: Inside the Lyme Epidemic*. New York: St. Martin's Griffin.

CHAPTER 10

Ecobiopolitics and the Making of Native American Reservation Health Inequities

Merrill Singer and G. Derrick Hodge

Introduction

Racism has a long environmental history in the United States. Its emergence and manifold expressions reflect the entwinement of four fundamental features of American society: cultural prejudice dating to the rise of the colonial encounter with indigenous peoples; structural inequality involving legal and everyday discrimination as social mechanisms that insure unequal access to wealth, status, and power; the spatial segregation of socially subordinate groups; and the externalization of key costs of capitalist industrial production onto vulnerable populations. Because the inherent and requisite inequalities of capitalism infiltrate every crevice of social and moral life, they are necessarily embodied in society's and the economy's relationship to the natural world (see Harvey 1997). Since at least the 1970s, activists and scholars have recognized that one way in which inequality is manifest (and reproduced) in the United States is via the targeted use and misuse of natural resources (cf. Environ. Summit II 2002; United Church of Christ 1987), and detailed analyses have demonstrated that this is

A Companion to the Anthropology of Environmental Health, First Edition. Edited by Merrill Singer.

the result of the process of production and consumption under capitalism (Schnaiberg 1980; Schnaiberg and Gould 1994).

Yet race is also a factor, whether as cause of, or merely justification for, health disparities and environmental injustices. Whether race or class is the primary driver of environmental inequality, Native American peoples have been the recipients of both class- and race-based violence, and have faced "an unfair burden of environmental justice issues" (Bienkowski 2012; see also LaDuke 1999). Historically, these issues are products of the fact that (a) reservations were often located by the government on what was deemed less valuable land; (b) some reservations were sparsely populated; (c) poverty and government pressure pushed some tribal governments to seek brokered deals with various polluting industries; (d) regulatory chicanery made some reservations exempt from many environmental laws and not fully under indigenous control; and (e) the hindered sovereignty of reservations left them vulnerable to environmental degradation including illicit toxic waste dumping (Brook 1998). Scholars and activists have labeled the result "ecocide" (Grinde and Johansen 1995). Unsurprisingly, this differential burden of environmental degradation has resulted in higher rates of morbidity and mortality among first nations (for one of many examples, see Williams and Collins 1995).

The following analysis demonstrates that the *ecobiopolitical* model of critical medical anthropology can illuminate the social origin of environmental threat and morbidity on Native American reservations. This approach is informed by a synthetic and holistic exploration of the linkages between power and social structure, nature–society relations, and health and the environment. The label "ecobiopolitics" draws needed attention to the complex entwinements across conceptual domains that underlie the making of human health and disease in the contemporary world.

Following a discussion of the ecobiopolitical model, we examine the historical and statistical profile of poor health and land-use conflicts on Native American reservations in the United States. The analysis then identifies three sources of environmental health threats: the location of polluting industries on or near reservations, the use of reservations for "legal" hazardous waste disposal, and covert waste dumping on tribal lands. We propose that the ecobiopolitical model within the critical medical anthropological paradigm can bridge the gap, decried by Brulle and Pellow (2006), between the known history of environmental racism and known health disparities among Native American communities.

The Ecobiopolitics and Environmental Racism

Central to the ecobiopolitical model is an historical understanding of the relationship between ecology and politics in the making of health. A key aspect of this relationship emerges from the ways that politics shapes control over land and resources, as well as how land (or place) is culturally constructed. This approach incorporates analyses of the economic requirements of capitalism and public-policy implementation (i.e., political economy). Health, in turn, is powerfully influenced directly by political economy (e.g., unequal access to food or medicine) and indirectly as mediated by socially impacted environments (e.g., industrial pollution; see Peet, Robbins, and Watts 2011).

Eric Wolf developed the concept of "ecobiopolitics" in 1972, integrating ecology and political economy in order to assess the "constantly shifting dialectic between society and land-based resources, and also within classes and groups within society itself" (Blaikie and Brookfield 1987: 17). During the 1980s cultural ecologists, ecological anthropologists, and rural development specialists used Wolf's ideas to develop the multidisciplinary approach of ***political ecology***. The contemporary economic system of concern to political ecology is late global capitalism, characterized by (a) a tiny but super-rich elite that controls most of the wealth; (b) a myopic capitalist focus on the ever-expanding treadmill of production and ceaseless profit making; (c) a governance structure that serves to enhance the wealth of the elite while controlling popular unrest using both stick and carrot mechanisms; (d) discursive and hegemonic cultural production that embeds ideologies and stereotypes into the dominant cultural logic; (e) the spatial segregation of socially subordinate groups that serves to warehouse or isolate surplus labor; and (f) the drive to externalize real production costs, according to which the burden of pollution and waste are primarily experienced by governments and by powerless communities (Baer, Singer, and Susser 2013). Thus, contemporary capitalism requires aggressive and often reckless and underregulated resource extraction, which in turn produces a constantly growing volume of toxic waste; this then requires the identification of dumping grounds for convenient waste product disposal, and media disinterest in identifying capitalist wealth and power as the actual source of much ill health.

What emerges from the ecobiopolitical perspective is recognition that health and well-being result from the interaction of physical bodies with hierarchical social bodies and environmental conditions. This understanding is based on structurally multisided or interscaler analysis of the linkages between micro settings and macro structures by way of intersectorial processes (Neumann 2005). Uniting ecological, political, and health factors into a single theoretical model facilitates an understanding of health as a reflection of the ways that social structures of inequality reshape environments that are detrimental to the health of subordinate populations, a patterns that well reflects environmental health patterns on Native American reservations.

Environmental racism involves two components. First, hazardous siting decisions are driven by economic factors and market dynamics: such facilities tend to be placed on cheap land, which, as a consequence of displacement and discrimination, is disproportionately occupied by low-income communities (Espeland 1993; Checker 2005). Second, marginalized communities, having been limited from full political participation by past and prevailing policies and practices, are less likely to launch effective resistance. And, because it often comes with some amount of desperately needed economic benefit, they may even welcome hazardous facilities (Scheer and Moss 2010).

The "racism" framing has proven useful – since it invokes ideals of justice that are well rooted in the American imaginary and that have considerable traction in both law and public morality – but its use has not been uncontested. Scholars have argued that "race" is not exclusively or even primarily the *cause* of the unequal distribution of toxic dumping or the (re)location of vulnerable populations. Rather, insatiable economic production processes in late capitalism create waste which is dumped in areas where communities have little political power to avoid it (see Beck 1995; Gould, Schnaiberg, and Weinberg 1996). Poor communities – *of whatever ethnicity* – are prime targets for these economic decisions.

Historical Background: Health and the Reservation Environment

The many factors that impact the health of over one million indigenous people living on reservations in the United States – poverty, discrimination, adverse coping mechanisms, and limited access to health care – have been the subject of a mountain of social scientific and medical research. Yet the impacted environment is a critical element that often is overlooked in assessments of Native American well-being. For example, the US Department of Health and Human Service's "Health Characteristics of the American Indian or Alaska Native Adult Population: United States, 2004–2008" (Barnes, Adams and Powell-Griner 2010) focuses on the effects of sociodemographic characteristics (e.g., education, poverty, health insurance), health-related behaviors (e.g., smoking, drinking, obesity), and health care utilization (e.g., contact with health care providers, immunizations) but fails to mention environmental (let alone political-ecological) factors in Native American health. The same pattern is found in literature reviews like Sandefur, Rindfuss, and Cohn's (1996) analysis of key trends in Native American health.

Clearly, material deprivation has been a dominant form of stratification under which indigenous American populations have suffered enormously. The median income of Native American households is $35,192 compared to $50,502 for the United States as a whole (American Community Survey 2011). The overall percentage of Native Americans living below the federal poverty line is 29.5 percent (American Community Survey 2011), making them among the poorest populations in the country. On reservations, the rate of poverty is even greater, reaching 35.7 percent (National Center for Education Statistics 2008). Living conditions on reservations are often severe, with 14 percent of homes lacking electricity, 20 percent lacking indoor plumbing, and 53 percent lacking telephone service (US Census Bureau 1995). Moreover, about 40 percent of on-reservation housing is structurally inadequate (Housing Assistance Council 2006).

This material inequality produces health disparities. In 2006 Native Americans had the second highest infant death rate in the country: 48.4 percent greater than the rate among white mothers (CDC 2012a). Further, Native American infants are two to three times more likely to die from sudden infant death syndrome (SIDS) than other infants (Office of Minority Health [OMH] 2005).

Several potentially lethal diseases are disproportionate among Native Americans. Indigenous people are twice as likely to die from diabetes, 60 percent are more likely to have a stroke, 30 percent are more likely to have high blood pressure, and 20 percent are more likely to have heart disease (OMH 2012). While the overall diabetes rate is 7 percent in the US population, it is 12.8 percent among Native Americans, with rates as high as 27.6 percent among Native Americans in southern Arizona (OMH 2005). A significantly higher percentage of Native Americans (36%) with heart disease die before the age 65 compared to only 15 percent among Caucasians (OMH 2012). Indigenous people also have disproportionately high death rates from liver disease and hepatitis and are four times more likely to die from tuberculosis than Caucasians (Jones 2006). Native adults are 30 percent more likely to have asthma than non-Hispanic whites (CDC 2012b). Treatment disparities related are also higher than for other US Americans (Indian Health Service 2013). As a result of these health deficits, Native American life expectancy is 4 years shorter than the national average (Sarche and Spicer 2008; Indian Health Service 2013).

The specific contribution of environmental factors in the health profile and health disparities of Native Americans, as well as of other poor communities in the United States, remains understudied (Brulle and Pellow 2006). The following discussion indicates that multiple industrial leaks, intentional dumping, and toxic emissions have poured massive quantities of hazardous materials onto reservations, producing a disproportionate burden of disease. As the ecological condition of the globe continues to deteriorate, struggle over natural resources continues to be a critical factor in indigenous health (Barboza 2013). The deadening effects of modern American capitalism are disproportionately distributed, just as are its benefits.

Indian Removal and the Siting of Reservations

The toxic and poor land quality of Native American lands is neither an historical accident nor the result of any cultural deficiency on their part, but rather is the result of aggressive westward economic expansion (Kahn 2012: 205). This process was calculated and unconcerned with indigenous well-being:

> When they withdraw themselves to the culture of a small piece of land, they will perceive how useless to them are their extensive forests, and will be willing to pare them off from time to time in exchange for necessaries for their farms and families. To promote this disposition to exchange lands, which they have to spare and we want, for necessaries, which we have to spare and they want, we shall push our trading uses, and be glad to see the good and influential individuals among them run in debt, because we observe that when these debts get beyond what the individuals can pay, they become willing to lop them off by a cession of lands. (Jefferson 1803)

Aside from the obvious intention to use debt manipulation to gain access to Native lands, implied in this letter is the idea that emergent capitalist society more effectively uses nature than do indigenous communities, providing a rationale for relocating Native Americans to less desirable land with presumably more limited resource potential. Thus, federal policy, including the Indian Removal Act of 1830, was designed to displace Native Americans from coveted land and to relocate them to areas seen as relatively "valueless by nineteenth-century standards" (Lewis 1994). Moral justifications were encoded into law.

Regulatory policies, and many treaties between the federal government and Native American peoples, reflect an American obsession with trying to reconcile economic and military conquest with an avowed respect for law. Military victories over Native Americans were routinely followed by "the charade ... of signing treaties that made the land transfers appear to be mutually agreed transactions" (Foner 2006). The internal colonialism that swept westward, destroying human communities, animal populations, and forestland, was not an accident of history, nor a singular unfortunate event; rather, it was the inevitable consequence of the economic logic that gripped that nation at that time and that continues to guide both domestic and foreign policy today.

Ideologies of Land

This logic finds expression as an ideology of nature that is antithetical to idea systems found among Native Americans (Hanlon 2008). Exemplary of this conflict, Nader and Gusterson (2007: 307) note a critical distinction between traditional Navajo understanding of the natural world and the views promoted by the nuclear industry which operates uranium mines on or near a number of reservations: "For the Navajo the land is sacred, life giving and sustaining ...; for the nuclear industry [Navajo] land ... is a wasteland ... Places the Navajo use for medicine and sacred ritual the nuclear industry classifies as wastelands."

In the same vein, Winona LaDuke (2010) has contrasted the capitalist industrial worldview with that of indigenous North American cultures. First, while many indigenous peoples hold that natural laws are preeminent, industrial capitalist ideology claims that humans are *entitled* to full dominion over the environment; though motivated by the needs of capitalist expansion, the colonizers justified this ethic with recourse to the creation account of Genesis, in which humanity is instructed to "subdue" and "dominate" all of creation (Genesis 1:28). Second, while indigenous societies view natural patterns as cyclical, capitalist industrial society is characterized by linear thinking and an endless commitment to growth. Third, while indigenous societies tend to see humans as *part* of nature, industrial society places humans outside of nature, and sees the latter as something that must be struggled with, conquered, and put to productive and profitable use. In the industrialist ethos, indigenous peoples were usually defined as a "barrier" to progress that must be removed, tamed, isolated, and controlled (Jacobs 2014). Finally, while indigenous societies often practiced some form of "conspicuous (re) distribution" (e.g., gaming traditions among many tribes), industrial society emphasizes accumulation.

Capitalism and Toxicity

Reservations as Wastelands: Externalizing Corporate Costs

The dominant economic model of neoliberalism provides disincentive: the producers of externalities lack an incentive to consider the adverse effects of their actions on others. One illustration is the health crisis facing the Keweenaw Bay Indian Community of the Lake Superior Band of Chippewa who live on the L'Anse Reservation on Michigan's Upper Peninsula. At issue for the Community is the Eagle Project, a nickel and copper mine being dug by the transnational Kennecott Utah Copper, part of the Rio Tinto Zinc conglomerate. The Eagle Project mine is on 1600 acres of land now owned by Kennecott that was part of lands given up by the Chippewa under pressure from the US government in 1842 (although the Chippewa retained the right to continue hunting, fishing, and gathering on the ceded land). Tribal concerns about water pollution from the mine stem from the method, sulfide mining, which extracts metals from sulfide ores. When the ores are crushed, the sulfides are exposed to air and water, catalyzing a chemical reaction that produces highly toxic sulfuric acid. The acid then drains into nearby rivers, lakes, and groundwater sources – a phenomenon called acid mine drainage (Bienkowski 2012). As a consequence of corporate lack of interest in health and government deregulation, "Native Americans have to contend with some of the worst pollution in the United States" (Bullard 2001).

A similar cause for concern for the Keweenaw Bay Community is found in the corporate despoiling of the St. Lawrence River in upper New York state and its impact on the indigenous Mohawk people. In the 1950s, various industries were attracted to the banks of the St. Lawrence because of the low-cost energy made available by the Moses–Sunders Power Project constructed by the US Army Corps of Engineers assigned to the Robert Moses–Robert H. Saunders Power Dam. Companies like Reynolds Metals, General Motors, and ALCOA – all of which make extensive use of carcinogenic and teratogenic polychlorinated biphenyls (PCBs) produced by the Monsanto Chemical Company – established factories along the river. Construction of the dam began with the eviction (in some cases by force) of 6500 predominantly Akwesasne Mohawks, and the flooding of six villages and three hamlets. Over time, the companies dumped thousands of pounds of toxic PCB contaminants into the St. Lawrence. Additionally, aluminum refining processes used along the river produced various other toxic substances, such as fluoride, which were emitted into the air through unfiltered smokestacks. General Motors ultimately was found by the Environmental Protection Agency (EPA) to be the largest PCB polluter, with 10 dump sites along the river within the company's 210-acre riverfront property. Unfortunately, even when gross negligence and civil or even criminal liability are established in court, the current "pro-business" mood of most state and federal legislators mean that corporations are not held responsible.

At the same time, General Motors also built open pits for depositing PCBs and other toxic chemicals. According to Christopher Amato, then assistant attorney general of New York, "The entire GM facility was utilized for dumping – they dumped all over the place … They never got permits from the state for these facilities" (quoted in Rae and Witherspoon 2001: 6a). PCBs released in water collect in fish species like salmon, bass, sturgeon, pike, and perch, longtime sources of protein among reservation residents. As a result, the area ultimately was designated as a "Great Lakes Area of Concern" – one of 43 toxic hotspots identified in a water quality agreement between the United States and Canada. Some areas along the St. Lawrence were designated Superfund sites, which ranked them among the nation's most hazardous spots. These include the Reynolds Metals and the ALCOA sites (EPA 2012a, 2012b). Over time, people living on the reservation began to link their rising incidence of illness with fish they ate from the now-polluted river. According to reservation resident John Bigtree, "Years ago … I raised 10 kids and we fished a lot. Then they got sick. They got upset stomachs, and some of them were throwing up. And I said, 'That's it.' We stopped eating fish out of the river" (quoted in Rae and Witherspoon 2001: 6a).

The Akwesasne have experienced various health consequences because of their prolonged exposure to PCBs. A study by Schell *et al.* (2008), for example, demonstrated a reduction in thyroid function among Akwesasne Mohawk youth directly related to serum levels of PCBs. Akwesasne men exposed to PCBs also have lower testosterone levels (Goncharov *et al.* 2009). Other, longer term consequences of PCB exposure, such as asthma and diabetes, continue to mount in the Akwesasne population because of the enduring presence of industrial pollutants on their reservation.

In the Pine Ridge Oglala Lakota Reservation in South Dakota, environmental threat comes from the combined impact of industrial, agricultural, and military sources:

> Many wells and much of the water and land on the Reservation are contaminated with pesticides and other poisons from farming, mining, open dumps, and commercial and governmental mining operations outside the Reservation. A further source of contamination is buried ordnance and hazardous materials from closed U.S. military bombing ranges on the Reservation … Scientific studies show that much of the High Plains/Oglala Aquifer [which begins underneath the Pine Ridge Reservation] has been contaminated with farming pesticides and commercial, factory, mining, and industrial contaminants. (Schwartz 2006)

As many as 14 percent of wells that tap the High Plains/Oglala Aquifer contain one or more pesticide or other industrial farm chemicals, most commonly altrazine, a herbicide used on cornfields that is a known hormone disruptor. Five percent of aquifer wells contain nitrate levels that exceed Environmental Protection Agency safety standards (Bair 2011).

The health threats of uranium mining represent particularly egregious expressions of this pattern of lack of interest in the health of Navajo land and peoples. During the Cold War, the United States government energetically encouraged uranium production as part of the nuclear arms race with the Soviet Union. Native knowledge about the environment was used to identify potential mine sites, and a number of corporations soon discovered large uranium deposits on and near a Navajo reservation, Although the Navajo were not warned of its radioactivity or its significant health risks, for over 42 years Navaho mine workers (paid at or below minimum wage) toiled as blasters, timber men, muckers, transporters, and millers. Their labor enabled the extraction of approximately four million tons of uranium ore from mines on the reservation, most of which was used to make nuclear weapons (beginning with the Manhattan Project) and produced significant profits for private corporations.

As the Cold War came to an end, most of the mines were abandoned, workers were laid off, and corporations left the area. Unfortunately, discarded radioactive materials were also abandoned:

> The companies often left behind radioactive waste piles and open tunnels and pits. Few bothered to fence the properties or post warning signs. Federal inspectors seldom intervened. Over the decades, Navajos inhaled radioactive dust from the waste piles, borne aloft by fierce desert winds. They drank contaminated water from abandoned pit mines that filled with rain. They watered their herds there, then butchered the animals and ate the meat. Their children dug caves in piles of mill tailings and played in the spent mines. (Pasternak 2006)

Such corporate behavior – and government indifference – is not the result of one or two irresponsible corporations; rather, it is part and parcel of the system of neoliberal industrial extraction and production. When Kerr–McGee shut down its uranium milling factory in Shiprock, New Mexico, "it left behind some 70 acres of raw uranium tailings containing approximately 80 percent of the original radioactivity found in uranium ore" (Johnston, Dawson, and Madsen 2007: 104). Abandoned tailings were piled in mounds within 60 feet of the San Juan River, the primary source of water for 15,000 people living in the Shiprock area. Other water sources also were put at risk. At Rio Puerco, the failure of a dam caused 93 million gallons of radioactive water and 1000 tons of contaminated sediment to be released into the river. At least 1700 reservation residents were affected by the severe contamination of the sole water source (Johnston, Dawson, and Medsen 2007).

Despite existing knowledge about the health risks of exposure to uranium, neither the mining companies nor the United States Atomic Energy Commission informed workers about the dangers. Neither did they implement safety procedures or provide protective equipment to minimize contamination (Brugge and Goble 2002; Panikkar and Brugge 2007). Nor were miners told about a 1950 Public Health Service study that had issued an ominous warning to uranium mine workers. That study, jointly initiated by the Colorado, Utah, New Mexico, and Arizona Health Departments, found that levels of radon in the Navajo region "exceeded expectations and concluded that results presented a rather serious picture" (Panikkar and Brugge 2007: 126). Mine owners had insisted that researchers who carried out the study should *not* inform workers of their findings. Moreover, in the early years of mine operation, few Navajo miners spoke English and few had had formal education, rendering them unable to learn from or contribute to mounting discussion of the health risks of radiation in the wider society. Navajo miners were not given preemployment health screenings, nor was there a medical program for the workers (Johnston, Dawson, and Madsen 2007).

Further, research has shown that radon accumulates in uranium mines, and its decay products (called "radon daughters") become lodged in workers' lungs, conveying large amounts of carcinogenic radiation to surrounding tissues. As a result of exposure and lack of protection, "Many miners died from radiation-related illnesses; some, unaware of harmful health effects, hauled contaminated rocks and tailings from local mines and mills to build homes for their families," thus resulting in further exposure (Frosch 2009). In other cases sand and crushed rock from uranium mines was used as flooring in Navajo homes (Pasternak 2006). The cancer death rate on the Navajo Reservation – which historically had been considerably lower than that of the general US population – began to increase in the 1960s and doubled from the early 1970s to the late 1990s (Gilliland *et al.* 2000). Over 500 Navajo uranium miners died of lung cancer from 1950 to 1990 as miners ran a risk of developing lung cancer at a rate that was 28 times greater than that of Navajos not exposed to uranium (Mulloy *et al.* 2001; Daitz 2003). A population-based case-control study by Samet *et al.* (1984) assessed the relationship between uranium mining and lung cancer by examining 32 cases of lung cancer in Navajo men listed with the New Mexico Tumor Registry between 1969 and 1982. For each case two controls with nonrespiratory cancer were recruited. Among the 32 Navajo lung cancer patients, 72 percent had been employed as uranium miners, whereas none of the control cases had worked in this industry. The researchers concluded that their findings "demonstrate that in a rural nonsmoking population most of the lung cancer may be attributable to one hazardous occupation" (Samet *et al.* 1984: 1481).

Lung cancer among miners was not the only health cost of uranium mining on the Navajo Reservation. Heightened levels of miscarriages, cleft palates, and other birth defects have been associated with exposure to a uranium polluted-environment. A study of birth defects, stillbirths, and other adverse birth outcomes among over 13,000 Navajos born at the Public Health Service/Indian Health Service Hospital in Shiprock, New Mexico (Shields *et al.* 1992) found a statistically significant relationship between uranium operations and unfavorable birth outcomes among mothers living near mine tailings or dumps. Birth defects were also significantly higher when either parent worked in the Shiprock electronics assembly plant. The morbidity and mortality that occurred on the Navajo Reservation at the hands of the uranium industry, and as a consequence of government indifference, could have been significantly lessened had Navajo miners not been perceived as cheap disposable labor and their land (aside from the uranium) as essentially worthless wasteland.

It is not just the type of material that is toxic, but also the manner of its extraction. Hydraulic facturing (fracking) emerged in the 1940s as means of extracting "extreme energy" (fossil fuels that could not be obtained with conventional drilling methods) and has led to the widespread use of this technology in energy production on Native American land and elsewhere. In North Dakota, for instance, fracking has produced an energy boom but also, as elsewhere, concerns about environmental damage and associated health consequences. Chemical fluids used for fracking have the potential to enter potable water sources, and through chemical spills and evaporation of wastewater escape into the air. An investigative reporter at the *New York Times* (Urbina 2011) obtained thousands of internal documents from the Environmental Protection Agency, state regulators, and fracking companies showing that the dangers to the environment and health are significantly greater than is usually reported. The documents indicate that among other environmental risks, fracking waste, discharged into rivers that supply drinking water, contains radioactivity at levels far higher than federal regulators maintain is safe. Cancer-causing chemicals like naphthalene, benzyl chloride, and formaldehyde have been found to be in use at about one-third of fracking sites (Darling and SkyTruth.org 2013).

Release of this kind of information has given credence to apprehensions on reservations like Fort Berthold, home to Mandan, Hidatsa, and Arikara peoples in western North Dakota. The Fort Laramie Treaty of 1851 created a 12 million-acre reservation, but continual appropriatation has dwindled its extent to only 400,000 acres, on which there are now 500 oil wells. Conventional extraction methods cannot access all of the reservation's Bakken Shale oil, an enormous deposit trapped between layers of rock two miles below the surface. But fracking has suddenly made this arid reservation land potentially valuable again. According to Marilyn Hudson, head of the Three Affiliated Tribes Museum, because of the wells "the relationship to the land is being destroyed. We are looking at the death of our tribal society as we knew it" (quoted in Gibson 2012a; also see Gibson 2012b).

Of special concern from the standpoint of the environment is the so-called Halliburton loophole, named after the corporation that patented an early version of hydraulic fracturing. Enacted during the George W. Bush administration, the loophole exempts the oil and gas industry from the requirements of the Safe Drinking Water Act. The Environmental Awareness Committee (2011), formed by concerned residents of the Fort Berthold Reservation, has filed a human rights brief with the United Nations asserting:

> The environmental dangers that have come with the oil drilling are evident throughout the reservation with spills, leaks and accidents already occurring everywhere ... [Having] no current environmental department in place to monitor and regulate the oil industry has led to illegal dumping of wastewater in several areas of the reservation with minimal to no fines being issued ... The Mandan, Hidatsa and Arikara peoples have suffered tragedy after tragedy over the course of the past few centuries and yet we remain here today, struggling to keep our culture and traditions intact. But now our water is at stake. Water is life.

Toxic Trade and Reservation Poverty

In addition to toxic emissions, a significant source of environmental health risk on reservations is their use as waste disposal sites. A growing body of research shows that living near a toxic waste site is a critical health threat

(Chatham-Stephens *et al.* 2013). The Nuclear Information and Resource Service (2006), a networking center for citizens and environmental activists, notes:

> Low-income and minority communities are disproportionately targeted with facilities and wastes that have significant and adverse human health and environmental effects. This places the burdens of society on those who are most vulnerable. These communities are at a tremendous economic and political disadvantage over the decision-making process that is dominated by large, wealthy corporations and/or government agencies.

Reservations are appealing hazardous waste disposal sites because indigenous Americans have less access to the political and economic power needed in order to effectively resistance dumping. Corporate interest in hazardous waste disposal on reservations has indeed elicited interest among some tribal leaders and other reservation residents, but poverty, unemployment, and other pressing social problems have hampered these efforts. Further, some corporations have coopted reservation heads with private financial entitlements, and a number of tribal governments have embraced the idea of generating revenue through brokered deals with the government, waste companies, and polluting industries. As Lopez (2004) asserts with specific reference to nuclear waste, however, in the view of tribal and other opponents to such a course, "No matter how pretty a picture the government paints about their [*sic*] "benevolent" efforts to improve the economic development of the reservations, this policy is virtually a bribe to try to coerce Native tribes into taking nuclear waste [off] of the hands of the government."

In recent years, corporations have courted tribal governments by coopting the green movement's language about mitigating global warming through the use of alternative energy sources. In part, this new approach involves proposals for waste incinerators labeled as "renewable energy" and "recycling projects." Various companies seek Native American partners for the use of pyrolysis, gasification, and plasma arc technologies as a way to (allegedly) eliminate and recycle all types of waste as a source of renewable energy. Promoters claim that these approaches are pollution free, since they do not produce emissions and hence are a "green" alternative to polluting waste incineration. Environmentalists have rejected such claims by arguing that they are merely thinly veiled "green washing" and that "these technologies are 'incinerators in disguise' that heat the waste materials and then burn the gases that are called 'syngas.' This combustion process is the incineration that results in emissions of toxic and criteria pollutants into the air, including dioxins, highly toxic chemicals linked to a wide range of illnesses including cancer [and] reproductive, developmental and immunological diseases" (Norrell 2011).

Thus, through rhetorical and financial manipulation, corporations who wish to externalize the real costs of their toxic waste are able to silence what little resistance Native Americans might otherwise offer.

Illegal Hazardous Dumping on Reservations

In addition to legal dumping schemes, the hindered sovereignty of reservations leaves them vulnerable to unauthorized and covert toxic waste dumping via midnight dumping or Native entrepreneurs (Brook 1998). "Midnight dumpers" are corporations and individuals who secretly deposit waste on Native American lands without seeking or receiving tribal approval or even notifying indigenous residents. An example of this was Ford Motor Company's dumping of paint sludge and other chemicals from its factory in Mahwah, in northern New Jersey, in a remote mountain section of Ringwood that is home to the Ramapough people. An investigative journalist located paint sludge near homes, in parks, in the watershed, and near public water supplies, and conducted house-to-house documentation of health complaints among the Ramapough. Laboratory tests found lead, arsenic, and xylenes in the sludge, in some cases 100 times the levels the federal government deems safe. Tests indicated that the contamination was spreading (Barry *et al.* 2005).

The area in which the Ramapough live was so contaminated with industrial waste that during the 1980s the EPA designated the Ringwood Mines landfill as a Superfund site. Initial cleanup efforts were so inadequate that the area subsequently had to be returned to the Superfund list. In late winter 2006, 600 Ramapough, led by Wayne Mann, filed a mass tort suit (*Mann vs. Ford*) against the Ford Motor Company, its contractors, and the Borough of Ringwood. Having used its deep corporate pockets to extend an expensive legal process, Ford eventually settled the suit with the Ramapough for a meager payout of $12.5 million, though legal observers had assumed that the liability would be in the billions (Exposed 2011).

Even companies with legal contracts for industrial or municipal waste disposal sometimes use reservations as unauthorized dumpsites. On the Torres Martinez Cahuilla Indian Reservation in the Coachella Valley of California, illegal dumping eventually reached

> crisis levels as unscrupulous waste haulers used the open desert land as a dumping ground outside the reach of state regulatory agencies. Illegal dump operators burned massive amounts of waste, creating plumes of smoke that clouded the skies and forced schools to close. New dumpsites appeared overnight on remote reservation roads. Despite persistent efforts, the tribe's staff were unable to stem the tide of trash. (EPA 2008)

The second type of illicit dumpers identified by Brook (1998) are tribal members motivated by private profit or personal convenience, as in the enormous unofficial dump that developed on the Navajo reservation near the airport in Window Rock, Arizona after World War II. Eventual cleanup of the site involved the removal of 400 cubic yards of trash composed of everything from thousands of disposable diapers, to broken televisions and refrigerators, to two cars dating to the 1930s. The dump contained multiple layers of garbage in a ravine 40 feet deep and 100 feet long. It is estimated that the site is one of over 400 illegal dumps on the reservation (Donovan 1997).

A third category that we would add to Brook's typology is illicit government dumping, such as the Cold War era Department of Defense disposal of 1500 55-gallon drums filled with military materials (e.g., incinerated metals) and explosive devices into Lake Superior, near the home of the Red Cliff Band of Lake Superior Chippewa. The drums had been taken by barge onto the lake and pushed into the water where they lay on the lake bottom for many years. Efforts to remove the drums by the Red Cliff Band were severely hampered by the high cost of such removal (Simonson 2013).

In addition to the multiple health risks created by the various forms of toxic waste dumping, this activity threatens tribal sovereignty by delegitimizing the right of tribes to set their own internal policies, and by providing a pretext for paternalistic federal government intervention to address tribal failure to maintain health and safety. Since the government itself has engaged in such dumping while also hampering the ability of reservations to control their borders, the dilemma of illicit dumping exemplifies the broader ecobiopolitics confronting indigenous peoples.

Resilience, Reworking, and Resistance

Another aspect of environmental racism is the pattern of participatory injustice according to which, in the case of Native Americans, some people are accorded little say in what happens to environmental conditions. "Past development in Indian Country was the old formula where companies came in and built projects, but only leased the land and did not include the tribe as equity partners … That old paradigm left us with all the social and environmental costs and none of the economic benefits" (David Lester, a member of the Muscogee Creek Tribes, quoted in Paskus 2010). A similar pattern prevails in federal regulation of environmental conditions on Native American reservations. For example, Kloeckner (2012: 10057), observes that the partnership between the United States and Native America tribes "in regulating pesticide pollution in Indian country under the Federal Insecticide, Fungicide, and Rodenticide Act is weak, dysfunctional, and dominated by the federal government."

One consequence of the layered history of physical, discursive, and structural violence endured by indigenous people is that they can be forced into no-win situations in which they must make choices among a very narrow set of potentially ominous possibilities. While it is critical to pay close attention to "human agency in the transformation of the complex, interacting web that characterizes the environment" (Turshen 1989: 17), decisions often are not made under optimal conditions. Political arrangements, "including the force of structural factors (such as structural violence or the social construction of 'risk environments'), do not always allow people to act in accord with their [best] intentions [or interests]. Rather, they select behaviors among those that are possible within structurally imposed constraints, some of which may be quite risky" (Baer, Singer, and Susser 2013: 291).

Coe and Jordhus-Lier (2011) label this "constrained agency," based on the distinction made by Katz (2004) between resilience, reworking, and resistance strategies of structurally subordinated populations. "Resilience" refers to the small acts of "getting by" that help both individuals and groups cope with everyday burdens but do not directly challenge existing unequal social relations (e.g., kin networks that assist family members through economic and personal crises). "Reworking" refers to an intermediate strategy that reflects people's struggles to improve their material conditions, such as the health, dental, social, and development services funded by gaming in the Shakopee Mdewakanton Sioux Community in Minnesota. Like resilience, reworking – or what Baylor (2007) has called "normal politics" – does not challenge reigning structures but rather seeks small realignments in power relations that facilitate a somewhat fairer access to resources (Singer 1995). In the case of the Shakopee Mdewakanton Sioux (2012), tribal monies are even used to fund development initiatives in neighboring non-Native communities. Finally, "resistance" refers to direct challenges to dominant power relations, such as the 1972 seizure of the Bureau of Indian Affairs national headquarters, the 1969 occupation of Alcatraz Island, and the 1973 uprising at Wounded Knee.

Native American resistance in defense of traditional lands can be seen at multiple sites. In Florida, the Miccosukee Tribe has been engaged in a pitched legal struggle to protect their 9-mile tract of the Everglades from efforts by the South Florida Waste Management District and the State of Florida to pump phosphorous-rich water (from fertilizer runoff from sugar fields) into swamplands. The Miccosukee are aware of a study by the Centers for Disease Prevention and Control to measure the correlation between fish consumption from local waters and high levels of mercury in Native Americans' blood. One hundred adult tribal representatives were found to have mercury levels ranging between 0.2 and 13.8 µg/L (compared to a baseline of 0.5 µg/L in unexposed individuals). Mercury in the Everglades is largely the result of emissions of coal- and oil-fired electrical power plants, municipal solid waste incinerators, medical waste incinerators, and coal-fired cement kilns (Roe 2003). Miccosukee concern about phosphorous is based on studies showing that it has been found to increase the proliferation of cattails that push out other plants and make the area uninhabitable by many animal species, and, in this way, threaten the Miccosukee way of life as Everglade dwellers. Despite threats from Governor Jeb Bush while he was in office, the Miccosukee remain on their land, which they continue to attempt to protect from the ongoing degradation of the Everglades.

Across the country from the Everglades, the Moapa Band of Paiutes living on the Moapa River Reservation in Arizona have been subjected to the health and lifestyle impacts of coal-ash air pollution emitted by the Reid Gardner coal-fired power plant. The plant with its giant smokestacks billowing various contaminants and particulate matter is sited just 400 yards from the reservation. Residents complain of breathing and other health-related problems, and of being imprisoned in their homes when the ash is flowing over the reservation. In the words of Chairman of the Band William Anderson, who has led resistance to the Reid Gardner plant, "Our children are losing more than their health because of the power plants; they're losing their culture … There are too many mornings when our elders can't have a morning walk outside, too many afternoons when our kids stay indoors because of bad air" (Anderson 2011).

In 2005, the Onondaga Nation filed a case against New York arguing that the state had repeatedly violated treaties signed with the Onondaga, resulting in the extensive loss of land (from 2.5 to 6900 acres) and massive environmental pollution. A core issue of this filing was the pollution of Onondaga Lake, which has become one of the most polluted inland bodies of water in the United States. From 1946 until the 1970s, the lake, which is located northwest of Syracuse and is deemed sacred among the Onondaga, was a dumping ground for mercury by the Honeywell corporation, known for its production of home thermostats. Sediments at the bottom of the lake have been found to be contaminated with polychlorinated biphenyls, pesticides, creosotes, heavy metals, polycyclic aromatic hydrocarbons, chlorinated benzenes, and BTEX compounds like benzene. Unsafe levels of pollution in the lake led to the banning of ice harvesting at the beginning of the twentieth century, with swimming being banned in the 1940s, and subsequently fishing as well (Matthews, Effler, and Matthews 2000). The Onondaga case was dismissed, as were their appeals to the Second Circuit Court and the Supreme Court. Denied all options by US courts aligned with the notion of supreme power being invested in the nation/state, and treaties notwithstanding, the Onondaga filed a petition, now pending, with the Inter-American Court of Human Rights, the human rights arm of the pan-regional Organization of American States (OAS). According to Traditional Chief of the Onondaga Nation, Todadaho Sid Hill, "We understand that the U.S. does not adhere to the OAS … But I don't know where we go. We've exhausted our avenues" (quoted in Tullo 2014).

Another expression of Native America resistance to ecocide by the energy industry is Diné Care, a Navajo nongovernmental organization that works with several Navajo communities. Exemplary was the group's struggle against the Desert Rock coal-fire plant in collaboration with another Navajo group called Doodá Desert Rock. According to Elouise Brown, president of Doodá, the purpose of the group is "to defend and preserve our lands, water, air and people – not for ourselves but for generations to come. Our core philosophy is to protect our future from within – not with corporate bias, political influence or self-destructive economic development" (Brown 2007).

The struggle at Desert Rock dates to the 1970s when the Peabody Western Coal company bought land in the Black Mesa area of Arizona to develop a coal mine. The deal was engineered by a former US attorney who officially represented the Hopi but was covertly working for Peabody (Paskus 2010). The result was that 10,000 people were displaced from their homes on the land designated for the strip mine. To meet its needs, the mine annually pumped over 4000 acre-feet of groundwater, sending coal slurry 273 miles by pipeline to the Mohave Generating Station. Such a quantity of water extraction dropped the water level in the Navajo aquifer and dried up local wells.

The genesis of the Desert Rock plant was a Navajo desire to control energy development on the reservation in order to avoid cases like Peabody. The 1500 megawatt Desert Rock facility was intended to produce a significant amount of electricity for the reservation and for sale to others. The tribe was to own up to half the plant, the other half being owned by Sithe Global, an international company engaged in the construction, acquisition, and operation of electric generation facilities. Yet from the beginning, "the Navajo tribal government's approach did little to reassure community members that Desert Rock would be different from past projects involving outside companies" (Paskus 2010).

Diné Care and other reservation activists organized demonstrations, including a blockade of Sithe vehicles and occupation of a protest camp at the plant's building site. Despite this activism and continued grass-roots opposition, in July 2008 the EPA concluded that Desert Rock would not worsen pollution in the Four Corners area, and therefore issued an air quality permit. This decision reflects what the Environmental Research Foundation has referred to as the "regulatory-industrial complex." In the assessment of the Foundation (1991), "there is not a venal uncaring waste industry being held in check by a government that is aggressively protecting the environment. There is in fact a venal uncaring waste industry being supported and assisted by the federal government."

Perhaps in response to Native activism, after the announcement of the EPA decision the state of New Mexico, which opposed the project, pointed out that the region already had three coal plants and tens of thousands of oil and gas wells. The health impacts of these facilities have been witnessed over the years by health care providers like Adela Begaye:

> Today, we count four decades that contaminants from these three big coal plants have been pouring into the air in our region.... Today we have Head Start teachers asking for training to administer asthma medications to three- and four-year-olds. Today we have respiratory issues as a top reason for local hospital emergency room visits in a very rural area. (Begaye 2012)

Within a year of its initial decision, the EPA withdrew its air permit. Shortly thereafter, the Bureau of Indian Affairs similarly withdrew its support for the facility. As a result of continued protest and in light of these setbacks, the Desert Rock power plant lost its momentum and was terminated.

As this case and multiple others demonstrate, not all Native Americans have responded passively to environmental racism. In different times and places, tribes have variously used resilience, reworking, and resistance strategies, as well as a combination of these, sometimes in partnership with environmental and non-reservation citizen groups. These confrontations constitute contemporary expression of a 400-year multisited struggle for the integrity of their land by indigenous people.

Conclusion: Anthropology and the Ecobiopolitics of Indian Reservations

Health on Native American Reservations – as elsewhere – is the product of complex interactions of multiple factors. On the surface, these are environmental, biological, social, historical, racial, and political, but beneath these is the economic imperative to accumulate wealth through dispossession, differentiation, and uneven geographical development (Smith 1992, 1996, 2008; Harvey 1997). Analyses of any form of stratification, especially race, ethnicity, and geography, must first consider the requirements of contemporary American capitalism – the urgent need for constant expansion in order to avoid economic crises, the frantic search for new resources, and the desire to obscure the true environmental consequences of corporate behavior through covert dumping practices and the externalization of costs. We have argued that environmental racism certainly does take full advantage of race-based divisions in order to accumulate wealth, but its primary engine is not some nebulous and unexplained cultural phenomenon of racism, but rather the economic imperatives of late capitalist accumulation.

To date, however, most assessments of health on reservations and causal factors shaping the health characteristics of Native Americans have been limited to consideration of poverty and health care utilization, lifestyle and personal behavior (e.g., drinking and drug use, diet and exercise, sexual activity, automobile accidents, interpersonal violence), and mental health issues (e.g., psychological distress, suicide, homicide). This is to be expected, as the dominant ideology of individualism causes even well-intentioned people to search for causes in personal decisions and not in structural constraints. Thus, the roles of structured power relations, the decimation of the environment, and collaborative government/corporate actions – as well as the inherent environmental racism that has justified such iniquities, even when it has not motivated them – have not been primary or even secondary objects of consideration.

The analytic concept of ecobiopolitics accentuates the deep impress of political economy on health as mediated by the environment, drawing attention to critical factors whose influences are often overlooked, understudied, or elided. It is surely not an overstatement to assert that health is at once always environmental, always biological, and always political – and above all, always economic. In the case of Native Americans, ecobiopolitics has entailed a prolonged struggle for land and sovereignty in which public discourses about, and treatment of, Native American land has been a critical health determinant.

REFERENCES

American Community Survey. 2011. "Selected Population Profile in the United States." American Fact Finder. US Bureau of the Census. http://factfinder2.census.gov/faces/tableservices/jsf/pages/productview.xhtml?src=bkmk.

Anderson, W. 2011. "Pollution Is a Fact of Life When Living next to the Reid Gardner Plant." By William Anderson, chairman of the Moapa Band of Paiutes. Western Environmental Law Center, November 6. http://www.westernlaw.org/article/pollution-fact-life-when-living-next-reid-gardner-plant-william-anderson-chairman-moapa-band (accessed December 2, 2015).

Baer, H., Singer, M., and Susser, I. 2013. *Medical Anthropology and the World System*. Westport, CT: Greenwood.

Bair, J. 2011. "Running Dry on the Great Plains." *New York Times*, op-ed, November 30 http://www.nytimes.com/2011/12/01/opinion/polluting-the-ogallala-aquifer.html?_r=0 (accessed December 2, 2015).

Barboza, T. 2013. "Water War between Klamath River Farmers, Tribes Poised to Erupt." *Los Angeles Times*, May 7. http://www.latimes.com/news/local/la-me-klamath-20130507,0,1265691.story (accessed December 2, 2015).

Barnes, P., Adams, P., and Powell-Griner, E. 2010. *Health Characteristics of the American Indian or Alaska Native Adult Population: United States, 2004–2008*. National Health Statistics Report No. 2010. Washington, DC: US Department of Health and Human Services.

Barry, J., Layton, M.J, Nussbaum, A., Trombone, T., Washburn, L., Williams, B., and Franklin, T.F. 2005. "The Feds, the Mob: Making a Wasteland." *The Record*, October 2. http://www.northjersey.com/news/environment/specialreports/Making_a_wasteland_Ford_the_feds_the_mob.html (accessed December 2, 2015).

Baylor, T. 2007. "The American Indian Movement's Strategic Choices: Environmental Limitations and Organizational Outcome." Proceedings of the Seventh Native American Symposium, November 1–2. Southeastern Oklahoma State University. http://www.se.edu/nas/files/2013/03/NAS-2007-Proceedings-Baylor.pdf (accessed December 8, 2015).

Beck U. 1995. *Ecological Enlightenment: Essays on the Politics of the Risk Society*. New York: Humanities Press.

Begaye, A. 2012. "40 Years of Coal-Burning Power Plants on Navajo Land." *Indian Country*, April 27. http://indiancountrytodaymedianetwork.com/2012/04/27/40-years-coal-burning-power-plants-navajo-land (accessed December 8, 2015).

Bienkowski, B. 2012. "Pollution, Poverty and People of Color: A Michigan Tribe Battles a Global Corporation." *Scientific American*. http://www.scientificamerican.com/article.cfm?id=pollution-michigan-tribe-battle-global-corp&page=2 (accessed December 2, 2015).

Blaikie, P. and Brookfield, H. 1987. *Land Degradation and Society*. London: Routledge.

Brook, D. 1998. "Environmental Genocide: Native Americans and Toxic Waste." *American Journal of Economics and Sociology*, 57(1): 105–113.

Brown, E. 2007. "Doodá Desert Rock!" *Earth First Journal*. http://earthfirstjournal.org/article.php?id=288.

Brugge, D. and Goble, R. 2002. "The History of Uranium Mining and the Navajo People." *American Journal of Public Health*, 92(9): 1410–1419.

Brulle, R.J. and Pellow D. 2006. "Environmental Justice: Human Health and Environmental Inequalities." *Annual Review of Public Health*, 27: 103–124.

Bullard, R. 2001. "It's Not Just Pollution." Poverty, Health and the Environment. http://www.ourplanet.com/imgversn/122/bullard.html (accessed December 2, 2015).

CDC (Centers for Disease Control and Prevention). 2012a. *American Indian and Alaska Native Populations. Minority Health*. http://www.cdc.gov/minorityhealth/populations/REMP/aian.html (accessed December 2, 2015).

CDC (Centers for Disease Control and Prevention). 2012b. *Summary Health Statistics for U.S. Adults*. http://www.cdc.gov/nchs/data/series/sr_10/sr10_252.pdf (accessed December 2, 2015).

Chatham-Stephens, K., Caravanos, J., Ericson, B., Sunga-Amparo, J., Susilorini, B., Sharma, P., Landrigan, P., and Fuller, R. 2013. "Burden of Disease from Toxic Waste Sites in India, Indonesia, and the Philippines in 2010." *Environmental Health Perspectives*. doi: 10.1289/ehp.1206127.

Checker, M. 2005. *Polluted Promises: Environmental Racism and the Search for Justice in a Southern Town*. New York: New York University Press.

Coe, N. and Jordhus-Lier, D. 2011. "Constrained Agency? Re-Evaluating the Geographies of Labour." *Progress in Human Geography*, 35(2): 211–233.

Daitz, B. 2003. "A Doctor's Journal; Navajo Miners Battle a Deadly Legacy of Yellow Dust." *New York Times*, May 13. http://www.nytimes.com/2003/05/13/health/a-doctor-s-journal-navajo-miners-battle-a-deadly-legacy-of-yellow-dust.html?pagewanted=all&src=pm (accessed December 2, 2015).

Darling, D. and SkyTruth.org. 2013. "Cancer-Causing Chemicals Used in 34% of Reported Fracking Operations." Indigenous Environmental Network. http://www.

ienearth.org/cancer-causing-chemicals-used-in-34-of-reported-fracking-operations/ (accessed December 2, 2015).

Donovan, B. 1997. "Navajo Tribe Embarks on a Long-Term Cleanup." *High Country News*, August 18. http://www.hcn.org/issues/112/3563 (accessed December 2, 2015).

Environmental Awareness Committee. 2011. Fort Berthold – Three Affiliated Tribes Environmental Awareness Committee brief to Catarina de Albuquerque. http://treaty council.org/PDF/MHA%20Nation%20EAC%20submission%20to%20the%20UN%20 Rapportuer%20on%20Water%20%5BFinal%5D.pdf.

Environmental Research Foundation. 1991. "The Poisoners Invade Indian Country." *Rachel's Hazardous Waste News* #239. http://www.ejnet.org/rachel/rhwn239.htm (accessed December 2, 2015).

EPA (Environmental Protection Agency). 2008. *Pacific Southwest, Region 9: Tribes.* http://www.epa.gov/SoCal/tribes.html.

EPA (Environmental Protection Agency). 2012a. *Reynolds Metals Company. Region 2 Superfund.* http://www.epa.gov/region2/superfund/npl/reynoldsmetals/.

EPA (Environmental Protection Agency). 2012b. *Aluminum Company of America. Region 2 Superfund.* http://www.epa.gov/region2/superfund/npl/aluminumcompany/.

Espeland, W. 1993. "Power, Policy and Paperwork: The Bureaucratic Representation of Interests." *Qualitative Sociology*, 16(4): 297–317.

Exposed. 2011. "The Cochran Firm Defrauds Native American Clients to Save Ford." http://freespeakblog.blogspot.com/2011/08/cochran-firm-defrauds-native-american. html (accessed December 2, 3015).

Foner, E. 2006. "Review of *How the Indians Lost their Land: Law and Power on the Frontier.*" *London Review of Books*, February 9. http://www.ericfoner.com/reviews/ 020906lrb.html (accessed December 2, 3015).

Frosch, D. 2009. "Uranium Contamination Haunts Navajo Country." *New York Times*, July 26. http://www.nytimes.com/2009/07/27/us/27navajo.html?_r=0 (accessed December 2, 3015).

Gibson, J. 2012a. "Shale Oil Boom in North Dakota is Impacting Native Americans Especially Hard." *Indigenous Environmental Network*, December 3. http://www.ienearth. org/shale-oil-boom-in-north-dakota-impacting-native-americans-especially-hard/

Gibson, J. 2012b. "How the North Dakota Fracking Boom Shook a Family." *Guardian Environmental Network*, December 4. http://www.guardian.co.uk/environment/ 2012/dec/04/north-dakota-fracking-boom-family (accessed December 2, 3015).

Gilliland, F., Hunt, W. Pardilla, M., and Key, C. 2000. "Uranium Mining and Lung Cancer among Navajo Men in New Mexico and Arizona, 1969–1993." *Journal of Occupational and Environmental Health*, 42: 278–283.

Goncharov, A., Rej, R., Negoita, S., Schymura, M., Santiago-Rivera, A., Morse, G., the Awkwesasane Task Force on the Environment, and Carpenter, D. 2009. "Lower Serum Testosterone Associated with Elevated Polychlorinated Biphenyl Concentrations in Native American Men." *Environmental Health Perspectives*, 117: 1454–1460.

Gould, K., Schnaiberg, A., and Weinberg, A. 1996. *Local Environmental Struggles: Citizen Activism in the Treadmill of Production.* Cambridge: Cambridge University Press.

Grinde, D. and Johansen, B. 1995. *Ecocide of Native America: Environmental Destruction of Indian Lands and Peoples.* Santa Fe, NM: Clear Light.

Hanlon, S. 2008. "A Non-Indian Entity is Polluting Indian Waters: 'Water' Your Rights to the Waters and 'Water' Ya Gonna Do About It." *Montana Law Review*, 69(1): 174–226.

Harvey, D. 1997. *Justice, Nature, and the Geography of Difference.* Malden, MA: Blackwell.

Housing Assistance Counci.l 2006. *Housing on Native American Lands.* http://www. dcat.net/workshoptoolkit/Workshop_Toolkit/Assistance_files/NativeAmerInfo Sheet.pdf (accessed December 2, 2015).

Indian Health Service. 2013. *Indian Health Disparities.* http://www.ihs.gov/factsheets/index.cfm?module=dsp_fact_disparities (accessed December 2, 2015).

Jacobs, D. Trend Four Arrows. 2014. "The Continuing Saga of Anti-Indianism in America: Critique of a Bestseller and the Reviewers Who Praise It." TruthOut. http://www.truth-out.org/opinion/item/26675-the-continuing-saga-of-anti-indianism-in-america-a-critique-of-drury-and-clavin-s-bestseller-and-the-reviewers-who-praise-it (accessed December 2, 2015).

Jefferson, T. 1803. President Thomas Jefferson to William Henry Harrison, Governor of the Indiana Territory. http://courses.missouristate.edu/ftmiller/Documents/jeffindianpolicy.htm.

Johnston, B.R., Dawson, S., and Madsen, G. 2007. "Uranium Mining and Milling: Navajo Experience in the American Southwest." In B.R. Johnston (Ed.), *Half Lives & Half-Truths: Confronting the Radioactive Legacies of the Cold War* (pp. 97–116). Santa Fe, NM: School for Advanced Research.

Jones, D. 2006. "The Persistence of American Indian Health Disparities." *American Journal of Public Health*, 96(12): 2122–2134.

Kahn, B. 2012. "Separate and Unequal: Environmental Regulatory Management on Indian Reservations." http://environs.law.ucdavis.edu/volumes/35/2/kahn.pdf (accessed December 2, 2015).

Katz, C. 2004. *Growing Up Global: Economic Restructuring and Children's Everyday Lives.* Minneapolis, MN: University of Minnesota Press.

Kloeckner, J. 2012. "Sovereignty: Establishing Tribal Pesticide Programs That Recognize Inherent Tribal Authority and Promote Federal-Tribal Partnerships." *Environmental Law Reporter*, 42: 10057–10077.

LaDuke, W. 1999. *All Our Relations: Native Struggles for Land and Life.* Cambridge, MA: South End.

LaDuke, W. 2010. "Our Home on Earth." In J. Walljasper (Ed.), *All That We Share: A Field Guide to the Commons.* New York: New Press.

Lewis, D. 1994. "Essay on Native American Environmental Issues." In M. Davis (Ed.), *Native America in the Twentieth Century: An Encyclopedia.* New York: Garland.

Lopez, B. 2004. "Radioactive Reservations: The Uphill Battle to Keep Nuclear Waste Off Native American Land." Nuclear Age Peace Foundation. http://www.wagingpeace.org/articles/2004/09/01_lopez_radioactive-reservations.htm.

Matthews, D., Effler, S., and Matthews, C. 2000. "Ammonia and Toxicity Criteria in Polluted Onondaga Lake, New York." *Water Environment Research*, 72(6): 731–741.

Mulloy, K., James, D., Mohs, K., and Kornfeld, M. 2001. "Lung Cancer in a Nonsmoking Underground Uranium Miner." *Environmental Health Perspectives*, 109(3): 305–309.

National Center for Education Statistics. 2008. *Status and Trends in the Education of American Indians and Alaska Natives.* http://nces.ed.gov/pubs2008/nativetrends/tables/table_1_6c.asp (accessed December 2, 2015).

Nader, L. and Gusterson, H. 2007. "Nuclear Legacies: Arrogance, Secrecy, Ignorance, Lies, Silence, Suffering, Action." In B.R. Johnston (Ed.), *Half-Lives and Half-Truths: Confronting the Radioactive Legacies of the Cold War.* Sante Fe: SAR.

Neumann, R. 2005. *Making Political Ecology.* London: Hodder.

Norrell, B. 2011. "Greenwashing: Corporates Target Indian Country with Scams." *The Narcosphere*, August 2. http://narcosphere.narconews.com/notebook/brenda-norrell/2011/08/greenwashing-corporations-target-indian-country-scams (accessed December 2, 2015).

Nuclear Information and Resource Service. 2006. "Radioactive Racism: The History of Targeting Native American Communities with High-Level Atomic Waste Dumps." Public Citizen. http://www.nirs.org/radwaste/scullvalley/historynativecommunities nuclearwaste06142005.pdf (accessed December 2, 2015).

OMH (Office of Minority Health). 2005. *Health Status of American Indian and Alaska Native Women.* Washington, DC: US Department of Health and Human Services.

OMH (Office of Minority Health). 2012. *American Indian/Alaska Native Profile.* http://minorityhealth.hhs.gov/templates/browse.aspx?lvl=2&lvlID=52.

Panikkar, B. and Brugge, D. 2007. "The Ethical Issues in Uranium Mining Research in the Navajo Nation." *Accountability in Research*, 14: 121–153.

Paskus, L. 2010. "The Life and Death of Desert Rock." *High Country News*, August 16. http://www.hcn.org/articles/the-life-and-death-of-desert-rock (accessed December 2, 2015).

Pasternak, J. 2006. "A Peril That Dwelt among the Navajos." *Los Angeles Times*, November 19. http://www.latimes.com/news/la-na-navajo19nov19-story.html (accessed December 2, 2015).

Peet, R., Robins, P., and Watts, M. 2011. *Global Political Ecology.* New York: Routledge.

Pulido, L. 2000. "Rethinking Environmental Racism: White Privilege and Urban Development in Southern California. *Annals of the Association of American Geographers*, 90: 12–40.

Rae, L. and Witherspoon, R. 2001. "Mohawk Way of Life Befouled by PCBs." *The Journal News*, November 5, pp. 1a, 6a–7a.

Roe, A. 2003. "Fishing for Identity: Mercury Contamination and Fish Consumption Among Indigenous Groups in the United States." *Bulletin of Science, Technology & Society*, 23(5): 368–375.

Samet, J., Kutvirt, D., Waxweller, R., and Key, C. 1984. "Uranium Mining and Lung Cancer in Navajo Men." *New England Journal of Medicine*, 310: 1481–1484.

Sandefur, G., Rindfuss, R., and Cohn, B. 1996. *Changing Numbers, Changing Needs American Indian Demography and Public Health.* Washington, DC: National Academy Press.

Sarche, M. and Spicer, P. 2008. "Poverty and Health Disparities for American Indian and Alaska Native Children: Current Knowledge and Future Prospects." *Annals of the New York Academy of Sciences*, 1136: 125–136.

Scheer, R. and Moss, D. 2010. "Earth Talk." http://www.emagazine.com/earth-talk-archive/week-of-02-21-10 (accessed December 2, 2015).

Schell, L., Gallo, M., Denham, M., Ravencroft, J., DeCaprio, A., and Carpenter, D. 2008. "Relationship of Thyroid Hormone Levels to Levels of Polychlorinated Biphenyls, Lead, p,p'- DDE, and Other Toxicants in Akwesasne Mohawk Youth." *Environmental Health Perspectives*, 116(6): 806–813.

Schnaiberg A. 1980. *The Environment: From Surplus to Scarcity.* New York: Oxford University Press.

Schnaiberg, A. and Gould, K. 1994. *Environment and Society: The Enduring Conflict.* New York: St. Martin.

Schwartz, S. 2006. "The Arrogance of Ignorance: Hidden Away, Out of Sight and Out of Mind." http://www.nativevillage.org/Messages%20from%20the%20People/the%20arrogance%20of%20ignorance.htm (accessed December 2, 2015).

Shakopee Mdewakanton Sioux. 2012. "Shakopee Mdewakanton Release *Omakatoh Wowapi* Four Year Report." http://www.shakopeedakota.org/4yrReport.html (accessed December 2, 2015).

Shields, L., Wiese, W., Skipper, B., Charley, B., and Banally, L. 1992. "Navajo Birth Outcomes in the Shiprock Uranium Mining Area." *Medical Physics*, 63(5): 542–551.

Simonson, M. 2013. "Red Cliff Band Hopes to Remove Explosive Barrels." *Wisconsin Public Radio News*, March 7. http://news.wpr.org/post/red-cliff-band-hopes-remove-explosive-barrels.

Singer, M. 1995. "Beyond the Ivory Tower: Critical Praxis in Medical Anthropology." *Medical Anthropology Quarterly*, 9(1): 80–106.

Smith N. 1992. "Geography, Difference and the Politics of Scale." In J. Doherty, E. Graham, and M. Malek (Eds.), *Postmodernism and the Social Sciences* (pp. 57–79). New York: St. Martin's.

Smith N. 1996. *The New Urban Frontier: Gentrification and the Revanchist City.* New York: Routledge.

Smith N. 2008. *Uneven Development: Nature, Capital, and the Production of Space*, 3rd ed. Athens: University of Georgia Press.

Tullo, M. 2014. "U.S. Tribe Looks to International Court for Justice." http://www.truth-out.org/news/item/23191-us-tribe-looks-to-international-court-for-justice (accessed December 2, 2015).

Turshen, M. 1989. *The Politics of Public Health.* New Brunswick, NJ: Rutgers University Press.

United Church of Christ's Committee on Racial Justice. 1987. *Toxic Wastes and Race in the United States.* http://www.ucc.org/about-us/archives/pdfs/toxwrace87.pdf (accessed December 2, 2015).

United States Bureau of the Census. 1995. *Housing of American Indians on Reservations: Statistical Brief.* Washington, DC.

Urbina, I. 2011. "Regulation Lax as Gas Wells' Tainted Waters Hits Rivers." *New York Times*, February 26. http://www.nytimes.com/2011/02/27/us/27gas.html?_r=0 (accessed December 2, 2015).

Williams, D. and Collins, C. 1995. "U.S. Socioeconomic and Racial Differences in Health: Patterns and Explanations." *Annual Review of Sociology*, 21: 349–386.

Wolf, E. 1972." Ownership and Political Ecology." *Anthropological Quarterly*, 45(3): 201–205.

PART III The Political Ecology of Health

CHAPTER 11

Water, Environment, and Health: The Political Ecology of Water

Linda M. Whiteford, Maryann Cairns, Rebecca K. Zarger, and Gina Larsen

Introduction

Water, a life-sustaining necessity, seems to be disappearing, or at least being radically changed. To some, water is thought of as scarce and almost magical; to others it is an underappreciated, plentiful resource. Whether through the creation of dams, increased groundwater pumping, or changing water allocation among states and regions, water is moving due to human intervention. This movement has disparate effects on human populations and their health and well-being. In this chapter we employ a political ecology perspective to understand how flows of water impact environments and human health. We present three case studies that apply a political ecology framework to clarify invisible relations and hidden agendas that shape water use and practice. Throughout this chapter, examples of unintended consequences stemming from changes to water systems, power-laden decision making related to water rights and ownership, and politicized water management practices provide a look into the complex and uneven outcomes that emerge due to particular choices about where water flows, who has access to it, and the quality of available water. Drawing on

A Companion to the Anthropology of Environmental Health, First Edition. Edited by Merrill Singer.

ecological theorizing from Muir to Bateson, Robbins argues that "any tug on the strands of the global web of human–environment linkages reverberates through the system as a whole" (2004: 5). In this chapter, we examine varied ways in which a "tug" on how people perceive and use water changes the systems in which they are embedded, and, furthermore, how this impacts human health. We provide ways to engage with the idea of a "web" of human–environment linkages, and encourage investigating the unexpected relationships between water and the social and environmental spheres that tether its use.

Theorizing a Political Ecology of Water and Human Health

Whether referred to as a "waterscape" (Strang 2004), a "waterworld" (Hastrup 2009), or a "hydro-social cycle" (Swyngedouw 2004, 2009), one thing is clear: water is fundamental to the human experience. The need for water is all encompassing. Simply put, "water is life." Orlove and Caton (2010) use Mauss's idea of a "total social fact" to discuss water's ubiquitousness to both social and physical life. For anthropologists, research on water has focused on a variety of topics including water management institutions (Trawick 2003; Wutich 2011), meanings and cultural significance of water (Strang 2004), links between water access and health (Ennis-McMillan 2006; Whiteford and Whiteford 2005), politics of water distribution, privitization, and scarcity (Johnston and Donahue 1998; Barnes 2013), gender and water (Whiteford 1997), and water sustainability (Orlove and Caton 2010), just to name a few important thematic areas. What foundational questions have anthropologists and others asked around human connections to water? How are the politics of water tied to human health in tangible ways? The relationships are, admittedly, incredibly complex, but the case studies we analyze in this article illustrate just how fundamental an anthropological approach to understanding such links can be. The politics of waterscapes impact everyday lives around the globe. Here we provide a short synopsis of a broad theoretical lens, political ecology, before moving on to discuss the connections between politics of access and control over water resources with human health and well-being.

A growing number of scholars have drawn from the interdisciplinary theoretical framework of political ecology, a sometimes frustratingly broad field of inquiry that emphasizes the ways politics and power shape and redefine human relations with nonhuman "nature" (for an engaging introduction, see Robbins 2012). A foundational premise that arises from a political ecology perspective is that what was often conceptualized as "pristine" nature has in fact been socially constructed over centuries through "Western" and European worldviews (Cronon 1995; Moran 2006). The term "political ecology" was coined by Eric Wolf (and others) in the 1970s, combining political economy with a more explicit focus on the environment. Political ecology analyses, which grew exponentially between the 1990s and 2000s, address "comparative anatomies of networks" (Robbins 2004: 212) to reach explanations for historical and present connections between actors (such as farmers, consumers, transnational lending banks, and national governments) as they rework the landscape to fit their own needs – or are prevented from doing so by those who are more powerful. Attention to the negotiations between local social and ecological processes and global hierarchies of power is another hallmark of the approach (Paulson, Gezon, and Watts 2005).

By unpacking simplistic, ahistorical, and apolitical explanations for why a particular landscape looks the way it does, or how one group of people came to be marginalized from vital resources they depend upon while others benefit, the tools of political ecology provide a way to "challenge dominant interpretations of the causes of environmental degradation and contest prevalent prescriptions for solving such problems" (Gezon and Paulson 2005: 2). Gezon and Paulson (2005) argue that political ecology has been from its inception an applied field, with researchers often working collaboratively with local people, nongovernmental organizations (NGOs), or other institutions to address inequitable environmental change. With the emergence of political ecology in fields such as geography, anthropology, and development studies, researchers turned their attention to focal resources as components of local ecosystems in order to trace the links to political and economic processes at multiple scales. These resources include forests, agricultural practices, and water (which we focus on here). Early anthropological research in political ecology of water included studies of the politics of water and health in Honduras (Stonich 1998), water scarcity in the US southwest (Sheridan 1998), and hydropolitics in Zimbabwe (Derman 1998).

As Swyngedouw has argued, a political ecology of water suggests that "transformations of, and in, the hydrological cycle" are closely correlated to power relations at local, regional, and global scales (2009: 56). In what he terms the "hydro-social cycle," it is impossible to separate out the social from the biophysical when considering the circulation of water, and nor should we attempt to do so. Furthermore, water environments are "actively and historically produced" such that they should no longer be viewed as "natural" (2009: 56). This is an important point: once the social and hydrological are conceptualized as mutually constituted, a political-ecological analysis of water flows becomes possible. So, for example, water demand and scarcity can be viewed as culturally constructed and changes in cultural practices can be seen when conflicts over competing uses for water emerge (Johnston 2003). Decisions to divert or restrict the flow of water in response to flooding or hurricanes are not natural at all – they are power-laden and political (Zarger 2009). However, water scarcity is a "life-threatening reality" for millions who "suffer from diseases linked to contaminated water" (Johnston 2003: 75). For these reasons, there is a renewed urgency to understand how social power relates to water management, infrastructure, supply, quality, and redistribution.

One of the key concepts that has emerged from work in the political ecology of water is the need to understand the social, political, and historical situatedness of water access, rights, and control. Who decides where a community or a city's water comes from is a pressing question that multi-scale ethnographic research can address. This can also be extended to wastewater if water resources are viewed in a holistic feedback loop. Access to water is essential for survival and watery landscapes typically hold significant meaning across cultures, carrying with them rules of access that affect who can use particular water sources (Strang 2004). These rules – whether spoken, unspoken, written, or codified into complex regulations – often have demonstrable linkages to human health (Singer and Evans 2013).

Orlove and Caton (2010: 404) suggest that an anthropological analysis of waterworlds might consider "five principal themes: value, equity, governance, politics, and knowledge." Each of these areas links water, environment, and health, as illustrated by the case studies in this chapter. In Bolivia, social categories of difference, community politics, and hybrid knowledge systems created by engineers and local residents collide around management of water and wastewater treatment systems. Water governance can have a direct relationship to water quality and waterborne disease such as cholera, which is illustrated in the case study from Ecuador. Values ascribed to particular landscapes, such as the wetlands and lakes of south-central Florida, drained by groundwater pumping from the aquifer, can have a measurable impact on individual emotional distress. Each of these cases provides insight into how waterworlds are intimately linked to human health and well-being and the urgent need to consider these intersections in future research.

Case Study: Political Ecology and Piped Water in Alto Beni, Bolivia – Water Infrastructure and Management

Water and sanitation (WatSan) development has been a key goal of development agencies in Bolivia since the 1990s. The United States Agency for International Development (USAID) and allied US-based development agencies such as ACDI/VOCA (acronym only) have collaborated with local communities with the aim of constructing piped, potable water systems, sometimes combined with sewage/wastewater treatment systems. The provision of WatSan technology in this fashion is labeled as "transnational development," and in Bolivia, WatSan cannot be removed from discussions of the impact of international aid, government relationships with international donors, US-based development through NGOs, or human rights (Goodale 2009). It is also strongly tied to local perceptions, abilities, and practices related to water use and management. These political, social, and environmental factors all have an influence on the construction and maintenance of WatSan development. Through an anthropological approach, this case study presents a portion of a project that linked these various levels of influence to an assessment of long-term efficacy of a WatSan project in the Alto Beni region of Bolivia. This project was part of a larger interdisciplinary grant at the University of South Florida.[1]

The project chose to focus on the position of one rural community in the Alto Beni region that had a comprehensive WatSan system (potable water, sewage, and wastewater treatment). The WatSan project that provided this infrastructure, initiated in 2007 and completed in 2009, was an example of a collaboration in which community members worked with US-funded aid groups to construct the infrastructure itself and to design the long-term management of the system. The system was implemented by ACDI/VOCA, funded by USAID, and approved by the vice-ministry of Coca and the Fondo Communitario de Desarrollo Integral [Essential Community Development Fund] or FCDI (Vargas-Carlos 2008; Fuchs and Mihelcic 2011). Labor and counterpart payments (days of work, materials) were supplied by the community, and they had a voice in design choices and construction practices.

Political ecology framed the research, and focused the researcher on the politics that bring particular water systems into play – that is, the complex international political system surrounding WatSan provision – and the actual organizations that put these systems into place in the field site. It also considered community-negotiated relationships with water resources and community impact on ecological resources. The project investigated the intersection of the political and the environmental, where transnational aid has worked with local agencies to construct new WatSan systems that change resource use practices, and where local communities are in the process of adapting to or resisting these changes. Social and environmental outcomes from the system were just beginning to emerge. It is at this intersection that political ecology provided a way to examine marginalization, health risk and behavior, land and resource ownership, and infrastructure in terms of an environmental system (water). The study was completed in agreement with the idea that there is a benefit to addressing and presenting "global, regional, and local scales and perspectives" in comparison to and in light of one another in order to proffer full understanding (Svarstad, as cited in Gezon and Paulson 2005: 14). For the research in Bolivia that meant starting from the politics that drive ecological action (in this case "transnational development") and moving to the organization and adaptation seen in local groups using a WatSan system.

The research methods included semi-structured interviews with development professionals (n = 11), focus groups (n = 4), semi-structured interviews with community members (n = 32), structured, systematic sample surveys (n = 138), community member-led mapping (n = 7), and participant observation (Cairns 2014). As an example of one of the ways in which the complex relationship between transnational and regional aid agencies and local practices was seen in this specific context, focus was given to individual relationships with the piped drinking water system. In the town the drinking water came from four different springs high in the nearby mountains, and was piped down through several communities. The springs that fed the water system were perceived by the community to provide good, "sweet" water. The water tasted great, and was often lauded as the "best water around." It was also perceived as plentiful, except for a short dry season. Aid agencies were concerned about pathogens in the water and implemented chlorination at the tank for treatment. While some (although not all) individuals within the town believed that the water was being treated with chlorine at the tank, it was actually not being treated. While the operator did receive formal training from the aid agency on how to treat with chlorine, he did not feel he was fully able to treat the water safely, and was concerned about doing harm to the community if he did it incorrectly. This unexpected choice to not use the treatment system spurred further analysis of the issue of water potability and water treatment practice in the town.

The study results suggest that there was a complex relationship between how individuals perceived the potable water infrastructure, the management of the system's water treatment/potability function (chlorination), and individual water treatment practices. There was an overall trust in the appropriateness and effectiveness of the infrastructure itself, and a general trust that the infrastructure was sustainable and well-implemented by the aid agencies (at least in the short term). Of those surveyed, when asked directly, 89.9 percent of individuals felt that the water system was worth what they paid for it. As well, 89.9 percent of individuals felt that the system would still be working in two years, 79.0 percent felt that the system would still be working in five years, and 58.7 percent felt it would be still be working in ten years. There was an understanding that the system (for now at least) worked and worked well (62.3% of respondents found the water quality "good to very good" and 33.3% found it "neutral"). However, only 33.3% felt the water was safe to drink without boiling it (although, qualitatively, many admitted to drinking water without boiling it on occasion, especially while working or when they were tired) (Cairns 2014). Some individuals were aware that the water that passed through the piped system was not treated correctly. Others were not. Either way, individuals acted on their perceived knowledge.

Qualitative results suggested that some residents wanted the water to be chlorinated, and trusted it as a treatment process. Others were concerned about chlorination as a potentially negative process rather than a positive one, arguing that it made the water taste bad and was potentially hazardous to their health. Some individuals felt that the water was safe naturally, and so to chlorinate was an unnecessary risk – both to human health and to the watershed. Others just preferred to treat the water by boiling or filtering – not with chemicals. Some people just boiled the water because the aid agencies told them to. These differing views represent tensions between the perceived and actual effectiveness of the water system, expectations of chlorination treatment, and perceptions of "natural" water quality. (Strang discusses a similar tension between perceptions of "natural" water and "unnatural" chlorinated water from her work in the UK; 2004: 114–117.) In the Bolivian case, trust in the water system, relationship with the water source, and effective treatment were all negotiated in a dialogue between development agencies' training, local understandings of what constitutes "sweet" water, and relationships with WatSan infrastructure over time. Who knew the water's actual safety, and who was able to treat it properly based on that information, was varied and not transparent. Some individuals were acting on incorrect or unclear information and thus had less ability to ensure that their water was truly safe to drink.

Regardless of perception of water treatment effectiveness or actual practice, most people in the sample recognized the improvement in water technology and drinking water safety since the implementation of the system. No one yearned for the days without piped water or the days when the pipes were made of metal instead of plastic – in fact 87.3 percent of individuals felt that their health had improved due to the implementation of the potable water system. In reality, though, whether individuals were actually fully aware of the safety of their water varied. Individuals' perceptions of the new drinking water infrastructure, their perceptions of chemical treatment, their understanding of waterborne disease, and their trust in externally designed WatSan systems and NGO practices all moderate their use of and expectations surrounding their drinking water. The most divisive factors in individuals' choices about how to handle their drinking water were whether or not they believed in the "pure" quality of their drinking water source, and whether or not they trusted chlorination as a treatment practice. Various iterations of these perceptions caused diverse actions on the part of individual community members.

The central tension of "who gets to decide" on questions of water provision and water system maintenance is key to sorting out conflicting views on water potability. The production of potable water systems is a dynamic relationship between US-based NGOs, the Bolivian state, and local communities. It was the agencies who chose the chlorination system – and it was the operator who chose not to manage the system due to his own concerns (and those raised by some community members). These decisions impacted local residents directly – but these choices were not fully transparent or collaborative at either level (although we do want to stress that both choices were made with the community's best interest at the core). While local residents were supportive of the water system infrastructure, many were less trusting overall of the treatment technologies for potable water. On the community's part, the lack of understanding related to chlorination safety, lack of certainty on the operator's choices related to chlorination, and long-held perceptions of the safety of natural water sources led to differing practices in in-home drinking water treatment. This muddled relationship with the system's treatment infrastructure mitigates the effectiveness of the system as a whole in relation to potential positive health outcomes, which was a main reason for the system's implementation in the first place. Until there is more dialogue between development agency processes for design of water treatment and local perceptions, there will be tension between ideas of "natural" versus piped water, and untreated versus treated potable water, and this could have negative or marginalizing impacts.

NGOs and community members could work together to address concerns about the maintenance of the WatSan system. Training on chlorination and its health benefits (and explanations of its safety for consumption) should be designed and/or repeated. Implementing more user-friendly chlorination practices for the operator could also be useful (and were recommended by development professionals interviewed for the study). In addition, NGOs would be well advised to understand local resistance/concerns related to treatment technologies like chlorination, especially those that stem from local understandings of environment and water resources. Attention should be paid not only to the perceived health impacts of the system (e.g., the number of people who think their health has improved), but also to the more specific goal of ensuring full health benefits (whether or not they are actually drinking safe water in practice).

WatSan infrastructure development changes local ecosystems and changes water use practices – all with the aim of imparting benefit to humans. In order to have this aim fully realized, we must make sure that infrastructure is working to the best of its ability in the time, culture, and place where the infrastructure is constructed. Political ecology provides a frame from which one can look at the politics surrounding potable water practices at a variety of levels, within different social groups, and with a focus on constructive critique of power relationships and transnational decision making. Using this frame, political ecologists can elicit the ways in which perceptions of the natural environment constrain practices related to use of WatSan infrastructure.

Case Study: The Political Ecology of Water – The Case of Cholera

This case study uses the example of a bilateral behavior change intervention during the 1992 cholera pandemic to demonstrate the efficacy of the political ecology of water framework. Behavior change projects require the understanding of immediate and proximate stimuli of the behavior that is sought to be changed. In the case of the cholera pandemic, behavior change occurred because the intervention considered the local environment, the larger, regional political history, and the global economic shift toward neoliberalism in its design. Cholera is caused by bacteria (*Vibrio cholerae*) in food, water, feces, and other substances. With a short incubation period, the bacteria produce a toxin that activates enzymes in the intestines, causing copious amounts of watery diarrhea, vomiting, and muscle cramps. Cholera can quickly result in severe dehydration and death if left untreated. It is particularly deadly among children and the elderly, or anyone immunologically compromised or nutritionally stressed, and in the past has been called "the blue death," because patients nearing death from cholera can turn a shade of blue or gray from the loss of fluids in their bodies (Kiple 1976). Once the cholera bacteria are introduced into human hosts, disrupting transmission is dependent on a complex array of environmental, political, and cultural factors. A political ecology framework captures each of these variables and, therefore, is particularly useful in understanding patterns of waterborne illnesses.

The spread and severity of cholera outbreaks are directly related to human activities (e.g., hand washing, defecation disposal, food sharing), and environmental factors (e.g., water source, proximity to animal or human activities). Patterns of water usage, and thus disease risk, are further shaped by cultural beliefs, gender-based labor patterns, history, politics, and ecology. In much of the world, access to employment opportunities, out-and-return migration, lack of water infrastructure such as water filters and disinfectants, and a lack of sanitation infrastructure combined with the practice of open-air defecation all exacerbate issues related to transmission of this disease (Whiteford, Laspina, and Torres 1996).

In 1991 a cholera outbreak in Peru and Ecuador became an epidemic, spreading throughout Central and South America, killing more than 9000 people and infecting many more (Whiteford and Vindrola Padros 2015). In the Ecuadorian case, governmental and international health authorities were able to control the outbreak in the urban centers within the first 15 months of the initial epidemic. However, the rural, dispersed, and indigenous communities of the Andean highlands continued to suffer from ongoing deaths due to the disease. A bi-national team from the Ecuadorian Ministry of Health and USAID worked together to try to understand the epidemic and to develop a health behavior intervention to stop the spread of cholera in the highlands. The team included a physician, a medical anthropologist, and a nonformal educator, who over a period of 12 months helped the local communities reduce and then avoid cholera. The intervention was successful in first controlling and then eliminating the disease from the intervention communities because the framework employed allowed for incorporation of local beliefs and behaviors related to water and the environment, as well as biomedical views of disease transmission.

The two Ecuadorian mountain states where the research and subsequent intervention occurred had the highest ongoing rates of cholera (Chimborazo and Cotopaxi). They were also the states with the largest concentration of indigenous people. These states, along with the state of Imbabura (where the intervention did not occur) were areas rich in indigenous traditions, festivals, food sharing practices, and water handling behaviors. They were also overwhelmingly poor, politically underrepresented, had substandard water and sanitation infrastructure, open-air aqueducts, and depressed economies which necessitated labor out-migration. By employing a political ecology perspective to understanding water handling practices, several key issues critical to the design of the subsequent interventions emerged.

The two most crucial issues found were the geophysical and political isolation of the at-risk population and the related lack of water and sewerage infrastructure. The Ecuadorian government had not provided sufficient water and sewerage infrastructure in the highlands – in part, because the communities were dispersed and the terrain rugged, but also because the indigenous communities had histories of oppositional relations with the national government. Thus, decisions related to provision of water and sanitation systems were not just environmental – they were political. In addition to these difficulties, the availability of a reliable source of water from the mountains provided the misleading image that the water was clean (a theme also noted in the Cairns case study in Bolivia). However, the water in open aqueducts is easily contaminated and, in this case, was contaminated by a local upstream hospital treating cholera patients and dumping waste into the aqueduct. The result was that water in the downstream communities became contaminated. The failure of the national government to provide effective water and sanitation infrastructure meant that few attempts were made to chlorinate or otherwise decontaminate the water supply.

The second key issue was women's perception of, and use of, water. Both in the household and extra-household contexts, gender roles shape water handling practices and reflect the culturally determined ethnoecology of water (Whiteford 1997; Whiteford and Vindrola Padros 2011). In the Ecuador case, women made decisions about how to use water (for drinking, cooking, washing, feeding the animals), and those decisions were shaped by access to water and their perceptions of its cleanliness. Water use and reuse (e.g., hand washing, dishwashing) were implicated in the spread of the disease.

Another, related issue was male labor out-migration. In many highland communities, men migrated to urban areas for work and then returned home to participate in traditional festivals. This labor pattern further compounded the communities' increased risk of cholera. During seasonal rituals and ethnic festivals, food was prepared, served, and shared among large groups, and eaten with hands. Return labor migration for festivals that resulted in changes in food handling practices was consistently associated with spikes in the epidemiological rates of cholera (Whiteford, Laspina, and Torres 1996). Men returning from urban areas may have been exposed to the disease in their work sites (for instance, in the large port city of Guayaquil where cholera was endemic), and thus returned to their communities carrying and sharing the *Vibrio cholera* bacterium.

The bi-national research team identified the following variables that directly and indirectly facilitated the spread of cholera: (a) political marginalization; (b) lack of adequate water and sanitation infrastructure; (c) hygiene related to hand washing; (d) water insecurity; (e) defecation in fields or other areas close to water sources or households; (f) consumption of food prepared and served by street vendors; (g) communal food preparation and consumption during religious and community festivals.

In the areas most heavily affected by the Ecuadorian cholera epidemic women were in charge of the household water supply, as they were for food handling and meal preparation. The research strongly suggested that water handling behavior, like food handling practices and sanitation and hygiene behaviors, were patterns created as cultural responses to the environment. When water is scarce, people use it sparingly, and often do not wash their hands, and rarely use soap when they do. In the fields, hands may come into contact with cholera-infected feces and transport the vibrios to the next host. When hands are not washed frequently and are used to reach into common food bowls, others sharing the food may also become infected. But the political ecology framework allowed for inclusion of variables beyond the household and community, and we found that disease transmission in the highlands was impacted by the national politics of international trade and changing global lending policies. In the 1990s, many countries like Ecuador reduced their focus on the needs of the rural, indigenous communities (such as those in the highland states), and instead turned their attention to global trade. World Bank policies that, for instance, mandated decentralization of services resulted in the transfer of the financial burden for maintaining water systems from the national government to local and state governments. That placed the responsibility on local communities to provide the resources for developing or maintaining the water and sanitation infrastructure, rendering the provision of adequate water and sanitation almost impossible for many highland communities.

Defecation in open fields is a response to living without access to latrines or sanitation systems. In much of the world, human and animal feces are used to fertilize crops. Sometimes feces are buried or turned under the ground, thus removed from people coming into contact with them. However, if the feces are not buried, and if they carry the cholera bacterium, then the disease can be spread by contact, resulting in fecal–hand–oral transmission. Likewise, in much of the world, water systems are limited to freshwater aqueducts, rain barrel water collection, or water that is trucked in from a distance. Water in such systems is rarely assessed or disinfected; thus once the cholera vibrio is introduced, it can spread easily.

What we see in this case study of the cholera epidemic in Ecuador is the necessity to embed health research (such as epidemiological research) in the larger political ecology frame that incorporates local beliefs, gender roles, economic isolation, and the consequences of neoliberal reforms. In this case, the beliefs and behaviors of individuals in the most highly affected highland communities were relatively clearly identified. As well, community support for health was evident even before the health behavior change intervention. Some people recognized ways to change their own practices to reduce the likelihood of contacting and spreading the disease. What they needed was support from beyond their community so that they could pay for soap, chlorine, and household water-storage tanks. The findings from the study allowed the communities to identify some of the specific barriers to controlling the spread of waterborne disease (points (a) to (g) above). Once these barriers were identified and understood, local communities could create actions to overcome these barriers, such as changing behaviors related to food handling and water and sanitation practices. Home water storage and treatment became key to modifying water consumption practices and improving food safety. Enhanced understanding of cholera transmission facilitated changes in defecation and removal practices. Within two years of the political ecology of water and behavior intervention, the local communities had succeeded in controlling, and finally eradicating, cholera. As one of the community members told us: "We learned how to change the way we think and act; the [cholera] project has been good for the community."

Case Study: The Political Ecology of Water Scarcity and Emotional Distress – "It hurts my heart because this is where I was born and raised"

When one hears the term "water scarcity," Florida does not come immediately to mind. Florida is touted as being a luxurious paradise surrounded by water. The rainy season brings copious amounts of rainfall to the region. How could water shortage be a problem for Floridians? The truth is that water scarcity has been and still is a problem in many parts of Florida, particularly the Tampa Bay area (Rand 2003). Water scarcity does not simply reflect supply and demand of the resource, but also how water is valued and the degree of control there is over water resource management and distribution (Johnston 2003). In the Tampa Bay region, the relevance of a political ecology of water analysis might be less apparent than in other parts of the world, but it is no less present. The politics behind the way water is pumped and distributed and the effects of those political choices on the local landscape is a major concern of affected residents. In west-central Florida, water is often pumped from underground aquifers (called groundwater pumping) in rural regions and delivered to urban centers. This movement of the water resource has historically left behind a wake of environmental degradation in the form of dried-up wetlands, diminishing lakes, and even more numerous sinkholes for rural residents. Legal battles and environmental movements surrounding water have been prominent in the Tampa Bay area for decades. Issues such as groundwater pumping, wetland and lake degradation, drought, and pollution of water resources are only a few of the ways in which water scarcity and the political ecology of water are manifested in the Tampa Bay area. Some Tampa Bay residents' connection to water and local landscapes can be powerful enough to evoke deeply emotional memories and feelings surrounding the disappearance or destruction of cherished water bodies and ecosystems (Larsen 2012).

In 2011, an interdisciplinary team of researchers at the University of South Florida began conducting research on public perceptions of the water distribution system in Tampa Bay.[2] The overarching goals of the project were to gain an understanding of where local residents believed their water came from, what they thought of the politics behind the way water is distributed, and if they had noticed any changes in local wetlands or lakes due to groundwater pumping or development (Lewis *et al.* 2013). Over the course of interviewing residents about their experiences, something unexpected happened. The participants began to share very emotional stories about their experiences of seeing personally treasured local landscapes disappear due to groundwater pumping or development and urban sprawl. One of the most moving interviews was with a man who reminisced about a lake he used to visit as a child. He vividly described what the lake used to look like and how he interacted with the lake before it was over-pumped and destroyed. Before he could finish the story, the man's eyes welled up with tears and he chose to change the course of the conversation.

After talking with local residents about their experiences of environmental degradation in the region due to groundwater pumping and development and seeing the emotional responses residents gave regarding their feelings about the loss of their valued landscapes, a related study was embarked upon to measure the mental and emotional effects of landscape degradation on Tampa Bay residents (for a more complete treatment of this case study, see Larsen 2012). The topic of distress tied to environmental change has rarely been studied in academic and research sectors, especially in the United States. Due to the exploratory nature of the topic, the focus moved to Tampa Bay residents who were also members of environmental organizations as a pilot group for studying the relationships between stress and environmental change. Twenty-one participants were interviewed, all of whom were members of at least one of five different local environmental organizations, about their interactions with their local environment, personal connections to natural spaces, and experiences witnessing local landscape change over time. In addition to the interviews, two different stress scales (the Hopkins Symptom Checklist 10 and the Environmental Distress Scale, both described in more detail below) were used with each of the participants to quantitatively measure distress experienced from local environmental change. The results from the study showed a correlation between environmental degradation and emotional distress and suggest a need for more research on the topic of environmental destruction in all of its forms and its effects on human well-being.

In general, the results from the individual interviews showed that the research participants had strong personal connections with their local environment, often stemming from childhood. When asked explicitly if they had a personal connection with the natural environment, all 21 participants said yes. The most commonly given answer was "absolutely" (Larsen 2012). The environmental changes the participants noticed most often in their local environments over time included increased development activities and changes in water resources. The participants also discussed the ways in which they experienced mental and emotional distress tied to environmental change and shared that local environmental change caused them stress (in both negative and motivating ways). Participants further argued that their well-being was impacted by environmental change, primarily through air and water pollution. When asked to quantify the amount of stress out of their total life stressors that local environmental change caused the participants, the results varied. One participant believed that only 1 percent of her total life stressors were due to local environmental change, while another participant claimed 90 percent of his total stress was the result of local environmental change. There was considerable variability between the two extreme numbers, with most percentages falling between 20 percent and 60 percent (Larsen 2012).

Though the results of the interviews and stress scales spanned a number of topics, including childhood memories, increased local development, and concern for future generations, one of the clearest themes raised by the research participants as a whole was the destruction of water bodies such as lakes and wetlands due to groundwater pumping and development, and the emotions surrounding those water-related environmental changes. The participants most often discussed changes they had noticed in local lakes, ponds, and the Hillsborough River (a well-known river in the Tampa Bay region that is part of the water supply), but also talked about the ocean and wetlands in the Tampa Bay region. Though not all changes in water resources mentioned were negative (some participants talked about the increased health of the ocean locally and the Hillsborough River over time), participants frequently discussed their concerns seeing lakes and ponds dry up over the years, and their fears surrounding diminishing water table levels and the Floridian aquifer. Most of the research participants were unsure what was causing lake levels and the water table to diminish. When asked how seeing changes in local water bodies made them feel, approximately two-thirds of the research participants used the words "sad" or "sadness," along with "worried," "powerless," "disgusted," "discouraged," and "angry." In general, participants used negative words to describe their feelings toward changes in water resources (Larsen 2012).

Not only did the participants express negative feelings toward changes in local water resources during the interviews, it appeared that they also experienced emotional distress due to these changes as measured by the Environmental Distress Scale (EDS). The EDS is an indicator of the biopsychosocial cost of ecosystem destruction and seeks to measure distress caused by various forms of environmental change (Higginbotham *et al.* 2007). The EDS, originally developed by Higginbotham *et al.* for use in an Australian mining community, was adapted to Tampa Bay and administered during each of the 21 interviews. Some of the water-related statements on the 91-item Likert scale EDS that the research participants scored the highest, which correlated to high distress, included "I am saddened when I look at degraded local landscapes and damaged wetlands and lakes," "It is stressful for me personally seeing lake levels decrease," and "It is stressful for me personally seeing wetlands dry up" (Larsen 2012).

The sample of results discussed here show how the political ecology of water framework can be used to understand impacts on local residents in Tampa Bay, Florida. Though not all changes in water resources are caused by human activities (unpredictable rainfall patterns and drought can also negatively impact local water resources), human-induced environmental changes in Tampa Bay cannot be overlooked. Political influence over where development takes place in the area, whether it results in the destruction of wetlands or the bulldozing of forested areas, clearly affects citizens. Residents may use those spaces for recreation or might have a personal or spiritual connection to those spaces and feel a sense of place within those areas. Also, the decisions behind water management and distribution, and where water is pumped from, can have both ecological consequences, such as lakes and wetlands drying up, and emotional consequences for some residents in the Tampa Bay region.

The destruction of ecosystems due to top-down forces such as political will and profit-driven decisions about where development takes place and where groundwater water is pumped from, and subsequent human distress are not obvious connections to most. However, the distressing effects of ecosystem destruction are tangible. While no broad generalizations about environmental destruction and distress can be made from this case study, this topic is ripe for exploration. By understanding how the politics of environmental change, in the United States and globally, affects people emotionally, anthropologists and other social scientists can begin to understand whether and how various populations value local landscapes and are emotionally affected by environmental change and destruction. Through this approach, the political ecology of ecosystem and water resource destruction can be addressed, including understanding why political leaders, developers, water managers, and other key stakeholders make the decisions they do about development and groundwater pumping and how that changes local ecology and the lives of affected residents. Only after comprehensive research on the link between environmental destruction and human well-being with a variety of populations can the problem of environmental destruction and human distress be properly addressed and solutions created that benefit humans and the environment upon which they depend.

Conclusion

These three case studies from anthropological fieldwork in Bolivia, Ecuador, and Florida demonstrate the utility of employing a political ecology framework when looking at interstices among environment, human behavior, and health. Each case raises questions about the "disconnect" between politics, policies, and their local applications. Whether the disconnects are related to groundwater pumping in Florida and loss of waterscapes that occurs as water is pumped out of rural communities and into other more politically powerful urban communities, or the disconnect between the neoliberal reforms in Bolivia and Ecuador that privilege the reallocation of responsibilities from the central government to those communities and individuals least able to shoulder them, the underlying theme is of political power used to alter waterscapes, and thus, human lives.

As we acknowledge at the beginning of this chapter, political ecology has been critiqued as being too diffuse and unfocused, as well as privileging politics over ecology (Vayda and Walters 1999). However, more recent syntheses of the field argue that despite the variability in approaches to the field, it is well positioned for "meaningful engagement" (Robbins 2012: 252) with the most pressing problems of global environmental change (Baer and Singer 2009). With this in mind, we argue that a political ecology of water can and should be more explicitly linked to human health and well-being. As such, the cases described illustrate how such a framework can be effectively applied to unpacking complex multi-scale scenarios that attend to the importance of politics over an increasingly scarce or valuable resource. For instance, understanding how well-intentioned international aid in water and sanitation projects fails at the local level for want of sustained education and training, or how lost landscapes imprinted from childhood memories are invisible to water boards and policy makers, or how gender and geography shape disease transmission, requires flexibility of perspective that enhances the overall analysis. Water – its use, meanings, distribution, cost, and control – is a critical global issue with a rapidly increasing urgency. Political ecology offers a framework that validates both the global and the local, and when applied to waterscapes, connects the two in intellectually challenging and meaningful ways. Beyond this, we are also reminded that "these discussions are part of a quest to find ways of asking questions and gathering information to facilitate struggles for greater social and environmental justice" (Paulson *et al.* 2005: 212) and thus we encourage fellow scholars to apply similar analyses more broadly in other spheres and locations. As we further engage theoretically informed critique of pressing human problems we can perhaps anticipate the unintended impacts of change in water practices and policies in meaningful and actionable ways.

NOTES

1 This material is based upon work supported by the National Science Foundation under Grant No. 0908425 (PI: James Mihelcic). Any opinions, findings, and conclusions or recommendations expressed in this material are those of the author and do not necessarily reflect the views of the National Science Foundation.

2 This material is based upon work supported by the National Science Foundation under Grant No. 0948986 (PI: David Lewis). Any opinions, findings, and conclusions or recommendations expressed in this material are those of the author and do not necessarily reflect the views of the National Science Foundation.

REFERENCES

Baer, H.A. and Singer, M. 2009. *Global Warming and the Political Ecology of Health.* Walnut Creek, CA: Left Coast Press.

Barnes, J. 2013. "Water, Water Everywhere, But Not a Drop to Drink: The False Promise of Virtual Water." *Critique of Anthropology,* 33(4): 371–389.

Cairns, M. 2014. "WatSan Processes and Critical Infrastructure: Environment, Rights, and Waste in Bolivia." Doctoral dissertation, University of South Florida.

Cronon, W., 1995. "The Trouble with Wilderness or, Getting Back to the Wrong Nature." In W. Cronon (Ed.) 1995. *Uncommon Ground: Toward Reinventing Nature.* New York: W.W.Norton.

Derman, B. 1998. "Balancing the Waters: Development and Hydropolitics in Contemporary Zimbabwe." In J.M. Donahue and B.R. Johnston (Eds.), *Water, Culture, and Power: Local Struggles in a Global Context.* Washington, DC: Island Press.

Ennis-McMillan, M.C. 2006. *A Precious Liquid: Drinking Water and Culture in the Valley of Mexico.* Belmont, CA: Cengage Learning.

Fuchs, V.J. and Mihelcic, J.R. 2011. "Analysing Appropriateness in Sanitation Projects in the Alto Beni Region of Bolivia." *Waterlines,* 30: 122–134.

Gezon, L. and Paulson, S. 2005. "Place, Power Difference: Multiscale Research at the Dawn of the Twenty-first Century." In A. Escobar, A. Gardner, and M. Brodgen (Eds.), *Political Ecology across Spaces, Scales, and Social Groups* (pp. 1–16). New Brunswick, NJ: Rutgers University Press.

Goodale, M. 2009. *Surrendering to Utopia: An Anthropology of Human Rights.* Stanford, CA: Stanford University Press.

Hastrup, K. 2009. "Waterworlds: Framing the Question of Social Resilience." In K. Hastrup (Ed.), *The Question of Resilience: Social Responses to Climate Change.* Copenhagen: Royal Danish Academy of Science and Letters.

Higginbotham, N. Connor, L., Albrecht, G., Freeman, S., and Agho, K. 2007. "Validation of an Environmental Distress Scale." *Ecohealth,* 3: 245–254.

Johnston, B.R. 2003. "The Political Ecology of Water: An Introduction." *Capitalism Nature Socialism,* 14: 73–90.

Johnston, B.R. and Donahue, J.M. 1998. "Introduction." In J.M. Donahue and B.R. Barbara Rose Johnston (Eds.), *Water, Culture, and Power: Local Struggles in a Global Context.* Washington, DC: Island Press.

Kiple, K. 1976. *Blacks in Colonial Cuba, 1774–1899.* Gainesville, FL: University of Florida Press.

Larsen, G. 2012. "Wetland and Lake Destruction, Development and Mental/Emotional Distress Among Residents of Tampa Bay, Florida." Graduate School Theses and Dissertations. http://scholarcommons.usf.edu/etd/4356.

Lewis, D., Zarger, R., Landry, S., Rains, M., Akiwumi, F., Crisman, T., Bell, S., and Treittin, C. 2013. "Urban Development, Power Relations, and Water Redistributionas Drivers of Wetland Change in the Tampa Bay Region Socioecosystem: ULTRA-Ex Final report to the National Science Foundation." http://www.research.gov.

Moran, E.F. 2006. *People and Nature: An Introduction to Human Ecological Relations.* Malden, MA: Blackwell.

Orlove, B. and Caton, S.C. 2010. "Water Sustainability: Anthropological Approaches and Prospects." *Annual Review of Anthropology*, 39: 401–415.

Paulson, S., Gezon, L.L., and Watts, M. 2005. "Politics, Ecologies, Genealogies." In A. Escobar, A. Gardner, and M. Brodgen (Eds.), *Political Ecology across Spaces, Scales, and Social Groups*. New Brunswick, NJ: Rutgers University Press.

Rand, H. 2003. *Water Wars: A Story of People, Politics, and Power*. United States of America: Xlibris Corporation.

Robbins, P. 2004. *Political Ecology: A Critical Introduction*, 2nd ed. Oxford: Blackwell.

Robbins, P. 2012. *Political Ecology: A Critical Introduction*, 3rd ed. Oxford: Blackwell.

Sheridan, T. 1998. "The Big Canal: The Political Ecology of the Central Arizona Project." In J.M. Donahue and B.R. Barbara Rose Johnston (Eds.), *Water, Culture, and Power: Local Struggles in a Global Context*. Washington, DC: Island Press.

Singer, M. and Evans, J. 2013. "Water Wary: Understandings and Concerns about Water and Health among the Rural Poor of Louisiana." In H. Kopnina and E. Shoreman-Ouimet (Eds.), *Environmental Anthropology Tomorrow*. New York: Routledge.

Strang, V. 2004. *The Meaning of Water*. Oxford: Berg.

Stonich, S. 1998. "Water, Power, and Environmental Health in Tourism Development: The Bay Islands, Honduras." In J.M. Donahue and B.R. Johnston (Eds.), *Water, Culture, and Power: Local Struggles in a Global Context*. Washington, D.: Island Press.

Swyngedouw, E. 2004. *Social Power and the Urbanization of Water: Flows of Power*. New York: Oxford University Press.

Swyngedouw, E. 2009. "The Political Economy and Political Ecology of the Hydro-Social Cycle." *Journal of Contemporary Water Research and Education*, 142: 56–60.

Trawick, P. 2003. *The Struggle for Water in Peru: Comedy and Tragedy in the Andean Commons*. Stanford, CA: Stanford University Press.

Vargas-Carlos, M. 2008. "Analisis Ambiental de Zonas de Conservacion Para la Provision de Agua (ZOCOPA) Sistema Sapecho." Unpublished report.

Vayda, A.P. and Walters, B. 1999. "Against Political Ecology." *Human Ecology*, 27(1): 167–179.

Whiteford, L.M. 1997. "The Ethnoecology of Dengue Fever." *Medical Anthropology Quarterly*, 11: 202.

Whiteford, L.M., Laspina, C., and Torres, M. 1996. "Cholera Control in Ecuador: Behavior-based Control Activities Environmental Health Project." Unpublished report. CDM, Arlington, VA.

Whiteford, L.M. and Vindrola Padros, C. 2011. "The Medical Anthropology of Water." In M. Singer and P. Erickson (Eds.), *Blackwell Medical Anthropology Companion*. Malden, MA: Blackwell Publishers.

Whiteford, L.M. and Vindrola-Padros, C. 2015. *Community Participatory Involvement: A Sustainable Model for Global Public Health*. Walnut Creek, CA: Left Coast Press.

Whiteford, L.M. and Whiteford, S. 2005. *Globalization, Water, & Health: Resource Management in Times of Scarcity*. Santa Fe; NM: School of American Research Press.

Wutich, A. 2011. "The Moral Economy of Water Reexamined: Reciprocity, Water Insecurity, and Urban Survival in Cochabamba, Bolivia." *Journal of Anthropological Research*, 67: 5–26.

Zarger, R.K. 2009. "Mosaics of Maya Livelihoods: Readjusting to Global and Local Food Crises." *Annals of Anthropological Practice*, 32: 130–151.

CHAPTER 12 Remembering the Foundations of Health: Everyday Water Insecurity and Its Hidden Costs in Northwest Alaska

Laura Eichelberger

Introduction

"People from outside have come to Qimmiurat with lots of negative thoughts that we can't afford the water and sewer in the future," Audrey,[1] a single mother and manager of the utility, told me when I asked her about the progress of the Iñupiaq village's piped water and sewer project. Qimmiurat's project would provide running water and sewerage to households of this water-insecure village of just over 450 people. It would also decommission the existing sewage lagoon located in the middle of the community that overflows every spring during the annual flood. The project had been delayed for over a decade, however, by funding shortages and disagreements between the community, government agencies, and engineering firms. As with all rural water and sanitation projects in Alaska, one of the primary concerns had been, and continues to be, sustainability: whether Qimmiurat would be able to operate, maintain, and recover the costs associated with this expensive development project.

A Companion to the Anthropology of Environmental Health, First Edition. Edited by Merrill Singer.

Audrey: I tell them that we're already paying a lot to keep our environment clean, and because we have to go to the doctor and other stuff … We've beat that subject to death with them. They keep telling us that it's not worth the investment because people aren't going to be able to afford the water and sewer when the project is done. … Someone just got Hep. A this fall. I told [the environmental health agency responsible for the project]; they didn't want to hear it. They were startled. We don't have real ways to stay clean and you get sick. Someone I think got it last year too. We're seeing one case a year or every other year.

Laura: How did they respond?

Audrey: They were startled. You know, they were here. They come out on trips and they stay here, but I don't think they understand how hard it is here. Especially people at the top. How difficult it is to try to maintain your health with limited water. They go home and can wash themselves.

Residents in this Arctic Alaska Native village I call Qimmiurat know firsthand the hidden costs of water insecurity and the invisibility of their experiences of water-washed disease. Like one-third of households in remote Alaskan Native villages that lack running water and sewer services (Hennessy *et al.* 2008), Qimmiurat residents experience the consequences of inadequate water access and sanitation every day. Yet development policies place priority on economic sustainability in ways that erase these experiences and public health needs, even where improving public health through water and wastewater infrastructure is the stated objective of such projects.

Bartram and Cairncross (2010), two prominent public health advocates for improved drinking water sources and sanitation, have characterized hygiene, sanitation, and water (HSW) as the "forgotten foundations of health." They note that while some claim that the benefits of investing in HSW are not substantiated, there is ample evidence that improving HSW has far reaching benefits not captured by disease-specific statistics. These include reducing malnutrition caused by diarrhea and associated long-term sequelae, health costs at household and national levels, and the economic impact of time involved in water collection. In contrast to concerns about whether investing in water and sanitation is cost effective, studies that account for this wide range of benefits estimate a net benefit of US$3–46 per $1 invested (Hutton, Haller, and Bartram 2007; Bartram and Cairncross 2010). Further, they argue that universal piped water and sanitation within homes, schools, and workplaces must be the ultimate goal of development policies because of the demonstrated significantly higher benefits associated with this level of service (Bartram and Cairncross 2010).

Why, given the overwhelming evidence, has the public health importance of HSW been "forgotten"? I argue that, in addition to the focus on disease-specific statistics (primarily focused on children's health), their importance has been largely rendered invisible through neoliberal policies that look to market solutions to environmental health problems. These policies end up prioritizing economic considerations and render daily experiences of water insecurity invisible, regardless of the intentions of the agencies and organizations involved.

A plethora of invisibilities remain around water and sanitation needs, including those of people living within "developed" countries and the Far North. Based on ethnographic data collected over 18 months between 2008 and 2009, in this chapter I describe the everyday struggles, hidden costs, and myriad health concerns borne by Iñupiaq communities living in water insecurity in Alaska's Northwest Arctic. Two of the questions this chapter addresses through ethnographic description are what everyday water insecurity looks like in Arctic Alaska Native villages, and what it is like to live with enough clean water to drink, but not to meet your other everyday needs.

Background

Water insecurity has been variably defined in terms of poor quality, inadequate access to improved water sources, seasonal fluctuations in available sources, and the subsequent effects of these conditions on daily practices, hygiene, and health (Ennis-McMillan 2001; Howard and Bartram 2003; Whiteford and Cortez-Lara 2005; Wutich and Ragsdale 2008). Drawing on this literature, I define water insecurity as the conditions of long-term or periodic scarcity of clean water and wastewater services that lead to inadequate clean water access, poor sanitation, and exposure to pathogens and contaminants, all of which affect how people use water and put these populations at higher risk of disease. Under these conditions, people might have enough clean water to drink, but not for hygiene. Their daily activities are likely to revolve around how and when they will access water (Ennis-McMillan 2001; Bartram and Cairncross 2010). Further, they are at higher risk of diseases associated with inadequate HSW, as well as associated long-term health sequelae (Bartram and Cairncross 2010).

My analysis of water insecurity and its hidden costs is influenced by insights from the political ecology of health and water, as well as discussions around structural violence. The political ecology of health examines the historical political economy of disease, as well as institutional and local discourses of disease and suffering, and considers disease and "the places of disease" as outcomes produced by and productive of social relations and power dynamics over time and at multiple scales (Baer 1996; Mayer 1996; King 2010, 49).

From this perspective, water insecurity is not a priori natural. Rather, it results from the intersection of ecological factors, inequalities of power, and economic disparities that intersect over time (see also Bakker 2004; Johnston 1998, 2005; Whiteford and Cortez-Lara 2005). Neoliberal policies, for example, have failed to achieve equitable water access and have in many cases created or exacerbated water insecurity (Derman and Ferguson 2003; Ferguson 2005; Johnston 2005; Whiteford and Whiteford 2005).

Further, experiences of water insecurity and its hidden costs and health risks are not evenly distributed across populations. Rather, they vary by social circumstances and positionalities such as gender (Ferguson 2005; Sultana 2009). Finally, the literature on structural violence and vulnerability (Farmer 1996, 2004; Quesada, Hart, and Bourgois 2011), which examines the indirect forces of oppression embedded within a social system that produce suffering, questions assumptions of local agency to mitigate suffering and provides a lens for understanding how experiences of water insecurity and its hidden costs are erased.

Water Insecurity in Remote Alaska Native Communities

Water insecurity is a problem that remote Alaska Native communities share with millions of people worldwide. Despite a tremendous amount of money spent on improving safe water and sewerage infrastructure, today approximately one in three households continues to lack running water and sewer services (Hennessy *et al.* 2008). Several studies have focused on the many environmental, economic, and social factors that hinder access to water and sewer services. These include high water tables, permafrost, seasonal flooding, the remoteness of villages, small populations that increase per-household costs, limited cash economies and poverty, and cultural differences and miscommunications between agencies and communities (Tussing 1982; Huskey 1992; EPA 1995; Berardi 1998b, 1998a; Wiita and Haley 2003). Less well understood is how water insecurity fits into a larger historical set of political and economic forces that intersect with ecologic factors. Understanding this history is key for understanding how daily water insecurity is rendered invisible today.

Briefly, the problem of water insecurity emerges from the history of the creation of permanent settlements beginning in the late nineteenth century. Missionaries and the US Bureau of Education encouraged the once semi-nomadic Iñupiat (along with other Alaska Native peoples) to settle in these permanent villages both by coercion and by the availability of medicines during a period of devastating epidemics of novel infections introduced by the influx of Russians and Americans (Ducker 1996; Berardi 1999).

The creation of permanent villages, combined with the availability of pharmaceutical medicines during devastating epidemics, reduced infant and child mortality. They thus contributed to a dramatic increase in children (Chance 1990) and produced a need for water and waste management not previously experienced (Berardi 1999). Infectious epidemics continued to be a problem in the nascent villages well into the twentieth century, in part due to overcrowding in dwellings, poor ventilation in households, and inadequate clean water and sanitation (Lantis 1963; Blackman 1992).

In 1954, the Village Sanitation Aide Program began training local men as sanitarians, while also installing safe water points throughout the participating villages (Morley 1954; Rogers 1956; Lantis 1962). The Village Safe Water (VSW) Act of 1972 replaced this program, and established a state-run program "to provide safe water and hygienic sewage disposal facilities" that would "be available for use by the public and ... designed to assure year-round use" (Alaska State Legislature 1972).

The development of village infrastructure, including water treatment and wastewater systems, occurred in tandem with the growth of Alaska's petrol economy following the construction of the Trans-Alaska Pipeline in 1977. The sudden influx of oil revenue funded development projects throughout the state (Leask 1983; McBeath and Morehouse 1994; Mitchell 2001). This huge influx of state capital enabled rural growth, including services and projects that would otherwise have been unaffordable in communities with limited tax bases (Leask 1983).

The influx of capital investment during this period, combined with decreased mortality rates from treated water (US Congress 1994), led again to an increase in village populations. Alaska Natives, who had been migrating out of villages in the 1950s and 1960s, began moving back into remote communities partially because of the new availability of employment and public services supported by the transfer economy, and in part to qualify for Native corporation dividends under the Alaska Native Claims Settlement Act (ANCSA) (Leask 1983; Kruse and Foster 1986; Berardi 1999). The economies of rural municipalities that resulted from this sudden growth in government (including local employment) became dependent on state subsidies for their operations (Leask 1983; Knapp and Huskey 1988).

Contributing to the problem was the fact that growth in populations and public services were not considered when the Bureau of Education chose village sites. In the latter half of the twentieth century, it became apparent that their ecological conditions were largely unsuitable for providing adequate clean water and sewerage using modern technologies to the growing populations (Berardi 1999). Environmental challenges to the operation and maintenance of water and sanitation systems have only become worse with climate change. Increasing rates and severity of flooding, erosion, and the melting of permafrost threaten the integrity of these expensive infrastructures, and at the same time decrease water quality (Brubaker *et al.* 2011). Thus, VSW's founding goal of establishing safe water and sewage disposal facilities "designed to assure year-round use" has yet to be realized. The question today voiced by politicians, environmental health agencies, and even some Iñupiaq leaders has become whether the money has been well spent, and how to more efficiently allocate limited funds.

Economic concerns around safe water and sewage disposal facilities began shortly after this historical surge in construction projects. By the mid-1980s, the world price of oil upon which Alaska's economy depended was falling, and the state of Alaska began reconsidering its role in subsidizing village governments (Knapp and Huskey 1988; Flanders 1989; Dombrowski 2001). At issue was whether communities had a right to treated water infrastructure, because, as one report framed the problem, the widely held perception was that "rights are not limited by costs" that led to unsustainable spending (Knapp and Huskey 1988: 33). The costs and benefits of rural public services were called into question in ways that reduced rural water and sanitation to an issue of expectations (Kruse and Foster 1986), not public health.

The effect of recent fluctuations in the world energy market on clean water access in remote Alaskan villages illustrates the public health significance of the water-energy nexus, a term used to describe the relationship between water security and energy security (Eichelberger 2010). The sudden rise in the global price of oil from around $54 per barrel in January 2007 to over $133 in June 2008 (US Energy Information Administration 2016) led to a dramatic increase in energy prices that affected household access to water, as well as the operations and maintenance of safe water and wastewater systems (Eichelberger 2010). Between June 2014 and December 2015, the global per barrel price of crude oil plummeted from over $105 to just under $40 (US Energy Information

Administration 2016). Fluctuations in the price of crude oil have dramatic effects in petro-economies, such as that of Alaska (McBeath and Morehouse 1994). In 2015, Iñupiaq leaders reported a decrease in already limited funding available for village capital projects, including water and sewerage.

In this economic climate, the question of the costs of clean water and wastewater infrastructure has taken on a new urgency (Eichelberger 2012). In 2008, both state and federal agencies involved in the funding and construction of water and sewage disposal facilities were increasingly requiring that villages demonstrate "sustainability" prior to the approval of projects and allocation of funds. In this political and economic climate, policies related to clean water and sewerage define sustainability largely in terms of economic criteria.

The sustainability of villages is assessed by the Rural Utility Business Association (RUBA), and their reports have become key documents through which villages compete with each other for limited water and sanitation project funding. RUBA assessments use sustainability indicators that include an 80 percent collection rate on water and sanitation user fees that can be as high as $150 per month, creating local incentive for households to disconnect from their only source of treated water. Although agencies officially evaluate project proposals based on public health needs, village populations are too small to produce disease- and village-specific statistics to demonstrate their need for these expensive facilities. In contrast, RUBA assessments include village-specific economic data that are easier to collect and use in comparing one community proposal to another (Eichelberger 2012, 2014).

This situation underscores contemporary concerns about the sustainability of water and sanitation infrastructures. Indeed, the rationale of sustainability, which emphasizes efficiency and full-cost recovery, has largely (though not officially) replaced public health concerns related to the treatment and distribution of water, and wastewater management. Whereas it has been widely recognized that the state-funded construction of water treatment and wastewater facilities improved Alaska Native health (US Congress 1994), today economic criteria take a higher precedence in the allocation of project funding (Eichelberger 2012, 2014). The emphasis on economic sustainability contributes to an erasure of the daily experiences and hidden costs of water insecurity, local inequalities of clean water access, as well as public health needs.

Everyday Water Insecurity and Hidden Costs

In late January, with the temperature well below –20 °F, I watched a boy, perhaps 11 or 12 years old, slowly drive his four-wheeler away from the washeteria up the road. He stopped several times to steady the 32-gallon bucket, steering with one hand while holding onto the bucket with the other, carefully maneuvering the vehicle around bumps in the frozen road. This scene played out every day in Qimmiurat until very recently, when the village completed the initial construction of an in-home piped water and wastewater system to which households are still being connected. Many households, however, have yet to be connected to the system and must still haul their own water.

As in other communities worldwide characterized by water insecurity (Ennis-McMillan 2001), daily life in Qimmiurat is largely organized around obtaining water. Nowhere is this more evident than the washeteria, where the gendered social relations of water insecurity play out and their hidden costs become visible. At the time of my fieldwork, all households in this village of just fewer than 500 people hauled water from the washeteria, which combines the only public (for fee) showers, laundry, and clean water access in the community. Water plant operators pump raw water from the river to the washeteria, where they treat it and store the "safe water" in a tank. Residents then haul treated water from an external access point to their homes.

The washeteria is busy from the time it opens at eight in the morning to the time it closes at night, which varies according to the seasons, availability of water, and decisions of the water plant operators. On one side of the wall, the male water plant operators operate the water treatment facility; on the other, women and girls spend many hours doing laundry. The phone in the washeteria rings frequently with people, usually women and girls, calling to see how long the line is for a washer. With only four functioning washing machines to serve a community of over 450 people, the line is usually long, especially on the weekends.

Outside the washeteria there is often a line of four-wheelers, snow machines, and the occasional dog sled. Boys and men, and to a lesser extent girls and women, await their turn at the only water access point to fill containers varying in size from 5-gallon "jerry jugs," to 32-gallon trashcans with lids, to large tanks towed behind four-wheelers (Figure 12.1). Those with larger containers struggle

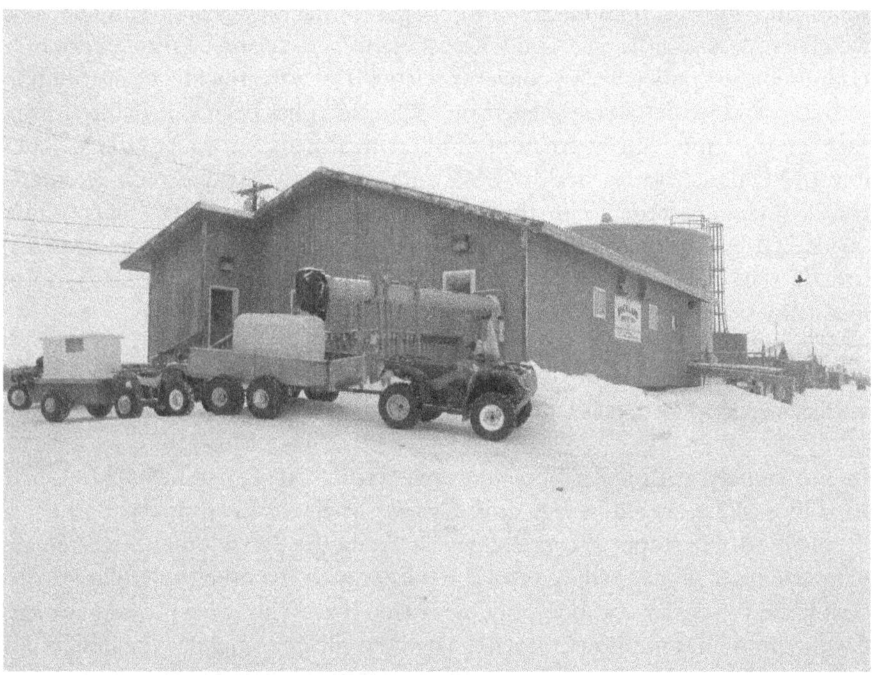

Figure 12.1 Qimmiurat's washeteria.

during the winter to navigate around the stalagmite of ice that forms below the hose in order to get their vehicle close enough. Those with smaller containers struggle to get enough water to last through the day.

With few exceptions, the majority of Qimmiurat households use 5-gallon "honey buckets" lined with trash bags and topped with a toilet seat as toilets. Households place full bags of sewage outside their homes on the side of the road, often in cardboard boxes, and the City of Qimmiurat hauls the bags of sewage to the dump (or more recently, the new sewage lagoon). These bags of sewage often break open while awaiting collection. Honey buckets constitute a significant health risk because of cross-contamination – the distribution of fecal bacteria throughout the community and into homes by boots and tires (Chambers *et al.* 2008, 2009). Researchers studying one Alaska Native village lacking in-home piped water and sewerage have found fecal bacteria in hand washing basins, on dippers used to access water from storage buckets, as well as kitchen counters and floors (Chambers *et al.* 2008).

Based on survey data collected between January and May of 2009, the average water consumption in Qimmiurat was 2.4 gallons per capita per day (gal/c/d) (see Eichelberger 2010 for full description). Residents reported spending anywhere from 15 minutes to almost an hour hauling water, often making multiple trips a day. These numbers stand in stark contrast to the minimum daily per capita consumption recommended by the World Health Organization of 13.2 gal/c/d, a tap within 100 meters of a home, and collection time not to exceed five minutes. As studies elsewhere have documented, one significant hidden cost of water insecurity is time lost to accessing water (Bartram and Cairncross 2010).

Further, the type of household system, availability of the washeteria, combined with household costs associated with hauling water (detailed below) and social axes of insecurity such as gender and wealth (Farmer 1996), mean that water consumption rates vary by household and fluctuate throughout the year. Between 2008 and 2009, when I conducted field research, approximately eight households had flush-haul systems. These homes had one or two in-home taps, a shower, and a flush toilet, and used 200- or 300-gallon storage tanks in heated sheds to store their self-hauled treated water. Flush-haul households reported an average consumption rate of 4.8 gal/c/d, with the largest reported consumption rate being 7.1 gal/c/d. Households that were plumbed for flush-haul but which no longer used their systems, owing to the energy and maintenance costs involved as well as the smell, consumed an average of 2 gal/c/d. "Honey bucket" households, by contrast, stored treated water in 32-gallon trashcans with lids (locally referred to as "buckets"). Self-reported water consumption in these households ranged from 0.4 gal/c/d to 3.5 gal/c/d, with an average water consumption of 1.6 gal/c/d (Eichelberger 2010).

Water-Energy Nexus and Social Axes of Water Access

Three household characteristics stand out in the 11 Qimmiurat households that reported the lowest consumption rates of domestic water. All were honey bucket households; three were headed by single employed mothers with young children;

and three reported that they did not have regular access to a vehicle. Indeed, gasoline, diesel, and other externally priced commodities are a major component of safe water production and distribution.

Because residents haul water themselves, access to a gasoline-powered vehicle is one of the largest determinants of how much water a household can access. The weight of water, the significant distance from the access point to each home, and the time involved in hauling water contribute significantly to the fact that vehicles are central to determining household water consumption. The simple fact that a gallon of water weighs 8.35 pounds per gallon makes hauling adequate domestic water too costly in terms of time for single mothers with young children who do not have vehicles, and physically impossible for the disabled. A 5-gallon jug of water, which is the lowest reported volume of water people hauled, weighs 42 pounds. The World Health Organization's recommended domestic water consumption rate of 13.2 gal/c/d weighs 110.2 pounds. This contributes to the lower consumption rates among single women with young children and the disabled (often the situation of elders), particularly if they lack a vehicle.

Household composition further affects water consumption, and shapes water insecurity in gendered ways. Male kin may not reside at home for many reasons. In these villages, local jobs are few, seasonal, and depend on infrastructure projects. With few opportunities and self-reported high stress, turnover in these positions can be high. Employment opportunities are greater outside the village, at Red Dog Mine or as far away as Anchorage or Fairbanks, but these require the separation of families for extended periods of time. Further, most of the permanent positions in villages are occupied by women: administrators, community health aides, and other office-based employment. As of the 2000 Census, 29 percent of households in Northwest Alaska were headed by women and the number of elder women living alone has risen since 1994 (AFN 2004; Goldsmith *et al.* 2004).

The hidden costs of not having a vehicle or kin who can haul water, aside from the lower access to water and the associated risks to health, include having to pay others to help haul water. On a daily basis in Qimmiurat, someone would make an announcement over the VHF (the community CB radio) that they could haul water for $10, sometimes $20, per haul. Other times, I heard women announcing that they would pay someone to haul water for them.

Household costs of living, already high before the energy crisis of the mid-2000s, play a significant role in safe water access. Between 2000 and 2006, utility costs in remote regions rose by 50 percent. By 2006, the median share of income for utilities among the poorest 20 percent households in remote areas was 33 percent (Saylor and Haley 2007). Thus, Qimmiurat residents were increasingly faced with choosing between purchasing domestic water (including showers and laundry), purchasing gasoline at as much as $10 per gallon, or paying utility bills (Eichelberger 2010).

One employed mother of four described the choices she faces between paying bills and purchasing water for her household of six: "I figure we spend about 320 to 500 [a month] on laundry, hauling water, showering, gas to haul the water … Sometimes I have to put off showers and laundry so I can pay my bills! … It's becoming harder and harder to live here because of the water thing."

Inclement weather, such as extremely cold temperatures and seasonal flooding, can make hauling water difficult if not impossible. Sitting in the City Office on a cold day in January, one single mother described to me how difficult getting water had been during a recent cold snap over the Christmas and New Year's holidays (when I had been visiting my family in Fairbanks):

> *Martha*: It was like 40 to 50 below for the last two weeks. You're lucky you weren't here! It was hard to haul water because the snow machines and Hondas wouldn't start. I noticed people around town were starting to look a little dirty.

She chuckled as she described how the lack of water affected people's access to water and showers, including herself. Her desk is often abuzz with people who come in to purchase shower and laundry tokens for the washeteria and she noted that they had been purchasing fewer tokens during that time.

> *Martha*: People weren't washing because it was hard to get water.
> *Laura*: Did you also ration water?
> *Martha*: I tried to save it for cooking so I didn't use it to clean at all. I didn't wash my hair for a long time, until my head started to hurt.

Indeed, most Qimmiurat residents reported that it was more difficult to haul water in the winter rather than the summer, in part because their vehicles often cannot start in temperatures below –35.

> *Aaron*: It's dangerous to get water in the winter. There's a big hill [of ice that sits under the watering point] that gets slick and high. [My wife's] brother got a concussion from slipping on it.

The washeteria's fluctuating hours of operation affect domestic water access. The external safe water access point is always available unless the water plant operators cease pumping and treating water. Water plant operators close the washeteria, including the external access point, due to inclement weather such as extremely cold temperatures (in order to conserve the clean water available because they cannot pump during cold snaps), a lack of parts to repair or materials necessary to maintain the system (such as shortages of gas), and environmental conditions such as flooding or turbid river water.

For employed women, and mothers of young children in particular, doing laundry (and even showering) can be a time-consuming task only achieved on weekends or late into the night. When the water plant operators close the washeteria early, or shut off the electricity in the middle of the night to conserve energy or to discourage use of the facilities, it is the women who are most affected. This is where the gendered division of labor and the fact that most water plant operators are men creates a situation of unequal control of access to water that affects women's daily lives.

Women are uniquely affected by limited water in other, subtle ways. Women largely occupy the limited permanent local employment opportunities within the villages. Government administrators, clerks, storekeepers, and health aides are predominantly women, while men are more likely to be employed as water plant operators and in seasonal construction. With limited employment opportunities and great demand, rumors regarding those who hold these coveted positions abound. More than once, in different villages, a female head of a honey bucket household told me stories of someone having reported them to their boss for using water available at their employment or for showering during office hours.

These accounts illustrate how struggles around water access – including limited washeteria hours, access to a vehicle and male kin, the weather, and the ability to pay for water – affect all residents, but individuals are affected in particular ways according to their age, gender, kin network, employment, and age of their children. These social axes shape how the hidden costs of water insecurity are experienced differentially. In contrast, policies related to water and sanitation infrastructure development consider neither these hidden costs, nor local inequities of safe water access and sanitation. Further, as Bartram and Cairncross (2010) have likewise noted, the focus on disease-specific statistics fails to recognize the widespread economic and health consequences of water insecurity.

Health Consequences

A Qimmiurat teacher, in February 2009, described the consequences of lack of access to water as follows:

> There's never a point when everyone's healthy ... One student of mine has been in and out of school for weeks because they keep getting sick. Most parents do a good job. They spend a lot of time at the washeteria doing clothes. But it has to do with the trouble it is to wash your hands without running water ...
>
> ... There are definitely times when only a few kids are in class. When strep starts going around ... you start to notice a pattern. When strep is going around, we up the awareness in the school. We remind the kids how to sneeze, how to cough ... but there are times of the year when we say, "Why? Why do we have strep? Why do we have stomach problems?"
>
> ... After Christmas, I don't know why, kids start dropping like flies. And there are some that say it's because of their sleeping schedule over the holiday, but still. You get the goopies, the strep, the stomach problems ...There's been a lot of stomach stuff lately. I have a lot of kids using the bathroom regularly and I don't know why.
>
> ... Right behind the school in the summer time, it's full of water. And they've tried to drain it out, but it doesn't work. It's full of water, and the honey buckets from the houses there ... well, not all of [the sewage] always makes it to the dump. That water is always dirty. And the kids skip rocks, play around, and splash in it. It's water; they want to play in it.

Water insecurity in these communities has critical public health consequences, including a higher incidence of lower respiratory and skin infections (Hennessy *et al.* 2008; Chambers *et al.* 2009; Wenger *et al.* 2010). In villages where less than 10 percent of households have in-home piped water, children suffer some of the highest rates of invasive pneumococcal infection worldwide (Wenger *et al.* 2010). These statistics, however, do not capture residents' daily and seasonal experiences of disease and struggles to mitigate the risks of infection.

Qimmiurat's K–12 school is a site at which the community-wide health effects of water insecurity are visible on a daily basis, as it is the single place where the majority of the population spends the most hours together. As is true of villages across the region, a large proportion of Qimmiurat's population is school-aged children and schools are one of the primary employers in the community. Further, children are at the greatest risk for water- and sanitation-related disease, particularly young children who crawl on the floor and put things such as toys in their mouths (Chambers *et al.* 2009, 2008). When a disease outbreak occurs in the community, the school is one of the first places to experience its effects.

One of the health consequences of inadequate water access that schools regularly contend with is lice infection, which is highly communicable. Although not widely recognized as associated with water insecurity, the recommended preventatives measures along with teacher accounts illustrate how inadequate water access can contribute to lice infestations. According to the Centers for Disease Control and Prevention (CDC), "getting head lice is not related to cleanliness of the person or his or her environment" (CDC 2013). However, the CDC recommends prevention and control measures that include machine washing and drying clothing, linens, and other items worn or used by the individual with head lice. One Qimmiurat teacher described how lice and water insecurity go hand in hand: "You pick and choose what you can afford to wash. [So] they probably won't wash their pillowcases that they sleep on every night. Kids sleeping over spreads it."

Lice are also highly stigmatizing. Teachers and residents reported that those children who are found to have lice will often burst into tears. One teacher described the social effects of lice on her students:

> Lice, or *kumak*, have become a big problem recently. It stays in the bedding ... It's a self-esteem thing. There's a lot of teasing. It's an embarrassing thing. The children cry after the nurse identifies them as having lice. The other day, a girl scratched her head during my class, and I saw two girls sitting behind her look at each other. [She raised her eyebrows to demonstrate.]

Female heads of households with small children were most concerned about what they classified as strep throat, pneumonia, impetigo, and "bad stomach," an illness characterized by symptoms of gas, diarrhea, and sometimes vomiting that was more likely to be experienced by adults. These concerns were confirmed by community health aide practitioners at the clinic:

> We see lots of viral infections: colds, sore throats, strep – both viral and bacterial. There needs to be more hand washing. The clinic encourages hand washing, but we don't know how often people are changing their basin water. It's recommended that you change it every hour. Kids get lots of illnesses. They crawl on the floor and put things in their mouth. We see a lot of kids with respiratory diseases. About every other month someone is referred out to Anchorage or Quag˙aq, mostly kids.

Illness can constitute a significant social and economic strain on a household, evident in the hidden costs of a child's illness. Mothers, or grandmothers if they are the caretakers of their grandchildren, bear the brunt of work related to caring for sick children and mitigating the health risks associated with inadequate water and sanitation.

In addition to the time they spend at the washeteria doing laundry, mothers are usually the ones who accompany a sick child to the clinic or to the hospitals in Quag˙aq or Anchorage. In Qimmiurat, parents and community health aides reported that many children are sent to Anchorage or Quag˙aq because of pneumonia, tonsil removal due to strep throat, or to have tubes put in their ears because of repeated otitis media infections.

Even in communities with running water and wastewater systems, periodic service interruptions combined with disparities in service levels create conditions ripe for water-washed diseases, and their accompanying hidden costs. Accompanying a sick child to the doctor outside the village can constitute a significant strain on the family, as this mother in Ilavut described:

> *Reagan*: We have to ration our water in the spring, after the ice departs, because of all of the debris and dead animals in the water. The City issues a boil water notice then. About 3 months ago [in wintertime] the clinic ran out of Tylenol. The water was bad because it was turning into springtime. Everyone had diarrhea and vomiting. There was a boil notice. Everyone starting buying bottled water from the store ... Pneumonia is recently a problem. My one-month-old baby got it. Lots of babies were sent to the hospital [in Quag˙aq] in April. It's tough on the family when the baby goes with the mom. The mother goes to Quag˙aq with the baby, and no one cares for the kids. It takes a lot away from the family.

Although some local tribal councils[2] have travel monies available, their financial resources are finite and not all are able to support their members' travel for medical visits. Those who do not qualify for Medicare, Denali KidCare,[3] or who cannot obtain tribal support have to pay for their travel themselves, a hidden cost of illness that is directly related to the cost of fuel.

Risk Mitigation: Public versus Professional Responses

The everyday experiences of water insecurity and its hidden costs, along with struggles to prevent and treat illnesses, often stand in contrast to the visible public health responses to water-wash diseases and messages regarding their mitigation. In February 2009, after an extended closure of the washeteria due to the freezing of the water intake line, a public health information sign was posted in the Post Office. It warned residents that infections of strep throat and pertussis were increasing in the region, and advised two risk reduction measures: avoiding crowds and crowded places, and hand washing under hot running water with soap. This set of instructions made little sense in a community without an in-home piped running water system that was experiencing a housing shortage such that in some cases two or more families would share one small home. Indeed, the poster illustrates the contradictions between local experience and a generalized public health response to disease infection. Similar public health notices advising preventative actions that were unfeasible in Qimmiurat appeared around the community throughout the year.

This disconnect between the health education materials and the reality on the ground points to the silences that occur around suffering. Few data exist that public health officers and policy makers can use to accurately depict and respond to the situation of water insecurity and related diseases at the local level. The small size of village populations makes epidemiological studies of infectious diseases difficult, while the rare case or outbreak of devastating infections give the false impression that sanitation-related disease is relatively under control. This epidemiologic invisibility (Eichelberger 2014) contributes to the erasures of public health needs related to HSW.

The chasm that exists between the public health advisories and the reality of water insecurity shape the lay epidemiology that surrounds infectious disease, water, and sanitation. Avoiding infections is a daily concern for those living without adequate access to water, and especially in communities where honey buckets are hauled through the village to the sewage lagoon.

Asked what protective measures they take to avoid illness in their households, female heads of household reported what someone working in public health would hope to hear. For example, when I conducted an initial survey in Qimmiurat women told me that they change the washbasin water regularly (sometimes hourly), they make their children wash their hands when they come in to the house, they tell their children to avoid areas of town known to be contaminated with honey bucket waste, they spend hours every week doing the family laundry, and they use a clean dipper to obtain water from their 32-gallon water bucket. Notably, in contrast to the public health poster described above, no one ever told me that they avoid crowded places or wash their hands with hot running water.

However, subsequent observational data and interviews revealed that these self-reported protective measures are neither always followed nor feasible. For example, households do not always have control over whether their honey buckets are taken to the sewage lagoon before the bags break open and spill their contents. Washbasins are more likely to be changed after the water has become visibly dirty. In addition, dippers used to scoop treated water from the buckets in which it is stored were often 2-cup measures not kept in sanitary locations, and are therefore one likely source of contamination.

Finally, despite stated intentions at both the local and regional levels, at the time of my fieldwork sewage handlers in Qimmiurat had not been trained in how to avoid cross-contamination, or in cleanup procedures. Individual households did report several risk mitigation strategies, such as avoiding areas of town that smelled, pouring bleach in areas contaminated by sewage, or putting gasoline in stagnate puddles and setting them alight.

Water Insecurity and Health over the Life Course

Although children are at a higher risk of many diseases associated with inadequate clean water access and poor sanitation (Chambers *et al.* 2008, 2009; Bartram and Cairncross 2010), water insecurity, its health outcomes, and its hidden costs are experienced throughout the broader community and across lifespans. As the previous ethnographic accounts detail, a child's illness and the hidden costs of water insecurity affect the larger household. Further, epidemiologic evidence suggests that particular infections in early childhood associated with inadequate clean water and sanitation produce adverse health outcomes throughout life.

For example, among Alaska Native populations the risk of invasive pneumococcal disease (IPD), a precursor to many otitis media infections (OM, middle ear infections), is disproportionately higher than among non-Alaska Native children (Davidson *et al.* 1994). This increased risk of IPD has been linked to a lack of in-home piped water in these populations, and has not been decreased by the introduction of the 7-valent pneumococcal conjugate vaccine (Wenger *et al.* 2010). As a cluster of overlapping diseases,[4] OM's long-term effects on health and well-being include hearing loss, speech delay, and learning problems, as well as increased mortality from brain abscesses and meningitis (Qureishi *et al.* 2014). Further, OM is one of the most common reasons for antibiotic use and surgery among children, leading to concerns related to antibiotic resistance, health care costs, and surgery-related complications (Qureishi *et al.* 2014).

On a worldwide scale, one of the primary health concerns related to water insecurity is diarrheal disease. Repeated diarrhea-associated dehydration and malnutrition in the first 2 years of life, when the human body undergoes critical growth and development, put children at risk for several disability outcomes that outweigh statistics on mortality from diarrheal disease alone (Guerrant *et al.* 2002). The consequences of these repeated insults on the body include fitness impairment, stunting, cognitive impairment, and lower school performance (Guerrant *et al.* 2002, 2008; Bartelt *et al.* 2013).

Indeed, the health effects of water insecurity are not limited to childhood, but can manifest throughout the life course. Growing epidemiologic evidence links infection by the bacterium *Helicobacter pylori* (*H. pylori*) to conditions that characterize water insecurity, including untreated water and a lack of a fixed hot water supply (Mendall *et al.* 1992; Frenck and Clemens 2003; Bellack *et al.* 2006; Khalifa, Sharaf, and Aziz 2010). Infection by the bacterium causes anemia, chronic gastritis, peptic and duodenal ulcers, and stomach cancer (Brown 2000; Khalifa, Sharaf, and Aziz 2010; de Martel *et al.* 2012; de Martel, Forman, and Plummer 2013).

Such living conditions during childhood have been linked to increased risk of *H. pylori* infection (Mendall *et al.* 1992). A widely accepted hypothesis states that early childhood infection might lead to a low-grade chronic inflammatory state of the gastric mucosa that leads to a higher risk of stomach cancer later in life (Frenck and Clemens 2003; Correa and Houghton 2007). Indeed, stomach cancer has been shown in many geographic contexts to be associated with unimproved drinking water supplies (Haenszel *et al.* 1976; Risch *et al.* 1985; Boeing *et al.* 1991; Tran *et al.* 2005; Eichelberger *et al.* 2015). Other possible non-infectious risk factors for stomach cancer include exposure to nitrate-contaminated water, which can leak into drinking water sources from sewage, fertilizers, and natural erosion (IARC 2010).

Inadequate clean water sources and poor sanitation thus present multiple health risks, both infectious and non-infectious, that can have serious long-term health consequences. Although children are at a higher risk of many diseases associated with inadequate clean water access and poor sanitation (Chambers *et al.* 2008, 2009; Bartram and Cairncross 2010), attention should also be paid to long-term morbidity and hidden costs across the life course. These combined experiences of acute and chronic outcomes over the lifespan contribute to the everyday struggles around water insecurity.

Conclusion

These ethnographic data demonstrate how water insecurity is experienced in Arctic Iñupiaq villages on a daily and seasonal basis, how these experiences are affected by the water-energy nexus and vary by social axes, and how people struggle to mitigate the risks associated with water insecurity in the face of public health responses that are inappropriate for water insecure communities. As Audrey described at the beginning of this chapter, Qimmiurat's residents and other Iñupiat living without adequate clean water and sanitation across the region recognize that their experiences are largely invisible. The few cases of Hepatitis A that might occur in one village in a year are not enough to elicit a public health response that overcomes economic concerns driving water treatment and wastewater project funding decisions beyond hygiene promotion.

The chapter began by describing how water insecurity can be produced and reproduced as a consequence of policies and interventions with ostensibly positive objectives of improving local health and well-being. "Sustainability," for example, is a goal shared by both local communities and state agencies (Eichelberger 2014). However, sustainability policies are in fact guided by neoliberal principles of efficiency and full-cost recovery, which supersede the public health importance of clean water and wastewater infrastructure. Such neoliberal policies thus erase the daily struggles around water and health, the hidden costs of water insecurity, and its long-term health sequelae. This is how, in the words of Bartram and Cairncross (2010), HSW have been "forgotten" as the foundations of health.

Anthropologists are well situated to provide rich ethnographic data that can inform interventions and public health-centered policies. For example, hygiene and sanitation promotion have proven in many contexts to be among the most cost-effective interventions to control disease (Bartram and Cairncross 2010). Yet such programs run the risk of reproducing paternalistic assumptions of local ignorance and, as public health officers characterized the problem for Alaska Natives in the mid-twentieth century, indifference to sanitation (Buck and Hays 1943). As this chapter has demonstrated, the Iñupiat recognize the importance of hygiene, sanitation, and water, but their ability to adhere to hygiene promotion standards is severely limited by access to clean water. Ethnographic data on clean water access, uses, and how these might fluctuate by seasons and according to social axes can help tailor such interventions to their local contexts.

Further, as I have described elsewhere (Eichelberger 2012, 2014), small population sizes limit a community's ability to demonstrate statistically the validity of their health concerns in order to substantiate investment in water treatment facilities. As Bartram and Cairncross (2010) have also noted, the focus on disease-specific statistics belies the broader benefits of HSW, contributing to the epidemiologic invisibility of the needs of small populations (Eichelberger 2014).

The consequences of water insecurity, both epidemiologic and economic, need to be considered beyond disease-specific statistics and include the myriad hidden costs and long-term health consequences experienced by those living with inadequate clean water and sanitation. Water insecurity is a problem facing millions of people worldwide. An estimated 780 million people globally live without access to an improved drinking water source, and sanitation service coverage continues to trail the benchmarks set by the Millennium Development Goals (Bartram and Cairncross 2010; WHO and UNICEF 2012). Further, an estimated 80 percent of the world's population is at risk for water insecurity, and this problem is expected to grow with increasing demand for water and diminishing water resources due to climate change (Hope *et al.* 2012). Though often considered a problem of low-income countries, this case study as well as the recent highly publicized water contamination in Flint, Michigan illustrate the importance of understanding water insecurity in wealthy countries such as the United States.

Anthropologists can contribute significant data detailing the hidden costs and long-term consequences of water insecurity beyond disease-specific statistics and extreme events, such as cholera epidemics. Further, we can contribute much-needed data on how energy issues affect access to clean water, and how water insecurity fluctuates and is experienced differentially according to social axes over the life course. To do so, we need to pair our efforts with those of epidemiologists and others to engage in mixed-methods research that reaches across disciplinary boundaries. This is particularly important as we increasingly see the effects of climate change on health and water resources worldwide, and as neoliberal policies continue to be touted as the solution to water insecurity. By helping to bring the wide-ranging consequences of water insecurity out of epidemiologic invisibility, anthropologists can contribute to a remembering of HSW as the foundations of health.

NOTES

1 In order to protect the anonymity of the residents in these small communities, I have given each informant and village a pseudonym.
2 Most Alaska Native villages have a state-charted city government and a federally recognized tribal council. Residents of one village may be members of a tribal council in another village.
3 Denali KidCare is Alaska's Medicaid program for children under 18 years old and pregnant women.
4 Different types of OM include acute OM (AOM), acute suppurative OM (a subtype of AOM), OM with effusion (OME), and chronic suppurative OM (CSOM). Although generally treated as distinct diseases, Qureishi and colleagues (2014) describe OM as a "continuum/spectrum of diseases" with substantial overlap.

REFERENCES

AFN. 2004. *Our Choices, Our Future: Analysis of the Status of Alaska Natives Report 2004.* Anchorage, Alaska: Alaska Native Policy Center.

Baer, H. 1996. "Toward a Political Ecology of Health in Medical Anthropology." *Medical Anthropology Quarterly*, 10(4): 451–454.

Bakker, K. 2004. *An Uncooperative Commodity: Privatizing Water in England and Wales.* Oxford: Oxford University Press.

Bartelt, L. A., Lima, A. A., Kosek, M., Penataro Yori, P., Lee, G., and Guerrant. R.L. 2013. ""Barriers" to Child Development and Human Potential: The Case for Including the "Neglected Enteric Protozoa" (NEP) and Other Enteropathy-associated Pathogens in the NTDs." *PLoS Neglected Tropical Diseases*, 7(4): e2125. doi: 10.1371/journal.pntd.0002125.

Bartram, J. and Cairncross, S. 2010. "Hygiene, Sanitation, and Water: Forgotten Foundations of Health." *Plos Medicine*, 7(11). doi: 10.1371/journal.pmed.1000367.

Bellack, N. R., Koehoorn, M.W., MacNab, Y.C., and Morshed, M.G. 2006. "A Conceptual Model of Water's Role as a Reservoir in Helicobacter Pylori Transmission: A Review of the Evidence." *Epidemiological Infection*, 134(3): 439–449. doi: 10.1017/S0950268806006005.

Berardi, G. 1998a. "Application of Participatory Rural Appraisal in Alaska." *Human Organization*, 57(4): 438–446.

Berardi, G. 1998b. "Natural Resource Policy, Unforgiving Geographies, and Persistent Poverty in Alaska Native Villages." *Natural Resources Journal*, 38(1): 85–108.

Berardi, G. 1999. "Schools, Settlement, and Sanitation in Alaska Native Villages." *Ethnohistory*, 46(2): 329–360.

Blackman, M.B. 1992. *Sadie Brower Neakok: An Inupiaq Woman.* Seattle: University of Washington Press.

Boeing, H., Frentzel-Beyme, R., Berger, M., Berndt, V., Gores, W., Korner, M., Lohmeier, R., Menarcher, A., Mannl, H.G., Meinhardt, M., and *et al.* 1991. "Case-control Study on Stomach Cancer in Germany." *International Journal of Cancer*, 47(6): 858–864.

Brown, L.M. 2000. "Helicobacter Pylori: Epidemiology and Routes of Transmission." *Epidemiological Review*, 22(2): 283–297.

Brubaker, M., Berner, J., Bell, J., and Warren, J. 2011. *Climate Change in Kivalina, Alaska: Strategies for Community Health.* Anchorage, Alaska: Center for Climate and Health, Alaska Native Tribal Health Consortium.

Buck, C.E. and Hays, G. 1943. "Public Health Needs in Alaska." *Alaska's Health*, 1 (Special Edition): 3–15.

CDC (Centers for Disease Control and Prevention). 2014. *Head Lice: Epidemiology & Risk Factors.* http://www.cdc.gov/parasites/lice/head/epi.html (accessed December 4, 2015).

Chambers, M.K., Ford, M.R., White, D.M. Barnes, D.L., and Schiewer, S. 2008. "Distribution and Transport of Fecal Bacteria at Spring Thaw in a Rural Alaskan Community." *Journal of Cold Regions Engineering*, 22(1): 16–37.

Chambers, M.K., Ford, M.R., White, D.M. Barnes, D.L., and Schiewer, S. 2009. "Transport of Fecal Bacteria by Boots and Vehicle Tires in a Rural Alaskan Community." *Journal of Environmental Management*, 90(2): 961–966.

Chance, N.A. 1990. *The Iñupiat and Arctic Alaska: An Ethnography of Development.* Case Studies in Cultural Anthropology. Fort Worth, TX: Holt Rinehart & Winston.

Correa, P. and Houghton, J. 2007. "Carcinogenesis of Helicobacter pylori." *Gastroenterology*, 133(2): 659–672. doi: 10.1053/j.gastro.2007.06.026.

Davidson, M., Parkinson, A.J., Bulkow, L.R., Fitzgerald, M.A., Peters, H.V., and Parks, D.J. 1994. "The Epidemiology of Invasive Pneumococcal Disease in Alaska, 1986–1990 – Ethnic Differences and Opportunities for Prevention." *Journal of Infectious Diseases*, 170(2): 368–376.

de Martel, C., Ferlay, J., Franceschi, S., Vignat, J., Bray, F., Forman, D., and Plummer, M. 2012. "Global Burden of Cancers Attributable to Infections In 2008: A Review and Synthetic Analysis." *Lancet Oncology*, 13(6): 607–615. doi: 10.1016/S1470-2045(12)70137-7.

de Martel, C., Forman, D., and Plummer, M. 2013. "Gastric Cancer: Epidemiology and Risk Factors." *Gastroenterology Clinics of North America*, 42(2): 219–240. doi: 10.1016/j.gtc.2013.01.003.

Derman, B. and Ferguson, A. 2003. "Value of Water: Political Ecology and Water Reform in Southern Africa." *Human Organization*, 62(3): 277.

Dombrowski, K. 2001. *Against Culture : Development, Politics, and Religion in Indian Alaska, Fourth World Rising Series.* Lincoln, NB: University of Nebraska Press.

Ducker, J.H. 1996. "Out of Harm's Way: Relocating Northwest Alaska Eskimos, 1907–1917." *American Indian Culture and Research Journal*, 20(1): 43–71.

Eichelberger, L. 2010. "Living in Utility Scarcity: Energy and Water Insecurity in Northwest Alaska." *American Journal of Public Health*, 100(6): 1010–1018.

Eichelberger, L. 2012. "Sustainability and the Politics of Calculation: Technologies of 'Safe Water', Subject-Making, and Domination in Alaska." *Journal of Political Ecology*, 19: 145–161.

Eichelberger, L. 2014. "Spoiling and Sustainability: Technology, Water Insecurity, and Visibility in Arctic Alaska." *Medical Anthropology*, 33(6): 478–496.

Eichelberger, L., Murphy, G., Etemadi, A., Abnet, C.C., Islami, F., Malekzadeh, R., and M Dawsey, S.M. 2015. "Risk of Gastric Adenocarcinoma by Water Source in the Golestan Gastric Cancer Case-Control Study". *PLOS One* 10(5): e0128491.

Ennis-McMillan, M.C. 2001. "Suffering from Water: Social Origins of Bodily Distress in a Mexican Community." *Medical Anthropology Quarterly*, 15(3): 368–390.

EPA (Environmental Protection Agency). 1995. *Federal Field Work Group Report to Congress on Alaska Rural Sanitation.* Seattle WA: US Government Printing Office, Environmental Protection Agency Water Division.

Farmer, P. 1996. "On Suffering and Structural Violence: A View from Below." *Daedalus*, 125(1): 261–283.

Farmer, P. 2004. "An Anthropology of Structural Violence." *Current Anthropology*, 45(3): 305–325.

Ferguson, A. 2005. "Water Reform, Gender, and HIV/AIDS: Perspectives from Malawi." In L.M. Whiteford and S. Whiteford (Eds.), *Globalization, Water, and Health: Resource Management in Times of Scarcity* (pp. 45–66). Santa Fe, NM: School of American Research Press.

Flanders, N. 1989. "The Alaska Native Corporation as Conglomerate: The Problem of Profitability." *Human Organization*, 48(4): 299–312.

Frenck, R.W., Jr. and Clemens, J. 2003. "Helicobacter in the Developing World." *Microbes Infect*, 5(8): 705–713.

Goldsmith, S., Angvik, J., Howe, L., Hill, A., and Leask, L. 2004. *The Status of Alaska Natives Report 2004* Vol. 1. Anchorage, AK: University of Alaska, Institute of Social and Economic Research.

Guerrant, R.L., Kosek, M., Lima, A.A., Lorntz, B., and Guyatt, H.L. 2002. "Updating the DALYs for Diarrhoeal Disease." *Trends in Parasitology*, 18(5): 191–193.

Guerrant, R.L., Oria, R.B., Moore, S.R., Oria, M.O., and Lima, A.A. 2008. "Malnutrition as an Enteric Infectious Disease with Long-Term Effects on Child Development." *Nutrition Review*, 66(9): 487–505. doi: 10.1111/j.1753-4887.2008.00082.x.

Haenszel, W., Kurihara, M., Locke, F.B., Shimuzu, K., and Segi, M. 1976. "Stomach Cancer in Japan." *Journal of National Cancer Institute*, 56(2): 265–274.

Hennessy, T.W., Ritter, T., Holman, R.C., Bruden, D.L., Yorita, K.L., Bulkow, L., JCheek, J.E., Singleton, R.J., and Smith, J. 2008. "The Relationship between In-Home Water Service and the Risk of Respiratory Tract, Skin, and Gastrointestinal Tract Infections among Rural Alaska Natives." *American Journal of Public Health*, 98(11): 2072–2078.

Hope, R., Hansen, K., Mutembwa, M., and Schlessinger, S. 2012. *Water Security, Risk and Society – Key Issues and Research Priorities for International Development*. Synthesis report submitted to UK Collaborative on Development Sciences by Oxford University Water Security Network, June 2012.

Howard, G. and Bartram, J. 2003. *Domestic Water Quantity, Service, Level and Health*. Geneva: World Health Organization.

Huskey, L. 1992. *The Economy of Village Alaska*. Anchorage, Alaska: University of Alaska, Institute of Social and Economic Research.

Hutton, G., Haller, L., and Bartram, J. 2007. "Global Cost-Benefit Analysis of Water Supply and Sanitation Interventions." *Journal of Water and Health*, 5(4): 481–502. doi: 10.2166/Wh.2007.009.

IARC. 2010. "IARC Monographs on the Evaluation of Carcinogenic Risks to Humans. Ingested Nitrate and Nitrite, and Cyanobacterial Peptide Toxins." *IARC Monographs on the Evalation of Carcinogenic Risks to Humans*, 94: v–vii, 1–412.

Johnston, B.R. 1998. "Culture, Power, and the Hydrological Cycle: Creating and Responding to Water Scarcity on St. Thomas, Virgin Islands." In J.M. Donahue and B.R. Johnston (Eds.), *Water, Culture, and Power: Local Struggles in a Global Context* (pp. 285–312). Washington, D : Island Press.

Johnston, B.R. 2005. "The Commodification of Water and the Human Dimensions of Manufactured Scarcity." In L.M. Whiteford and S. Whiteford (Eds.), *Globalization, Water, & Health: Resource Management in Times of Scarcity* (pp. 133–152. Santa Fe, NM: School of American Research Press.

Khalifa, M.M., Sharaf, R.R., and Aziz, R.K. 2010. "Helicobacter Pylori: A Poor Man's Gut Pathogen?" *Gut* Pathology, 2(1): 2. doi: 10.1186/1757-4749-2-2.

King, B. 2010. "Political Ecologies of Health." *Progress in Human Geography*, 34(1): 38–55.

Knapp, G. and Huskey, L. 1988. "Effects of Transfers on Remote Regional Economies: The Transfer Economy in Rural Alaska." *Growth and Change* (Spring): 25–39.

Kruse, J. and Foster, K. 1986. "Changes in Rural Alaska Settlement Patterns." *Alaska Review of Social and Economic Conditions*, 23(1): 1–19.

Lantis, M. 1962. *The Alaska Native Village Sanitation Program at the end of five years*. Anchorage, Alaska: Arctic Health Research Center.

Lantis, M. 1963. "Acculturation and Health" (revised by the author, February 1963). In *Alaska's Health, A Survey Report (1954)*, ed. Parran Committee: The Graduate School of Public Health, University of Pittsburgh.

Leask, L. 1983. "Effects of Oil Revenues on State Aid to Local Government in Alaska." *Alaska Review of Social and Economic Conditions*, 20(4).

Mayer, J. 1996. "The political Ecology of Disease as One New Focus for Medical Geography." *Progress in Human Geography*, 20(4): 441–456.

McBeath, G.A. and Morehouse, T.A. 1994. "Political Economy: Myths and Realities." In *Alaska Politics & Government* (pp. 51–74). Politics and governments of the American states. Lincoln: University of Nebraska Press.

Mendall, M.A., Goggin, P.M., Molineaux, N., Levy, J., Toosy, T., Strachan, D., and Northfield, T.C. 1992. "Childhood Living Conditions and Helicobacter Pylori Seropositivity in Adult Life." *Lancet*, 339(8798): 896–897.

Mitchell, D. 2001. *Take My Land, Take My Life : The Story of Congress's Historic Settlement of Alaska Native Land Claims, 1960–1971*. Fairbanks, AK: University of Alaska Press.

Morley, L.A. 1954. "Suggest Plan to Train Villagers as Sanitation Aides in Their Own Communities." *Alaska's Health*, 11 (April): 3–4.

Quesada, J., Hart, L.K., and Bourgois, P. 2011. "Structural Vulnerability and Health: Latino Migrant Laborers in the United States." *Medical Anthropology*, 30(4): 339–362. doi: 10.1080/01459740.2011.576725.

Qureishi, A., Lee, Y., Belfield, K., Birchall, J.P., and Daniel, M. 2014. "Update on Otitis Media – Prevention and Treatment." *Infectious Drug Resistance*, 7: 15–24. doi: 10.2147/IDR.S39637.

Risch, H.A., Jain, M., Choi, N.W., Fodor, J.G., Pfeiffer, C.J., Howe, G.R., Harrison, L.W., Craib, K.J., and Miller, A.B. 1985. "Dietary Factors and the Incidence of Cancer of the Stomach." *American Journal of Epidemiology*, 122(6): 947–959.

Rogers, G.W. 1956. "Water Development Projects are Begun in Three Alaska Villages." *Alaska's Health*, 13(June): 1, 7.

Saylor, B. and Haley, S. 2007. *Effects of Rising Utility Costs on Household Budgets, 2000–2006*. Anchorage: University of Alaska, Institute of Social and Economic Research.

Alaska State Legislature. 1972. *Village Safe Water Act*.

Sultana, F. 2009. "Fluid Lives: Subjectivities, Gender and Water in Rural Bangladesh." *Gender, Place, and Culture: A Journal of Feminist Geography*, 16(4): 427–444.

Tran, G.D., Sun, X.D. Abnet, C.C., Fan, J.H., Dawsey, S.M., Dong, Z.W., Mark, S.D., Qiao, Y.L., and Taylor, P.R. 2005. "Prospective study of Risk Factors for Esophageal and Gastric Cancers in the Linxian General Population Trial Cohort in China." *International Journal of Cancer*, 113(3): 456–463. doi: 10.1002/ijc.20616.

Tussing, A.R. 1982. *Alaska: Precarious Riches and Stubborn Poverty*. Anchorage, Alaska: University of Alaska, Institute of Social and Economic Research.

US Congress. 1994. *An Alaskan Challenge: Native Village Sanitation*. Washington, DC: Office of Technology Assessment, US Government Printing Office.

US Energy Information Administration. 2016. *Petroleum and Other Liquids: Spot Data* (Monthly). http://www.eia.gov/dnav/pet/pet_pri_spt_s1_m.htm (data released January 27, 2016).

Wenger, J.D., Zulz, T., Bruden, D., Singleton, R., Bruce, M.G., Bulkow, L. Parks, D., Rudolph, K., Hurlburt, D., Ritter, T., Klejka, J., and Hennessy, T. 2010. "Invasive Pneumococcal Disease in Alaskan Children: Impact of the Seven-Valent Pneumococcal Conjugate Vaccine and the Role of Water Supply." *Pediatric Infectious Disease Journal*, 29(3): 251–256.

Whiteford, L.M. and Whiteford, S. 2005. "Paradigm Change." In L.M. Whiteford and S. Whiteford (Eds.), *Globalization, Water, & Health: Resource Management in Times of Scarcity* (pp. 3–23). Santa Fe, NM: School of American Research Press.

Whiteford, S. and Cortez-Lara, A. 2005. "Good to the Last Drop: The Political Ecology of Water and Health on the Border." In L.M. Whiteford and S. Whiteford (Eds.), *Globalization, Water, & Health: Resource Management in Times of Scarcity* (pp. 231–254). Santa Fe, NM: School of American Research Press.

WHO (World Health Organization) and UNICEF. 2012. *Progress on Drinking Water and Sanitation: 2012 Update*. United States of America: WHO/UNICEF Joint Monitoring Programme for Water Supply and Sanitation.

Wiita, A. and Haley, S. 2003. *Evaluation of the U.S. Army Corps of Engineers' Water and Sanitation Project in the Village of Buckland, Alaska Phase 2*. Anchorage, Alaska: Anchorage, AK: University of Alaska, Institute of Social and Economic Research.

Wutich, A. and Ragsdale, K. 2008. "Water insecurity and Emotional Distress: Coping with Supply, Access, and Seasonal Variability of Water in a Bolivian Squatter Settlement." *Society of Scientific Medicine*, 67(12): 2116–2125. doi: 10.1016/j.socscimed.2008.09.042.

CHAPTER 13 Food Security: Health and Environmental Concerns in the North

Kirsten Hastrup, Anne Marie Rieffestahl, and Anja Olsen

Introduction

In this chapter, we focus on environmental challenges to health in the global North. Our main cases derive from the Nordic countries and some of their indigenous populations in the Arctic regions, but our message is truly global. The point is that food security no longer is an exclusive issue for the global South – not having enough to eat – but a pervasive global issue of unsafe food, resulting in a virulent spread of "northern" diseases related to obesity, Type II diabetes, and cardiovascular diseases. In addition to the globalization of overeating, the world is also facing a truly boundless risk of contamination of even the most local of foods. Let us start by tracing this development in broad strokes.

The United Nations was created in the 1940s to secure an international balance between nation-states, some of which had been at war with each other, while others were emerging in the process of decolonization. Under the new UN umbrella several organizations were designed to look into particular areas of concern; among them were the World Health Organization (WHO) and the

A Companion to the Anthropology of Environmental Health, First Edition. Edited by Merrill Singer.

Food and Agriculture Organization (FAO). The concerns of these organizations were, and still are, global health and food security, the latter defined as "the reassurance that all people at all times have both the physical and economic access to the food they need for an active, healthy life. This means that food itself is safe, nutritionally adequate and culturally appropriate and that this food be obtained in a way that upholds basic human dignity" (WHO 2006). The issue of food safety is our main concern here, in line with the definition provided by FAO (2001: 58), which stresses people's "access to sufficient, safe and nutritious food that meets their dietary needs and food preferences for an active and healthy life."

While food is a biological necessity, hunger is a hard social fact (Hastrup 1993). This is evident even as we consider earlier discussions of food security; postwar and postcolonial realities gradually raised a new kind of awareness about the social and political dimensions of hunger that eventually was to transform the issue from being simply a matter of local food shortages keeping population numbers in check, as Malthus had suggested in 1798 (1970: 242). Yet, in the 1940s when the WHO and FAO were first set up, the priority was simply (and importantly) to increase food supply in impoverished regions. This sufficiency perspective was still dominant in the postcolonial times of the 1970s, exemplified by the 1974 World Food Conference in Rome. The conference took place in the wake of a devastating famine in Bangladesh, and the government attendees to the conference made the proclamation that "every man, woman and child has the inalienable right to be free from hunger and malnutrition in order to develop their physical and mental capacities," as stated in the first clause of the resulting *Declaration on the Eradication of Hunger and Malnutrition* (UN Resolution 3348, 1974). The goal was to eliminate hunger, food insecurity, and malnutrition within a decade, a matter pertaining to the impoverished global South.

An important step toward a new understanding of famine was taken by Amartya Sen (later a Nobel Laureate in economics), who doubted the general proposition that famine was a direct outcome of food shortage. Some famines, he argued, occurred during periods of peak food availability for the economy as a whole, as was the case for the 1974 famine in Bangladesh (Sen 1987: 7). As he succinctly suggested, "starvation is the characteristic of some people not *having* enough food to eat. It is not the characteristic of there *being* not enough food to eat" (Sen 1981: 1). Food sufficiency remained at the core of food security, but politics and distribution were now seen by many to be very much part of the problem. This recognition precipitated a process during which the hard fact of hunger gradually moved beyond measuring individual intakes of calories and weight to the food-related social experience of well-being and belonging. In addition to the matter of basic sufficiency and entitlement to food, there emerged an explicit acceptance of entitlement to *safe* and nutritional food, as mentioned above.

However, when the UN Millennium Development Goals to be reached by 2015 were set up, "to end poverty and hunger" was still the top priority as Goal 1. This reflects the sad fact that, even by the turn of the millennium, the international community could hardly keep up with multiple emergencies of famine, among other issues (e.g., Singer 2011). On the verge of 2015, the set date, even some of the more modest targets within the ambitious goal have become subverted by a runaway world of crisis, financial as well as environmental. This is underscored by Goal 7, "to ensure environmental sustainability," where the issue of access to safe drinking water is aligned with biological degradation of the living environment and increasing patterns of slums in the new mega-cities of the world. While this is not our primary concern here, the history of global industrialization did introduce a major imbalance between the rich and the poor, which included an unequal distribution of health hazards (Beck 1998). Now, the bill is being sent back to the North, where even the most prosperous states face new concerns about public health.

While hunger and poverty have not been obliterated from the world, the connotations of food security (and its opposite, food insecurity) have multiplied and now reflect a global situation that radically departs from the post-World War II scenario. On a truly global note, it is increasingly clear that climate change has serious implications for food safety, and always has had (Hassan 2002; FAO 2008a, FAO 2008b; Ringler, Biswas, and Cline 2010). Part of the problem is related to demographic changes and environmental migration, part of it to shifting resource bases (Lobell and Burke 2010; Hastrup and Olwig 2012). On another level, we find an increasing challenge to food safety from environmental contaminants, as well as changing microbiological regimes, including genetically modified organisms, chemical additives to processed food, and new scientific knowledge about the health hazards presented by quite ordinary (processed) food items, on which we elaborate below. Along with global health problems of obesity and Type II diabetes, all of these developments move the problem of food security from being a problem exclusively in the global South to also embracing the global North.

In an inverse movement of this global process, a stress on local food as more wholesome than imported food is taking root in the North in response to a new call for consumer-citizenship (see e.g., Meneley 2008; Mol 2009; Paxson 2010). Another reaction is found in the grass-roots movements against GMOs (genetically modified organisms) that are seeking to retain at least some control over consumption in an age of food scares (Whatmore 2002: 120–145). While there need not be any scientific guarantee that local produce is healthier than imported, an Australian study suggests that people have a habitual trust in their local food governance and assume food supply to be safe unless (or until) they have evidence to the contrary; at the same time they are prepared to disclaim foreign food more or less wholly (Henderson *et al.* 2012). The sense of trust is significant, particularly when it is notably absent, for instance in regions or states that cannot support an infrastructure guaranteeing healthy produce, as suggested for Georgia (Dunn 2008), and by the repeated food scares such as the BSE (bovine spongiform encephalopathy) outbreaks in Britain (Caplan 2000).

In short, a new and comprehensive sense of food insecurity is emerging, and among certain groups of people a new risk-awareness affects both their sense of well-being and their trust in the future. In the Nordic countries, which are among the most privileged countries on the globe with general social security, including free medical care for all, and a relatively high life expectancy, people are increasingly concerned about the vast number of chemicals, heavy metals, artificial hormones, and so forth that demonstrably affect health in general and human reproduction in particular. These well-known health threats link the privileged North directly to the less privileged parts of the world; the contamination of the environment is indeed global, irrespective of origin and historical imbalances. Globally, one could also add the new risks posed by the acidification of the sea (see Singer, this volume), the desertification of large areas, and the swamping of agricultural lands from melting glaciers and rising seas, all of them affecting the accessible resources (see IPCC 2007 for a general overview). Along with the general challenges posed by climate change, more localized processes of environmental degradation and depletion of particular resources aggravate social stress and entail poorer health prospects (Confalonieri *et al.* 2007).

In this chapter, we examine a broad spectrum of uncertainty that is pushing the concern about food security toward increasing focus on the issue of food safety. In turn, this may contribute to the charting of new areas of unease, and hence of new avenues for action. We start, in the first section, with a discussion of emerging fears as traditional food items are increasingly seen as unsafe, and point to the fact that these fears may lead to new forms of social suffering on the margins of the Nordic welfare states. These issues are explored through an examination of two cases. The first case is a hunting community in northwest Greenland facing a series of worrying developments with respect to their traditional dietary habits. A new study of health in the region points to the fact that their fears for the future as well as past experiences of (possible) exposure to nuclear radiation have a negative health impact. The second case is the Sami of northern Sweden and Norway, who likewise find themselves on the edge of tradition, both in the sense that they may now choose between traditional and modern food, and in a fearsome past experience of nuclear contamination in the wake of the Chernobyl disaster. Both cases emphasize well-being and food preferences as a comprehensive social, cultural, and historical fact, now under siege by environmental changes whose effects are barely known as yet.

In the second section, we move into a discussion of dietary requirements and recommendations as set up by the health authorities, and as accepted, contested, or explicitly disregarded by the general public in the Nordic countries, where people often take the management of food risk in their own hands. This discussion shows how science-based health campaigns are not directly translatable into practice, because people are always acting upon socially negotiable notions of risk, while also responding to the increasingly individualized management of food safety (Halkier and Holm 2006). Even when people choose very strict health regimes beyond the official health advice, and thus demonstrating (individual) determination to fight for their own health, lapses occur for a number of good (social) reasons. For others, risk management mainly consists in doing what feels right; "rightness" again is subject to social situation, and the general point about dietary preference and eating habits as embedded in social settings is further confirmed – which somewhat tempers the notion of a truly individual responsibility for food safety.

Knowing the health risks associated with particular food items – and acting upon this knowledge – becomes even more complicated when we move to the third section of this chapter, which takes us into the molecular constituents of carbohydrate-rich food items that have been shown to contain acrylamide after heating. Acrylamide has been classified as a carcinogen, and a correlation between high exposure to acrylamide and certain forms of cancer has been established. The discussion therefore takes us to the heart of a pervasive food insecurity of a new – and invisible – kind. By contrast with the case of heavy metals in marine mammals, traditionally constituting the basic food item in northwest Greenland, which may lead to public health advisories that people should eat less of it, exposure to acrylamide is much more covert and tricky, because it is present everywhere, for instance in coffee, bread, breakfast cereals, roast potatoes, and much more. This calls for a new kind of awareness of health hazards and food safety, both in the North and elsewhere, and also for a rethinking of balancing information and dosing advice in innovative ways, so as to inspire trust in food governance.

The macro-ecological environmental degradation visible in many regions, and as discussed in many chapters in this book, is thus accompanied by micro-biological health hazards, increasingly distributed across the globe along with industrial food items, replacing or supplementing previously home-grown supplies. This is what makes the issue of food safety truly global, something we aim at showing below.

Local Tradition: Food Preferences and Fear

On the fringe of the Nordic welfare states, some of their Arctic populations already face some of the direr consequences of the global development, having democratized risk in the sense that the bill for industrial development in the global North has now been distributed to all, not least in terms of environmental degradation. The Arctic Monitoring and Assessment Programme (AMAP), for example, regularly publishes disturbing findings about diet and contaminants. In 2009, AMAP documented that sweet and fatty store-bought food had become the main source of energy for children in the region (especially in North America, but also in the Arctic more generally), and that "the decreasing proportion of traditional foods in the diet has had negative impact on the intakes of most nutrients," while still contributing positively to the intake of vitamin C, folate, and possibly calcium (AMAP 2009: 21). What is also apparent is that "dietary exposure to persistent contaminants and metals in Arctic indigenous communities is higher than in neighboring non-indigenous communities. The main explanation is that indigenous populations consume tissue from marine top-predators that are not normally eaten in other parts of the world" (AMAP 2009: 21–22). With the rather dramatic anthropogenic environmental changes in the Arctic in the wake of global warming, living conditions are further deteriorating with new problems of storage (now that the natural deep freezer is switching off) of more obviously sick and polluted animals, and of intensified zoonotic disease frequencies (see e.g., Hovelsrud *et al.* 2012). All of this again is related to the general environmental changes in the region, including the thinning of sea ice, the reduction of snow cover, the thawing of permafrost, and the related changes in floral and faunal distribution.

This takes us to a hunting community in northwest Greenland (Avanersuaq), where we find one of the last truly High Arctic hunting communities, numbering some 800 people in a vast territory, until recently ice-covered for most of the year, now melting rather rapidly. While in some – maybe not too distant – future, the warming may open up entirely new economic possibilities, at present the economy is entirely dependent on the living resources and hunting, which is becoming increasingly precarious. The hunters and their families are all too aware of their shrinking opportunities and of the need to monitor the sea ice very closely, whenever they go out; a proper reading of the ice is a matter of life and of remaining self-sufficient (Hastrup 2009a, 2013a). The environmental degradation (by comparison even with the recent past) has also contributed to new concerns about health in this northernmost (inhabited) region of Greenland.

Greenland nowadays has self-rule, but it is still part of the Danish kingdom and is closely monitored in terms of health and well-being; generally, the country finds itself between a traditional subsistence economy based on hunting, fishing, and some sheep rearing (in the south), and a modern economy, accompanied by a modern outlook and very much shaped by Nordic values and horizons. It is estimated (by the Greenlandic Board of Nutrition and Environment) that on average one-quarter of the food intake in Greenland consists of traditional food, while the remaining three-quarters are imported; in small towns and even smaller settlements, the proportion of traditional food is higher, but everywhere there is a fragile balance between two health regimes to be maintainted (Bjerregaard and Mulvad 2012). Generally, local, traditional food is deemed healthy – in spite of the problem of heavy metal contamination in both marine mammals and in polar bear – the latter now a less prominent part of the local food than before. The point is that among the food options available, local food is the most nutritional, if in important ways apparently less "safe," and not compliant with the fiber recommendation (Jeppesen and Bjerregaard 2012). There is thus a tension between food preferences and food safety, and a potential loss of self-reliance if the hunters are advised against seeking to sustain their own subsistence as they have done since time immemorial – dwelling within a forbidding landscape.

The questionnaire-based Survey of Living Conditions in the Arctic (SLICA) shows how a large proportion of people in the Arctic still perceive traditional food as an important part of their diet, not only in terms of nutrition as such but also as part of general well-being (Poppel *et al.* 2007). The statistics on food choices provided by the survey match the experience in Avanersuaq, where for all festive occasions traditional Greenlandic food is served and offered to anyone from the community who cares to come. Eating this food gives people a sense of continuity and belonging, by celebrating their traditional hunting life and also by sharing. People also say that they need to have *mattak* (narwhal blubber) stored for the winter as a remedy against depression (Hastrup 2009b). They know about pollution and have been targeted by health campaigns over many years, warning about the accumulation of heavy metals in marine mammals, and advising people to eat variedly and to avoid older seal and bear where the contaminants are more concentrated than in younger animals. This public health advice is most emphatically directed at pregnant women.

However, even here the case is not as clear as one would think. In one study, the conclusion was that while the accumulation of heavy metals etc. may have some harmful effects, it seems that the particular kind of fat in these animals goes a long way toward protecting people against cardio-vascular diseases (Hansen 2000). Also, in actual fact the alternatives are few. The further north one goes, the less choice of diet there is, because all provisions beyond the local resources have to be flown or sailed in from far away and are consequently priced beyond the economic capacity of most households. This effectively leaves large groups of people at a loss; if no longer able to hunt, they have to resort to industrialized food that contains high levels of sugar and low levels of protein and vitamin. The challenge, which is professionally addressed in Greenland, is to design health campaigns with an innovative approach to traditional foods in combination with a new "cuisine" (Bjerregaard and Mulvad 2012).

If we zoom even closer in on the health of the population in Avanersuaq, one notes a significant development in local perceptions of health and risk. This development is heavily influenced by an event that took place in 1968, when an American B-52 plane crashed in the region and caused a degree of plutonium pollution. People's subsequent fear of environmental radiation has negatively affected their sense of self-reliance and safety; this example testifies to the oft-noted point that singular dramatic events can contribute to long-term anxieties (e.g., Harries 2008). This was one of the reasons behind a recent (2010) study of health in the region, centered on the town of Qaanaaq with some 600–700 inhabitants (Bjerregaard and Dahl-Petersen 2010). The study was based on both qualitative and quantitative methods, and found some highly interesting trends in relation to the issues of safety we are discussing here.

The study documented that while people in Qaanaaq generally felt more exposed to contamination and subjectively considered themselves to be more afflicted by illness than people further south, there were no epidemiological indications that they were in fact more affected by either radiation or diseases related to earlier exposures than their compatriots further south. Yet there were significant differences in their perceptions of health; generally the northerners saw themselves as much more vulnerable, not only because of their own health condition, which they evaluated negatively, but also because of a greater prevalence of infected and therefore inedible game. The environmental threat became very conspicuous in the malformation of fish and game and was further intensified by the presence of a US airbase.

One reason given by study participants for the apparent sense of actual or pending illness was a pervasive sense of fear, which links up with the new global realities of invisible contamination and long-distance effects of industrial (including military) developments. In a follow-up study in 2011, based on a new set of interviews with people in Qaanaaq, the findings of the previous study were confirmed and elaborated in terms of policy issues (Den individuelle helbredsundersøgelse 2011). One conclusion was that more reliable information from the authorities was needed to empower people and to downscale their, partially unfounded, worries about contamination; this information should range from actual dietary and lifestyle factors, on the one hand, to larger issues of wildlife management and environmental changes, on the other. While the local food options are few, a measure of trust in food governance may still be established, alleviating individuals from making an impossible choice. Of note, in a recent published study of an Australian indigenous community, where health was significantly better than in comparable communities, it was convincingly argued that through a sustained, productive interaction with both neighbors and government agencies, people had been able to uphold a degree of collective efficacy in relation to their land (Anderson and Kowal 2012). By contrast, the isolation and lack of agency in the face of major environmental threats in Avanersuaq entails a greater sense of health risk; there is less possibility for resource diversification. This is where we possibly need to theorize a new notion of "community food security" (Anderson and Cook 1999).

What we are getting at here is the fact that people across the globe are living with multiplying "liquid fears" (Bauman 2006). They are *liquid* because they seep into the everyday and greatly affect the sense of self and safety; as *fears* they are distinct from risk as we (following Bauman) use these terms in this paper. Risks are identifiable and something to be managed, while fears are unknown both in origin and scope. The concept of risk makes sense only in a routinized world, where one may calculate risks with reference to precedents (Bauman 2006: 10, 98ff.). Beyond the presumably calculable risks are those dangers that are noncalculable, because they belong in a setting that is irregular in principle, and where non-repetition is the rule. It seems that the distinction between known or at least identifiable *risk* and unknown and even unknowable sources of danger and *fear* is socially very important when current ideas of food safety are discussed. The implied sense of uncertainty takes fear beyond anything that can simply be managed, which is underscored by uncertainty about the impacts of future climate change, among other adverse anthropogenic environmental changes.

On the Arctic margins of the Nordic welfare states, where access (physically or economically) to modern, mass-produced food supplies are unstable, and where there is still a strong preference for local food items that may no longer be healthy, people are left to negotiate their fears as best they can. Trude Giernes (2008) has shown how in northern Norway the Sami see their whole way of life as under threat and how Sami women respond to health challenges with a keen eye for social needs and cultural security. Medical discourses never totally replace local moral discourses, which is also evident from Lena M. Nilsson's work on Sami lifestyle and health in northern Sweden. Interestingly, what is most highly acclaimed as being of cultural importance today was not of most obvious importance traditionally (Nilsson *et al.* 2011: 315), even cultural security changes over time. These studies temper any facile equation between what is signposted as "traditional food" and health, while also (in the Sami case) pointing to a broader choice over the years than in Avanersuaq. In the Swedish study, a weak increase in mortality patterns among men claiming continued adherence to a traditional Sami diet may even be explained by an underreporting of the actual volume of fatty fish and berries in the past, as well as the inverse, that is, a non-acknowledgment of increased consumption of red meat, and a less physically demanding work life nowadays (Nilsson *et al.* 2012).

In the Sami case, it is evident that cultural food preferences shifted, but also that there is no easy way to explain Sami health by reference to food alone. They did not suffer like the people of Avanersuaq from dietary changes per se, maybe because their lifestyle actually no longer differed very much from other groups' in northern Sweden. But like the people in Avanersuaq, they had earlier been subject to almost limitless fear in the wake of the nuclear fallout from Chernobyl in 1986, which contaminated the lichen in vast areas of the Sami region in Sweden and Norway, and hence also the reindeer herds eating the lichen. In consequence, large herds were slaughtered, while freshwater fish, wild berries, and other natural resources were deemed out of bounds for years. This set the stage for the development of nostalgia for the past, and an overemphasis on traditional food in earlier times, when the world was pure. Along with changes to the landscape, due to the shrinking of the permafrost, this has precipitated a new sense among the Sami that, to survive, they must once again be allowed to move their herds about freely (Reinert *et al.* 2009). Beyond the political message and the appeal to Sami-ness there is an indication also of a wish to reconnect to a traditional lifestyle, now mainly connected to herding, even though recent analysis shows that this was just one among many economic strategies, where found at all (Bjørklund 2013).

It seems that the current "liquid times" (Bauman 2007) incorporate people all over the globe into a unified world, equally exposed to contamination and to environmental degradation seeping in from unknown directions. In other words, along with the global environmental challenges, in terms of both global warming and heavy pollution, there is no way in which "local" food can be seen as inherently safe, even if the appeal to local tradition also serves as a vehicle of nostalgia for a pure past.

Social Action: Dietary Choice and Risk Handling

Climate change may come at a different pace in regions at lower latitudes than the Arctic, but it still has potential health impacts that are beginning to show (Lake *et al.* 2012). Extreme weather events and the production of biofuels may reduce cereal production for consumption, elevated temperatures may lead to an increase of pathogens in food, and pathogens and chemicals in food may be globally transmitted, to mention but a few examples (ibid.). In short, climate change may affect diet in the North too, and calls for new risk identification systems (Marvin *et al.* 2009).

If fear, in the terminology adopted in this chapter, relates to the unknown nature of a dangerous agent, risk points toward something believed to be manageable. This places risk squarely in the social domain (Douglas and Wildavsky 1983). As such, risk has been claimed to be a more or less constitutive factor in the global era (Beck 1998). Until recently, the Nordic countries were seen as societies where food security could be taken for granted, certainly if it were only a matter of there being "enough" food. However, in the present era, and in the global North as well as in the global South, food security – and food safety, in particular – also relates to the proper selection among the abundance of food available on the market, often of unknown provenance and little control.

Traditionally, the Nordic household economy reflected an age-old economic diversification of strategies of farming, husbandry, fishing, hunting, and gathering, which largely remains basic even today. Farming itself was internally diversified, embracing both cattle breeding and agriculture, the latter reflecting the fact that the Nordic countries were just that: Nordic, and thus favoring rye and barley over wheat and other more southerly products. Barley was mostly consumed in fluid form, as barley soup (gruel) or beer. By contrast, rye was eaten in lumps of bread with salted bacon or herring. Cooking and local food preferences are not independent of the physical environment and the economic opportunities, of course, but it is also closely linked up with a sense of belonging and not least with a set of social relations that qualify propriety and value. Thus we know that in southern Europe, where wheat dominated, rye was seen as a poorer cousin in the family of grain; it was something that might avert famine, but certainly not something one would choose for its taste (Braudel 1981: 109ff.). The natural resources is one thing, "taste" quite another. Meals carry important cultural messages, as do drinks. And they have a remarkable tenacity, even when other matters change. With industrialization and, lately, with environmental changes, new challenges to healthy life have emerged, and risk handling has become part of an ongoing negotiation of long-lingering social norms and ambivalent experiences of modern everyday life (Halkier 2004). Everyday strategies for managing risk are based on a complex set of considerations, including equal amounts of evidence and intuition, and influenced by trust in health advice on the one hand and tradition on the other (Zinn 2008). The final choice involves weighing possible courses of action against one another, on the basis of a composite assessment of danger, pleasure, well-being, identity, social situation, and morality. In these assessments, matters of taste and social norms play an important part.

Some people subscribe to a moral domain, embedded in particular social obligations, and demonstrate the "right" values through their dietary choice (Raisborough 2007: 25). Such "rightness" is explicitly appraised by some families, who focus on the exclusion of particular food products in order to gain what they believe to be a healthier life. They may follow a particular dietary regime called Super-Healthy Family that was introduced in Denmark in 2007 by a journalist (Mauritson 2007). At the opposite end of the spectrum, other people engage in voluntary risk taking by dissociating themselves from the advice given and finding their own way in the jungle of health advice and health hazards. While in the Arctic, where food choice traditionally was limited, there was a call for more exact advice to help people negotiate a circumscribed arena of food choice, in the more southerly Nordic regions there is too much, or possibly too detailed, information in the public sphere, which makes people deaf to most of it. This has become clear in a study of blue-collar men in Nordic countries (Rieffestahl n.d.). On the basis of interviews with groups of working-class Danish, Icelandic, and Swedish men, the study clearly showed that they hardly followed any health advice given.

The overload of information confuses people, who discern manifest disagreements between health experts, which again create even more insecurity in society (Beck 1993; Tulloch and Lupton 2003: 3). Both adherents to a strict – and allegedly super-healthy – regime and the men who choose to distance themselves from any advice actually turned down the public health campaigns. Part of the explanation may rest with the design of the campaigns, being based on a view of social agents as inherently rational individuals, who just need to be educated to act in their best interests. This view of rationality as located in individual reasoning is challenged by the fact that there see to be many reasons for people to suspend particular courses of action for other, equally good reasons. The challenge in health policy is to take the situational nature of rationality into account, and not to connect it with any particular regime (Lupton 1996: 151).

The challenge manifests itself when people try to transform their knowledge into practice. Modern people would like to be rational, and to exercise self-control and self-discipline, but also to retain a space for giving in to impulses and to express their feelings, which in the arena of food consumption is often connected with eating for pleasure and forgetting themselves (Kristensen 1999: 75). As a result of this ingrained schism, people have a hard time following public health advice to the letter. The Super-Healthy Families take to a ready-made and very strict doctrine, as an explicit response to their growing insecurity about what they should do, given their duty to take responsibility for their own health as consumers (Halkier 2003: 204). The responsibility may become so burdensome that their choices, doubts, and reflections upon food entail a focus on the food products as such, completely shunning the sensory experience and the pleasure of sharing a meal (Rieffestahl 2014). This means that experience-based knowledge about food and eating has become a minor part in everyday life (Christensen 1999).

Meanwhile, changes are taking place in the industrial nations where the bulk of the population is no longer directly involved in producing food. According to Goody (1982), it is a shift that gives cooking a special quality in urban Western society because people are partly dissociated from the preparation of food and even more separated from its production. The ingredients arrive already prepared. The result is a homogenization of taste, as processed food is more or less the same in Reykjavík and in Copenhagen, for instance. In other words, the northerners are left with not much local environmental flavor to their food, and with no proper yardstick of their own ability to assess the nature of "good" food.

This points to a distance between producer and consumer, implying that the consumers in many cases have no clue about the origin and production of the food they buy and eat (Fischler 1988; Halkier 2004). It is therefore increasingly difficult to assess what one eats, because the food producers are able to make substitutes that are close to the authentic food items (Fischler 1980: 986). This is where the issue of trust as a reflexive act again becomes pertinent (Luhmann 2000); different groups of people may have different degrees of trust in science and public food governance, but everybody relies to some degree on an element of trust, because they cannot know for certain what's what (Henderson *et al.* 2012). Food labeling, for instance, is often seen as a short cut to trust, as it supports people in making a healthy choice without demanding too much factual knowledge. The problem is that such practices often confuse people further, because there are too many messages on offer. The drawback of labeling (for all its merits) is not only that people may lose their own sense of what is healthy food, but also that the messages often are perceived as contradictory and never address the *social* nature of eating. Evidently, new habits may take root, and labels may point some consumers in the right direction, but we must not forget the social nature of any action, and the complexity of "rational" choice (Christensen 1999).

An interesting response to the illegibility of public health advice is the upsurge of particular dietary regimes setting a strict, uniform course to be followed. One example is found in the above-mentioned health concept Super-Healthy Family, based on excluding cow's milk, gluten, and sugar, because these products are believed to be detrimental to body and mind. Adherents consider these food products to be toxic because of their concern about chemical additives in processed food, and this worry becomes the major issue in their everyday life. Instead, it is recommended that people opt for alternatives such as rice drink and soy products, as these are considered healthier to digest (Rieffestahl 2014). Here the environment creeps back into the discussion of health – but negatively so, as we shall see, rice and soy being nonlocal foods.

Adhering to a strict dietary regime provides families following the super-healthy plan with an easy gateway to improved health, it seems, and offers a sense of self-control, which may create a feeling of pleasure and well-being. Control implies pleasure because it steers families toward a healthy body; it may also imply a sense of restriction and loss, but as we know from Simmel, the "negative" does not necessarily lead people away from their values. On the contrary, the so-called negative may lead people closer to the positive, while positing meals on a spiritual and more meaningful level than merely alleviating hunger (Simmel 1998: 142–143). However, the very sense of control, as embedded in the exclusion of traditional food items such as cow's milk, gluten, and sugar, makes the dietary regime a daily struggle for some families. They experience difficulties in everyday life due to grocery shopping and taking part in social events where food is included. Also, ideally the family should make home-cooked meals in order to know what they eat, which clashes with their busy everyday life.

In Denmark, there is a long history of agriculture and production of various food products from farming. In addition to the "pure" products such as milk and flour, many processed food items also contain cow's milk, sugar, and cereals containing gluten. Even though the variety of food options increases all the time, the "forbidden" items are essential ingredients in various dishes, and they are a central part of a long Danish food tradition (Troels-Lund 1969: 14–17). By their choice of diet, the Super-Healthy Family alienates itself from the social convention of sharing meals by their stressing of so-called nontraditional food items, at the expense of conventional Danish foods (Rieffestahl 2014). As a result, the adherents do not succeed in managing the perceived risks for long. Relapses occur quite quickly, because the concept is too foreign to their familiar, historically produced food habits and takes too much effort to follow. It also undermines the sense of social belonging, by dissolving social relations (Douglas 1992). Perceptions of what is the "natural" (local) food and social well-being go together.

The self-declared super-healthy strategy is, as mentioned, not the only response to the overflow of health information, of course, nor the only scale upon which to balance putative bodily health with social well-being. There is a significant alternative in not caring at all, or in resorting to an unmediated sense of what "feels right." The Nordic blue-collar men in the study introduced above seem to have dissociated themselves from active risk handling; in general, such conduct may result in a poorer health among men (Halkier 2003: 205). Through the interviews, it became clear that these men did not follow the advice given and they explained that they did not consider themselves to be a target group and could not relate to the health advice because it was too far removed from their habits; furthermore, they found it contradictory and confusing, and largely chose to ignore it.

Moreover, they viewed health information as rules that had to be followed at all times, which was socially impossible. The general problem is that health authorities relate food directly to nutrition, while consumers implicitly and explicitly relate food to social events and relationships (Halkier 2004). This obviously causes some misunderstanding between the two groups, a fact which clearly influenced the men's attitude. The expert expectation that individual consumers should take responsibility for their own health clashes with the sense of belonging to a social group where certain things are done and eaten in particular circumstances, and are not to be regimented by external agents who are perceived as different by education and class background.

Significantly, the participants in the study stressed that they did not want anybody to "dictate" to them. They preferred to find their own way and believed that this was possible simply by using their common sense. They stressed that food habits should not become a science. However, in the course of the interviews, the men actually did express quite solid knowledge about health, which somehow redeems the Nordic health policy advisory system after all. The influence from the larger society upon their lifestyle was implied in their descriptions of their ways of living; they knew that they had to choose vegetables instead of French fries and they got a bad conscience from time to time if they ate too much candy or junk food. Still, as long as they felt fit and well, they would eat what they preferred and did not acknowledge any need to change their eating habits; this would be too time consuming, anyway.

However, several men voiced a latent fear of getting a disease; somewhat paradoxically, this fear kept them away from the doctor because they could not cope with the fact that they might be ill. Nevertheless, they would not change their eating habits or lifestyle until they had a diagnosis, and preference, taste, time, and food price stood out as having the highest priority in their choice of what and when to eat. Some of the men had taken health checks, when offered them at work, and saw it as an alternative to public health advice and food labeling; the health check was seen as a kind of personal guidance that they could relate to. The men rarely discussed health among themselves, but the competitive atmosphere that was created among them on the job through measurements of weight, blood pressure, and physical fitness rating motivated them to lose weight or see the doctor. Compared to the Super-Healthy Families, these men lived by a much broader definition of healthy living, and they implicitly and explicitly located their health within a larger field of social relations. Within that field they knew what was right or wrong, and it was not exclusively related to the foodstuff as such, but also to moments and pleasures of eating together.

One important lesson from the discussion in this section is the realization that the handling of risk, including the risks associated with unhealthy eating habits, is always a *social* action. This implies that choices are made with a view to many other sentiments and relations than one's relation to one's own body. In the North, where the occurrence of obesity and Type II diabetes is rising alarmingly, very few can claim total ignorance about the correlation between food and health. Even so, in many situations people choose to disregard their knowledge for other, and immediately more important, social reasons.

Another lesson is that in spite of the fact that the "environment" is significantly downplayed in discussions of food and health in Denmark (Lassen and Korzen 2009), it is still implicitly present in the sense that food items belonging to the local environment are more natural underpinnings of social life. This is increasingly supported by a growing awareness of the water footprints made by the North, importing fruit and vegetables from the South, and contributing further to the depletion of water resources in faraway regions (Hoekstra 2008; Meissner 2012). Once again, northern health concerns are closely linked with global conditions.

Hidden Knowledge: The Microbiology of Health

Even people who are able to grasp and to act upon science-based information about healthy food choices and to consider issues of water footprints are occasionally faced with challenges, especially when nutritional advice clashes with toxicological knowledge. The main challenge rests with the complexity of toxicological issues, which are still only partly known and documented by scientists, and certainly not an easy matter to handle in everyday lay practice. It becomes more complicated to act upon precisely because of the fine-grained nature of the scientific knowledge, and no less because of its sometimes counterintuitive nature.

Even food items that are generally deemed healthy or harmless may, under certain circumstances, become harmful and even constitute a threat to health. Thus, in a recent study of coffee consumption and cancer risk from Sweden it has been demonstrated that the brewing method (filtered or boiled) has an impact on the cancer risk. For instance, it was shown that for breast cancer, boiled coffee was associated with reduced risk, while it was positively associated with risk of respiratory cancer (Nilsson *et al.* 2010). Clearly, given such findings, people would find it hard to play it safe, as it were. Not only is this kind of knowledge hidden from ordinary people (if not by design, then at least by implication, because it is imbued with contradictory messages that will not appeal to the media), it is also fraught with paradoxes upon which it is impossible to act – and even to talk about.

Some of the most obvious quandaries between nutrition and toxicology concern fish, fruit, and vegetables, however. These food groups constitute the backbone of nutritional recommendations in most Western countries and populations are encouraged to let them constitute a substantial part of the daily diet. A high intake of fish has in some, but not all, studies been related to lower rates of heart disease and colorectal cancer, favorable neurodevelopment, and a range of other positive health outcomes, but fish also contains substances with known harmful effects including mercury, dioxins, and polychlorinated biphenyls (PCBs) (Mozaffarian and Rimm 2006). These conflicting messages on benefits and risks of fish leave the public in confusion regarding the role of fish in their daily diet (Verbeke *et al.* 2005) – as we saw above for the marine resources in Greenland, contaminated by heavy metals and other pollutants in the sea (see also AMAP 2002). There, the pollution was explicitly related to the fact that the marine mammals were last in the food chain; in the Nordic fisheries the problem with harmful substances is less pronounced but still women of childbearing age are advised to limit their intake of salmon caught in the Baltic Sea due to the identified high content of dioxins.

The complexity of the microbial realities of allegedly healthy food is also increasingly apparent when we move out of the sea and onto the land in the case of gardening and agriculture. Fruit and vegetables are possibly the food items most strongly advocated by health authorities, but even they are not without controversy. Consumers are repeatedly faced with the discussion of pesticides used during plant growth, and it is (almost) common knowledge that remains of pesticides have been identified in fruits and vegetables sold in general stores. What is less clear is how these pesticides may or may not have a negative impact on consumers' health and possibly on future generations. When the toxicology and tolerable dose of a pesticide is evaluated, effects on lifespan, reproduction (both ability to reproduce and birth defects), cancer development, and hormonal disruption in rats are among the factors considered. Though these tests seem reassuring, knowledge of how pesticides affect human health is often scarce (Damalas and Eleftherohorinos 2011). Small wonder that some people simply turn a blind eye to this kind of knowledge, which therefore remains if not directly hidden, then at least deliberately overlooked.

The tale of acrylamide is a third example of the clash between nutrition and toxicology. Acrylamide is a polymer that is widely used in industrial settings – it is for example, the main ingredient of acrylic sealer – and has been a well-known environmental problem for decades. In 1994, the International Agency for Research on Cancer classified acrylamide as being a probable human carcinogen (group 2A) (IARC 1994). In 2002, however, acrylamide was detected in various foods by researchers from the University of Stockholm (Ahn *et al.* 2002). It turned out that acrylamide was formed as a byproduct of the Maillared reaction, that is, the browning reaction that occurs through interaction of proteins or amines with carbohydrates facilitated by heating. In the formation of acrylamide, the involved components are the amino acid asparagine and reducing sugars (fructose, glucose, etc.) heated at temperatures above 120°C (Blank *et al.* 2005). The name "asparagine" reflects the fact that this amino acid was first detected in asparagus, but the combination of asparagine and reducing sugars is present in many of the most commonly eaten plant based foods worldwide, including potatoes, cereals, soy beans, and corn.

This implies that acrylamide is formed in industrial settings when coffee beans are roasted and potato chips are deep fried, but also in ordinary households where the roasting of potatoes and baking of bread forms acrylamide. Thus we are faced with basically armless substances that constitute natural parts of commonly eaten foods, but which are transformed into carcinogenic substances by ordinary food processing. This is obviously a difficult message for the general population to deal with; but also, food authorities and researchers have been challenged by the fact that a proven human carcinogen has suddenly been identified in a variety of foods. Besides those mentioned above, high amounts are also found in breakfast cereals, crisp bread, French fries, crisps, cocoa, and cookies.

The expected carcinogenic prospects of acrylamide are brought up in the media on a regular basis when new – and so far always inconclusive – research is released. It has not yet been possible to perform research projects that provide final answers on how acrylamide from foods affects human health; on one hand, no one can offer conclusive assurance that acrylamide is unproblematic from a public health point of view; on the other hand, no one wants to strongly advise against basic foods like potatoes, bread, and coffee. This leaves the handling of risk in people's own hands, potentially resulting in a deliberate negligence of any health advice, as noted above for working-class Nordic men.

With regard to fish, toxicological concerns have been integrated in the official recommendations, advising against very high intake especially among pregnant women, reminding us of the plight of the north Greenlanders. But with regard to fruits, vegetables, and acrylamide, the authorities disagree on the health impacts of the unwanted contents, leaving the final risk evaluation to the consumers.

The list of potential negative substances inherent in commonly eaten foods is much longer, including, among many others: remains of medication feed to cattle in meat and cow's milk, cadmium in seeds and whole grain cereals, mycotoxins in cereals and nuts as well as potential unwanted effects of genetic modified plants introduced to the food chain (Tally 1999; Julin *et al.* 2012; Bawa and

Anilakumar 2013; Ostry, Malir, and Ruprich 2013). Common to all the unwanted substances are that they are invisible, and due to their diffusion it is impossible to avoid them all; they are even found in the very foods the authorities recommend we should increase our intake of. This is a challenge for the population but certainly also for those formulating health advice.

Divergence is an inherent issue when it comes to evaluating associations between foods and human health; the tricky matter is how to handle these dilemmas. The solution can be looked for in tradition, where the Greenlandic hunter retains marine mammals as his primary food source because culture posits this as the right way to live. The answer can also be sought in dietary regimes, like Super-Healthy Family, where strict, but very clear, rules for dietary practice remove the responsibility from the individual. A third strategy is to trust the authorities. In the Nordic countries the health authorities are, to a large extent, independent of interests other than insurance of public health. The best strategy, at least in those countries, may therefore be to rely on the official statements when told that, overall, fish are healthy for most people, but that women of childbearing age should avoid eating large amounts of certain types; that remains of pesticides in fruits and vegetables are regulated to a reasonable extent; and that formation of acrylamide in commercially produced foods will be acted upon if acrylamide is confirmed to be a relevant public health problem.

While on the negative side of new micro-biological knowledge about health risks is the inherent impossibility of avoiding all toxicants, on the positive side it is now possible to identify biomarkers that testify strongly to the beneficial effects of particular food items that have a long pedigree in northern Europe, namely whole grain wheat and rye intake (Landberg 2009). Whole grain consumption is now recognized worldwide as a healthy choice, and most often it is easily accessible – at least in the global North. Among the more spectacular findings is a clear association between a high intake of such fiber with a reduced risk of colorectal cancer (Aune *et al.* 2011; Tjønneland and Olsen 2011).

What these positive results share with the more controversial negative findings on toxins within fish, fruit, and vegetables is their being deeply ingrained in the microbial realities of the human body and in food items. These realities remain hidden from most people, and are often controversial among specialists. The question is how it may be translated into functional knowledge, by which people may confidently live without necessarily understanding the nitty-gritty of scientific discussion. Whatever the answer, we have a new and deeper sense of the microscopic environment affecting health as deeply as the changing landscapes and seas around us.

Concluding Remarks: Food Safety in Changing Environments

In this chapter we have triangulated emergent challenges to food safety worldwide, not least those that are related to environmental concerns. These concerns are multiplying as well-known landscapes and resources are destabilized in the wake of climate change and other anthropogenic degradations. The result is found in emerging "food wars" in the global community (Lang and Heasman 2004), and in increasing uncertainties about food safety in people's everyday lives.

While food security – in the sense of all people getting sufficient nutrition to lead active and healthy lives – has not nearly been achieved in spite of long-term international efforts, an even more complex issue of safety is creeping up on the global community, North and South alike. New patterns of disease, including dramatic increase in Type II diabetes, in obesity, in certain forms of cancer, and in cardiovascular problems, testify to a global malaise that is not easily countered by simple advice, because of its very complexity. Meanwhile, people's general fears of the unknown multiply, as scientific knowledge deepens and the hidden threats from microbiological realities surface, yet remain incomprehensible. Thus, what is called the "gluten syndrome," comprising a variety of allergic responses to gluten, seems to be on the increase, and scientists are now suggesting natural therapies, among which are epigenetic intervention or RNA interference (Rustgi *et al* 2014). For the non-scientist, this demands a lot of trust in techniques bordering on the unfinished GMO debate, and replacing one set of unknowns with another.

Our tour around a rethinking of food safety started with the macro-ecological problems facing the hunting communities of the Arctic that leaves them with no real choice of a healthy diet, while all too aware of the pollution of their environment. A brief comparison with Sami diets and lifestyle was made, confirming that fears of the unknown did not abate with more knowledge. We then, in the second section, visited consumers in the Nordic countries and saw how the multiplicity of choices did not necessarily entail a healthy lifestyle, but potentially drew people toward rather militant dietary regimes entailing a degree of alienation from the social community. Ever more substantiated advice from health authorities induced others, men in particular, to disregard any dietary advice, because they saw it as socially destructive. In the third section, we explored some of the recent findings on carcinogens in very common food items, processed in ordinary ways, and concluded that even foods acclaimed by health authorities, for all their merits, are not beyond suspicion. All of them are products of an environment that is increasingly polluted and that harbors as yet unknown toxins.

What has become clear over the last two decades is that humanity may be facing a dietary revolution that will be greater than the revolution in eighteenth-century Europe that saw new food items making headway into the Old World – potatoes, rice, and maize, to mention just a few staples (see Braudel 1981). It took a long time, however, and the ancient food regimes of wheat and wine in southern Europe, and of rye, barley, and beer in the Nordic countries, were not disbanded even while gradually being supplemented by new items in the wake of multiplying colonial relations that were to separate the global North and from the global South for a long time. Now that global climate changes reunite the globe, and gradually shift the resource bases around in a new way, North and South alike face health consequences. They certainly share the concerns about food security (FAO 2008b).

This is where anthropology's commitment to understanding what climate change means to the everyday lives of people across the globe becomes expedient (Hastrup 2013b; Hastrup and Rubow 2014). The new anthropological interest in nature embraces both health and environment, and directs our attention to the complex relations between social and natural developments (Hastrup 2014).

In closing the argument, it is apt to return to FAO and relate a recent call to prepare for a new management of food safety:

> Emerging food safety risks may require a change to the "old" way of doing things – both in terms of industry food safety management programmes and public sector food safety activities, including the development of guidance of industry on "good practice". A better understanding of changes that might arise is an essential first step to ensuring preparedness for those changes. (FAO 2008a: 6)

In fact, we hope to have contributed to a better understanding of the changes that take place and affect everybody, and we urge policy makers to put a strong effort into improving food production in the North no less than in the South, and demand a greater responsibility from industrial and food-handling companies, thus inspiring more trust in consumers, who are presently bewildered by the illegibility of the state. In that respect our ambition resembles Florence Sabin's public health campaign in the United States in the 1940s, where she struggled to regulate the entire milk industry – instead of simply educating housewives to prevent disease (Dunn 2011).

In the larger scheme of global food security, it is expedient to rethink issues of safety with a view to new environmental challenges that affect the entire world and give rise to new fears of invisible and largely unknowable threats to human health and social life worldwide.

ACKNOWLEDGMENTS

The authors would like to acknowledge their inspiration from the Nordforsk project: HELGA. Nordic Whole Grain, of which they were all part. The project also (partly) funded the research made by Anne Marie Rieffestahl and Anja Olsen. Kirsten Hastrup further wants to acknowledge the European Research Council for funding her research in climate change generally and fieldwork in Greenland more particularly, within the project Waterworlds.

The authors also want to thank the editor of this volume, Merrill Singer, for his highly perceptive and productive comments on the first draft.

REFERENCES

Ahn, J.S., Castle, L., Clarke, D.B., Lloyd, A.S., Philo, M.R., and Speck D.R. 2002. "Verification of the Findings of Acrylamide in Heated Foods." *Food Additives and Contaminants*, 19(12): 1116–1124.

AMAP. 2002. *Persistent Organic Pollutants in the Arctic*. Oslo: Arctic Monitoring and Assessment Programme.

AMAP. 2009. *Human Health in the Arctic*. Oslo: Arctic Monitoring and Assessment Programme.

Anderson, H. and Kowal, E. 2012. "Culture, History, and Health in an Australian Aboriginal Community: The Case of Utopia." *Medical Anthropology*, 13(5): 438–457.

Anderson, M.D. and Cook, J.T. 1999. "Community Food Security: Practice in Need of Theory?" *Agriculture and Human Values*, 16: 14–1150.

Aune, D., Chan, D.S., Lau, R., Vieira, R., Greenwood, D.C., Kampman, E., and Norat, T. 2011." Dietary Fibre, Whole Grains, and Risk of Colorectal Cancer: Systematic Review and Dose-Response Meta-Analysis of Prospective Studies." *British Medical Journal* (November 10) 343: d6617.

Bauman, Z. 2006. *Liquid Fear*. Cambridge: Polity.

Bauman, Z. 2007. *Liquid Times: Living in an Age of Uncertainty*. Cambridge: Polity.

Bawa A.S. and Anilakumar K.R. 2013. "Genetically Modified Foods: Safety, Risks and Public Concerns – A Review." *Journal of Food Science and Technology*, 50(6): 1035–1046.

Beck, U. 1993. *Risk Society: Towards a New Modernity*. London: Sage.

Beck, U. 1998. *World Risk Society*. Cambridge: Cambridge University Press.

Bjerregaard, P. and. Dahl-Petersen, I.K. 2010. *Sundhedsundersøgelsen I Avanersuaq 2010*. Statens Institut for Folkesundhed. SIF's Grønlandsskrifter nr.23.

Bjerregaard, P. and Mulvad, G. 2012. "The Best of Two Worlds: How the Greenland Board of Nutrition Has Handled Conflicting Evidence about Diet and Health." *International Journal of Circumpolar Health*, 71: 185–188.

Bjørklund, I. 2013. "Domestication, Reindeer Husbandry and the Development of Sámi Pastoralism." *Acta Borealia: A Nordic Journal of Circumpolar Societies*, 30(2): 174–189.

Blank, I., Robert, F., Goldmann, T., Pollien, P., Varga, N., Devaud, S., Saucy, F., Huynh-Ba, T., and Stadler, R.H. 2005. "Mechanisms of Acrylamide Formation: Maillard-Induced Transformation of Asparagine." *Advances in Experimental Biology*, 561: 171–189.

Braudel, F. 1981. *The Structures of Everyday Life: Civilization & Capitalism 15th–18th Century*, vol. I. Translated from French by M. Kochan and S. Reynolds. London: Collins.

Caplan, P. 2000. "'Eating British Beef with Confidence': A Consideration of Consumers' Responses to BSE in Britain." In P. Caplan (Ed.), *Risk Revisited* (pp. 184–203). London: Pluto Pres.

Christensen, G. 1999. "Næring og nydelse i oplysningstiden. Diskursiv regulering af mad- og spisevaner 1936–1985." *Mad og drikke. Tidsskriftet Antropologi*, 39: 95–108.

Confalonieri, U., Menne, B., Akhtar, R., Ebi, K.L., Hauengue, M., Kovats, R.-S., Revich, B.., and Woodward, A. 2007. "Human Health. Climate Change 2007: Impacts, Adaptation and Vulnerability." Contribution of Working Group II to the *Fourth Assessment Report of the Intergovernmental Panel on Climate Change*, edited by M.L. Parry, O.F. Canziani, J.P. Palutikof, P.J. van der Linden, and C.E. Hansen (pp. 391–431). Cambridge: Cambridge University Press.

Damalas, C.A. and Eleftherohorinos, I. G. 2011. "Pesticide Exposure, Safety Issues, and Risk Assessment Indicators." *International Journal of Environmental Research and Public Health*, 8(5): 1402–1419.

Den individuelle helbredsundersøgelse af beboerne i Avanersuaq i April–May 2011. Departementet for Sundhed, Grønlands Selvstyre 2011. www.nanoq.gl.

Douglas, M. and Wildavsky, A. 1983. *Risk and Culture*. Berkeley, CA: University of California Press.

Douglas, M. 1992. *Risk and Blame: Essays in Cultural Theory.* London: Routledge.

Dunn, E.C. 2008. "Postsocialist Spores: Disease, Bodies and the State in the Republic of Georgia." *American Ethnologist*, 35(2): 243–258.

Dunn, E.C. 2011. "The Pasteurized State: Milk, Health and the Government of Risk." *Endeavour*, 35(2–3): 107–115.

FAO (Food and Agriculture Organization). 2001. *The State of Food Insecurity in the World.* Rome: Food and Agricultural Organization of the United Nations.

FAO (Food and Agriculture Organization). 2008a. *Climate Change: Implications for Food Safety.* Prepared by L.-A. Jaykus, M. Woolridge, J.M. Frank, M. Miraglia, A. McQuatters-Gollop, C. Tirado, R. Clarke, and M. Friel.

FAO (Food and Agriculture Organization). 2008b. *Climate Change and Food Security: A Framework Document*, edited by W. Killmann.

Fischler, C. 1980. "Food Habits, Social Change and the Nature/Culture Dilemma." *Social Science Information*, 19(6). London: Sage.

Fischler, C. 1988. "Cuisines and Food Selection." In D.M.H. Thomson (Ed), *Food Acceptability.* London: Elsevier.

Giernes, T. 2008. "Perceptions of Risk and Uncertainty among Sami Women Involved in Reindeer Herding in Northern Norway." *Health, Risk & Society*, 10(5): 505–516.

Goody, J. 1982. *Cooking, Cuisine and Class: A Study in Comparative Sociology.* Cambridge: Cambridge University Press.

Halkier, B. 2003. "Mad, risiko og hverdagens politik." In L. Holm (Ed.), *Mad, mennesker og måltider – samfundsmæssige perspektiver.* Copenhagen: Munksgaard.

Halkier, B. 2004. "Handling Food-related Risks: Political Agency and Governmentality." In M.E. Lien and B. Nerlich (Eds.), *The Politics of Food.* London: Berg.

Halkier, B. and Holm, L. 2006. "Shifting Responsibilities for Food Safety in Europe: An Introduction." *Appetite*, 47(2): 127–133.

Hansen, J.C. 2000. "Grønlandsk kost. En miljømedicinsk vurdering." *Dike/Inussuk – Arktisk Forskningsjournal* 2.

Harries, T. 2008. "Feeling Secure or Being Secure? Why It Can Seem Better Not to Protect Yourself Against a Natural Hazard." *Health, Risk & Society*, 10(5): 479–490.

Hassan, F.A. 2002. *Droughts, Food and Culture: Ecological Change and Food Security in Africa's Later Prehistory.* New York: Kluwer.

Hastrup, K. 1993. "Hunger and the Hardness of Facts." *Man. Journal of the Royal Anthropological Institute*, 28: 727–739.

Hastrup, 2009a. "The Nomadic Landscape. People in a Changing Arctic Environment." *Danish Journal of Geography*, 109(2): 181–189.

Hastrup, K. 2009b. "Arctic Hunters. Climate Variability and Social Flexibility." In K. Hastrup (Ed.), *The Question of Resilience. Social Responses to Climate Change.* Copenhagen: The Royal Danish Academy of Sciences and Letters.

Hastrup, K. 2013a. "Anticipation on Thin Ice: Diagrammatic Reasoning Among Arctic Hunters." In K. Hastrup and M. Skrydstrup (Eds.), *The Social Life of Climate Models. Anticipating Nature* (pp. 77–99). London: Routledge.

Hastrup, K. 2013b. "Anthropological Contributions to the Study of Climate: Past, Present, Future." *WIREs Climate Change.* doi: 10.1002/wcc.219.

Hastrup, K. (Ed.) 2014. *Anthropology and Nature.* London: Routledge.

Hastrup, K. and Rubow, C. (Eds.) 2014. *Living with Environmental Change. Waterworlds.* London: Earthscan.

Hastrup, K. and Olwig, K.F. (Eds.) 2012 *Climate Change and Human Mobility. Global Challenges to the Social Sciences.* Cambridge: Cambridge University Press.

Henderson, J.A., Ward, P.R., Coveney, J.D., and Meyer, S.B. 2012. "Trust in the Australian Food Supply: Innocent Until Proven Guilty." *Health, Risk & Society*, 14(3): 257–272.

Hoekstra, A.Y. 2008. "The Water Footprint of Food." In J. Förare (Ed.), *Water for Food* (pp. 49–60). Stockholm: The Swedish Research Council.

Hovelsrud, G.K., Poppel, B., van Oort, B.E.H., and Reist, J.D. 2012. "Arctic Societies, Cultures, and Peoples in a Changing Cryosphere." In *Snow, Water, Ice and Permafrost in the Arctic (SWIPA): Climate Change and the Cryosphere.* Oslo: Arctic Monitoring and Assessment Programme (AMAP).

IARC (International Agency for Research on Cancer). 1994. *Monographs on the Evaluation of Carcinogenic Risks to Humans – Some Industrial Chemicals.* International Agency for Research on Cancer; 1994 February 22. Report No. 60.

IPCC. 2007. "Climate Change 2007: Impacts, Adaptation and Vulnerability." Contribution of Working Groups II to the *Fourth Assessment Report of the Intergovernmental Panel on Climate Change*, edited by M.L. Parry, O.F. Canziani, J.P. Palutikof, P.J. van der Linden, and C.E. Hansen. Cambridge: Cambridge University Press.

Jeppesen, C. and Bjerregaard, P. 2012. "Consumption of Traditional Food and Adherence to Nutrition Recommendations in Greenland." *Scandinavian Journal of Public Health*, 40(5): 475–481.

Julin B., Wolk A., Bergkvist L., Bottai M., and Akesson A. 2012. "Dietary Cadmium Exposure and Risk of Postmenopausal Breast Cancer: A Population-Based Prospective Cohort Study." *Cancer Research*, 72(6): 1459–1466.

Kristensen, S.T. 1999. "Sult, appetit og mæthed. Mellem biologi og kultur." *Mad og drikke. Tidsskriftet Antropologi*, 39: 65–80.

Lake, I.R., Hooper, L., Abdelhamid, A., Bentham, G., Boxall, A.B.A. Draper, A., Fairweather-Tait, S., Hulme, M., Hunter, P.R., Nicholls, G., and Waldron, K.W. 2012. "Climate Change and Food Security: Health Impacts in Developed Countries." *Environmental Health Perspectives*, 120(11): 1520–1526.

Landberg, R. 2009. "Alkylresorcinols as Biomarkers of Whole Grain Wheat and Rye Intake." Doctoral thesis (no. 2009: 11), Swedish University of Agricultural Sciences, Uppsala.

Lang, T. and Heasman, M. 2004. *Food wars. The Global Battle for Mouths, Minds and Markets.* London: Earthscan.

Lassen, J. and Korzen, S. 2009. "The Environment Overlooked? The Role of the Environmental Concerns in Organic Food Discourses." *Anthropology of Food.*

Lobell, D. and Burke, M. (Eds.) 2010. *Climate Change and Food Security: Adapting Agriculture to a Warmer World.* New York: Springer.

Luhmann, N. 2000. "Familiarity, Confidence, Trust: Problems and Alternatives." In D. Gambetta (Ed.), *Trust: Making and Breaking Cooperative Relations.* Oxford: Blackwell.

Lupton, D. 1996. *Food, the Body and the Self.* London: Sage.

Malthus, T.R. [1798] 1970. *An Essay on the Principle of Population*, edited by A. Flew) Harmondsworth, UK: Pelican.

Marvin, H.J.P., Kleter, G.A., Prandini, A., Dekkers, S., and Bolton, D.J. 2009. "Early Identification Systems for Emerging Food-Borne Hazards." *Food and Chemical Toxicology*, 47: 915–926.

Mauritson, N.-B. 2007. *Kernesund Familie Sådan!* JP/Politikens Forlagshus A/S.

Meissner, S. 2012. "Virtual Water and Water Footprints: Global Supply and Production Chains and Their Impacts on Freshwater Resources." In P. Hahn, K. Cless and J. Soentgen (Eds.), *People at the Well: Kinds, Usages and Meanings of Water in a Global Perspective* (pp. 44–64). Frankfurt: Campus.

Meneley, A. 2008. "Oleo-Signs and Quali-Signs: The Qualities of Olive Oil." *Ethnos*, 73(3): 303–326.

Mol, A. 2009. "The Embodied Normativity of the Consumer-Citizen." *Journal of Cultural Economy*, 2(3): 269–283.

Mozaffarian, D. and Rimm, E.B. 2006. "Fish Intake, Contaminants, and Human Health. Evaluating the Risks and the Benefits." *Journal of the American Medical Association*, 296(15): 1885–1899.

Nilsson, L.M., Dahlgren, L., Johansson, I., Brustad, M., Sjölander, P., and van Guelpen, B. 2011. "Diet and Lifestyle of the Sami of Southern Lapland in the 1930s–1950s and Today." *International Journal of Circumpolar Health*, 70(3): 301–318.

Nilsson, L.M., Johansson, I., Lenner, P., Lindahl, B., and van Guelpen, B. 2010. "Consumption of Filtered and Boiled Coffee and the Risk of Incident Cancer: A Prospective Cohort Study." *Cancer Causes Control*, 2010: 1533–1544.

Nilsson, L.M., Winkvist, A., Brustad, M., Jansson, J.-H., Johansson, I., Lenner, P., Lindahl, B., and Van Guelpen, B. 2012. "Sami Diet and Mortality in a Northern Swedish Population." In L.M. Nilsson, "Sami Lifestyle And Health – Epidemiological Studies from Northern Sweden." Doctoral dissertation, Umeå University: Public Health and Clinical Medicine/Nutritional Research.

Ostry, V., Malir, F., and Ruprich, J. 2013. "Producers and Important Dietary Sources of Ochratoxin A and Citrinin." *Toxins*, 5(9): 1574–1586.

Paxson, H. 2010. "Locating Value in Artisan Cheese: Reverse Engineering *Terroir* for New-World Landscapes." *American Anthropologist*, 112(3): 444–457.

Poppel, B., Kruse, J., Duhaine, G., and Abryutina, L. 2007. *SLiCA Results*. Anchorage: Institute of Social and Economic Research, University of Alaska Anchorage.

Raisborough, J. 2007. "Contexts of Choice: The Risky Business of Elective Cosmetic Surgery." In J. Scott Jones and J. Raisborough (Eds.), *Risk, Identities and the Everyday*. London: Ashgate.

Reinert, E.S., Aslaksen, J., Eira, I.M.G., Mathiesen, S.D., Reinert, H., and Turi, E.I. 2009. "Adapting To Climate Change in Sámi Reindeer Herding: The Nation-State as Problem and Solution." In W.N. Adger, I. Lorenzoni, and K.L. O'Brien (Eds.), *Adapting to Climate Change: Thresholds, Values, Governance*. Cambridge: Cambridge University Press.

Rieffestahl, A.M. 2014. "Super-Healthy Families: Alternative Food Habits and their Social Implications." In *Food, Culture & Society*, 17(4): 615–627.

Rieffestahl, A.M. n.d. "Nordic Men's view on Food Habits and Health." Under review.

Ringler, C., Biswas, A., and Cline, S. (Eds.) 2010. *Global Change: Impacts on Water and Food-Security*. New York: Springer.

Rustgi, S., Wen, N., Osorio, C., Brew-Appiah, R.A.T., Wen, S., Gemini, R., Mejias, J.H., Ankrah, N., Moehs, C.P., and von Wettstein, D. 2014. "Natural Dietary Therapies for the 'Gluten Syndrome.'" *Scientia Danica. Series B, Biologica*, vol. 3. Copenhagen: The Royal Danish Academy of Sciences and Letters.

Sen, A. 1981. *Poverty and Famines: An Essay on Entitlement and Deprivation*. Oxford: Clarendon.

Sen, A. 1987. *Hunger and Entitlements. WIDER Research for Action*. UN University.

Simmel, G. [1910] 1998. *Måltidets sociologi. In: Hvordan er samfundet muligt? Udvalgte sociologiske tidsskrifter*. København: Gyldendal.

Singer, M. 2011. "Toward a Critical Biosocial Model of Ecohealth in Southern Africa: The HIV/AIDS and Nutrition Insecurity Syndemic." *Annals of Anthropology Practice*, 35(1): 8–27.

Tally, M.R. 1999. "The National Milk Safety Program and Drug Residues in Milk." *Veterinary Clinics of North America: Food Practice*, 15(1): 63–73.

Tjønneland, A. and Olsen, A. 2011. "Fibre and Prevention of Chronic Diseases. Fibre Specifically from Cereals and Whole Grains Is Most Effective at Reducing Risk." Editorial, *British Medical Journal*, 2011: 343:d6938.

Troels-Lund, T.F. 1969. *Dagligt Liv i Norden i det sekstende Århundrede. Fødemidler, Hverdag og Fest*, vol. 3. Copenhagen: Gyldendal.

Tulloch, J. and Lupton, D. 2003. *Risk and Everyday Life*. London: Sage.

Verbeke, W., Sioen, I., Pieniak, Z., Van Camp, J., and De Henauw, S. 2005. "Consumer Perception Versus Scientific Evidence about Health Benefits and Safety Risks from Fish Consumption." *Public Health Nutrition*, 8(4): 422–429.

Whatmore, S. 2002. *Hybrid Geographies: Natures, Cultures, Spaces*. London: Sage.

WHO (World Health Organization). 2006. *World Health Report*. Geneva.

Zinn, J.O. 2008. "Heading into the Unknown: Everyday Strategies for Managing Risk and Uncertainty." *Health, Risk & Society*, 10(5): 439–450.

CHAPTER 14

New Toxics Uncertainty and the Complexity Politics of Emerging Vapor Intrusion Risk

Peter C. Little

Introduction

The health–environment nexus is a vibrant domain of anthropological research that challenges researchers to grapple with the politics of uncertainty, facticity, and possibility, and to confront clashing contact zones of bodies and subjectivities, economies and ecologies, powerful corporations and distressed communities. Those working on the front lines of this nexus are generally dealing with an array of unknowns and situations of "toxic confusion" (Auyero and Swistun 2009: 11) that, instead of leading to scholarly surrender and research avoidance, attracts and intensifies critical thinking. Some have rightly noted that,

> Scholars working at the intersection of environment and health feel free to take the factuality of many hazards for granted: that Chernobyl and Bhopal did indeed kill many people, that urban pollution exacerbates asthma, that tropical environments cause sleeping sickness through tsetse flies. Historically, however, as each of these new certainties has crystallized, a multitude of new uncertainties has sprouted around them. Much history of environment and health is about what we don't, or don't quite, know. (Mitman, Murphy, and Sellers 2004: 12)

A Companion to the Anthropology of Environmental Health, First Edition. Edited by Merrill Singer.

This chapter explores one such "new uncertainty" circulating among some environmental and public health scientists, regulators, and concerned citizens living in contaminated communities: *vapor intrusion*. According to the United States Environmental Protection Agency (EPA), vapor intrusion occurs when volatile[1] organic chemicals (VOCs) from contaminated soil and groundwater vaporize and rise through gaps or pores in soil and foundations into homes and other buildings. A national effort spearheaded by the US EPA to better understand and revisit sites with a potential for vapor intrusion (VI) has been underway since the late 1990s, when the potential for significant human exposure was first recognized. According to the EPA:

> In extreme cases, the vapors may accumulate in dwellings or occupied buildings to levels that may pose near-term safety hazards (e.g., explosion), acute health effects, or aesthetic problems (e.g., odors). Typically however, the chemical concentration levels are low or, depending on site-specific conditions, vapors may not be present at detectable concentrations. In residences with low concentrations, the main concern is whether the chemicals may pose an unacceptable risk of chronic health effects due to long-term exposure to these low levels. A complicating factor in evaluating the potential chronic risk from vapor intrusion is the potential presence of some of the same chemicals at or above background concentrations (from the ambient (outdoor) air and/or emission sources in the building e.g., household solvents, gasoline, cleaners) that may pose, separately or in combination with vapor intrusion, a significant human health risk. (U.S. EPA 2002: 5)

I first learned about VI in 2002 while living in Endicott, New York, birthplace of International Business Machines (IBM) and the site of a contentious hazardous waste site that has become a "poster child" community for VI risk (see Little 2013, 2014). I attended a public meeting on VI and learned that a chemical spill from the former IBM plant had released a plume of chlorinated volatile organic compounds (CVOCs) into a residential area spanning nearly 300 acres. The main contaminant of concern was trichloroethylene (TCE), a dominant toxic substance at VI sites and a known cancer-causing chemical that has recently been determined by numerous epidemiological studies to be "carcinogenic to humans by all routes of exposure and poses a potential human health hazard for noncancer toxicity to the central nervous system, kidney, liver, immune system, male reproductive system, and the developing embryo/fetus" (Chiu *et al.* 2013:303). TCE was a heavily used solvent in chipboard manufacturing operations at the former IBM plant.

Witnessing agency responses to the VI threat in Endicott, I quickly learned that VI was an elusive and emerging environmental public health problem based on the complex science of an exposure pathway that was difficult for both citizens and scientists to fully understand and act on, especially because both VI science and regulation were still in the making. More recently, VI has become a contentious topic of environment law, leading affected citizens and their lawyers down an equally complex path of uncertain litigation. This set of circumstances was my introduction to the vibrant "political ecology of health" (Baer 1996; Baer, Singer, and Susser 1997; Harper 2002, 2004; Baer and Singer 2009;

Dietrich 2013) in general and the political ecology of vapor intrusion risk in particular. As defined here, the political ecology of health is a critical theory of environmental health problems that attends to both the intersecting politics of risk science and uncertainty and the lived experience of "toxic frustration" (Singer 2011). This chapter draws on this critical environmental health theory to analyze the complexities of VI risk.

I first provide a brief history of the development of VI, exploring how this new and uncertain toxic substance exposure topic became a public health risk and a focus of concern for government agencies and community organizations. This section is followed by a brief VI ethnographic case study exploring the above-mentioned politics of uncertainty common in sites of VI risk. Next, I explore the value of the political ecology of health perspective for teasing out the global environmental health risk and policy dimensions of this emerging toxics debate, exposing the complexities of contemporary risk management decisions in our late industrial age, and developing a critical approach to VI risk that addresses the trenchant politics of science, regulation, and law, all issues that more generally present challenges for critical medical anthropologists engaging the complex global and international environmental health dynamics of industrial pollution.

An Emerging Environmental Health Risk

While federal and state agencies in the United States have been aware of the potential for vaporized contaminants, especially volatile organic compounds (VOCs), to enter homes and buildings since the 1990s, scientists and regulators held that levels of indoor air contamination would not be of concern due to processes of dilution and attenuation. Environmental health scientists and engineers have only recently come to realize the actual potential for VI to result in widespread human exposures. Indoor air sampling at a vapor intrusion site in Colorado – the Redfield Site – in the late 1990s found significant levels of the contaminant trichloroethylene (TCE) in homes where a computerized exposure model recommended by the EPA had predicted little or no contamination (Folkes *et al.* 2009). This finding resulted in a national effort spearheaded by the EPA and state agencies to better understand VI risk and to revisit sites where cleanup had already occurred but the potential for VI remained high.

In most cases, the primary targeted chemicals of concern at VI sites are TCE, tetrachloroethylene (PCE), and trichloroethane (TCA), all chlorinated hydrocarbons. Each is highly volatile and associated with serious negative health impacts, such as cancer, organ damage, and/or birth defects. Policies to address vapor intrusion are still in the development stage. The New York State Departments of Environmental Conservation (NYDEC) and Health (NYDOH), as well as the EPA, have all issued draft guidance on the evaluation of vapor intrusion at contaminated sites, but none has been finalized. Much of the delay comes down to the fact that VI is a complex phenomenon that poses several concrete national environmental public health policy challenges. First, there is currently a lack of legally enforceable cleanup standards for toxic substances in residential indoor air. Second, it is difficult to accurately determine which sites and/or buildings in a community have the potential to be at risk of VI and which should be tested. Third, not being able to accurately "determine" VI risk makes it difficult to make decisions on whether to proceed with mitigation, further monitor the problem, or take no action. A fourth challenge is how to ensure the protection of public health over the long term, including the proper maintenance of mitigation systems and achieving full cleanup of contaminated sites. And finally, the persistent power of corporations and their influence on neoliberal deregulation further complicates the development of more protective VI environmental health policies. All of these issues, as will be discussed later, add to the dense crux that emerges when exploring the global dimensions of VI risk.

The discussion of the emerging threat of VI requires attention to a coevolving development that greatly informs debates over this new environmental health risk: controversy over the toxicity and regulation of TCE. For the past seven years, community leaders, scientists, public officials, and academics (myself included) have been fighting for better protection and better toxicological risk assessments for TCE. TCE first entered public debate as the culprit toxin involved in the Woburn, Massachusetts cancer cluster of childhood leukemia cases, which was the subject of the 1998 film *A Civil Action*. TCE is a chlorinated solvent once widely used as a metal degreaser and is a widespread groundwater contaminant found at hundreds of military bases and industrial sites throughout the United States. In addition to cancer, TCE causes harmful effects to the central nervous system, kidney, liver, immune system, male reproductive system, and the developing fetus (Chiu *et al.* 2013). In 1987, the EPA completed the first risk assessment for TCE and classified it a "probable" human carcinogen. The most recent human health risk assessment of TCE produced by the US EPA's Integrated Risk Information System (IRIS) program has determined that TCE is 5 to 65 times more toxic than previously estimated, resulting in TCE being "re-classified" as "carcinogenic to humans by all routes of exposure" (US EPA 2011; Chiu *et al.* 2013).

Until recently, citizens fighting for better protection from this harmful toxic substance have been stonewalled by the powerful influence of chemical industries in general, and the US Departments of Defense and Energy in particular. These two federal agencies alone are responsible for nearly 750 hazardous waste sites containing TCE. Citizens seeking greater protection were stymied by political blockades set up by the Bush administration, which forced the EPA to stall its TCE risk assessment. In addition, the administration silenced established TCE science in 2007 by exempting the military and certain industries from laws that would limit air emissions of TCE and other halogenated solvents, an exemption which was challenged in court by the Natural Resource Defense Council and other environmental groups. In 2009, President Obama agreed to reconsider the Bush-era air emission exemptions. Although the outcome of that process is still pending, a 2009 draft TCE assessment report did classify TCE as carcinogenic to humans by all routes of exposure, based mainly on its high risk of causing kidney cancers, non-Hodgkin's lymphoma, and liver cancer.

TCE activists have been able to prod the EPA to update their toxicological profile for TCE to better reflect the growth of TCE science over the past two decades. We wrote a letter to EPA Administrator Lisa Jackson, which was signed by nearly 40 citizens representing communities across the United States with water and/or air contaminated with TCE or similar toxic substances. The letter, sent on September 26, 2011, urged the EPA to finalize their TCE assessment and issue the updated version to establish more protective cleanup standards and TCE exposure limits nationwide. Just two days later, the EPA took an important step toward TCE regulation by releasing the finalized toxicological assessment reflecting the findings of the National Academy of Sciences, which was largely responsible for updating the most recent science on the health risks of TCE exposure.

Despite these developments, a federal TCE standard has yet to be reached, but action has been taken at the state level. For example, in 2003 the New York State Department of Health (NYDOH) established an air guideline for TCE of 5.0 micrograms per cubic meter (mcg/m^3). In 2005, the NYDOH issued a draft "Trichloroethylene Air Criteria Document" which explained in detail the scientific process that informed how the state's TCE guideline was derived. Shortly after the release of this document, the NYDOH convened a Peer Review Panel to review the "Criteria Document." While the Panel generally acknowledged that the NYDOH staff did a thorough review of the scientific literature, it made a number of recommendations that if adopted would extend the lower end of the range initially used, which was 1.0 to 10 mcg/m^3.

Furthermore, in the summer of 2005, the NYDOH, under the federal oversight of the Agency for Toxic Substances and Disease Registry (ATSDR), released a Health Statistics Review for the IBM-Endicott Superfund Site that documented elevated rates of testicular cancer, kidney cancer, and heart birth defects in the Endicott area. The review claimed that these elevated rates were statistically significant, meaning they were unlikely to be due to chance alone. The report never suggested that IBM's TCE plume was the culprit for these community health statistics. TCE epidemiology, like most environmental epidemiology, is tainted with ambiguity and "lack of knowledge." This epistemic vacuity theme appears up front in a 2006 report produced by the New York State Assembly Committee on Environmental Conservation entitled *Vapor Intrusion of Toxic Chemicals: An Emerging Public Health Concern*:

> Significant barriers hamper our ability to assess the toxic effects of chemicals on human health. As a result, the toxic effects of the majority of chemicals used in commerce are unknown, and debate persists over the toxicity of the small number of chemicals, like TCE, that have been well studied ... Environmental epidemiologic studies ... suffer from a high potential for false negatives due to the small size of most study populations and a long-standing scientific convention, which places greater weight on avoiding false positives than avoiding false negatives. Such studies are further limited by the presence of possible confounding factors, while animal toxicological studies are limited by the need to extrapolate from one species

> to another. Both types of studies are costly and time consuming. As a result, debate over the toxicity of TCE has persisted due to differing judgments regarding the strength, applicability, and interpretation of both human and animal studies. (DiNapoli 2006: 2)

The inherent ambiguity of risk science has been noted in many social science critiques of risk assessments (Cullen and Small 2004; Cummings 1981; Jasanoff 1998; Tesh 2000), leading some researchers to even argue "that an understanding of locations and topics about which knowledge is lacking can be just as important within a community as understanding what is known" (Dowty and Allen 2011: 203). Moreover, dealing with VI risk is tantamount to "dealing with the unknown … [which] demands clear recognition of and communication about the limits of knowing" (Bleicher and Gross 2011: 187). The current scientific discourse on VI is marked by ambiguity and "knowledge-gaps" (Frickel and Vincent 2011), which contribute to the complexity and "volatility" (Rolph, Torres, and Everett 2012) of both VI science and the existing VI regulatory environment. As will be discussed later, these politics of uncertainty are largely informed by precarious legal and regulatory structures and politics that further complicate attempts to understand the international environmental health risks of VI, at the same time that these very "politics" showcase a vibrant new area of political ecology of health analysis.

Uncertainty and Complexity

Added to the complexities involved in understanding the environmental epidemiology of TCE exposure, there are many unknowns when it comes to the science of investigating, evaluating, and mitigating exposures related to VI. In this way, VI science, like environmental science and knowledge itself, is "multiple, complex, and situated" (Goldman and Turner 2011: 19). While measuring indoor air concentrations generally produces the most accurate information for determining ***exposure point concentrations*** (i.e., what people are actually inhaling), VI scientists and engineers generally use what they call ***attenuation factors*** to estimate the amount of vapor that might be entering the building. While attenuation factors are usually determined by investigating the relationship between groundwater contamination and indoor air concentrations, it is generally more reliable to use soil-gas-to-indoor-air attenuation factors. Further, new sampling techniques for VI are also emerging. According to one VI expert: "sampling technologies, using sensors that can be pointed at potential pathways and sources, are a superior way of resolving where VOCs are coming from. To some degree, those technologies exist now, but the entire field of vapor intrusion investigation will be greatly enhanced when chip-based sensors become available in the not-too-distant future" (personal communication from Bill Wertz). Even if such high-tech sampling technologies could be employed at every site, it remains unknown how these technologies will benefit impacted residents who struggle with the public health concerns of VI exposure.

In an interview with a VI expert, it was brought to my attention that there are many challenges that come with studying what experts in this field call "the VI pathway," as it is a new exposure route that triggers new environmental health concerns. Yet, these challenges can be "rewarding" and exciting from a science practice perspective:

> From the technical perspective, VI is a very challenging path to understand. The groundwater path has its challenges, but it is relatively simple in terms of contaminant migration through aquifers. You can put in a relatively small number of wells and characterize the nature and extent of contamination that way and feel fairly confident that you can make good decisions. What we have seen with vapor intrusion is that the distribution of VOCs in the subsurface and beneath peoples' houses and then even the VOCs getting into their houses is much more variable. There is a lot of spatial variability in the distribution and temporal variability in terms of changes through time. They are much greater than a classic groundwater plume. So that presents some of the technical challenges of VI in terms of control and understanding the nature of the vapor contamination. It has been a challenge as well as a real rewarding experience. You feel like you are kind of at the cutting edge of what's going on.

The scientific complexity just discussed, of course, has compounded the challenge of developing national VI policy. Amid the scientific challenge is the fact that VI impacts many regulatory programs, including those dealing with Superfund sites and brownfield developments. The Interstate Technology and Regulatory Council (ITRC) is the primary network of experts assisting states as they develop VI policies, but some states, especially those with lax environmental policies, currently lack adequate protocols for VI (ITRC 2007). The VI pathway is becoming "an inevitable regulatory issue … Understanding the risk posed by this pathway on property use and protection of human health will be a complex learning process as the regulators, environmental professionals, attorneys, real estate developers, insurance carriers, and myriad of other stakeholders become better acquainted with this next *regulatory juggernaut*" (Brock 2009: 2, emphasis added).

Even amid the health uncertainties of VI exposures, environmental health experts at VI sites, as in other hazardous waste sites, use "uncertainty analyses" to make human health risk estimates to guide decision makers. According to a recent report of the Institute of Medicine of the National Academies,

> There are no simple rules to translate uncertainty information into a decision. However, a decision maker should be informed about and appreciate the range of uncertainty when making a decision. How uncertainty analysis is used will differ depending on the type of uncertainty under consideration. Uncertainty analyses in human health risk estimates can help decision makers to weigh the marginal decrease in risk against the effort made to reduce it. Uncertainty analyses in technology availability can help decision makers to differentiate between well-established technologies with reasonably well known costs and those that have not been used for the purposes at hand. Uncertainty analyses in cost–benefit analyses can inform decision makers about the disagreement among experts about the way regulations affect the economy, even when using similar models … The success of

> a decision in the face of uncertainty depends on the analysts having a good understanding of the context of the decision and the information needed by the decision makers and also the decision makers having a good understanding of the evidence on which to base the decision, including understanding the uncertainty in that evidence. (Institute of Medicine 2013: 7)

While ethnographic research has shown community "involvement" and "engagement" to be a serious challenge for environmental health agencies anchored to environmental epidemiological logics (Little 2009), scientists and regulators involved in VI science and policy also point to specific community–agency relations challenges at VI sites. During a plenary session at the EPA forum in Philadelphia in January 2009, David Polish (2009), Community Involvement Coordinator for the EPA's Region 3, discussed the challenges to community involvement at VI sites. He contended that regulators and scientists working on VI sites need to do a better job at community involvement, and that the nature of VI calls for new community involvement tactics. For community relations to improve, he explained, scientists and regulators need to make some key changes. Among them, researchers and officials need to promptly meet with residents and other community members, visiting as many homes, businesses, and schools as possible to "sit down with the people." Polish emphasized that it was important to "make a connection" with residents and community members impacted by VI and to explain its threat (or "the situation") in layperson's terms. Finally, he added that all data collected in VI sites should be shared with impacted residents and the "community of interest." These are laudable changes that expose some of the meaningful inroads for ethnographic research at VI sites both in the United States and abroad, and I will return to these later. Next, I explore some ethnographic findings from my research in Endicott, New York, a community that is both the birthplace of International Business Machines Corporation (IBM) and the site of the most scientifically studied VI risk sites in the world.

Ethnographic Case Study: The IBM-Endicott VI Site

As I have found in my own ethnographic research (Little 2012, 2013, 2014), the struggle for residents living with VI risk goes beyond a concern with health, beyond the probabilistic science of risk, which is itself vexed by uncertainty. On the other hand, that is not to say that residents living *in* and *with* Endicott's IBM TCE plume are not concerned about the health risks of VI or don't attempt to make sense of these risks based on their own life experience. Amid grass-roots efforts to create TCE risk standards based on "today's best science" or "sound science," residents also make sense of VI risk and the uncertainty of this emerging exposure science in their own terms and based on their own local knowledge and experience.

Lenny Siegel, an activist and technical advisor to communities coping with VI, has called VI science a "rocket science" that leaves many impacted residents confused and unsure of the "truth" of VI risk and even unsure of their own risk situation after mitigation. My ethnographic research in a community coping with VI risk, as described below, confirms this confusion and precarious exposure situation, yet the narratives also reveal some unexpected additives that expose and intensify the meaningful place of the political ecology of health perspective in emerging VI risk debates. My defense of ethnography departs here from the simple claim that while ethnographic research "cannot replace epidemiological studies … it sheds light on some of the biases that shape risk assessment and environmental science" (Checker 2007:113; see also Allen 2003). While it is true that these lived experiences of VI risk or the so-called "social effect of risk definitions … [are] not dependent on their scientific validity" (Beck 1992: 32), it is worth remembering that VI risk science is in the making, as are residents' own framings of VI risk. In fact, within many decision-making contexts, public or lay knowledge has often been proven to be as important and valuable as the systematic knowledge of experts (Wynne 1989; Jasanoff 1992; Lave 2012). What is most important here, I think, is that neither plume residents, nor public health experts, are claiming *absolute* knowledge about VI and TCE exposure risk, which in turn adds to the complexity of political ecology of health problems in general.

Turning an ethnographic lens on environmental health science and expertise exposes the fact that even the most seasoned environmental epidemiologists and public health toxicologists themselves rarely, if ever, work with sound scientific "proof" in their own scientific work (Little 2009). As an anthropologist interested in the political ecology of health, it is ethnography that best illustrates how VI risk is *experienced*, how this toxics risk is socially constituted and lived (Auyero and Swistun 2009; Singer 2011; Little 2014). In other words, VI risk narratives and understandings matter within current VI debates because these risks are "constantly constructed and negotiated as part of [a] network of social interaction and the formation of meaning" (Lupton 1999: 29). The lived struggle to understand VI risk is equally informed by the intersecting realities of "social suffering" (Kleinman, Das, and Lock 1997) and "environmental suffering" (Singer 2011). When studied ethnographically, VI risk experience is interactively understood and socially processed and judged. What follows are selected findings from ethnographic research carried out between 2008 and 2009 at the IBM-Endicott Superfund site in western New York state. The site encompasses a 300 plus acre residential area with over 1200 residents inhabiting a recognized zone of "significant" TCE contamination and VI risk.

Lived Experiences of VI Risk

At the IBM-Endicott VI Site, numerous residents have told me that despite the uncertainties of their own VI risk situation, they *know* neighbors or have family members with certain illnesses that leave them asking etiological questions, thus informing their public health risk perception. Local risk perception seems to be most conditioned by sociality – most notably intersubjective experience – rather than residents' beliefs about their own personal health problems. Knowledge of the health problems of others was a strong focus of survey respondents' perceptions of risk. For example, survey respondents added comments like, "My husband died two years ago with bone cancer. We had a bicycle shop in the basement for 15 years prior to this. I believe this TCE contributed to his cancer. He worked in the basement every day," or "My stepsons who grew up here were both born prematurely," or "My daughter all of a sudden has colds and stiffness. When she is not here, she is fine. This place seems to make her sick," or "We get the headaches. We get a lot of headaches from living here. We don't know what it is caused by. It could be a series of things. My doctor said this is not the healthiest area to live in. So, there is a problem here." While these brief comments of survey respondents can create a snapshot picture of how people feel and understand VI risk, I found that the narratives that emerged from my in-depth ethnographic interviews with plume residents illustrate in more detail the "social" risk understanding of people living with VI.

One resident I interviewed talked about how the environmental health risks of VI are, as she put it, "close to home":

> When it is so close to home, it really makes you think. I took care of my one dear friend; she was 85 years old. She was old. She was diagnosed in October of 2006 with the same cancer my husband had, and she was dead in February. They said it was a rare kind of lymphoma that she had. But, her house was one of the ones tested, and what they found on the basis of her house was high levels. I don't know the levels, but they were high. I went to one of the town meetings, and they said it was the law that every doctor has to report all cases of cancer. I said, "Well, then doesn't it make sense when you've got 12 cases of cancer in 16 homes." I mean, the young man next door was in his early 30s when he got it. His dad, maybe 15 years later, was diagnosed on a Monday with a stomach cancer, and by Friday, he was dead. That is why I question the idea that only the elderly are affected. I don't think a 30-year-old should go like that. On the house on the corner, the green house, his brother was 21 years old and died of brain cancer, and a year later their mom died with recurring breast cancer. We had a girl that lived across the street that died last May. She fought with breast cancer that went all through her. She left behind a four-year-old. This is just chance? I don't think so.

Shannon then went on to contest the fuzzy position of public health experts. She found it frustrating to have experts say that plume residents are living "within a safe range" even while reports are finding significant relations between TCE exposure and her husband's cancer:

> The reports said, "You don't have to worry about these, and this is what you have to worry about. You're within a safe range ..." [H]ow do they really know? ... Initially, they first told me, when I questioned it and I brought out the cancer and I brought out my husband, they said it publically at the meeting: "There was no connection between these chemicals and non-Hodgkins lymphoma." Not two weeks later there was a report put out in the paper, and they were finding a significant relation between this and non-Hodgkins lymphoma. You know ... it's kinda frustrating. It's frustrating to be laughed at ... I don't claim to know everything, but I'm not stupid. I think that is what I resent more than anything else. It is that what we thought were legitimate concerns have just been ignored.

Shannon experiences the same "double bind" situations in which many residents of contaminated communities find themselves caught. She is between messages, dealing with "a persistent mismatch between explanation and everyday life" (Fortun 2001: 13). Experts tell her the environmental health risks are slim, yet she knows certain things are present and true (Checker 2007). Regardless of the state of the science of TCE and the continued emergence of new research findings, there seems to be an enduring sense of helplessness among plume residents. Most plume residents understand that they inhabit both a fragile environment saturated with ambiguity and a social environment that can lead to frustrating interactions with government officials focused mostly on the "burden of proof" rather than the subjective proof of lived experience.

My ethnographic research at the IBM-Endicott VI site also taught me that not all residents living in VI sites are equally concerned about the health risks of VI. For example, Larry, Shannon's husband, is sure that he will never really know how he got cancer twice, but he does not rule out the "possibility" the plume has caused some local health problems:

> I had cancer twice. Non-Hodgkin's Lymphoma. Twice. The first time was in 1993, and the second time was in 2002. Nobody knows the cause of cancer. Could it have something to do with the toxins that are here? Sure, it could, but no one has proof. It is just really unproven. I mean you can't really, I mean, they know through lab tests and stuff like that TCE can cause cancer, but is that what my problem is? Well, that is something you'll never know.... We just don't know what the health effects are. There is just no conclusive proof that this is the culprit. The only thing they say they know about TCE is from studying its effects on rats. Well, what does that mean? It is certainly a possibility.

As mentioned earlier, ambiguity is a common source of struggle for residents of contaminated communities (Edelstein 2004) even if they are certain something is wrong (Checker 2007). The all too familiar theme is that environmental health etiologies are hard to prove, leaving many plume residents – even those with family members with specific cancers commonly the focus of environmental illness debates – feeling perplexed and stuck with concerns, questions, and the problem of not knowing. The following is just one example of this ambiguity mentioned by informants:

> When it comes to health, that stuff is hard to prove. That is really hard to prove. I mean personal activity plays a role. My brother got leukemia, and they couldn't prove that it was the water. He died in 1985 when he was just 39, and there were 18 cases of cancer on that street. The people that lived in the house before him died of cancer. Their dog even died of cancer. There were different forms of cancer on that street .... I just don't know what this stuff is doing to our health. That is the main concern. What about our health? You don't know what it is going to do to your health.

As Beck (1992: 27) has argued, risks associated with toxic plunder "completely escape human powers of direct perception. The focus is ... on hazards which are neither visible nor perceptible to victims." Residents coping with VI risk grapple with tough questions: What is really there beneath my home causing VI? What is the "net result" of local environmental health risk? Neither expert nor layperson will likely find satisfactory answers to these questions. In VI risk sites, scientists and residents alike know that cancer most likely has multiple "causal agents." The belief that "the possible is richer than the real" (Prigogine 1997) seems to fit well with the majority of plume residents' understandings and framings of the health risks of VI risk. Especially on the topic of cancer, talk of possibility was far more common than talk of certainty. Indeed, it is possible that TCE risk has "*different* meanings for *different* people" (Beck 1992: 26, emphasis in original) and similar meanings for similar people. Teasing out the international and global political ecology dimensions of VI risk, for example, in places like China where expansive development projects on soil-contaminated lands is beginning to raise concerns about food safety and other environmental health risks, requires greater attention to the diversity of emerging "riskscapes" (Morello-Frosch and Shenassa 2006) and the plethora of challenges these converging and diverging riskscapes present for critical environmental health researchers tracking "emerging" risks in the United States and their presence and source of citizen concern and scientific interest in countries with no current VI.

Future Global Political Ecologies of VI Risk

Attending to the *global* political ecology of VI risk calls for a serious discussion of context, for the very reason that "Context – the way political and economic context influences scientific inquiry – holds perhaps the most implications for the political ecology of global environmental problems" (Peet, Robbins, and Watts 2011: 39). In what follows, I explore how future political ecologies of VI risk will likely need to refocus on the ecologies of connection that, in effect, expose the global dimensions and politics of this newly emerging toxics uncertainty.

Most VI experts agree that VI can occur wherever there is contaminated soil and groundwater, so that the political-ecological approach to VI risk within anthropology must call for a perspective that looks beyond the social, economic, political, and legal context of the United States, where most, if not all, of the current debate over VI is occurring. In fact, in 2013, in an effort to improve guidance for states addressing emerging VI risk, the EPA has "recommended" that VI risks be evaluated for "reasonably expected future land use conditions including new building construction and new uses and occupants for the uninhabited buildings," thus requiring the need for VI assessment at *any* site contaminated with volatile organic substances.

China, for example, is one place where soil contamination science is on the upswing, making China a very likely site of massive VI risk assessment and possible mitigation. In the mid-2000s, just around the time that VI began to "boom" in the United States, scientific interests in soil pollution in China began to emerge. For example, in 2006, the State Environmental Protection Agency

(SEPA or the MEP) and the Ministry of Land and Resources (MLR) in China launched a three-year soil pollution survey to primarily focus on areas with heavy industry and grain production operations. Supported by a billion dollar budget, the survey targeted the Jiangsu and Zhejiang provinces in the Yangtze River Delta, Guandong Province in the Pearl River Delta, Liaoning Province in north-east China, and the Hunan Province in central China. While the soil pollution survey is complete, public release of the data has not occurred. Despite this lack of public knowledge, scientists with the Institute for Soil Science at the Chinese Academy of Sciences have begun to develop a strong scientific base for concerns about soil contamination risks in China (Xia and Luo 2006; Luo *et al.* 2007, 2008, 2009; Zhang, Wu, and Luo 2008). Exploring the possible VI risks associated with this soil contamination disaster would certainly call for building on already existing anthropological research addressing the health–environment nexus in China (Lora-Wainwright 2013; Tilt 2013). This research has shown that the lived experience of industrial pollution and environmental health risk in China involves much more than pollution (Lora-Wainwright 2013; Tilt 2007, 2013). According Lora-Wainwright,

> Pollution is only one part of their life experience, alongside finding work, negotiating compensation, securing enough resources to care for elderly parents and to support children's education and renovating one's home. This normalization is central to allowing the hegemonic view of industrialization as an inevitable development path to mould locals' expectations and leave pollution unquestioned. (Lora-Wainwright 2013: 15)[2]

This situated response to environmental health risk (and likely response to VI risk) actually reinforces one of the strongest dimensions of political ecology: its enduring "interest in the impacts (social and ecological) of the acceptance of certain knowledge constructs as 'universal truth' and their subsequent application in faraway places" (Goldman and Turner 2011: 19). The growing interrelationship between environmental science and ecopolitics is yet another active ingredient in forging a global political ecology of VI risk. "Environmentalist politics are inseparable from the practice and development of environmental science, whether arguing for the importance of protecting particular plants, animals, or landscapes, or proving the reality and implications of global climate change" (Choy 2011: 11). In China, as in the United States, we could say that the very political ecology of VI risk emerges *with* the slow development of VI science in tandem with emerging environmental laws and regulations (Palmer 1998; Alford and Liebman 2001; Beyer 2006; Tilt 2007, 2013; Stern 2011).

The crippling ambiguities that arise in communities where VI risk has been identified has also resulted in a "volatile" environment of litigation. According to some environmental law specialists, VI "has become a hot topic amongst legal practitioners" (Rolph, Torres, Everett 2012: 107). These authors add that "[t]he attention and concern arises largely from the uncertainty surrounding vapor intrusion – an uncertainty that pervades real estate transactions, contaminated site cleanups, toxic tort suits, and class action litigation" (2012: 107–108). One lawyer working on VI cases explains that "The uncertainty about basic scientific and regulatory conclusions is not easy to counsel your clients through" (Distler *et al.* 2013: 100–110). It turns out that the environmental regulation and litigation politics informing the complexities of VI risk (e.g., building-by-building exposure variation) reflects a more general problem confronted by environmental lawmakers and regulators. According Kysar (2010), "environmental lawmakers and regulators not only must assess and manage threats of an unknown magnitude but they also must do so within the context of numerous overlapping dynamic systems, each of which is characterized by such perplexing features as extreme sensitivity to minor variations in condition, [and] irreducible levels of uncertainty" (Kysar 2010: 73). The continued struggle for residents at VI sites who have taken legal action is that relying on the nature and extent of the VI source, potential exposure pathways, human health exposures, and risk data as evidence for their cases is difficult for lawyers to work with. In other words, it is the combination of scientific uncertainty and "regulatory knowledge gaps" (Frickel and Vincent 2011) that presents an enduring and tormenting pivotal point in VI litigation.

Finally, the growth in VI science and regulation has spawned a specialized vapor intrusion consulting industry. The rise in environmental science and technology consulting firms offering sampling, monitoring, mitigation, and remediation services for communities and residents dealing with VI risk is yet another key area of VI risk to track. Such a focus will compel a more fully articulated political economy of VI science and the "co-production" (Jasanoff 2004) of VI science, government regulation, and a developing VI risk management sector which is a highly specialized sector of techno-scientific expertise. Moreover, focusing on how VI science and knowledge circulates amid this evolving consulting sector requires close attention to the networks of expertise shaping VI knowledge-production processes (Goldman 2011: 203), processes that will eventually help internationalize the VI science consulting industry. In the US context, the ITRC is largely dominated by consultants and industry representatives. How this techno-scientific consulting industry will spread and take shape in other countries is currently unknown, but one neoliberal theme can be expected to inform future VI science and regulation: "On the cultural terrain of neoliberalism, experts do not merely reassert their authority on the basis of their mastery and infallibility in technical matters. Rather, they find new grounds for claiming expertise, building their authority on claims to be responsible" (Ottinger 2013: 26).

Conclusion

In addition to exposing lived experiences of "contested environmental illness" (Brown 2007) and engaging the social, health, and environmental politics of corporate accountability and regulatory action (and inaction), the anthropology of environmental health is also about critically tracking the complexities and contested nature of new toxics uncertainty. This chapter has argued that attending to the political ecology of emerging VI risk not only helps to illustrate the "toxic frustration" (Singer 2011) experienced by residents living with VI risk, but also highlights the complex politics of scientific uncertainty, regulation, and law leading to difficult, yet important, discussion of the possible *global* political ecology of VI risk. Political ecology of health theory in critical medical anthropology is broadly interested in showing how power and inequality, including epistemic disputes between experts and nonexperts, figure in environmental health risk debates (Baer 1996; Baer, Singer, and Susser 1997; Harper 2002, 2004; Little 2009, 2013). It seeks to intensify our understanding of "contested environmental illness" (Brown 2007), of contested exposures, and helps us rethink VI risk "as an experiential state" (Harper 2002: 27). It confronts the ambiguities and contestations of risk analysis and assessment, and for VI debates in particular, it attends to situated and lived experiences of toxics suffering, trying to better understand the sciences, cultures, and economies of expertise that currently dominate discourse on this emerging environmental health risk.

Furthermore, this theory honors the meshed political nature of risk and risk mitigation. While numerous tests show that the mitigation of volatile organic compound (VOC) vapor intrusion can be effective and relatively inexpensive (Folkes and Kurz 2002; Folkes 2003; Folkes *et al.* 2009), as my ethnographic research has shown (Little 2012, 2014), even "mitigated" residents remain skeptical of the conclusion that they no longer need to worry about the possible health risks of TCE exposure. Trust in mitigation is a topic that needs further attention, especially if VI mitigation strategies become the national standard and become exported to places like China where growing soil contamination studies could lead to an expansion of VI debates. Furthermore, as anthropologists working in China have pointed out, there is a highly clandestine regulatory environment that directly sustains environmental health uncertainty (Tilt 2007; Lora-Wainwright 2013), resulting in perhaps an even more potent political ecology of VI risk than that witnessed in the United States.

VI debates are elusive and saturated with ambiguity, and the public health implications of VI exposure and litigation options for impacted residents are just beginning to be explored in the United States (DiNapoli 2006; Distler *et al.* 2013; Siegel 2007, 2008), but the *global* environmental health dimensions of VI risk have yet to be explored. In the United States, risk assessment and policy regarding VI is in its infancy, and citizen involvement has played a relatively minor role in decision making, even though a national stakeholder's coalition has made serious efforts to inform VI risk governance. On the national level, this is difficult enough, so efforts to generate international environmental health policies for VI risk management will be met with an avalanche of challenges conditioned largely by cultural, political, economic, bureaucratic, and legal variation.

In light of the pithy insight of Fortun (2001), critical questions anchor political-ecological critiques of this emerging environmental health risk: What is vapor intrusion said to mean? What does vapor intrusion risk stand for or evoke? My own ethnographic research on VI has helped me realize that political ecology not only provides sufferer voice and analytic detail to lived experiences of VI risk, showing how VI risk goes *beyond* health and toxic substance exposure, but also honors the contested grounds from which theses risks are "experienced, narrated, and known" (Reno 2011: 527). Of course, ethnography enriches political ecology of health analysis, for it "produces both situated and comparative insight, is able to see across scale, and leverage different analytic lenses. It can draw out nested and proximate systems, sensitive to their similarities, differences, and synergisms" (Fortun 2012: 451). Studying the complexities of VI riskscapes calls for a similar ethnographic approach, even if designing and carrying out a global VI risk study is met with a plethora of research challenges and vibrant cultural, political, economic, and regulatory disconnects.

While VI risk, as discussed here, opens up new conversation between anthropology and environmental public health, this new toxics uncertainty also calls for new anthropological engagements with environmental and property law, both of which are slowly dominating and conditioning VI risk assessments, regulatory guidance, and litigation. We should continue to take seriously environmental public health science approaches to toxics risk, but also endorse a "broader view that encompasses the other confounding variables that are at play in the production of environmental health issues" (Whiteford and Hill 2005: 234). In light of this insight, a critical understanding of VI risk knowledge production calls for building awareness of the broader neoliberalization of environmental knowledge production (Lave 2012). As Lave (2012: 29) points out,

> neoliberal science regimes' privileging of privatized and commercializable knowledge has also generated a big boost in the credibility of extramural science and the people who produce it, with contradictory effects. On the one hand, commercial knowledge claims are no longer seen as potentially compromised by conflicts of interest, but instead as legitimized by market forces. On the other hand, environmental consultants [e.g., VI consultants] have been able to establish serious scientific credibility in startling upsets of the traditional [state] construction of scientific legitimacy ... [and] [c]itizen scientists (of the activist persuasion) are now accorded a place at the table in many regulatory decisions (Brown and Mikkelsen 1990; Cohen and Ottinger 2011; Frickel *et al.* 2010; Moore *et al.* 2011; Ottinger 2009).

VI science is equally informed by these neoliberal science and knowledge production trends. First, VI consultants play a powerful role in shaping the VI science that is in turn informing the development of VI law and regulation, and the impact of the ITRC is but one clear example of this. Second, the increasing role of "community stakeholders" at national EPA VI forums is a telling sign of increased public involvement in VI policy, but the "scientific" impact of "citizen science" at VI sites remains a contentious issue. This is primarily because even VI consulting scientists themselves, who have advanced degrees in volatile organic compound analysis, are confronted with legitimate "site-specific" sampling and risk prediction challenges.

Finally, attending to the global dynamics of VI risk sets in bold relief discursive cruxes and politics that can emerge when challenged to think "comparatively" about VI risk, when comparing what are usually highly variable exposure scenarios and contexts. There is a sort of volatile political ecology that emerges with VI risk debates, for these toxics debates are debates with "discursive gaps, and discursive risks" (Fortun 2012: 452). In other words, a truly *political* ecology of health perspective, one that recognizes and confronts its own instability, ought to think seriously about the very real challenge of articulating the environment–health nexus in general and new toxics uncertainties in particular. In this way, Fortun (2012) may be a helpful theoretical guide for those intrigued by precariously emerging toxics debates and risks like VI: "Discursive gaps emerge when there are conditions to deal with for which there is no available idiom, no way of thinking that can grasp what is at hand. Discursive risks emerge because of a tendency to rely on established idioms and ways of thinking, nonetheless" (Fortun 2012: 452). As a critical theory of health–environment relations, the analytic purchase of the political ecology of health perspective is enriched by its very ethical stance on and attachment to *known* politics of knowledge and epistemic confusion, politics of regulation and legal volatility, and the ground-level politics of complexity and possibility that people living in and with contamination struggle to deal with and understand.

NOTES

1 In chemistry and physics, volatility refers to the tendency of a substance to form vapors, which are molecules in a gaseous state, and escape from a liquid or solid. Volatility is directly related to a substance's vapor pressure, Henry's law constant, and is indirectly related to a substance's molecular weight (i.e., substances with lower molecular weights tend to volatilize more readily than substances with similar molecular structures that have higher molecular weights).

2 This normalization is, in many ways, internalized and "individualized" (Tilt 2013) in this cultural and political economic context, which only further complicates the possible study of VI risk in China.

REFERENCES

Alford, W.L. and Liebman, B.L. 2001. "Clean Air, Clear Processes? Struggle over Air Pollution Law in the People's Republic of China." *Hastings Law Journal*, 53(3): 703–748.

Allen, B.L. 2003. *Uneasy Alchemy: Citizens and Experts in Louisiana's Chemical Corridor Disputes.* Cambridge, MA: MIT Press.

Auyero, J., and Swistun, D.A. 2009. *Flammable: Environmental Suffering in an Argentine Shantytown.* Oxford: Oxford University Press.

Baer, H.A. 1996. "Toward a Political Ecology of Health in Medical Anthropology." *Medical Anthropology Quarterly*, 10(4): 451–454.

Baer, H.A., and Singer, M. 2009. *Global Warming and the Political Ecology of Health: Emerging Crises and Systemic Solutions.* Walnut Creek, CA: Left Coast Press.

Baer, H.A., Singer, M., and Susser, I. 1997. *Medical Anthropology and the World System.* London: & and Garvey.

Beck, U. [1986] 1992. *Risk Society: Towards a New Modernity.* London: Sage.

Beyer, S. 2006. "Environmental Law and Policy in the People's Republic of China." *Chinese Journal of International Law*, 5(1): 185–211.

Bleicher, A, and Gross, M. 2011. "Response and Recovery in the Remediation of Contaminated Land in Eastern Germany." In R.A. Dowty and B.L. Allen (Eds.),

Dynamics of Disaster: Lessons on Risk, Response, and Recovery (pp. 187–202). London: Earthscan.

Brock, C. 2009. "Is Vapor Intrusion the Next Regulatory Juggernaut?" *Seattle Daily Journal*, July 30, p. 2.

Brown, P. 2007. *Toxic Exposures: Contested Illnesses and the Environmental Health Movement.* New York: Columbia University Press.

Brown, P. and Mikkelsen, E. 1990. *No Safe Place: Toxic Waste, Leukemia, and Community Action.* Berkeley: University of California Press.

Checker, M. 2007. "'But I Know It's True': Environmental Risk Assessment, Justice, and Anthropology." *Human Organization*, 66(2): 112–124.

Chiu, W.A., *et al.* 2013. "Human Health Effects of Trichloroethylene: Key Findings and Scientific Issues." *Environmental Health Perspectives*, 121(3): 303–311.

Choy, T. 2011. *Ecologies of Comparison: An Ethnography of Endangerment in Hong Kong.* Durham, NC: Duke University Press.

Cullen, A.C. and Small, M.J. 2004. "Uncertain Risk: The Role and Limits of Quantitative Assessment." In T. McDaniels and M.J. (Eds.), *Small Risk Analysis and Society: An Interdisciplinary Characterization of the Field* (pp. 163–212). Cambridge: Cambridge University Press.

Cummings, R B.1981. "Is Risk Assessment a Science?" *Risk Analysis*, 1(1): 1–3.

Dietrich, A.S. 2013. *The Drug Company Next Door: Pollution, Jobs, and Community Health in Puerto Rico.* New York: New York University Press.

DiNapoli, T.P. 2006. *Vapor Intrusion of Toxic Chemicals: An Emerging Public Health Concern.* New York State Assembly Report. New York: Committee on Environmental Conservation.

Distler, Mark, *et al.* 2013. "Vapor Intrusion: The State of the Science and the Law." *Environmental Law Reporter*, 43(1): 5–15.

Dowty, R.A. and Allen, B.A. 2011. "Afterword." In R.A. Dowty and B.L. Allen (Eds.), *Dynamics of Disaster: Lessons on Risk, Response, and Recovery* (pp. 203–207). London: Earthscan.

Edelstein, M.R. 2004. *Contaminated Communities: Coping with Residential Toxic Exposure.* Boulder, CO: Westview.

Folkes, D. 2003. "Design, Effectiveness, and Reliability of Sub-Slab Depressurization Systems." http://www.envirogroup.com/publications/folkes_epa_seminar.pdf (accessed August 15, 2015).

Folkes, D. and Kurz, D.W. 2002. "Efficacy of Subslab Depressurization for Mitigation of Vapor Intrusion of Chlorinated Organic Compounds. http://www.envirogroup.com/publications/effi cancyofslab.pdf (accessed August 15, 2015).

Folkes, D., Wertz, W., Kurtz, J., and Kuehster, T. 2009. "Observed Spatial and Temporal Distributions of CVOCs at Colorado and New York Vapor Intrusion Sites." *Ground Water Monitoring and Remediation*, 29(1): 70–80.

Fortun, K. 2001. *Advocacy After Bhopal: Environmentalism, Disaster, New Global Orders.* Chicago: University of Chicago Press.

Fortun, K. 2012. "Ethnography in Late Industrialism." *Cultural Anthropology*, 27(3): 446–464.

Frickel, S., *et al.* 2010. "Undone Science: Social Movement Challenges to Dominant Scientific Practice." *Science, Technology & Human Values*, 35(4): 444–473.

Frickel, S. and Vincent, M.B. 2011. "Katrina's Contamination: Regulatory Knowledge Gaps in the Making and Unmaking of Environmental Contention." In R.A. Dowty and B.L. Allen (Eds.), *Dynamics of Disaster: Lessons on Risk, Response, and Recovery* (pp. 11–28). London: Earthscan.

Goldman, M.J. 2011. "Circulation of Environmental Knowledge: Networks, Expertise, and Science in Practice." In M.J. Goldman, P. Hadasdy, and M.D. Turner (Eds.),

Knowing Nature: Conversations at the Intersection of Political Ecology and Science Studies (pp. 1–24). Chicago: University of Chicago Press.

Goldman, M.J. and Turner, M.D. 2011. "Introduction." In M.J. Goldman, P. Hadasdy, and M.D. Turner (Eds.), *Knowing Nature: Conversations at the Intersection of Political Ecology and Science Studies* (pp. 1–24). Chicago: University of Chicago Press.

Harper, J. 2002. *Endangered Species: Health, Illness, and Death Among Madagascar's People of the Forest*. Durham, NC: Carolina Academic Press.

Harper, J. 2004. "Breathless in Houston: A Political Ecology of Health Approach to Understanding Environmental Health Concerns." *Medical Anthropology*, 23(4): 295–326.

Institute of Medicine. 2013. *Environmental Decisions in the Face of Uncertainty*. Washington, DC: The National Academies Press.

ITRC (Interstate Technology and Regulatory Council). 2007. *Vapor Intrusion Pathway: A Practical Guideline. ITRC Technical and Regulatory Guidance Document*. Washington, DC: Interstate Technology and Regulatory Council.

Jasanoff, S. 1992. "Science, Politics, and the Renegotiation of Expertise at EPA." *Osiris*, 7(2): 195–217.

Jasanoff, S. 1998. "The Political Science of Risk Perception." *Reliability Engineering and Systems Safety*, 59(1): 91–99.

Jasanoff, S. 2004. *States of Knowledge: The Co-Production of Science and Social Order*. London: Routledge.

Kleinman, A., Das, V., and Lock, M. 1997. *Social Suffering*. Berkeley, CA: University of California Press.

Kysar, D. 2010. *Regulating from Nowhere: Environmental Law and the Search for Objectivity*. New Haven, CT: Yale University Press.

Lave, R. 2012. "Neoliberalism and the Production of Environmental Knowledge." *Environment and Society: Advances in Research* 3:19–38.

Little, P.C. 2009. "Negotiating Community Engagement and Science in the Federal Environmental Public Health Sector." *Medical Anthropology Quarterly*, 23(2): 94–118.

Little, P.C. 2012. "Another Angle on Pollution Experience: Toward an Anthropology of the Emotional Ecology of Risk Mitigation." *Ethos*, 40(4): 431–452.

Little, P.C. 2013. "Vapor Intrusion: The Political Ecology of an Emerging Environmental Health Concern." *Human Organization*, 72(2): 121–131.

Little, P.C. 2014. *Toxic Town: IBM, Pollution, and Industrial Risks*. New York: New York University Press.

Lora-Wainwright, A. 2013. "The Inadequate Life: Rural Industrial Pollution and Lay Epidemiology in China." *The China Quarterly*, 213: 1–19.

Luo, Yong-ming. 2008. *Soil Environmental Problems and Solutions in China*. Nanjing, China: Hohai University Press.

Luo, Yong-ming, *et al.* 2007. *Hong Kong Soils and Environment*. Science Press.

Luo, Yong-ming, *et al.* 2009. *Soil Environment and Ecological Safety*. Science Press.

Lupton, D. 1999. *Risk*. New York: Routledge.

Mitman, G., Murphy, M., and Sellers, C. 2004. "Introduction: A Cloud over History." In G. Mitman, M. Murphy, and C. Sellers (Eds.), *Landscapes of Exposure: Knowledge and Illness in Modern Environments* (pp. 1–17). OSIRIS 19.

Moore, K., *et al.* 2011. "Science and Neoliberal Globalization: A Political Sociological Approach." *Theory and Society*, 40(5): 505–532.

Morello-Frosch, R. and Shenassa, E.D. 2006. "The Environmental 'Riskscape' and Social Inequality: Implications for Explaining Maternal and Child Health Disparities." *Environmental Health Perspectives*, 114(8): 1150–1153.

Ottinger, G. 2009. "Epistemic Fencelines: Air Monitoring Instruments and Expert-Resident Boundaries." *Spontaneous Generations*, 3(1): 55–67.

Ottinger, G. 2013. *Refining Expertise: How Responsible Engineers Subvert Environmental Justice Challenges.* New York: New York University Press.

Palmer, M.1998. "Environmental Regulation in the People's Republic of China: The Face of Domestic Law." *The China Quarterly*, 156: 788–808.

Peet, R., Robbins, P., and Watts, M.J. 2011. *Global Political Ecology.* London: Routledge.

Polish, D. 2009. "Community Involvement Challenges at Vapor Intrusion Sites." Paper presented at the Environmental Protection Agency National Forum on Vapor Intrusion, Philadelphia, PA, January 12–13.

Prigogine, I. 1997. *The End of Certainty: Time, Chaos, and the New Laws of Nature.* New York: Free Press.

Reno, J. 2011. "Beyond Risk: Emplacement and the Production of Environmental Evidence." *American Ethnologist* 38(3): 516–530.

Rolph, C. G., Torres, V.E., and Everett, J.W. 2012. "The 'Volatile' World of Vapor Intrusion: Understanding Vapor Intrusion Regulation and the Potential for Litigation." *Pace Environmental Law Review*, 30: 107–139.

Siegel, L. 2007. "Report on the Albany Vapor Intrusion Activists' Meeting." Mountain View, CA: Center for Public Environmental Oversight.

Siegel, L. 2008. "Report on the National Stakeholders' Panel on Vapor Intrusion." Mountain View, CA: Center for Public Environmental Oversight.

Singer, M. 2011. "Down Cancer Alley: The Lived Experience of Health and Environmental Suffering in Louisiana's Chemical Corridor." *Medical Anthropology Quarterly*, 25(2): 141–163.

Stern, R.E. 2011. "From Dispute to Decision: Suing Polluters in China." *The China Quarterly*, 206: 294–312.

Tesh, S.N. 2000. *Uncertain Hazards: Environmental Activists and Scientific Proof.* Ithaca, NY: Cornell University Press.

Tilt, B. 2007. "The Political Ecology of Pollution Enforcement in China: A Case from Sichuan's Rural Industrial Sector." *The China Quarterly*, 192: 915–932.

Tilt, B. 2013. " Industrial Pollution and Environmental Health in Rural China: Risk Uncertainty and Individualization." *The China Quarterly*, 214: 283–301.

US Environmental Protection Agency. 2002. "OSWER Draft Guidance for Evaluating the Vapor Intrusion to Indoor Air Pathway from Groundwater and Soils (Subsurface Vapor Intrusion Guidance)." http://www.epa.gov/epawaste/hazard/correctiveaction/eis/vapor/guidance.pdf (accessed April 8.).

US Environmental Protection Agency. 2011. "Trichloroethylene Toxicological Review and Appendices." http://www.epa.gov/iris/supdocs/0199index.html (accessed February 12).

Whiteford, L.M. and Hill, B. 2005. "The Political Ecology of Dengue in Cuba and the Dominican Republic." In G. Guest (Ed.), *Globalization, Health, and the Environment: An Integrated Perspective* (pp. 219–238). Lanham, MD: AltaMira.

Wynne, B. 1989. "Frameworks of Rationality in Risk Assessment." In J. Brown (Ed.), *Environmental Threats* (pp. 45–78). London: Frances Pinter.

Xia Jia-qi and Luo Yong-ming. 2006. "Definition and Three Evaluation Guidelines of Soil Contamination." *Journal of Ecology and Rural Environment*, 22(1): 87–90.

Zhang Chang-bo, Wu Long-hua, Luo Yong-ming. 2008. "Application of Robust Estimator in Source Identification of Soil Pollutants: A Case Study at a Heavy Metal Contaminated Site." *Environmental Science*, 29(3): 804–808.

FURTHER READING

Beck, U. 1998. *World Risk Society.* Cambridge: Polity.

Beck, U. 2006. "Living in the World Risk Society." *Economy and Society*, 35(4): 329–345.

Caldwell, I. and Wang, X. 2011. "A Hidden Problem: China's Contaminated Site Soil Pollution Crisis." Joint Research Project Paper. USAID, Asia. Vermont Law School.

Cohen, B. and Ottinger, G. 2011. *Technoscience and Environmental Justice.* Cambridge, MA: MIT Press.

Downey, G.l. and Dumit, J. 1997. *Cyborgs and Citadels: Anthropological Interventions in Emerging Sciences and Technologies.* Santa Fe, NM: School of American Research Press.

Hess, David J. 2007. *Alternative Pathways in Science and Industry: Activism, Innovation, and the Environment in an Era of Globalization.* Cambridge, MA: MIT Press.

Latour, B. 1987. *Science in Action: How to Follow Scientists and Engineers Through Society.* Cambridge, MA: Harvard University Press.

Mandel, J.H., Kelsh, M., Mink, P.J., and Alexander, D.D. 2008. "Trichloroethylene Exposure and non-Hodgkin's Lymphoma: Supportive Evidence." *Occupational and Environmental Medicine*, 65(2): 147–148.

CHAPTER 15

The Political Ecology of Cause and Blame: Environmental Health Inequities in the Context of Colonialism, Globalization, and Climate Change

Eleanor S. Stephenson and Peter H. Stephenson

INTRODUCTION

There is probably no more common contemporary trope for environmental degradation than "the tragedy of the commons" notion advanced by Hardin (1968) and subsequently refurbished (Hardin 2008). Hardin, followed by many other writers (see, e.g., Machan 2001), has argued that forms of individual self-interest, which override long-term group interests, inevitably deplete shared

A Companion to the Anthropology of Environmental Health, First Edition. Edited by Merrill Singer.

resources. It is an economic view of limitations that remains deeply entrenched in development discourses, including within the development and research communities. This reasoning serves an interventionist rationale promoting outside expertise (and hence outside "interests") that can easily become self-congratulatory wherever an intervention succeeds, and exculpatory should it fail. As such, it is a discourse serving the manifold global and regional interests of outside "experts" far more than the interests of local peoples, who can be blamed for their selfish pursuit of limited resources usually narrated as "environmental mismanagement" or "over-use."

In this chapter, we explore how similar tropes manifest themselves within environmental health: pervasive reasoning that ascribes blame to local cultures, values, and practices for environmental health problems ranging from food insecurity to toxic mold exposure effectively obscures systemic and distal drivers of poor health, thereby rendering marginalized groups as the authors and not the victims of population health inequities. Outside interventions that aim to improve environmental management, health, or both tend to manage for a limited scope of perceived causes, and if they fail, subsequently sanction patients/peoples who are seen as resistant to the imposition of (externally defined) solutions to poverty and environmental health inequities. In these narratives of failure, legacies of colonialism and external forces associated with globalization, contemporary political domination, and global environmental change are frequently ignored. Many Indigenous peoples and institutions worldwide are working to counterbalance and refute manifestations of such narratives. For example, a recent health report from Nunavut Tunngavik Incorporated, the land claims organization representing Inuit in Nunavut, Canada, explains the problems with this tendency:

> All too often, media and research fails to place health outcomes into the historical, political, and economic contexts in which they exist. Doing so can leave communities vulnerable to victim blaming without the necessary actions being taken to eliminate the structural inequities in place that often make it difficult for people to achieve health and wellness. (2013: 6)

We explore here the dynamics of these narratives of failure and victim blaming, illustrating them with key historical environmental health and environmental management examples, and examples from fieldwork conducted in diverse settings in Canada and Nepal. Combined, these distinct cases show how the views of powerful outside actors continue to define local people's environmental health problems as grounded in cultural inadequacy rather than external power relations, which have, in many cases, already extensively modified housing, land tenure, agriculture, work, and kinship, often in ways that serve outside or colonial interests far more than those of local people. These pervasive dynamics compound the injustice of environmental health inequities, and we argue they are all the more pressing in contexts of global climate change, and all the more pernicious in contexts of rapid globalization and economic integration pressures.

Environmental Mismanagement Tropes

We term this line of investigation the political ecology of cause and blame, drawing inspiration from political ecological work that makes legible the links between proximate environmental outcomes (including their implications for human health and well-being) and distal political and economic forces. There is a growing body of interdisciplinary work debunking environmental mismanagement tropes that ascribe blame to local populations; here we offer a brief review of this work before turning to the ramifications of this for health – for environmental conditions always have profound impacts on the health of human beings who live in complex ecological relationships, where they, perforce, play a crucial role in sustaining that which sustains themselves.

Examining evidence for community-based management, Ostrom's work (1990), among others, seriously critiques the idea of environmental depletion as a function of local actors in favor of the notion that local actors actually provide solutions to resource sharing, where and when permitted to do so. Ostrom finds, for example, that common pool resource management is often most successful when users manage, with some rights (e.g., to harvest) and the ability to make rules. At best, commons management actions and systems may not be readily legible to outside actors – government and development agents, professionals, and scientists – whose explanatory models miss local management practices. However, various forms of colonial enclosure, such as legislated restrictions on previously practiced land uses, occupancy, and hunting and fishing rights, have been legitimized in the name of purported overgrazing, overfishing, and overharvesting. As such enclosure movements circumscribe new property rights (alienation rights), they may undermine historical sustainable use regimes, in some cases overwriting former tenure regimes of hunter-gatherers, Indigenous peoples, swidden agriculturalists, and pastoralists (see e.g., Scott 2009), compromising health and contributing to narratives of mismanagement. Examples from the literature in political ecology, such as Blaikie's (1985) work on the politics of soil erosion, describe how colonial processes of land appropriation are essentially "misread" (to borrow Fairhead and Leech's term, 1996) in a revisionist fashion to support an explanatory model rooted in overexploitation by local farmers rather than colonialism, and as such advance colonial interests in securing land and resources.

Inaccurate assumptions about land use have, at times, produced staggering misreadings of various environmental "degradation" issues. For example, Fairhead and Leech's (1996) seminal analysis of deforestation in West Africa finds that twentieth-century deforestation in Sierra Leone, Liberia, Benin, and Togo is likely only one-third the rate estimated previously: existing models of deforestation presupposed a neo-Malthusian narrative, assuming that there was a total forest cover prior to agricultural expansion, and in so doing set inaccurate baselines. In fact, the authors find good evidence to suggest that islands of forest in the savanna may actually be anthropogenic plantations, not remnants of previous forest stands, and, indeed, that farming practices may promote afforestation. The authors find that while population growth, economic growth, and poor policy drives deforestation across West Africa, so too do systemic forces like poverty and land tenure insecurity. Misreading environmental conditions at a particular baseline, as in this case, can result in imposed (mis)management regimes that do not effect intended changes, causing both human and environmental collateral impacts. For example, Scott (2009) notes that sedentarization policies advanced in the name of controlling deforestation in upland Southeast Asia have in some cases actually exacerbated it, changing tenure regimes (through community forestry) and forcing forest inhabitants to reduce fallow periods. Reduced fallow exhausts soils, reducing yields, and may lead to dependence on the temporary inputs associated with agribusiness – dependence which in turn underwrites the inexorable trend toward further alienation of land from farmers.

These examples do not refute the idea that deforestation or land degradation can be driven by population growth or that local management decisions can affect, and at times compromise, sustainable land use; however, they illustrate that deforestation and afforestation are contingent and situated practices that cannot be divorced from socioecological and historical context, and bring into relief the importance of distal drivers of poor health associated with environmental degradation.

Turning to desertification, we see how a misreading of dynamic landscapes and land use practices can not only produce a misunderstanding, but reify a new degradation phenomena, commanding international concern and intervention. In the 1970s, desertification was invoked as a master disaster narrative of the threatening, creeping Sahara and other major deserts. Major conferences, including the United Nations Conference on Desertification in the 1970s, drew global attention to the problem and rendered dry land management – which had until this time been the concern of dry land populations – an issue of global concern. This fear was closely linked to how the great Sahelian droughts of the 1970s, which killed over 100,000 in famine, and were attributed in part to desertification and unsustainable local land management practices (Batterbury and Warren 2001). However, these early understandings of desertification are now thought to be ill founded. Research conducted in the 1990s (see e.g., Thomas and Middleton 1994) have improved our understanding of dry land geomorphology and showed that dune systems are inherently dynamic and may expand and retreat over time, and that they are subject to change at far greater scales than what local management can account for, for example from climate fluctuations (as was likely the case in the Sahelian droughts). This newer body of research suggests that traditional management regimes were not to blame for purported desertification (Barraclough 1995). Rather, the desertification narrative is in part explained by sociocultural attitudes toward environmental change. These include the political marginality of dry land populations and colonial attitudes to development, which attributed African environmental change to poor land management and population pressures (effectively a neo-Malthusian argument). This reasoning also overlooked local people's extensive ecological knowledge concerning dynamic geomorphological processes. This misstep arose not just out of colonial attitudes, but out of hubris in research claims, including short-termism and an attitude of seeing all change as degradation. Most of all, this reading invoked fear about the supposedly inhospitable desert – obscuring the fact that people have lived and sustained themselves in dry land ecosystems for millennia.

Narratives that overlook human ingenuity, survival, and persistence are rife in discourse around environmental mismanagement. These examples of environmental misreadings – and at times the imposed solutions that follow – are animated by pervasive development discourses that cast minority, Indigenous, upland, remote, and other populations as undeveloped or "backwards." Perhaps the best recent example of this discursive pattern comes from Diamond's 2005 popular work, *Collapse*, which advances ambitious historical reconstructions of past societies in order to demonstrate to us how we too can "choose to fail or succeed." Diamond's narrative, however, leaves out not only the impacts of colonization in creating societal collapse, but also contemporary Indigenous populations and decedents, including Easter island descendants, Australian Aborigines, descendants of the Maya and the Anasazi and their neighbors (Wilcox 2010). These types of discursive rewritings can be interpreted within a broader architecture of knowledge in which discourse is understood to both produce and constrain truths that are inseparable from the currencies of power (Foucault 1969) – in this case, writing in localized environmental mismanagement and writing *out* the Indigenous peoples who are paradoxically still held responsible for degradation. We suggest these discourses distance "ourselves" (as managers, scientists, researchers, outsiders) from susceptibility to the same forms of environmental mismanagement – while we perpetuate global environmental change at an unprecedented scale (Röckstrom *et al.* 2009).

Against these dominant narratives of local environmental mismanagement it comes as little surprise that environmental health issues in particular give rise to powerful misreadings and victim blaming; and that environmental illness is at times mobilized to support interventions that respond to proximate drivers at the expense of tackling their distal roots. We here characterize these disparities as environmental health inequities. Population health research examining the social determinants of health has furnished an increasingly robust body of work debunking the notion of individual determinism over health, showing how wider systemic conditions affect health, making legible the contexts of illness, and providing a basis for reconceptualizing illness in terms of health *inequities*: the underlying causes of unequal outcomes that may lie outside the domain of health entirely, in social, economic, and political realities (Adleson 2005). This lens may be particularly cogent for environmental health disparities, which are widely related to socioeconomic marginalization and poverty, tenure insecurity, and local manifestations of global environmental change.[1] To illustrate this, we now turn to two examples that bring together tropes of both environmental mismanagement and ill health: food insecurity (a case from upland Nepal) and potentially toxic mold exposure (a case from a Canadian Indigenous community). These examples show the breadth of this discourse of victim blaming, and some of the mechanisms through which it is perpetuated. The two examples are drawn from very different ecological zones and political-economic circumstances, but they share a pervasive and troubling reasoning, where external forces and interventions displace and transform local experience in ways that result in poor health for which local people are held to account.

Climate Change and Food Insecurity in Upland Nepal

Mountain regions, home to some 720 million people worldwide (Beniston 2003), are projected to experience disproportionate impacts of anthropogenic climate change (Beniston 2003; Yao *et al.* 2012; IPCC 2013), owing to both biophysical sensitivities and socioeconomic conditions. The latter include limited infrastructure, poor access to markets, and sociocultural marginalization, all of which contribute to higher levels of poverty and food insecurity relative to lowland populations, especially in least developed countries (Choudhary *et al.* 2013). However, upland populations also have longstanding social, cultural, and economic adaptations to the high levels of climatic and environmental variability found in mountainous regions (Stevens 1993), while outside interventions enacted by distant central state governments, development agencies, or outside experts may shift vulnerabilities with unpredictable side effects (Scott 2009). These conditions create something of a perfect storm for environmental health inequities to be misread by well-intended outside "experts," who may advance strategies for development and adaptation that are not well matched for local needs.

In working with local people in the Himalayan mountain region of Humla, Nepal (Figure 15.1) in 2012 as a multidisciplinary team of master's students (from the University of Oxford's Environmental Change Institute) and interpreters, we found divergences between local and outside opinions on the causes

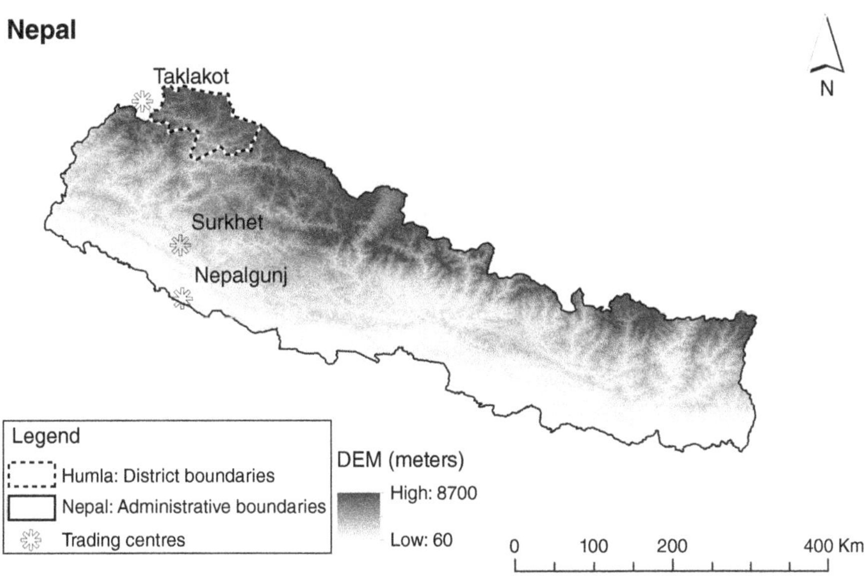

Figure 15.1 Humla District, Nepal (ArcGIS).

of and appropriate responses to food insecurity (Stephenson 2012). Located in the high Himalaya of northwestern Nepal and bordering the Tibetan Plateau, the people of Humla (Humlis) historically subsisted via a transhumance system of seasonal livestock migration, as Humli traders shuttled sheep and goat caravans between lower and upper pastures to exchange grain from Nepal's Terai lowlands with salt from Tibet, supplementing local harvests with grain obtained from a trade surplus (Bishop 1990). This adaptive system existed for a century and a half prior to the 1950s, when its stability is thought to have been disrupted by the Chinese annexation of Tibet, which restricted northward trade and access to pastures; and by long-term macroeconomic changes in the salt trade (Bishop 1990). Humlis' diversified livelihood strategies have nonetheless persisted in new forms, and today Humla exports medicinal plants, timber and wood products in exchange for imported rice, flour, alcohol, and a small selection of consumer goods (Bishop 1990; Roy 2010).

However, many Humlis have faced longstanding food insecurity and shortages, and Western Nepal as a whole ranks among the most food-insecure regions of the world[2] (Government of Nepal 2010). For the last four decades, Humla's local harvests have been supplemented with a national distribution program of subsidized rice, administered by the Nepal Food Corporation (NFC) in Simikot (District Development Committee 2066). In the 1990s, famine killed approximately 1500 people in the broader Karnali zone of western Nepal (Adhikari 2008), which may have been driven or exacerbated by government policies for community forestry which conserved forest resources, but limited access to pasture land, resulting in both less livestock for consumption or trade, and less means of transporting food (Panday 1999) – a recent example of an outside intervention enacted in the name of conservation and prevention of degradation with unexpected impacts for local people. As of 2008, following the Nepali civil war, the Hunger Index for the Mid-Western Mountain region (of which Humla is a part) ranked as "extremely alarming," on par with the Democratic Republic of Congo, the nation with lowest ranking food security of 88 countries ranked, and Humla required emergency food aid through the United Nations World Food Programme (Panday 1999: 90). Emergency humanitarian relief ceased following the war, but Humla's food security has remained tenuous, and food assistance distributed through the World Food Programme's "food assistance for assets" infrastructure development program and subsidized quotas from the national Nepal Food Corporation remain prominent sources of food grain, alongside local harvests and market-purchased imported food. As with other high mountain regions, Humla's rain-fed agricultural and pastoral systems may be particularly sensitive to early impacts of anthropogenic climate change (Thornton and Comberti 2013). To better understand this emerging vulnerability and existing food insecurity, 58 semi-structured and conversational interviews were undertaken in 2012 in three remote Humli settlements (two Nepali-speaking, one Tibetan-speaking, all approximately a 4-hour hike from the airstrip at the district capital of Simikot), as well as with centrally located policy makers and development workers in Kathmandu, Nepalgunj, and Simikot

(Stephenson 2012). Most of the 20 policy makers and development workers interviewed contrasted recent improvements in food security with an overarching decline. They explained longstanding food insecurity in Malthusian terms of overpopulation, lack of good land, and land degradation. They believed local people have become "dependent" on outside food assistance and consequently reduced their effort at agriculture, preferring to consume imported rice. They argued that increased food self-sufficiency is the path to food security, emphasizing the importance of a return to traditional crops and traditional diets, enhanced by some modern inputs like irrigation and better seed. They envisioned revitalized trade patterns with Tibetan markets once a road is constructed, allowing Humla to once again enjoy a trade surplus with the expansion of cash crop farming. A minority of development workers and researchers, especially within the World Food Programme (the organization most frequently blamed for creating dependency), suggested that food self-sufficiency is an unrealistic goal, and argued that food imports (including aid) must continue to support people as they improve agricultural yields for local consumption and, more crucially, develop other livelihoods such as cash crops, non-timber forest products, handcrafts, and tourism. They emphasized the need for interventions to educate farmers and overcome risk aversion that they believe may be hindering innovation. A small minority of outside experts identified climate change as an additional stressor contributing to food insecurity, but most emphasized rice preference, dependency, and "laziness."

In contrast, many of the 38 local farmers interviewed attributed food insecurity to changes in climate, including reduced precipitation and warming over the past several decades that compromises their ability to grow enough food, explaining that "they are planting but nothing is coming up." Farmers described how they have consequently diversified their livelihoods as a buffer against increasingly unpredictable rainfall. This is consistent with the findings of Thornton and Comberti (2012), whose concurrent work in the region found that 80 percent of farmers reported climatic changes, despite little to no local knowledge of anthropogenic climate change. This is also consistent with available climate data and projections for the region (ICIMOD 2011; IPCC 2013). Because of lack of regional data we cannot conclusively state that Humli farmers are experiencing impacts of anthropogenic climate change, but their experiences are consistent with projections for the region, and these conditions represent risks and constraints to future local food production. Already, these experiences of climatic change are spurring adaptation. In interviews, Humlis reported that the emerging development industry has allowed farmers to diversify their incomes and food supplies (as well as timber and non-timber forest products), so that "if it doesn't rain they don't depend on farming alone." Most expressed interest in being able to grow more of their own food, as they find this to be more nutritious and preferable to imported rice and flour, and wish to retain their way of life, stating, "If we could grow enough we'd never leave our home." However, many Humli farmers reported that the pursuit of agriculture must not come at the expense of other livelihood strategies.

Local responses and outlooks differed between communities, status groups, castes, occupational groups, and by age and gender. Some said they see potential for a brighter future in the provision of work from the growing NGO (nongovernmental organization) industry, road construction, and increased trade; others expressed unhappiness about relying on outside work, or fear that a planned road connection to Tibet will undermine livelihoods they have now through increased harvesting of forest products from outside traders entering from Tibet. Women reported increasing burdens of agricultural labor, while some men – especially those of higher caste and greater socioeconomic status – reported they were able to take advantage of new trade opportunities. While local farmers did not attribute declines in productivity to the availability of subsidized food or food assistance programs, members of the local elite (educators, and larger scale traders and shopkeepers) did, suggesting food aid must be withdrawn because it "makes people lazy" and has contributed to increasing gambling and drinking amongst men. Both homebrews and hard liquor imported from China are increasingly available, but while for outsiders concern about alcohol abuse plays into the dependency narrative, local respondents were more likely to describe alcohol use as a response to the hopelessness people feel as their crops fail, especially if they lack access to other livelihoods.

This gap in how local farmers and policy makers understand Humla's food insecurity may be understood as a misreading of local conditions by outside experts, who largely overlook climatic change or variability as a determinant of food insecurity. For example, development workers and policy makers routinely referenced seeing fields left fallow as evidence of a disincentive effect and dependency on food aid. Meanwhile, farmers reported that because they could no longer grow enough to meet their subsistence needs, they were leaving some of the least viable fields fallow to afford time to pursue work opportunities offered by development organizations or in trade. This misreading can in part be explained as a consequence of Humla's geopolitical and ecological conditions: rural Humla is geopolitically marginalized and isolated from the centers of decision making (Adhikari 2008; Bishokarma 2011), and the job posts of bureaucrats outside the district headquarters still remain unoccupied following Nepal's civil war (Government of Nepal 2010). District-level authorities, all based in the district capital of Simikot, confirmed in the interviews that they rarely visit rural areas, and rely on information relayed from NGOs that work in the villages, few of whom have a sustained presence. Instead, many NGOs rely on personal contacts and those few "model farmers" with whom they have the best working relationships and who are responsible for distributing benefits – often local elites who benefit most from development projects. As knowledge sharing occurs through these limited corridors, there are few opportunities to correct or revise interpretations.

In interviews, Humli farmers explained that they do use and want the materials, incentives, or employment opportunities provided by the NGOs most heavily advocating against dependency, suggesting there is also little incentive for local farmers to reject or speak up about development programs on the grounds that they are a poor fit for local needs (and regardless, project materials can often be redirected to meet local needs). However, labeling local people and their food habits and livelihood strategies as the problem also closes doors to productive engagement between outsiders and bottom-up community-based organizations like local women's groups and conservation groups who are actively seeking to improve their lives, and adds insult to injury as they do so. This misreading contributes to deteriorating relations between local people and outsider development professionals: in interviews, many respondents from within the development community expressed feelings of frustration over why interventions were not working, why materials were diverted from their intended purpose, and why Humlis were not more responsive to programs designed to help them. Humli residents were readily aware that the development community perceived them to be uncooperative and "lazy." This dependency narrative also effectively disavows responsibility for project failures, diverting blame to local farmers for their food insecurity and poverty, and obscuring governance problems and limitations (which gave rise to numerous local complaints about supply disruptions in subsidized food, poor coordination between different food assistance organizations, and the fairness of rice allocation quotas), as well as other distal concerns such as the potential for overharvesting of resources following road construction. Finally, "misreading" local conditions can result in maladaptive interventions: in the absence of safeguards to support diversified livelihoods and "climate-smart" agricultural interventions such as irrigation, expanding investment in subsistence agriculture in the name of agricultural self-sufficiency could ultimately further compromise food security if conditions of drought persist.

It is not novel that those of us who occupy positions of relative privilege legitimize social and economic status by casting the poor as indolent. The dependency discourse animates development interventions worldwide, and is particularly of concern in food assistance programs (Bishokarma 2011) where it is held as an antithesis to development goals of empowerment and self-sufficient resilience (Harvey and Lind 2009). Lentz, Barrett, and Hoddinot (2005) differentiate between positive dependency, where the alternative is destitution, and negative dependency, when meeting current needs undermines recipients' capacity to meet their own needs in the future. For many Humlis, food assistance likely constitutes a form of positive dependency, where the alternative is not greater self-sufficiency but rather greater food insecurity. We need not go far to find other purported cases of "dependency syndrome" that are not borne out by on-the-ground investigation. Bishokarma (2011), writing about neighboring Mugu province in Nepal, also finds no evidence for negative dependency, instead noting that food assistance is too unreliable for people to forgo growing what crops they can, but, as in Humla, water scarcity is a key constraint on agricultural production. Reviewing food assistance literature more widely, Lenze, Barrett, and Hoddinot (2005) urge caution when assessing dependency literature, noting that many studies asserting dependency rely on anecdotal evidence and presuppose a causal rather than correlative link between aid and negative dependency, failing to account for the targeting of aid to those households and communities already unable to meet their own needs. These cases of purported dependency syndrome speak to the pitfalls of blaming local, impoverished people for their condition. Doing so may disregard adaptive actions they take toward increased well-being, while glossing over other impediments they face, including those that have their origin in the actions of others beyond their communities. In this case, Humlis are navigating the complex conditions set in motion by exposure of climatic change and variability, integration into new markets, and novel interventions from the central Nepali state and development industry – with little to suggest that "laziness" and "dependency" motivates their actions.

In the example that follows, the ecological, cultural, economic, and political environment differs profoundly from this case in upland Nepal, but differs little in terms of the discourse, which ignores a critical examination of the role that a history of displacement and resource exploitation has played in producing health inequities.

Housing, Mold Exposure, and Industrial Development in a Canadian First Nations community

In working collaboratively with the Haisla, of the Central coast of British Columbia (Figures 15.2 and 15.3), to design culturally appropriate and environmentally sustainable housing designs as an interdisciplinary research group of independent architects, energy engineers and social scientists from the University of Victoria, we discovered that a major concern of community residents was the impact of mold in their current houses on the health of the community, especially children, many of whom used "inhalers" for the widespread diagnoses of asthma (Optis *et al.* 2012). Indeed, housing stock in many First Nations communities in Canada has been rendered uninhabitable – though, we stress, people still continue to live in these dangerous dwellings – by the extensive growth of mold. The health consequences can be profound. In a 2002–2003 survey conducted by the First Nations Centre and the National Aboriginal Health Organization, 44 percent of 10,616 respondents within reserve communities in Canada reported mold growth in their homes (First Nations Centre 2005). Similar accounts come from interviews conducted within specific communities (Berghout *et al.* 2005). The Kitamaat Band Council of the Haisla First Nation surveyed their community and informed us that 41 of 192 homes (21%) contained visible mold (MacTavish *et al.* 2012); additional internal mold may not be visible. The growth of mold in poorly ventilated, densely occupied houses can be rapid and represents multiple health risks including respiratory distress, vulnerability to infection by other agents, immune system disruption, cognitive problems (poor concentration) fatigue, and asthma. These are highly age related, generally affecting children more than adults (Optis *et al.* 2012).

The "housing problem" among the Haisla was often framed, in conversation with regional DIAND (Indian Affairs and Northern Development) bureaucrats, by the idea that "these people" (a frequently used phrase) just do not know how to care for their homes, in part because they were not allowed to own them as

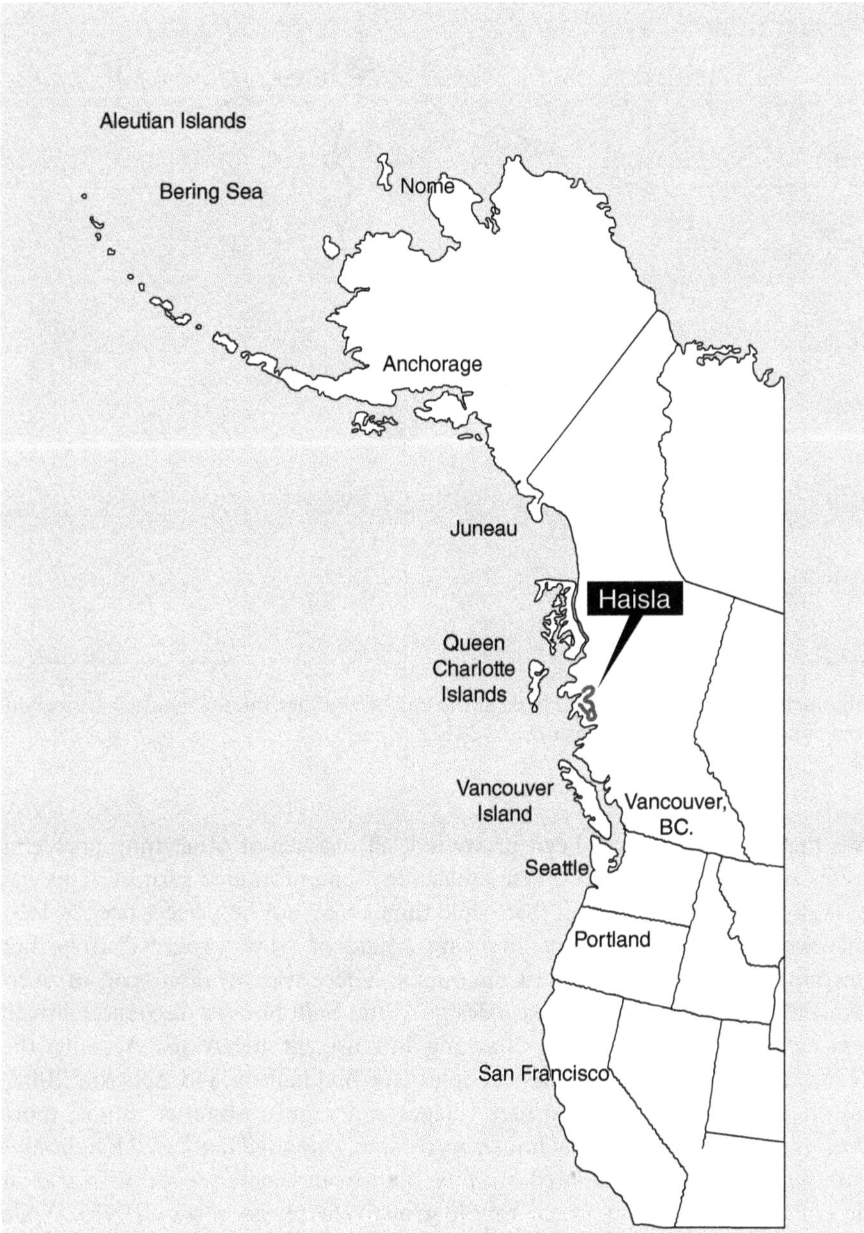

Figure 15.2 Location of the Haisla traditional territories within Western North America. Source: MacTavish *et al.* (2012).

individual property, and in part, it was often stated, because they just had "no concept of cleaning a modern house." It was also suggested in several interviews that until a century ago the population had moved frequently as a traditional way of life and lived in large traditional buildings that were probably filled with smoke from fire pits, thereby preventing mold growth. The implication of this

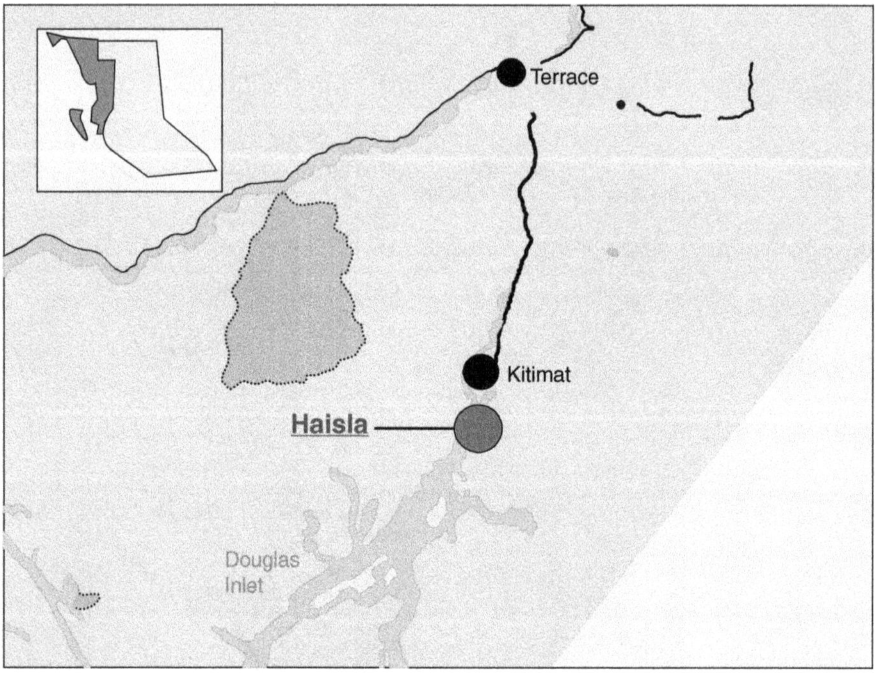

Figure 15.3 Location of the Haisla at the end of Douglas Inlet (Douglas Channel on some maps). Source: MacTavish *et al.* (2012).

was that while mold had been prevented, all manner of other lung problems were likely endemic due to smoke inhalation – an unfounded surmise. This was basically a way of suggesting that while things may not be perfect now, at least they were better than before, implying a kind of "slow progress" trope not uncommonly found in colonial discourses. There was no discussion of overcrowding in small, inappropriately designed and built houses: discussion instead was entirely oriented around changing intransigent behaviors. Actually, the Haisla, like all Northwest Coast Peoples (see Stephenson and Acheson 2003) historically had permanent winter villages and regular summer camps; more than a century ago traditional houses were large, extended kin-based longhouses with reasonably well-ventilated fire pits, built from cedar, a wood with a great deal of oil which helps to prevent mold growth (Stephenson *et al.* 1995). While some longhouses did remain well into the twentieth century, it is now predominantly a design used for community buildings, including schools and community halls. Following more permanent settlement around missions, many basic wood cabins were constructed, heated by wood stoves. These constructions tended to be well ventilated, because they were uninsulated and dry, due to the use of wood heat. These homes were mainly replaced between 1950 and the present with classic suburban-style bungalows made from inexpensive materials, including frames made from green (inadequately dried) timber (not cedar) frames, aluminum or synthetic siding, and occasionally stucco.

The construction of this kind of housing was contemporaneous with the wholesale movement of the Haisla community onto land about 12 km further down the channel, where they now live. This move was enforced by the provincial government, and acquiesced to by the federal government, in order to make way for a deep-water port at the end of Douglas Channel (the former village site), that was constructed to serve an aluminum smelter (both to offload bauxite and to ship out aluminum), and eventually the siting of other industries including pulp and paper manufacturing, wood processing, and potentially natural gas – some of which, we will suggest, may also be implicated in the creation of respiratory health inequities. The nearby town of Kitimat is the site of a major multinational corporation aluminum smelter (ALCAN), which receives massive amounts of electricity from subsidized hydroelectric power afforded by the Province of British Columbia, separately from the province's own electric utility. These power generation facilities are also the result of the alienation of First Nations land: the townsite and its industrial zone is the original site of the Haisla village. Prior to the move, the Haisla, like virtually all coastal First Nations in British Columbia, had suffered devastating population losses, particularly from smallpox and influenza (Stephenson and Acheson 2003). They had little capacity to resist the imposed move and even less provincial political power. The planned municipal town of Kitimat was built during the early 1950s after the provincial government of British Columbia "invited" ALCAN to develop hydroelectric facilities to support the aluminum smelting industry, which is one of the most intensive electrical power-using industries in the world (huge amounts of heat are required to smelt aluminum). So, with a promise of inexpensive power if they built a dam and power generation facility for their exclusive use, ALCAN decided to move to British Columbia. The company built a dam, a 16 km (10 miles) tunnel down and though a mountain to the generators, a power-generating facility, 82 km of transmission lines, a deep-sea terminal, and a smelter. The company also designed – and assisted with the initial construction of – the town. At the time, the combined development was widely considered to be among the most expensive projects ever attempted by private industry. It is important to recognize that the siting and construction of the smelter were done without any input from the local First Nation, who like all First Peoples in Canada did not even receive the right to vote until July 1, 1960 ("Dominion Day" as "Canada Day" was then called). The plans to build the dam on their traditional territory, the transmission lines, the smelter, and the entire town were completed without consultation at a time when the Haisla had no political rights whatsoever. The relocation and siting of the facility precipitated not only domestic air quality problems related to housing, but also industrial impacts: the known air quality impacts of aluminum smelting include nitrogen dioxide and sulfur dioxide emissions related to asthma and respiratory illness (Hunter 2013; ESSA Technologies 2013).

At the time the Haisla were (re)moved (in the middle of the twentieth century), new suburban-style housing was constructed on the new site of Kitamaat Village (as distinct from the Kitimat townsite) based on a design from Indian Affairs and Northern Development that is now found on many reserves in Canada: a small bungalow design which was popular in the 1950s and 1960s. The plan avoids construction of a basement, but entails downstairs, entry-level bedrooms and some storage, with an upstairs kitchen, living room, bedroom, and bathroom. Sometimes there is a deck off the living room/dining area. On reserves, these are often found to have unfinished ground floors due both to inadequate funds to complete the interior finishing of the building, and because the spaces are often used to store fishing and hunting equipment since many in the community are still engaged in a primary food economy. This type of equipment (nets, lines, etc.) is often wet, as are outboard motors, clothing, boots, and tools. The houses generally are constructed out of flimsy wallboard which is an excellent medium for the growth of mold, and they often do not have externally venting fans in kitchens and bathrooms, and instead outlet into the attic, or directly back into the kitchen which amplifies moisture rather than controlling it. Kitchens are also used to process wild foods in season (canning salmon, and berries, for example) in large amounts for family consumption, exchange, and feasting activities. Houses frequently have many more occupants than they were designed to hold because they were designed for people living in a non-Native nuclear family kinship system. In short, they are culturally inappropriate. These conditions – permanent dampness, overcrowding (hence increased CO_2 levels), heavy use of inadequately ventilated areas, and surfaces on which mold flourishes along with damaged and poorly built structures – have led to a serious set of health problems associated with mold. Houses built of traditional materials, using local labor and knowledge, and designed to meet the needs of extended families engaged in food procurement and processing, with sufficient outside storage, would mitigate the problem. Indeed, that is precisely what local people wish to have, and in our public design consultations with them, they were very specific in their recommendations for including all of these things (see MacTavish *et al.* 2012). A serious part of the problem is the externally mandated design, which is neither culturally appropriate, since it is designed for small nuclear families, nor environmentally sustainable, as it was designed for suburban commuters rather than rural fishing and hunting people also involved in forestry. Further, it usually is built with outside labor as well as imported materials.

This case is not unique: there is a long history of government neglect of First Nations housing in Canada, and, as in this case, it is often inextricably linked with the removal of local populations away from traditional areas of occupation to make way for resource extraction or outside settlement. A status report in 2006 from the auditor general of Canada stated that "problems with mold exist in many on-reserve houses [yet] no federal organization has taken responsibility for assessing the full extent of mold contamination and developing a strategy or action plan for addressing the problem" (Auditor General of Canada 2006). Following the auditor general's report, a First Nations indoor air quality committee was formed to develop a national strategy to address what it termed "the mold crisis." Its members included Indian and Northern Affairs Canada (INAC), Health Canada, and the Canada Mortgage and Housing Corporation in partnership with the Assembly of First Nations. The stated goal of the committee was to "develop sufficient awareness and capacity among First Nations home occupants, communities, and institutions so that they can prevent or remediate existing mold problems" (INAC 2008), clearly locating the problem at the local scale. To date, no publications or reports have yet been publicly released by the committee. This narrative advanced by the government effectively implies that the problem is intractable, and simply not their fault.

At the same time, Canada and the broader Canadian public remain beneficiaries of the dislocation that has contributed to this housing and mold crisis through existing and proposed industrial projects – projects that may also have implications for respiratory and environmental health. Today, sulfur dioxide emissions are poised to increase under a proposed expansion of the Rio Tinto ALCAN smelter, exacerbating chronic respiratory diseases such as asthma. The company estimates a 1 percent increase in the number of "restricted airway events" among the population with existing respiratory diseases, but suggests "reducing the level of physical activity, relocating indoors (where SO_2 levels should be lower) and through use of medication either before exercise or after symptoms are detected would be the recommended treatment" (ESSA Technologies 2013: 30) – all suggestions with further implications for respiratory health, and health and well-being more widely.

Beyond the existing aluminum smelter, Haisla territory has now become the primary site for slated for LNG (liquefied natural gas) export, using gas obtained from hydraulic fracturing of shale formations in British Columbia's Northeast. The operation is rapidly expanding, with the province aiming to increase natural gas production by more than 300 percent in less than a decade (BC Ministry of Energy and Mines 2012a, 2012b), with multiple export licenses now approved, including four facilities proposed in Kitimat. The townsite of Kitimat is also the designated terminus of the proposed Northern Gateway project. The Northern Gateway pipeline would carry DILBIT (diluted bitumen) a distance of 1177 km from Alberta's tar sands to Kitimat, in northwest British Columbia, where it would be loaded onto supertankers and shipped to Asia. It is expected to cost $7.9 billion and is supported by federal government, which has, according to the Supreme Court of Canada, a duty to consult First Nations over any resource development that might take place on their traditional lands.

These projects – to the degree they go ahead – will make Kitimat a hub for fossil fuel export of bitumen and LNG, and import of natural gas condensate, and will bring about new air pollution concerns from the terminals themselves and resultant shipping traffic. Local responses to these developments are mixed, ranging from partnership to rejection, in part due to environmental health concerns, and in part due to dissatisfaction with the consultation processes. The Northern Gateway pipeline has drawn strong and unanimous opposition from British Columbia First Nations that may impede its development entirely. It is beyond the scope of this chapter to detail the many failures of the current Canadian federal government to adequately consult with First Nations over resource development, but we can state that it is a duty observed more often in the breach than in the act. The federal government currently spends very large amounts of money ($106 million in 2012/2013 alone) settling litigation because it fails to consult, making perhaps a Faustian bargain that its fines and court activities will cost less than the scale of profits that will result should the projects go forward. Even strong supporters of the pipelines themselves, including a former federal cabinet minister, see the federal government's failure to consult as putting the pipelines at risk (McCarthy and VanderKlippe 2012). First Nations responses to LNG export have been more mixed: the Haisla are partnering in the construction of some LNG facilities, but the neighboring Gitga'at and coastal First Nations have raised apprehensions over air quality impacts from proposed LNG facilities. Legislative and policy changes have contributed to these concerns: initial plans from the province had called for LNG liquification and export facilities to be powered with renewable energy, minimizing air pollution (BC Ministry of Energy and Mines 2012a), but in 2013 the province, which faces limited hydroelectric capacity, revised the British Columbia Clean Energy Act to exclude LNG export facilities from its requirement for clean and renewable energy, allowing for facilities to be run by burning natural gas, thus contributing to increased emissions that threaten to undermine the billing of these facilities as clean energy projects (Stephenson and Shaw 2013), and to increase local air pollution (ESSA 2014).

Responding to growing concerns about air quality and respiratory health from cumulative industrial emissions, in 2013 the province announced it would fund a $650,000 study on LNG's potential impacts to air quality in Kitimat, examining the cumulative emissions of the existing ALCAN smelter, and the proposed oil refinery, crude-oil export facility, and LNG terminals under various scenarios (ESSA 2014); it had previously maintained that no such studies were required until *after* projects were approved (Hunter 2013). After delays and a fight to have the report released to the public, the final study has generated mixed responses. According to its press release, the province has drawn the conclusion that "there is lots of opportunity for industrial growth in the airshed if properly managed" (British Columbia Newsroom 2014), while opposition party critics have contested this characterization, suggesting it downplays human health and environmental impacts (Weaver 2014). The technical study itself indicates that under planned industrial developments, sulfur dioxide emissions will increase and may result in a small increase in respiratory incidents amongst those with existing respiratory conditions like asthma living in the near zone, including Kitimat townsite and Kitimaat Village (ESSA 2014: 81).

If indeed these industrial impacts on respiratory health are to be managed and mitigated as the province claims, further work is required. Unlike many British Columbia communities, to date Kitimat has no community air quality management plan in place (Hunter 2013), despite its constrained airshed and potential for cumulative impacts from proposed oil and gas facilities overlaid on emissions related to the existing aluminum smelter – and, of course, to domestic air quality concerns related, last but not least, to mold in housing. No known long-term research has been conducted to examine the implications of existing industrial air pollution for respiratory health in Kitimat. Attempts to gather such data have been impeded by the dispersal of patients amongst various area hospitals, and further impeded by confidentiality protocols that prevent researchers from amalgamating this data and interpreting it against residential information.

Therefore, we know little about possible contributions to respiratory illness from local industrial facilities that may compound domestic air quality concerns related to mold exposure. The example of mold growth, shoddy housing, and related poor health are generally framed within a discourse which circulates a set of assumptions that emphasize that changes in behavior, including attitudes toward cleaning and care, are required in order to mitigate the problem of mold growth, and in turn poor respiratory health. Overcrowding, inappropriate design, poor construction, a legacy of involuntary relocation resulting from highly profitable resource extraction and loss of land are not part of that discourse, although they are fundamentally causal.

Conclusion

Whether people live in the high altitude aridity of Humla, in Western Nepal, or coastal Kitamaat Village in British Columbia, Canada's temperate Pacific rainforest region, they share the same discursive environment – an environment within which blame and responsibility for health problems, ranging from food insecurity and malnutrition to asthma and chronic respiratory illness, is attributed local people's behavior and choices, while systemic factors are ignored. This blame shifts with local people's adaptations to externally imposed constraints and does not settle on those who have forced them to move, or to change in response to environmental problems originating a world away. In the context of increasingly rapid ecological change – from impending glacial retreat to sea-level rise in these two examples alone – the story of an imperiled common humanity is unfolding despite fragmented discourses of blame and responsibility which ignore distal and ultimate causes in favor of a continuing narrative of local inadequacy.

Today, such discourses remain motivated by colonial interests (maintaining legitimacy over rights to regulate land use and access), as well as contemporary non-state (neocolonial) interests in securing access to resources. In parallel, these narratives serve an exculpatory role against locating blame for distal drivers of global environmental change, such as anthropogenic climate change, pollution, and overconsumption, making these shifts in blame and attribution all the more pressing in contexts of global environmental change. Human intervention in ecological flows and processes to a degree that rivals geological forces (Steffen, Crutzen, and McNeill 2007) is trespassing on important planetary boundaries (Röckstrom *et al.* 2009). Never before could our ancestors change atmosphere and ocean chemistry on a global scale. Human appropriation of net primary productivity has increased such that humans now harness approximately 30 percent of global terrestrial net primary productivity, and by 2050 this is expected to reach 50 percent (Haberl *et al.* 2007). We are driving the sixth major extinction event (100–1000 times background levels). Steffen, Crutzen, and McNeill (2007) have suggested human intervention in the Earth system now amounts to a new epoch, the *Anthropocene* – a "no-analogue" world. These unprecedented distal drivers of environmental degradation – and resultant environmental health impacts – may be unintelligible from one another at times. While cautioning against crafting simple attributive links to environmental change (noting above the examples where doing so has proven a "misread" on causation), we also suggest that research has a key role to play here in identifying and interpreting environmental change across scales.

We suggest that these narratives are all the more pernicious in contexts of rapid economic change and globalization, and this research agenda is especially pressing in light of the increased economic integration being experienced by many of the same communities. Climate adaptation scholarship has theorized globalization and climate change as a "double exposure" (O'Brien and Leichenko 2000), with increased market integration pressures intersecting with environmental change. Peripheral regions especially are subject to economic transformations interlinked with ecological change (Thornton and Manasfi 2010; Peet, Robbins, and Watts 2011). Against this backdrop, there are unparalleled opportunities to alleviate poverty and reduce health inequities – however, at the same time, poor and marginalized communities and peoples remain the most deeply affected by poor environmental quality brought about by economic development, bearing the brunt of climate impacts, biodiversity loss, and pollution (addressed in several chapters in this volume). Climate change will frequently be experienced as an additional stressor among many, including contexts of political marginalization, poor health outcomes, legacies of colonialism, and poor environmental quality. We do not negate the agency and potential for local people to address and mitigate the burdens of poor environmental health, but rather draw attention to the systemic constraints they face in doing so, and the need to appropriately apportion responsibility for the origin of these environmental health inequities. We suggest that medical anthropology and health geography as well as related fields of research have a crucial role in opening a window not only on the real-world impacts of distal drivers like climate change and globalization, but also on how these impacts are conceptualized and "managed" by both local people and outside actors (Baer and Singer 2009, 2014).

While we have critiqued research that legitimates popularly held understandings of environmental illness that direct blame toward these impoverished or politically marginalized populations, or that presupposes local needs and forecloses pathways to adaptation, we want to conclude on a more optimistic note: while rooted in systemic issues, these tropes result in part from misunderstandings about the drivers and conditions of environmental health problems, and research can and does play a crucial role in addressing these dynamics. To this end, we call on the environmental health research community to interrogate discourses that add insult to injury by ascribing blame to local people for poverty, food insecurity, and poor environmental health – especially under conditions of unprecedented environmental and economic change. Health, development, and climate adaptation can all be theorized as discursive objects with the potential to be mobilized in support of both outsider and local priorities. Drawing attention to which priorities are served is a crucial role of research.

NOTES

1 Here, we use *global environmental change* to encompass not only global-scale changes like anthropogenic climate change, but also changes occurring at local scales that are so widespread that they constitute a global phenomenon, including biodiversity loss, land use change, deforestation, soil degradation, and pollution.

2 *Food security* is defined as a state "when all people, at all times, have physical and economic access to sufficient, safe and nutritious food to meet their dietary needs and food preferences for an active and healthy life (FAO 1996). The *food security* framing broadens the scope of inquiry beyond agricultural development, public health, or disaster management alone, encompassing different scales and sectors, chronic and acute crises, and environmental and socioeconomic drivers of change.

REFERENCES

Adhikari, J. 2008. *Food Crisis in Karnali Zone: A Historical and Politico-Economic Perspective.* Kathmandu: Chautari Books.

Adleson, N. 2005. "The Embodiment of Inequity: Health Disparities in Aboriginal Canada." *Canadian Journal of Public Health*, 95: S45.

Auditor General of Canada. 2006. *Status Report of the Auditor General of Canada.* Ottawa: Office of the Auditor General of Canada.

BC (British Columbia) Ministry of Energy and Mines. 2012a. *British Columbia's Natural Gas Strategy: Fueling B.C.'s Economy for the Next Decade and Beyond.* http://www.gov.bc.ca/ener/popt/down/natural_gas_strategy.pdf (accessed December 5, 2015).

BC (British Columbia) Ministry of Energy and Mines. 2012b. *Liquefied Natural Gas: A Strategy for B.C.'s Newest Industry.* http://www.gov.bc.ca/ener/popt/down/liquefied_natural_gas_strategy.pdf (accessed December 5, 2015).

British Columbia Newsroom. 2014. "Study Shows Kitimat Air Shed Can Handle New Industrial Development." July 18, 2014. http://www.newsroom.gov.bc.ca/2014/07/study-shows-kitimat-airshed-can-handle-new-industrial-development.html (accessed December 5, 2015).

Baer, H. and Singer, M. 2009. *Global Warming and the Political Ecology of Health: Emerging Crises and Systemic Solutions.* Walnut Creek, CA: Left Coast Press.

Baer, H. and Singer, M. 2014. *The Anthropology of Climate Change: An Integrated Critical Perspective.* London: Earthscan.

Barraclough, S. 1995. "Social Dimensions of Desertification: A Review of Key Issues." *Social Aspects of Sustainable Dryland Management*, 21–79.

Batterbury, S. and Warren, A. 2001. "The African Sahel 25 years after the Great Drought: Assessing Progress And Moving towards New Agendas and Approaches." *Global Environmental Change*, 11(1): 1–8.

Beniston, M. 2003. "Climatic Change in Mountain Regions: A Review of Possible Impacts." *Climatic Change*, 59: 5–31.

Berghout, J., Miller, J.D., Mazerolle, R., O'Neill, L., Wakelin, C., Mackinnon, B., Maybee, K. Augustine, D., Levi, C.A., Levi, C., Levi, T., and Milliea, B. 2005. "Indoor Environmental Quality in Homes of Asthmatic Children on the Elsipogtog Reserve (NB), Canada." *International Journal of Circumpolar Health*, 64(1): 2242–3982.

Bishokarma, M. 2011. *Assessing "Dependency": Food Security and the Impact of Food Aid on Livelihoods in Mugu.* Kathmandu: Vajra Publications.

Bishop, B.C. 1990. *Karnali under Stress: Livelihood Strategies and Seasonal Rhythms in a Changing Nepal Himalaya.* Chicago: University of Chicago.

Blaikie, P.M. 1985. *The Political Economy of Soil Erosion in Developing Countries.* London: Longman.

Choudhary, D., Ghosh, I., Chauhan, S., Bahti, S., and Juyal, M. 2013. "The Value Chain Approach for Mountain Development: Case Studies from Uttarakhand, India." ICIMOD Working Paper 2013/6. Kathmandu: ICIMOD.

Diamond, J. 2005. *Collapse: How Societies Choose to Fail or Collapse.* London: Penguin.

ESSA Technologies Ltd. 2013. "Sulphur Dioxide Technical Assessment Report in Support of the 2013 Application to Amend The -2-00001 Multimedia Permit for the Kitimat Modernization Project." Draft for Consultation. Volume 1: Executive Summary. Prepared for Rio Tinto Alcan, Kitimat, B.C.

ESSA Technologies Ltd. 2014. "Kitimat - Kitimat Airshed Emissions Effects Assessment." April 25, 2014. Final Report. Prepared for British Columbia Ministry of Environment. ESSA Technologies Ltd. Vancouver, BC. http://www.bcairquality.ca/airsheds/docs/ESSA-Kitimat-Airshed-Report_20140425.pdf (accessed December 5, 2015).

Fairhead, J. and Leech, M. 1996. *Misreading the African Landscape: Society and Ecology in a Forest-Savanah Mosaic.* Cambridge: Cambridge University Press.

FAO (Food and Agricultural Organization). 1996. *Rome Declaration on World Food Security.* Rome: FAO Corporate Document Repository. http://www.fao.org/docrep.

First Nations Centre. 2005. *First Nations Regional Longitudinal Health Survey (RHS) 2002/03.* Report on First Nations' Housing. Ottawa: National Aboriginal Health Organization.

Foucault, M. 1969. *Architecture of Knowledge* (2002 ed.). New York: Routledge.

Government of Nepal. 2010. *The Food Security Atlas of Nepal.* Food Security Monitoring Task Force, National Planning Commission.

Haberl, H., Erb, K.H., Krausmann, F., Gaube, V., Bondeau, A., Plutzar, C., and Fischer-Kowalski, M. 2007. "Quantifying and Mapping the Human Appropriation of Net Primary Production in Earth's Terrestrial Ecosystems." *Proceedings of the National Academy of Sciences*, 104(31): 12942–12947.

Hardin, G. 1968. "The Tragedy of the Commons." *Science (AAAS)*, 162(3859): 1243–1248.

Hardin, G. 2008. "Tragedy of the Commons." In D.R. Henderson (Ed.), *Concise Encyclopedia of Economics*, 2nd ed. Indianapolis: Library of Economics and Liberty.

Harvey, P. and Lind, J. 2009. *Dependency and Humanitarian Relief: A Critical Analysis.* London: Overseas Development Institute.

Hunter, J. 2013. "B.C. to Review Kitimat Air Quality in Light of LNG Development." *Globe and Mail,* October 3, 2013. http://www.theglobeandmail.com/news/british-columbia/bc-to-review-kitimat-air-quality-in-light-of-lng-development/article 14693489/ (accessed December 5, 2015).

ICIMOD/CBV/SNV. 2003. *Districts of Nepal Indicators of Development Update 2003.* Kathmandu.

ICIMOD. 2011. *Climate Change in the Hindu-Kush Himalayas: The State of Current Knowledge.* International Centre for Integrated Mountain Development. Kathmandu, Nepal. http://lib.icimod.org/record/9417/files/icimod-climate_change_in_the_hindu_kush-himalayas.pdf (accessed December 5, 2015).

IPCC (Intergovernmental Panel on Climate Change). 2013. "Climate Phenomena and their Relevance for Future Regional Climate Change." In *Climate Change 2013: The Physical Science Basis.* Contribution of Working Group I to the Fifth Assessment Report of the Intergovernmental Panel on Climate Change, edited by T.F. Stocker, D. Qin, G.-K. Plattner, M. Tignor, S.K. Allen, J. Boschung, A. Nauels, Y. Xia, V. Bex, and P.M. Midgley. Cambridge: Cambridge University Press.

INAC (Indian and Northern Affairs Canada). 2008. *Fact Sheet: National Strategy to Address Mould in First Nation Communities.* Ottawa, ON: Government of Canada.

Lentz, E., Barrett, C., and Hoddinott, J. 2005. "Food Aid and Dependency: Implications for Emergency Food Security Assessments." IFPRI Discussion Paper No. 12-2.

Machan, T.R. (Ed.) 2001. *The Commons: Its Tragedies and Other Follies.* Hoover Institutional Press Publication # 484. Stanford, CA: Stanford University Press.

MacTavish, T., Odile, M.-O., Optis, M., Stephenson, P., Shaw, K., and Wild, P. 2012. "A Participatory Process for the Design of Housing for a First Nations Community." *Journal of Housing and the Built Environment*, 27(2): 207–224.

McCarthy, S. and VanderKlippe, N. 2012. "Crucial Pipelines Jeopardized by Failure to Consult First Nations, Prentice Warns." *Globe and Mail*, September 27, 2012. http://www.theglobeandmail.com/report-on-business/industry-news/energy-and-resources/crucial-pipelines-jeopardized-by-failure-to-consult-first-nations-prentice-warns/article4572255/ (accessed December 5, 2015).

Nunavut Tunngavik Incorporated. 2013. *Annual Report on the State of Inuit Culture and Society 2011/12 – 2012/13: The Nunavut Inuit Health Survey: Understanding its Influence and Legacy.* http://www.tunngavik.com/files/2014/02/2011-12-12-13-SICS-Annual_Report-Eng.pdf (accessed December 5, 2015).

O'Brien, K.L. and Leichenko, R.M. 2000. "Double Exposure: Assessing the Impacts of Climate Change within the Context of Economic Globalization." *Global Environmental Change*, 10(3): 221–232.

Ostrom, E. 1990. *Governing the Commons: The Evolution of Institutions for Collective Action.* Cambridge: Cambridge University Press.

Optis, M., Shaw, K., Stephenson, P., and Wild, P. 2012. "Mold Growth in On-Reserve Homes in Canada: The Need for Research, Education, Policy, and Funding." *Journal of Environmental Health*, 74(6): 14–21.

Panday, D.R. 1999. *Nepal's Failed Development: Reflections on the Mission and the Maladies.* Kathmandu: Nepal South Asia Centre.

Peet, R., Robbins, P., and Watts, M. 2011. *Global Political Ecology.* New York: Taylor & Francis.

Pembina Institute. 2012. *Shale gas in Canada: Background Document for the Pembina Institute Thought Leader Forum. August 2012.* Pembina Institute, Vancouver, Canada.

Rockström, J. *et al.* 2009. "A Safe Operating Space for Humanity." *Nature*, 461(7263): 472–475.

Roy, R. 2010. *Contribution of NTFPs to Livelihood in Upper Humla, Nepal.* Asia Institute of Technology.

Scott, J.C. 2009. *The Art of Not Being Governed: An Anarchist History of Upland Southeast Asia.* New Havem CT: Yale University Press.

Steffen, W., Crutzen, P. J., and McNeill, J. R. 2007. "The Anthropocene: Are Humans Now Overwhelming the Great Forces of Nature?" *Ambio: A Journal of the Human Environment*, 36(8): 614–621.

Stephenson, E. 2012. "Food Security and Climate Change in Humla, Nepal: A Critical Ethnographic Approach." MSc dissertation, Environmental Change Institute, University of Oxford, UK.

Stephenson, E. and Shaw, K. 2013. "A Dilemma of Abundance: Governance Challenges of Reconciling Shale Gas Development and Climate Change Mitigation." *Sustainability*, 5(5): 2211–2232.

Stephenson, P., Elliott, S., Foster, L. and J. Harris. 1995. *A Persistent Spirit: Towards Understanding Aboriginal Health in British Columbia.* Western Geographical Series, Vol. 31. Vancouver: UBC Press.

Stephenson P. and Acheson S. 2003. "The Northwest Coast." In C.R. Ember and M. Ember (Eds.), *Encyclopedia of Medical Anthropology*, vol. 2 (pp. 890–902). Dordrecht, Netherlands: Kluwer.

Stevens. S. 1993. *Claiming the High Ground: Sherpas, Subsistence, and Environmental Change in the Highest Himalaya*. Delhi: Motilal Banarsidass Publishers.

Thomas, D.S. and Middleton, N. J. 1994. *Desertification: Exploding the Myth*. Chichester, UK: John Wiley & Sons.

Thornton, T.F. and Comberti, C. 2013. "Synergies and Trade-Offs between Adaptation, Mitigation and Development." *Climatic Change*, 1–14.

Thornton, T F. and Manasfi, N. 2010. "Adaptation Genuine and Spurious: Demystifying Adaptation Processes in Relation to Climate Change." *Environment and Society: Advances in Research*, 1(1): 132–155.

Weaver, A. 2014. "New Airshed Study Is a "nail in the coffin" for Government LNG Dreams in Kitimat." July 18, 2014. http://www.andrewweavermla.ca/2014/07/18/kitimat-airshed/ (accessed December 5, 2015).

Wilcox, M. 2010. "Marketing Conquest and the Vanishing Indian." *Journal of Social Archaeology*, 10: 92.

Yao, T., Thompson, L.G., Mosbrugger, V., Zhang, F., *et al.* 2012. "Third Pole Environment (TPE)." *Environmental Development*, 3: 52–64.

FURTHER READING

Appell, G.N. 1993. "Hardin's Myth of the Commons: The Tragedy of Conceptual Confusions." Working Paper 8. Phillips, ME: Social Transformation and Adaptation Research Institute.

Bishop, B.C. 1990. *Karnali under Stress: Livelihood Strategies and Seasonal Rhythms in a Changing Nepal Himalaya*. Chicago: University of Chicago.

Haun, B. 2008. *Inventing Easter Island*. Toronto: University of Toronto Press.

McAnany, P. and Yoffee, N. 2010. *Questioning Collapse: Human Resilience, Ecological Vulnerability, and the Aftermath of Empire*. Cambridge: Cambridge University Press.

CHAPTER 16 Political Ecology of a Drug Crop: The Intricate Effects of Khat

Lisa L. Gezon

Khat, a leafy bush whose leaves are chewed for a mild amphetamine effect, has been consumed in Ethiopia, Yemen, and Kenya for centuries in ritual and social contexts. In the last century, khat chewing has become more widespread in Africa as well as in the global North following the diaspora from Yemen and the Horn of Africa. In places where it is grown, this drug crop is the life's blood of local economies and, in some places, it is critical to the national economy, despite uneven legal status and sometimes strong public condemnation of the substance.

In this chapter, I argue that the effects of khat on environmental health are mixed. Khat contributes to improvements in health by providing an income to producers and traders. On the other hand, it detracts from overall environmental health by exposing people to pesticides, lowering water tables, and taking over land that could be used to grow food. In this way, it is similar to other agricultural commodities such as rice during the Green Revolution, whose large-scale production has had both positive effects of increasing food supplies and negative effects in terms of economic stratification, overall nutrition, and pesticide contamination (Kerr, Vardhan, and Jindal 2012).

This chapter presents a political ecology of drugs and health, using khat as an exemplar. It takes a commodity chain approach, presenting issues of consumption, trade, and production and their health effects. It considers the effects of

A Companion to the Anthropology of Environmental Health, First Edition. Edited by Merrill Singer.

the global war on drugs and general social disapprobation on the political silence surrounding the environmental and health challenges of khat production, arguing that drug crops present unique political-ecological dynamics compared with other commodities.

The connections between khat, environment, and health follow multiple strands, but they ultimately fit together into a political ecology of health, with multiple links between local and macro-structural constraints and opportunities. "Political ecology" is a term that has traditionally referred to an analytical approach that examines the intersections between "the social relations of power and the formation and functioning of ecologies and landscapes" (Rocheleau, Thomas-Slayter, and Wangari 1996). It has blended political economy with ecological perspectives in the context of the environmentalist movement and a concern for sustainability (Greenberg and Park 1994; Zimmerer and Bassett 2003; Robbins 2004; Paulson, Gezon, and Watts 2006; Biersack and Greenberg 2006). Critical scholars have broadened the political ecology perspective to consider issues of health (Baer and Singer 2009). As with ecological issues, broad-based political and economic dynamics of inequality shape the physical environments in which people face health opportunities and challenges.

With reference to khat – or any drug crop – a political ecology analysis reveals the importance of the biophysical environment to physical health. Legal and social disapproval, heavily influenced by the global politics of the "war on drugs," influences the ways in which drugs are produced, distributed, and consumed. Health and environment are connected through the opportunities and challenges this drug crop provides for mental and physical health. They are linked through the ways the plant provides income (increasing health for some) while putting pressure on critical resources such as land and water, which are essential to health as well as environmental sustainability. Health and environment are also related through national and international policies that shape how people discuss and take action regarding khat practices. This chapter provides an overview of the intersections between khat, environment, and health in the countries where the plant is produced and consumed. Original research conducted in Madagascar between 1990 and 2010 informs the analysis.

In examining physical health, this analysis focuses not on analyzing pharmaceutical effects on individual khat chewers, but rather on a political ecology of health, which evaluates consumption vulnerabilities and opportunities in the context of the broader political, economic, environmental, and health concerns. Scholarship on the political ecology of health has followed in the path of critical medical anthropology (Singer and Baer 1995), considering, for example, the spread of waterborne diseases such as cholera (King 2010). Baer and Singer (2009) have done an extensive analysis of the effects of global warming on such factors as climate-related shifts in subsistence strategies and nutrition and on the spread of vector-borne diseases and other epidemics in tropical areas. This entire volume presents a synthesis of approaches and presents new directions.

A political ecology of drugs is a direction within the political ecology of health that draws from a sensitivity to the role of anthropogenic environments in shaping the way people experience health opportunities and risks related to the production, trade, and consumption of psychotropic substances (Singer 2008; Page and Singer 2010; Singer, Tootle, and Messerschmidt 2013). Studies often focus on one aspect or another, especially when the processes are geographically far-flung: Sanabria (1993) did a political analysis of the social and economic impacts of coca farming in a Bolivian farming community as it became increasingly integrated into the international cocaine trade. On distribution, Chien, Conners, and Fox (2000) made an incisive critique of the war on drugs, and Bourgois (2002; Bourgois and Schonber 2009) studied street-level dealing. Other scholars have focused on the perspective of consumers, as in Singer's (2005) and Singer and Page's (2013) studies of heroin users. This study of khat provides a holistic attempt to tie the strands of the commodity chain together, identifying ways that they mutually constitute each other.

Consumption: Political Ecology of Drugs and Health

Khat has a long history of consumption in certain regions in Yemen (Weir 1985; Kennedy 1987) and Ethiopia (Gebissa 2004), where it is deeply engrained in ritual, social, and political contexts. Khat consumption has increased in the last decades within each of the countries that produce it and throughout the Horn of Africa and East Africa (Carrier 2007; Gebissa 2010c). Consumption has also grown globally, especially in countries where there are Somali immigrants, such as the UK, Australia, and the United States (Anderson and Carrier 2011; Osman and Söderbäck 2011; Feigin *et al.* 2012). In newer contexts of chewing, it has particularly taken hold with youth who use it socially as a way to pass time and as a stimulant to maintain alertness while working (Carrier 2005; Mbima 2006; Mains 2010).

Scientifically known as *Catha edulis Forsk*, khat is an amphetamine-like stimulant containing two alkaloids (cathinone and cathine), and tannins, with cathinone being the main psychoactive agent. Cathinone is unstable and breaks down into cathine after about 48 hours (Halbach 1972; Kalix 1992). Khat's active properties have been categorized as Schedule I and IV drugs by the World Health Organization. Cathinone has been listed as a Schedule I drug, along with substances of the highest risk and abuse potential and with no current medical use, including certain narcotics (including opium and heroin), LSD, and methamphetamine. After 24 to 48 hours, cathinone breaks down into cathine, which is a Schedule IV drug, defined as having low abuse potential, currently accepted medical use, with some risk of low-level dependence. Khat's active properties affect the central nervous system by stimulating the release of dopamine in the brain. This produces feelings of euphoria, which are often followed by a depression in mood. The mood depression, often associated with contemplation and reflection, is often welcomed as the final phase of a chewing session. Khat's maximum effect is reached about 2–2.5 hours after it is consumed (Cox and Rampes 2003; Odenwald 2007). Common side effects are loss of appetite, insomnia (note that sometimes this effect is sought out), and gastric disorders.

Consumption is linked to the environment in that supply – or the quantity of land and other resources used for its production – and consumer demand mutually influence each other. Aside from that, khat chewing is also linked to environment and health a less obvious way, in that fears about khat's health and social effects shape the ways in which policy makers address production- and consumption-related challenges and implement corrective strategies. An ambivalent silence shrouds khat-related health as well as agricultural issues, as efforts to eradicate and illegalize khat often take precedence over harm reduction measures through public health efforts.

Khat's relationship to health is highly debated and heavily politicized both because of its status as a Schedule I drug and because of concerns about khat consumption's social effects. Evaluations of khat's effects on physical health are frequently confounded with discussions of social and economic impacts of chewing. Based on a review of the literature, there is no conclusive evidence to support a claim that khat consumption has significantly deleterious physical health effects (Gezon 2013). Additional context-based research is needed, however, to know whether the manner of ingestion incurs negative effects. Preliminary observations, for example, suggest that chewing it after a large meal, and followed by milk (as it is traditionally done in Yemen), is likely healthier than not eating food and following it with the consumption of alcohol or cannabis to counter the effects of overstimulation, as is becoming more common in many newer contexts of chewing (Beckerleg 2010).

Assessments of khat's physical health effects are often intermeshed with evaluations of its effects on household and economic life, which I refer to as social health. Wherever it is chewed, khat's detractors accuse consumers of being lazy and avoidant of productive employment. Detractors often view problematic social factors such as unemployment and household instability as being caused by khat in a simplistic way, ignoring the broader contributing political and economic factors (Odenwald 2007; Armstrong 2008; Beckerleg 2008; Anderson and Carrier 2011; Gezon 2012c). Medical researchers Warfa *et al.* observe that debates about khat often carry a note of "moral panic" (2007: 309). According to pharmacologist Kalix, "the literature tends to either over indict the [khat] habit because it is strange and obvious, or to minimize its consequences in the view of its long-standing tradition and ethnological interest" (Kalix 1990 quoted in Odenwald 2007: 17).

It is naïve to blame khat for deeply rooted, historically entrenched poverty. The producing countries are among the poorest in the world. Yemen's per capita GDP (gross domestic product) ranks 189th out of 229 countries; Kenya ranks 198th; Ethiopia ranks 211th, and Madagascar ranks 218th.[1] The economic conditions of this global periphery were set in motion during the colonial era (Ferguson 1994; Wallerstein 2004; Escobar 2011) and have been perpetuated since then through excessive multilateral lending in the 1970s, which was then followed by bankruptcy and structural adjustment that began in the 1980s (Gezon 2006). Khat is an easy scapegoat, however, for people concerned about economic development. Because of its visibility, khat chewing is a tangible and morally provocative symbol. To see young men sitting around on the side streets who are laughing, chewing khat, and playing cards with their friends day after day incites disapproval and a sense that the chewers are willfully eschewing the kind of work ethic that observers imagine would allow the country to compete in the global capitalist economy.[2] Khat is also an easy target, since its consumption is a proximate cause of woes for many people who do not have adequate employment, who spend hard-earned money on khat, and who escape in the pleasure of chemically induced distraction, sometimes to the detriment of their families.

While it may be short sighted to trace a nation's poverty to khat chewing, khat's detractors do call attention to important factors that connect consumption to political economy, the environment, and health. Particularly amongst more recent communities of chewers, the despair that people feel from the lack of employment opportunities sometimes results in depression and may include escape-seeking behavior – in this case, in the form of khat. In many different contexts, scholars report that khat chewers enjoy the experience of dreaming about possibilities and making plans for bettering their lives – even though these plans rarely come to fruition, at least in part because the external conditions for realizing those dreams – including access to productive land and gainful wage employment – is lacking (Mbima 2006; Mains 2010). What is clear is that consumption of khat is not the decision of an individual in a vacuum. Rather, choices to consume are shaped by social, political, economic, and ecological contexts.

Humans have been known to use psychotropic substances for millennia, and it is not only the poor who consume them. Nevertheless, studies of social inequality reveal that the poor are often at the highest health risk for debilitating drug consumption and social risk of their drug habit disrupting their livelihood and that of those who are dependent on them. In the case of khat, expenditures for khat consumption often tax an already-thin household budget (Klein 2008), especially among the poor. Peer Gatter (2012) notes that a study of the relationship between khat chewing, poverty, and malnutrition in Yemen reported that poor households spend up to 39.3 percent of their earnings on khat, while it may cost wealthier households only around 8 percent of their household budget to satisfy their khat needs. Wherever khat is chewed, the economic drain of khat on consuming households arises, even if there are not statistics to support it. In addition to economic costs, there are additional social costs in the time it takes away from one's dependents (Pierre Mbima personal communication). Pharmacologists Nencini and Ahmed (1989) recognize that the general reaction against khat comes from this kind of social anxiety, as opposed to its inherent pharmaceutical effects. They wrote in their pharmacological review: "The most harmful effects of qat [khat] are probably in the realm of economics rather than in the realm of health" (1989: 27). While khat chewing has nowhere near the personal and social cost of a drug like heroin, it has disproportionately negative effects on the poor who are at greater pains to afford it and who have less access to health care in the case of any khat-related complications that may arise.

The next two sections trace the history of khat production and consider the implications of its expansion for the health of producers and consumers.

Production and Trade

The main centers of khat production in the world today are in Yemen, Ethiopia, and Kenya, but it also is grown in isolated areas within Madagascar, in eastern and southeastern Africa, Israel, and Saudi Arabia (Gatter 2012). In Ethiopia and Kenya, khat is an important export crop. Many tons of khat are sent to Djibouti and Somalia as well as shipped globally, often for the consumption of Somali migrants. The viability of khat as a cash crop in Ethiopia began when Ethiopian Airways was first established in the 1950s and could transport khat efficiently to Aden, or South Yemen, where khat production was low (Gebissa 2010b). Because khat's active biochemical property, cathinone, transforms into the less potent cathine within 24–48 hours, well-organized and rapid transport following harvest is critical. Production has increased dramatically in Ethiopia since the 1950s to meet a growing demand for khat in Aden and Somalia, and eventually to meet global demand in the UK and elsewhere. The Harerge highlands of eastern Ethiopia in particular saw an increase from 2996 hectares in khat production in 1954 to 112,206 in 2000 (Gebissa 2010a).

Catha edulis favors an altitude between 1500 and 2450 meters. It thrives under irrigated conditions, though it also grows in rain-fed conditions. To be maximally productive, it requires weeding and sometimes pest control, but it has no defined harvest period. Khat survives even with minimal care, though the quality and quantity of the khat harvest, the new leafy growth, will be higher where it has more water and is more consistently tended. Farmers often grow other crops in addition to khat. Feyisa and Aune (2003) report that khat is often intercropped with maize in the Habro district of eastern Ethiopia. Farmers prefer to have a diverse portfolio of crops in order to meet both subsistence and cash crop needs, as well as to maximize return throughout the year for crops that are harvested at different times. In Madagascar, for example, farmers with the means to do so may also grow corn, rice, grains, and vegetables in addition to khat.

In Yemen, most of the production is located in former North Yemen and relatively little is exported because of the high levels of consumption through the country. Some khat is, however, illegally exported to Saudi Arabia (Gatter 2012; Alsanosy, Mahfouz, and Gaffar 2013). Several factors contributed to the increase in khat production in Yemen, including motivation to find alternative sources of revenue when coffee exports were interrupted during the revolution of 1962 (Cassanelli 1986) and rising demand. A factor funding this increased demand was the remittances sent back by Yemenis who went to work in oil-rich Arab countries in the 1970s, which increased disposable income (Weir 1985).

Small-scale khat production has expanded to other countries, primarily for local consumption. Madagascar, where I have done fieldwork from 1990 to the present, is one of those countries and provides a valuable case study (Gezon 2006, 2012c).[3] Yemeni dockworkers brought khat to Madagascar around the turn of the twentieth century during the French colonial era. Those who settled in Madagascar began planting it in kitchen gardens for personal use. Demand increased as the Yemeni and Yemeni-descended population grew, and enterprising farmers began to plant it commercially on the fertile foothills of the northeast and east of Amber Mountain. Around the 1990s, consumption of khat began to increase in the general population. Taxi drivers are reputed to have been the first chewers, using the drug to help them stay awake during their long shifts. Others began chewing it socially and as a stimulant for increasing alertness at work. Similarly, khat first arrived in Uganda with Somali and Yemeni migrants. In the last decades, khat chewing has spread to many different regions of Madagascar (Beckerleg 2010).

Health Effects of Increased Purchasing Power for Farmers and Traders

Earnings from khat farming and trading provide an important source of income for many poor households – income that might be used to purchase healthy, nutritious foods and quality medical care. Given the intense poverty of the countries where khat is grown, the conversion of arable land for khat production has provided many people with a means to adapt flexibly to being at the margins of the global capitalist political economy. Profits from khat tend to be distributed widely throughout the farming and trading population. Throughout East Africa and Madagascar, khat is almost exclusively grown by smallholders, and socioeconomic differences between khat farmers, while existing, are small. Furthermore, even small fields provide enough return to alleviate poverty significantly. The case of Kenya is typical, where khat farms average about 3 acres, but farmers with even 1 acre can earn significantly from growing khat (Carrier 2007). According to Axel Klein (personal communication), there exist many viable small farms in East Africa and Madagascar because khat was never an integral part of elite culture as it has been in Yemen: it has always been a crop with only regional importance in Kenya and Ethiopia, and it is a relatively recent crop (decades as opposed to centuries) in Madagascar and Uganda.

In Yemen, however, the situation is more complex. There, khat chewing has a centuries-long history and has gained strong symbolic associations with Yemeni identity. It has become overtly appropriated in state-building projects, especially after the unification of Yemen in 1990 (Elie 2013b), and is omnipresent in social, political, and economic life. Khat production is similar in some ways to the African contexts, in that 90 percent of farmers own less than 1 hectare of land, and even that small amount of land is significant to household budgets. Many fields are largely dependent on rainfall. What makes Yemen different is that the remaining 10 percent of farmers are wealthy landowners with access to deep-water wells that provide year-round irrigation. Gatter (2012) reported that, in 2008, 64 percent of Yemen's khat was produced by 9 percent of khat farmers. Some of the nation's wealthiest people own these fields, including "affluent businessmen, influential members of Parliament, high ranking military officers, and powerful tribal shaykh families" (Gatter 2012: 28). Tremendous stratification between farmers exists within Yemen, owing in part to khat's high profile, given centuries' long use and contemporary political importance (Wedeen 2008), and in part to high demand in a country where 72 percent of men and 32 percent of women chew it (Gatter 2012) Nevertheless, khat production has helped to stem rural–urban migration among small-scale farmers in Yemen, since the price of khat is so much greater than that of cereals Gatter 2012: 22).

In the African contexts, trading khat happens at a small scale, and the distribution of khat is not monopolized by just a few wholesalers. Carrier (2007) writes that khat production and trade are characterized largely by trust and relations of affinity, and the same would be true for Madagascar. Carrier noted, however, that in the early 2000s, in light of the increasing international demand for khat, wealthy Somali traders rented some farms in one part of the khat-producing area. The farmers later complained about low returns from these renters as well as from other Somali buyers. It seems, however, that such Somali activity has abated in recent years (Carrier personal communication). Despite the Somali involvement, Carrier (2007) noted that even farmers with comparatively little land earned considerably more than by growing coffee, and ultimately profited from khat production.

The income provided by khat has a significant impact on the household budgets of both farmers and traders. Tefara and Start (2010) found that khat cultivation areas in Ethiopia correlate with a higher standard of living, as measured by the presence of irrigation, use of fertilizer and improved seed varieties, ownership of cattle for diary and oxen, ownership of small shops. Income for these amenities came from cash received from khat sales as well as from remittances from educated children. In Madagascar, while no thorough studies have been conducted, it was clear in the high khat production areas that people who owned fields tended to build homes made of durable materials, such as cement, have luxury items such as televisions, use satellite dish services, and some even own vehicles. In the main urban areas where khat was sold, many vendors expressed satisfaction with their earnings.

Higher household budgets tend to translate into higher health indicators, and, conversely, poverty correlates strongly with health measures such as life expectancy at birth and infant mortality, which are overwhelmingly due to preventable conditions such as malnutrition and waterborne diseases (Budrys 2003; Marmot 2005). In Ethiopia, Tefera *et al.* (2003) found a correlation between production of khat as a cash crop and several indicators, including food security and the long-term positive nutritional status of preschool children. While there are not good studies on the relationship between khat-related income and health, local research in Madagascar suggests that greater household incomes lead to higher quality health care and nutrition.

Data from my interviews conducted in 2010 suggest that being able to acquire high-quality Western biomedical health care services is a cultural value, and the ability to afford it is an important symbol of wealth and status. Educated, salaried professionals, as well as farmers and laborers with sufficient income, tend to go to private clinics, instead of the public hospital, which is less expensive but also more crowded and perceived as providing a lower quality service. People of all strata agree that having the money for purchasing (expensive) pharmaceuticals is important to good health, and people will even sell off investments (such as cattle) to afford medications. With regard to nutrition, a study of food consumption practices in the city of Diego Suarez revealed that prestige foods included fruits, vegetables, chicken, and beef, and that families with greater household income consumed these more regularly and had a more nutritionally rich diet overall (Gezon 2012c). Khat is a major source of earnings for households in both the rural and urban areas in northern Madagascar, affording many households access to nutritious foods.

In sum, khat has been a boon to farmers and traders, and while there has not been an abundance of research to support it, preliminary findings suggest that increased earnings permit people to afford higher quality health care and nutrition.

Production: Use or Misuse of Resources?

Despite the monetary benefits to farmers and traders, the proliferation of khat production has had mixed environmental effects, which have consequences for health. There are some concerns that it can put a stress on environmental resources, such as water and forest cover, and expose farmers to dangerous pesticides. Another concern is that it displaces food crops and threatens regional food security, and therefore nutritional health in the broader population. On the positive side, some argue that khat bushes are beneficial for stabilizing the soil and preventing erosion. As a crop, khat shares much in common with the challenges of other agricultural commodities. As a drug crop, however, it faces unique challenges. Because of its uneven legal status and because of often-pervasive moral disapproval of the substance, state-level agricultural extension services are often scarce to nonexistent. This increases people's vulnerability to negative health and environmental effects.

Water

Concerns about the effects of khat irrigation on water supplies have been voiced particularly for Yemen. Gatter (2012) writes that, "with its incentives and subsidies, the [Yemeni] government deliberately encouraged the cultivation of water-intensive crops" in the 1970s in the name of poverty alleviation and again in the 1990s after unification under the pro-khat regime (Elie 2013a). This dramatically increased khat production and extended it into areas that were once too arid for growing khat. Milich and Al-Sabbry (1995) report that boreholes with mechanized pumps have replaced many mountain springs in Yemen as sources of irrigation water. By the mid-1980s, over 80 percent of new wells were used to irrigate khat, and by the 1990s, some aquifers were depleted up to 7 meters. The authors mention that part of the problem is that the farmers do not see the relationship between overuse from boreholes and depletion of water from springs.

Access to irrigation is central to social differentiation among farmers of khat because the productivity of irrigated khat is considerably greater. Irrigation has also dramatically expanded the cultivable area into arid areas. While khat is drought resistant and can survive in low-rainfall conditions, it produces significantly more when it has steady access to water. This means that farmers with irrigated khat harvest all year round, which translates into significantly higher prices during the dry season when supply is low. Khat that is not irrigated does not produce well during the dry season.

Access to water is perhaps the most important factor differentiating khat farmers in Madagascar and Yemen. In Madagascar, those who have converted irrigated rice fields to khat production can harvest khat throughout the year. This contrasts with the majority, who plant on hillsides (including deforested patches) and depend on rainfall. In Yemen, the World Bank estimated that in the 1990s, only 20 percent of the water from wells benefited poor farmers, with the majority going to the wealthy (Gatter 2012). Farmers who own wells are at a particular advantage because of the low cost of fuel to operate the pumps and the lack of water-extraction fees owed to the government. Profits in the rain-fed areas are variable, depending on the amount of rainfall in any given year. Water is so critical to khat profitability that disputes over access to it have triggered considerable violence in Yemen (Gatter 2012: 236).

Water is a highly contested and politicized resource in many contexts globally (Donahue and Johnston 1997; Kane 2012), and access to quality water correlates with socioeconomic and health stratification. As Whiteford and Whiteford (2005) state, "[g]ood health, like access to clean water, is never randomly distributed across sectors of society but rather advantages certain groups," defined, for example by "[a]ge, wealth, ethnicity/race, and religion." In the case of khat, water is broadly relevant to health concerns because it is needed for drinking and sanitation, growing food, and keeping livestock. Water-related violence in Yemen has resulted in injury and even death for those involved. In this way, khat, as a water-consuming agricultural product, affects local health in ways that are not linked to its consumption as a drug or its earning potential for farmers and traders.

Pesticides

Pesticides pose a further threat to both farmers and consumers. Milich and Al-Sabbry (1995) report that in Yemen farmers use pesticides that, while water soluble, are sometimes applied right before harvest, before rain can wash the harmful chemicals off. Others have confirmed the potential health and environmental risks of pesticides that are being applied to khat in Yemen (Date, Tanida, and Hobara 2004; Gatter 2012; Masoud *et al.* 2012) and Ethiopia (Daba 2011). Pesticides are being used in Kenya, and they are encouraged by those supporting "modern" agricultural techniques, but many farmers and consumers prefer not to spray (Carrier 2007). In Madagascar, only a few of the wealthier farmers purchase pesticides to counteract insects, but many farmers are afraid of the side effects of pesticides and are hesitant to use them. Rumors about negative effects of pesticides frequently circulate, and consumers are less likely to want to purchase khat if they know pesticides have been applied.

Concerns with pesticides – as with water and forests – are not restricted to khat or any other drug crops, however. Rather, pesticides have been a major part of a global strategy for increasing food supply, and they contaminate most food sources (Daba 2011; Dowdall and Klotz 2014). This issue connects khat with broader agricultural concerns.

Forests and Soil

Clearing forests to create khat fields is another environmental concern in several places, including Madagascar and Ethiopia. Deforestion, or loss of access to forests, has been linked to health concerns, such as malaria and loss of access to important medicinal plants (Harper 2002). If khat production is connected with forest vulnerability or deforestation, then it may be contributing to health-threatening conditions. In Madagascar, in a survey of the area using satellite images and ground truthing to verify images, Gezon *et al.* (2005) report that there was little change in the landscape in the areas of highest khat production between 1972, the date of the earliest image examined, and the time of the ground survey in 2004. One exception was in an area that had had cyclone damage in 1984, which demolished many trees. After that, people cleared much of the destroyed forest land for khat fields. The overall low incidence of landscape change, despite the growth in khat production in the area, was most likely because most khat was grown on irrigated fields or on non-forested hills closer to existing areas of cultivation. Clearing forests to grow khat was a last resort, undertaken only by the poorest of newcomers to the region. Additional research is needed to determine the extent of clearing in the khat-producing areas of northern Madagascar since 2004.

Deforestation has also been noted in Ethiopia. In one study conducted in south central Ethiopia, Dessie and Kinlund (2008) found that an increase in khat production correlated with tree removal, but that the connection was not directly causal. They report that production of khat increased by 180 percent between 1991 and 2000, going from under 2 hectares of land under cultivation in 1991 to over 27 hectares in 2000. Many farmers have begun to grow khat in this region because of the hardiness of the plant and the relatively low labor input. Farmers also experienced high economic returns per hectare, with an overall 800 percent increase in revenue for farmers. Dessie and Kinlund (2008) found that, as in Madagascar, khat production resulted in the intensification of land use. Farmers planted the hearty, drought-resistant khat bushes on previously uncultivated lands. The availability of newly cultivable land also attracted immigrants to the region. Many of these newcomers have settled near forests, though they have not actually cleared trees to grow khat. Nevertheless, their presence contributes to pressure on forests from grazing, selective cutting for construction, and charcoal production. Despite these negative impacts, Dessie and Kinlund (2008) argue that the amount of land affected by khat is in comparison to the overall land in the region, and is therefore relatively insignificant.

Some have argued that khat is actually beneficial to forest and soil preservation. Based on his research in the Harer highlands of Ethiopia, where khat has traditionally been grown, Habtemariam Kassa (2010) has argued not only for the economic rationality of converting to khat, but also that khat production reduces soil degradation and erosion. In a 2012 interview with a journalist for the Center for International Forestry Research (CIFOR), Kassa, a CIFOR scientist, explained that farmers build terraces, improve the soil with manure, and keep cattle from grazing on the land where khat is growing. Thus, khat not only provides income for poor households, it also protects soil and forests (Rivera, Ortega-Huerta, Sarkar, and Rappole 2012).[4] Conservation agents in Madagascar also expressed to me that the threat of deforestation due to khat must be balanced with the way it reduces erosion through its root structure and that plantations near the protected forest of Mt. d'Ambre provide an important buffer for the forest.

Based on these findings, khat is not responsible for significant deforestation, but given the incentives for increasing land under khat cultivation, this may become an issue.

Food Security and Agricultural Priorities

In every locale, khat faces similar challenges in that it is a nonfood crop that competes with other crops for arable land and water resources. Taking away from food crop production could threaten regional nutrition and therefore be a threat to good health. A common concern in Madagascar is that khat production threatens the food supply of the surrounding area, based on the belief that khat is replacing some of the region's most fertile rice and vegetable fields (Minquoy 2006; Gezon 2012a). People suspect that farmers abandon food production because of the higher returns and lower labor inputs. Research between 2004 and 2010 revealed a situation much more complex. First, there was a significant decline in demand for vegetables since they were introduced in the colonial era to supply French colonists with food they were familiar with. Also, the irrigation and transportation infrastructure had deteriorated, making it difficult for farmers to deliver vegetables to points of sale.

Furthermore, the extent of land conversion in Madagascar was not as great as suspected, since much new production of khat occurred on previously uncultivated land, such as on unirrigated hillsides. Finally, many farmers did not actually abandon their rice and vegetables but strategically diversified their production portfolio to include khat. One wealthy and land-rich woman expressed local perspectives well when explaining why she grows vegetables and rice in addition to khat, despite the added labor of vegetable production. She said, "*samy am fotoany*," or, "everything in its own time." Because she has the means to do so, she grows vegetables in the early rainy season, when the prices for vegetables are high. Most farmers with a choice – those with adequate land, labor, water, and capital – choose to farm rice, vegetables, and other food crops. In sum, we determined that the reasons for the decline of food production in this region are complex and only minimally caused by the growing popularity of khat. On the contrary: khat provided a safety net for declining infrastructure and markets for vegetables (Gezon 2010, 2012a).

Fears about khat's role in supplanting other cash and food crops also exist in Ethiopia and Yemen. One concern is that such a strong emphasis on khat creates an unhealthy dependence (Elie 2013a). Khat is feared to displace cash crops (in particular, coffee) that provide export earnings. This is particularly the case in Yemen, where most khat is chewed internally and not sold internationally. Although it has been reported that farmers often prefer khat because it requires less work and yields a much higher profit than coffee (Weir 1985; Varisco 1997), Kennedy (1987) argued effectively that khat had not displaced coffee in Yemen. He explained that coffee and khat occupy different micro-ecological zones (Ward 1999) and so one does not easily substitute for the other. Coffee production had indeed declined, but it was not because khat has replaced it. In her study of khat in Yemen, Weir (1985) acknowledged that while khat did not displace coffee, it is likely to have replaced some grain farming, which brought back far less in profit.

In Ethiopia, on the other hand, khat has been an important source of governmental revenue. Between 1999 and 2004, the price of coffee fell from US$3 per kilogram to $0.86. Ethiopia's earnings from coffee went from 70 percent of exports to 35 percent of exports. During that same period, khat production doubled and became 13 percent of GDP. The price of khat rose to about $8 per kilogram, making it the logical choice of many farmers (Hailu 2010). In Madagascar, khat is neither exported nor even taxed (except within one municipality) by the government internally, and so it has no appeal at the national level as a boost to the overall economy.

While khat has contributed to Ethiopia's GDP, it has been identified as a threat to food production there. Because of the high costs associated with grain production, farmers had little incentive to grow available grains. Gebissa's edited volume (2010e) is dedicated to examining the relationship between food and khat in Ethiopia. He and his contributors point out some important reasons why many farmers have been both pushed and pulled into farming khat in Ethiopia. First, khat is well adapted to local environmental conditions. It can stand a certain amount of frost and drought, and its root system is useful in preventing erosion. Furthermore, while khat is growing to maturity, it permits intercropping, allowing farmers to earn a livelihood in the transitional period (Tefera and Start 2010). Second, regional demand for khat increased as transportation networks improved, and global demand for khat increased as Somali immigrants traveled abroad.

The third reason farmers have moved toward khat production is that, as in Madagascar, khat provided a solution to a local problem. In Ethiopia's case it was land scarcity associated with population increase and land concentration (Gebissa 2004, 2010b). Land is subdivided between inheritors, and immigrants have come to the region. This has reduced the average plot size (Kassa 2010) and increased the incidence of khat monocropping, due to khat's high return per unit of land. Gebissa (2010d) notes, however, that similar to Madagascar, farmers do not see monocrop khat production as an ideal. Most would prefer to grow vegetables and grain crops, as well as keep small livestock, alongside khat. Farmers are also well aware that khat has drawbacks, including some vulnerability to frost and fluctuating market prices (Tefera and Start 2010). As with khat everywhere, it also reduces their flexibility to adopt different crops because of the perennial nature of the khat bush.

Finally, and relatedly, khat is attractive to farmers because earnings from its sale provide capital for on-farm improvements and cash for purchasing food for consumption and other valuable services such as education and health care, thereby contributing to food security and overall health at the household level. Although khat is not a food crop, it is an important part of household food security for many. As scholars such as Oluyole *et al.* (2009), Thiengkamol (2011), and Maxwell and Wiebe (1999) have pointed out, growing subsistence crops is only one part of food security. Having a source of income from a product with high economic value, such as a recreational drug like khat, can be a critical component in providing cash for investing in food production in a balanced agricultural portfolio.

Similar issues arise cross-culturally with regard to khat production. In all locales, it is portrayed by some as a drug crop that competes with other crops for land and water and is accused of threatening food production. In each locale, the reasons for moving away from food production are complex, and it would be naïve to blame khat without examining the larger context of this transition. The correlation between declining food production and increased khat production does not take into account the possibility that khat expansion may well be an effect rather than a cause of that concern (Gezon 2012c). Blaming khat for reduced food production can be a red herring, taking attention away from larger concerns, such as the need for agricultural improvements.

Moving Forward with Production: Political Ecology of Silence

While khat has been beneficial to farmers and traders as a source of income, khat production is clearly not without problems such as the ones discussed above. One significant effect of khat's marginal status as a recreational drug is that in the place of proactive dialogue about khat's challenges and opportunities, there is relative silence on the part of state agencies.

In addressing their fears about food security, for example, the Ethiopian government introduced substantial assistance to farmers to encourage them to grow food crops. This included various extension services, including improved seeds and subsidized credit. But these initiatives did not address important reasons why farmers have reduced food production, such as the availability of khat combined with land scarcity. Despite state encouragement, few farmers decided to replace their khat with food crops. Gebissa (2010b) noted that despite the large-scale attention to agriculture in Ethiopia, khat has received virtually no consideration. This is also the case in Yemen and Madagascar. In writing about Yemen, Milich and Al-Sabbry (1995) note that even though donor nations have not sought eradication, as has been the case for coca in South America, donors have not developed initiatives to improve khat production.

In Yemen, Peer Gatter's (2012) extensive research reveals a history of state and donor silence on the topic of khat. In 1983, the Agricultural Research Authority (ARA) was formed for research and extension services. Despite khat's role as one of the most important crops to the Yemeni economy, it was excluded from ARA's activities and omitted from national statistics until 1997 (Gatter 2012). Even when donors began insisting on the inclusion of khat statistics, there was no sustained or well-funded support for research or agricultural extension. President Salih (president of unified Yemen from 1990 to 2012), while his regime encouraged khat production, avoided a discussion of water reforms or other agricultural extension activities because doing so would stir dissension and threaten his rule. Foreign donors had no interest in addressing khat proactively, either. The World Bank, the FAO, and the UN controlled the ARA's agenda and budget, and, according to Gatter: "[t]hese agencies would certainly not have consented to supporting research on making [khat] cultivation more productive and less water intensive – a crop that the World Health Organization had classified in 1980 as a drug of abuse" (2012).

Gatter describes a relatively short-lived governmental unit from 1998 to 2007 that attempted some research, but was not able to secure funding from either the government or donors for khat research and extension. Gatter concludes: "[U]ntil today Yemen has not developed any adequate strategy to address the pressing economic, social, environmental and health problems associated with [khat]. Instead, for long a blanket of silence has been laid over the issue" (2012: 234). Gatter reports that in the early 2000s, a Yemeni agency with a project to explore alternatives to pesticides in khat production could find neither donor nor government funding for this or any other of their relatively low-cost khat-related projects (2012).

The situation is similar in Madagascar, where there is frequent international NGO activity, often with governmental partnership, targeting individual farmers in promoting such activities as bee-keeping and improved fruit and vegetable growing. There are no efforts, however, at developing more efficient khat production or in facing the more macro-scale infrastructural (roads and canals) issues that would increase production of rice and vegetables as well as khat. Targeting khat as the cause of lowered vegetable and rice production while simultaneously ignoring it at the agricultural extension level obscures such local-level issues and will only further impoverish farmers. Ethiopia and Uganda have experienced similar silences, due in no small part to a history of colonial lack of interest and disapproval. Khat was first banned in British Somaliland (currently Somalia) in 1921. The first of several bans against it in Kenya occurred in 1934, though they were not strictly enforced until 1951. In French Somaliland (Djibouti), khat consumption was discouraged through high taxes (Gatter 2012).

Analysis of khat's agricultural issues and the silence that surrounds them ties into the tradition of political ecology. Political ecological analyses often point to the complexity of causation, where commonly assumed causes – often focusing on the responsibility of local actors – do not make sense when a broader political economic framework is considered. Scholars have analyzed such trenchant issues as erosion, deforestation, and overpopulation using this approach. In a seminal political ecology analysis, for example, Blaikie and Brookfield noted that "[l]and degradation should by definition be a social problem" (1987: 23), and not merely a technical problem of soil, climate, and geology. Ultimate causes of soil degradation can be found in social inequality and by examining the state and market pressures farmers face to intensify production.

Political ecologists have continued to seek explanations that analyze social inequalities and local ecological effects as embedded within broad political and economic dynamics. In a seminal study, Schmink and Wood (1987) demonstrated that it was not sufficient to identify local people as the cause of Amazonian deforestation. Rather, demands of expanding capitalism and state intervention unbalance subsistence-oriented agricultural systems and reorient them toward expansion. This encourages forest clearing by poor, small-scale, immigrant farmers, and ushers in highly capitalized actors with resources for extensive conversion of forests to agricultural fields.

Lucy Jarosz (1993) revealed a similar dynamic in the eastern rainforests of Madagascar, where local overpopulation is often blamed for deforestation. She points out that forest clearing is linked to colonial land appropriations and forced labor campaigns that resulted in mass flights of people into the fragile rainforest areas along the east coast. In an analysis of overpopulation, Campbell and Olson (1991) respond to neo-Malthusian fears that population pressure is the primary cause of the decline of the world's resource base. They point out that these fears ignore "the distribution of resources among regions and socioeconomic groups" (1991: 7). Their analysis proposes that high levels of consumption by the global elite provide at least as great a threat as population increase alone.

Critical analysis of political maneuvering and uneven access to resources in local practices are central themes in political ecology literature. In the case of khat, as this analysis has suggested, understanding why farmers increase their khat production to the detriment of food production, overuse water resources and pesticides, or remove forests to establish khat fields requires attention to broader political and economic issues. As a drug crop, khat faces unfavorable legal and moral standing in many contexts. And yet, despite this disapproval, scholars (Gebissa 2010a) and government officials alike realize that khat provides too much financial benefit to growers and traders to justify prohibition without a viable substitution. This ambivalence leads to a ripe silence that might be metaphorically referred to as "the elephant in the room," or, the overwhelming presence of something people pretend to ignore, but that has enormous effects nonetheless. An analysis of this silence reveals conditions that shape khat production and its lack of proactive oversight – and which, in turn, lay the framework for related health outcomes, including nutrition and access to health care.

State silence on the subject of khat in Africa has existed amidst vocal international debate as to its legality. Khat is legal in the major countries of production (Yemen, Ethiopia, Kenya, Madagascar), but it is illegal throughout most of

Europe and the United States, as well as in many countries in Africa and the Middle East (Anderson and Carrier 2013: 22). In many places, khat's legal status is complex or unclear (ACMD Recovery Committee 2103: 68), leading some to refer to it as a quasi-legal commodity (Cassanelli 1986). The Netherlands moved to ban khat imports in 2013. In July 2013, the UK announced that a ban would go into effect later in the year. Axel Klein (2013) noted that this decision contradicts the UK's expressed commitment to evidence-based policy making, pointing out that reports by the UK's Advisory Council on the Misuse of Drugs (ACMD) in 2013 and the World Health Organization in 2006 recommend against classifying the substance. As the UK is the major hub of khat distribution outside of its countries of production, the EU and other G8 countries – where khat is already illegal – have put the pressure on the UK to ban it. Klein argues that the social harm from banning the substance is greater than the benefit of giving in to this international pressure. Klein cites broader concerns that this move encourages the International Narcotics Control Board to ban international khat trade, which will "push the handful of producers – Kenya, Ethiopia, and Yemen – into an uncomfortable position" (Carrier and Klantschnig 2012: 8). These legal changes, if implemented, will dramatically impact East Africa, with the potential of impoverishing farmers and increasing violence related to illegal drug trade activity.

This trend toward illegalization fits the agenda of the global war on drugs, which was first announced by US President Richard Nixon in 1972 and enacted through prohibition and the disruption of supply chains (Carrier and Klantschnig 2012). Carrier and Klantschig have noted a more general use of the term to refer to "both prohibitionist policy towards drugs in general, and for a hegemonic way of thinking about various substances labelled as "drugs'" (ibid.: 3). Despite deep challenges to its effectiveness, the war on drugs continues to shape global policy today, as evidenced by the UK's recent ban on khat. Consequences of the war on drugs are smuggling, corruption, violence, and civil unrest, most dramatically as they have been experienced with coca in South America and heroin in Southeast Asia – not to mention the absence of harm reduction strategies that address health issues of consumers and sustainability initiatives that address environmental health.

Even though khat is legal in its major countries of production, it is politically sensitive for those governments to pay attention to khat, given the increasing condemnation of the substance by wealthy countries upon whom the khat-producing nations depend for aid and loans. In those places, khat has become a kind of "public secret," which Taussig has defined as "that which is generally known but cannot be spoken" (1999: 50). He explains that knowing what not to know is always strategic, and such is the case with khat and other drugs. Informally within Madagascar, for example, khat is known as the "green gold" of the north (Gezon 2012a) without which this region would be in far worse economic straits. And yet there are no public pronouncements on it, although in the mid- to late 2000s, there was an unsubstantiated rumor that the then president, Marc Ravaolmanana (president from 2002 to 2009), denounced khat consumption as bad for economic development. In 2008, a rumor spread that the government was considering making khat illegal, and it nearly incited a riot (Madagascar Tribune 2015). Since then, there have been no official pronouncements against khat, and very little talk of khat at all in public venues such as newspapers. Knowledge of the indispensable nature of khat to local economies paired with acute awareness of international censure keeps states strategically quiet.

As this section has revealed, the silence surrounding agricultural extension has effects on health in several important ways. Pesticides have harmful effects on consumers, and environmental health risks of consuming khat increase when agencies do not acknowledge and address the potential problem. Neglect of water issues has wide-ranging effects on health, from sanitation to agricultural food production. Ignoring khat also diminishes the search for alternative crops or activities that could earn farmers a comparable income. Khat consumption is linked with health and environment through the silence that prevents effective agricultural initiatives.

Conclusion

The strand that ties together a political ecology analysis of khat and health is its status as a controlled substance. Ideologies about "drugs" shape the ways in which it is produced, traded, and consumed, which in turn shape the environment in which people experience health risks and opportunities. To be more specific, silence associated with the war on drugs, as well as generalized ambivalence about the substance, combined with entrenched overall national poverty, shape the global footprint of khat and of many other drug crops.

Khat has had mixed effects. On the one hand, khat production is linked to overuse of water, negative health effects of pesticides, and the supply of a substance whose purchase poor households can ill afford. On the other hand, khat provides a significant income for farmers and traders. Given the intense poverty of the countries where khat is grown, the conversion of arable land for khat production has provided many people with a means to adapt flexibly to being at the margins of the global capitalist political economy. It has provided an alternative informal economy that has alleviated purchasing power distress for many individuals and households, thereby making more funds available for health care. Only the courage to face the khat situation as it is, with its opportunities and vulnerabilities, will lead to a positive outcome. Political ecology, with its focus on hierarchical and political access to health and environmental resources, can help pave the way for this to happen.

NOTES

1 Central Intelligence Agency, "The World Factbook," Central Intelligence Agency, https://www.cia.gov/library/publications/the-world-factbook/rankorder/2004rank.html.

2 The idea that individuals working hard will result in national global competitiveness has been criticized as naïve. See authors such as Escobar (2011) and Ferguson (1994) for critiques of economic development in the global South.

3 Regarding analysis of khat in Madagascar, much of the data was gathered by the author between 2003 and 2010. Field research was conducted for 6 months in 2004 and for a month at a time in the summers of 2005, 2007, and 2010. Over this time, observation and informal key informant interviewing were foundational methods. In addition, three different orally administered questionnaires were targeted at farmers, traders, and consumers in 2007 (Gezon and Totomarovario 2008); a questionnaire about urban food consumption accompanied by food diaries in 2005; and a smaller scale health care choice questionnaire was administered in 2010. Funding for this research was provided by the National Geographic Society (grant number 7413.03), the National Science Foundation (award number BCS-0318640), a US Department of Education Fulbright-Hays Faculty Research Abroad Fellowship, the University of West Georgia, and a Creative Residency at the Hambidge Center for the Creative Arts and Sciences.

4 Center for International Forestry Research, "Khat Cultivation in Ethiopia Fuels Economy, Reduces Deforestation," http://blog.cifor.org/8059/khat-cultivation-in-ethiopia-fuels-economy-reduces-deforestation.

REFERENCES

Agency, Central Intelligence. "The World Factbook." Central Intelligence Agency. https://http://www.cia.gov/library/publications/the-world-factbook/rankorder/2004rank.html.

Alsanosy, R.M., Mahfouz, M.S., and Gaffar, A.M. 2013. "Khat Chewing Habit among School Students of Jazan Region, Saudi Arabia." *PLoS ONE*, 8(6): 1–7.

Anderson, D.M. and Carrier, N.C.M. 2011. "Khat: Social Harms and Legislation a Literature Review." Home Office Occasional Paper 95.

Armstrong, E.G. "Research Note: Crime, Chemicals, and Culture: On the Complexity of Khat." *Journal of Drug Issues*, 38(2): 631–648.

Atroosh, K.B. and Al-Moayad, M.A. 2012. "Water Requirements of Qat (Catha Edulis) Cultivation in the Central Highlands of Yemen." *Journal of Scientific Research*, 4(1): 77–82.

Baer, H.A, and Singer, M. 2009. *Global Warming and the Political Ecology of Health: Emerging Crises and Systemic Solutions*, Vol. 1. Walnut Creek, CA: Left Coast Press.

Beckerleg, S. 2008. "Khat Special Edition Introduction." *Substance Use & Misuse*, 43(6): 749–761.

Beckerleg, S. 2010. "'Idle and Disorderly' Khat Users in Western Uganda." *Drugs: Education, Prevention & Policy*, 17(4): 303–314.

Biersack, A. and Greenberg, J.B. 2006. *Reimagining Political Ecology*. Durham, NC: Duke University Press.

Blaikie, P. and Brookfield, H. 1987. "Defining and Debating the Problem." In *Land Degradation and Society* (pp. 1–7). London: Methuen.

Bourgois, P. 2002. In *Search of Respect: Selling Crack in El Barrio (Structural Analysis in the Social Sciences)*. Cambridge: Cambridge University Press.

Bourgois, P. and Schonberg, J. 2009. *Righteous Dopefiend* (California Series in Public Anthropology). Berkeley: University of California Press.

Budrys, G. 2003. *Unequal Health*. Lanham, MD: Rowman & Littlefield.

Campbell, D.J., and Olson, J.M. 1991. "Framework for Environment and Development: The Kite." In Center for Advanced Study of International Development Occasional Paper No. 10. Lansing, MI: Michigan State University.

Carrier, N. 2005. "'Miraa Is Cool': The Cultural Importance of Miraa (Khat) for Tigania and Igembe Youth in Kenya." *Journal of African Cultural Studies*, 17(2): 201–218.

Carrier, N. 2007. "A Strange Drug in a Strange Land." In *Traveling Cultures and Plants: The Ethnobiology and Ethnopharmacy of Human Migrations*. New York: Berghahn.

Carrier, N. and Klantschnig, G. 2012. *Africa and the War on Drugs (African Arguments)*. London: Zed Books.

Cassanelli, L.V. 1986. "Qat: Changes in the Production and Consumption of a Quasilegal Commodity in Northeast Africa." In *The Social Life of Things: Commodities in Cutural Perspective* (pp. 236–257). Cambridge: Cambridge University Press.

Chien, A., Conners, M., and Fox, K. 2000. "The Drug War in Perspective." In J.Y. Kim, J.V. Millen, A. Irwin, and J. Greshman (Eds.), *Dying for Growth: Global Inequality and the Health of the Poor* (pp. 293–327). Monroe, ME: Common Courage Press.

Committee, ACMD Recovery. 2013. "What Recovery Outcomes Does the Evidence Tell Us We Can Expect?", 69. London: Advisory Council on the Misuse of Drugs.

Cox, G. and Rampes, H. 2003. "Adverse Effects of Khat: A Review." *Advances in Psychiatric Treatment*, 9: 456–463.

Daba, D., Hymete, A., Bekhit, A.A., Mohamed, A.M.I., and Bekhit, A.A. 2011. "Multi Residue Analysis of Pesticides in Wheat and Khat Collected from Different Regions of Ethiopia." *Bulletin Of Environmental Contamination and Toxicology*, 86(3): 336–341.

Date, J., Tanida, N., and Hobara, T. 2004. "Qat Chewing and Pesticides: A Study of Adverse Health Effects in People of the Mountainous Areas of Yemen." *International Journal of Environmental Health Research*, 14(6): 405–414.

Dessie, G. and Kinlund, P. 2008. "Khat Expansion and Forest Decline in Wondo Genet, Ethiopia." *Geografiska Annaler Series B: Human Geography*, 90(2): 187–203.

Donahue, J. and Johnston, B. (Eds.), *Water, Culture, and Power: Local Struggles in a Global Context*. Island Press.

Dowdall, C.M. and Klotz, R. 2014. *Pesticides and Global Health: Understanding Agrochemical Dependence and Investing in Sustainable Solutions* (Anthropology and Global Public Health). Walnut Creek, CA: Left Coast Press.

Elie, S.D. 2013a."From Ethnography to Mesography: A Praxis of Inquiry for a Postexotic Anthropology." *Qualitative Inquiry*, 19(3): 219–231.

Elie, S.D. 2013b. "State and Qāt Consumption in Yemen: A Cultural Means to Political Socialization." In *Working Paper Series*, 34.

Escobar, A. 2011. *Encountering Development: The Making and Unmaking of the Third World*. Princeton, NJ: Princeton University Press.

Feigin, A., Higgs, P., Hellard, M., and Dietze, P. 2012. "The Impact of Khat Use on East African Communities in Melbourne: A Preliminary Investigation." *Drug & Alcohol Review*, 31(3): 288–293.

Ferguson, J. 1994. *The Anti-Politics Machine: "Development," Depoliticization, and Bureaucratic Power in Lesotho*. Minneapolis, MN: University of Minnesota Press.

Feyisa, T.H. and Aune, J.B. 2003. "Khat Expansion in the Ethiopian Highlands: Effects on the Farming System in Habro District." *Mountain Research and Development*, 23(2): 5.

Gatter, P. 2012. *Politics of Qat: The Role of a Drug in Ruling Yemen (Jemen-Studien)*. Dr Ludwig Reichert Verlag.

Gebissa, E. 2004. *Leaf of Allah: Khat & Agricultural Transformation in Harerge, Ethiopia 1875–1991*. Oxford: James Currey.

Gebissa, E. 2010a. "Crop and Commodity: Economic Aspects of Khat Production and Trade." In *Taking the Place of Food: Khat in Ethiopia* (pp. 89–126). Trenton, NJ: Red Sea Press.

Gebissa, E. 2010b. "Keeping Tradition and Killing Time: The Use and Misuse of Khat of Ethiopia." In *Taking the Place of Food: Khat in Ethiopia* (pp. 57–88). Trenton, NJ: Red Sea Press.

Gebissa, E. 2010c. "Khat in the Horn of Africa: Historical Perspectives and Current Trends." *Journal of Ethnopharmacology*, 132(3): 607–614.

Gebissa, E. 2010d. "Leadership from Below: Farmers and Sustainable Agriculture in Ethiopia." In B.W. Redekop and S. Olson (Eds.), *Leadership for Environmental Sustainability*. Routledge Series in Business Ethics (pp. 158–169). New York: Routledge.

Gebissa, E. 2010e. *Taking the Place of Food: Khat in Ethiopia*. Trenton, NJ: Red Sea Press.

Gezon, L.L. 2006. *Global Visions, Local Landscapes: A Political Ecology of Conservation, Conflict, and Control in Northern Madagascar*. Lanham, MD: AltaMira.

Gezon, L.L. 2012a. "Drug Crops and Food Security: The Effects of Khat on Lives and Livelihoods in Northern Madagascar." *Culture, Agriculture, Food and Environment*, 34(2): 124–135.

Gezon, L.L. 2012b. "Drug Crops and Food Security: The Effects of Khat on Lives and Livelihoods in Northern Madagascar." *Culture, Agriculture, Food & Environment*, 34(2): 124–135.

Gezon, L.L. 2012c. *Drug Effects: Khat in Biocultural and Socioeconomic Perspective*. Vol. 3. Walnut Creek, CA: Left Coast Press.

Gezon, L.L. 2013. "Leaf of Paradise?: The Intricate Effects of Khat in Madagascar." *Drugs and Alcohol Today*, 13(3): 194–204.

Gezon, L.L. 2010. "Leaf of Paradise or Aid to Terrorism?: Cultural Constructions of a Drug Called Khat." In E.P. Durrenberger and S. Erem (Eds.), *Paradigms for Anthropology: An Ethnographic Reader* (p. 337). New York: Oxford University Press.

Gezon, L.L., Sweeney, S., Green, G., and Freed, B.Z. 2005. "Forest Loss and Commodity Chains in Northern Madagascar." *National Geographic Society*.

Gezon, L.L. and Totomarovario, A. 2008. "Encountering the Unexpected: Appropriating the Roles of Researcher, Teacher, and Advocate in a Drug Study in Madagascar." *Practicing Anthropology*, 30(3): 42–45.

Greenberg, J.B. and Park, T.K. "Political Ecology." *Journal of Political Ecology: Case Studies in History and the Social Sciences*, 1: 1–12.

Hailu, D. 2010. "Agrarian Debacle and the Spread of the Dollar Leaf in Northern and Southern Ethiopia." In E. Gebissa (Ed.), *Taking the Place of Food: Khat in Ethiopia*. Trenton, NJ: Red Sea Press.

Halbach, H. 1972. "Medical Aspects of Chewing of Khat Leaves." *Bulletin, World Health Organization*, 47: 21–29.

Harper, J. 2002. "Breathless in Houston: An Ethnography of Asthma." Paper presented at the Paper presented at the 62nd annual meeting of the Society for Applied Anthropology,, Atlanta, GA, 2002.

Jarosz, L. 1993. "Defing and Explaining Tropical Deforestation: Shifting Cultivation and Population Growth in Colonial Madagascar (1896–1940)." *Economic Geography*, 69(4): 366–379.

Kalix, P. 1990. "Pharmalogical Properties of the Stimulant Khat." *Pharmacology & Theraputics* 48(3): 397–416.

Kalix, P. 1992. "Cathinone, a Natural Amphetamine." *Pharmacology & Toxicology*, 70(2): 77–86.

Kane, S.C. 2010. *Where Rivers Meet the Sea: The Political Ecology of Water*. Temple University Press.

Kassa, H. 2010. "Khat and Livelihood Dynamics in the Harer Highlands of Ethiopia: Significance and Challenges." In E. Gebissa (Ed.). *Taking the Place Food: Khat in Ethiopia* (pp. 149–166). Trenton, NJ: Red Sea Press.

Kennedy, J.G. 1987. *The Flower of Paradise: The Institutionalized Use of the Drug Qat in North Yemen*. Norwell, MA: Kluwer.

Kerr, J., Vardhan, M., and Jindal, R. 2012. "Prosocial Behavior and Incentives: Evidence from Field Experiments in Rural Mexico and Tanzania." *Ecological Economics*, 73: 220–227.

King, B. 2010. "Political Ecologies of Health." *Progress in Human Geography*, 34(1): 38–55.

Klein, A. 2008. *Drugs and the World*. London: Reaktion Books.

Madagascar-Tribune.com. 2015. "Victimes Dâune Campagne De Dã©Nigrement." http://www.madagascar-tribune.com/Victimes-d-une-campagne-de,5322.html.

Mains, D. 2010. "Chewing and Dreaming: Youth, Imagination, and the Consumption of Khat in Jimma, Southwestern Ethiopia." In E. Gebissa (Ed.), *Taking the Place of Food: Khat in Ethiopia* (pp. 29–56). Trenton, NJ: Red Sea Press.

Marmot, M. 2005. "Social Determinants of Health Inequalities." *The Lancet*, 365(9464): 1099–1104.

Masoud, A.M., Al-Shehari, B.A., Al-Hattar, L.N., Altaezzi, M.A., Al-khadher, W.A., and Zindal, Y.N. 2012. "Alterations in Antioxidant Defense System in the Plasma of Female Khat Chewers of Thamar City, Yemen." *Jordan Journal of Biological Sciences*, 5(2): 129–133.

Maxwell, D. and Wiebe, K. 1999. "Land Tenure and Food Security: Exploring Dynamic Linkages." *Development and Change*, 30: 825–849.

Mbima, P.-E. 2006. "Place Du Français Et Pratiques Linguistiques Non Conventionnelles Chez Les Jeunes à Madagascar, Tome I." Doctoral dissertation, Nouveau Regime, Universite de la Reunion.

Milich, L. and Al-Sabbry, M. 1995. "The 'Rational Peasant' Vs. Sustainable Livelihoods: The Case of Qat in Yemen." *Development and Change*, 3: 43–46.

Minquoy, V. 2006. "Quand La Logique Dépasse L'éthique : Le Khat À Madagascar." *Les Cahiers d'Outre-Mer* 233 (Jan–March).

Nencini, P. and Ahmed, A.M. 1989. "Khat Consumption: A Pharmacological Review." *Drug and Alcohol Dependence*, 23(1): 19–29.

Odenwald, M. 2007. "Chronic Khat Use and Psychotic Disorders: A Review of the Literature and Future Prospects." *Journal of Addiction Research and Practice*, 53(1): 9–22.

Oluyole, K.A., Oni, O.A., Omonona, B.T., and Adenegan, K.O. 2009. "Food Security among Cocoa Farming Households of Onde, Nigeria." *Journal of Agricultural and Biological Science*, 4(5): 7–13.

Osman, F.A. and Söderbäck, M. 2011. "Perceptions of the Use of Khat among Somali Immigrants Living in Swedish Society." *Scandinavian Journal of Public Health*, 39(2): 212–219.

Page, J.B., and Singer, M. 2010. *Comprehending Drug Use: Ethnographic Research at the Social Margins*. New Brunswick: Rutgers University Press.

Paulson, S., Gezon, L.L., and Watts, M. 2006. "Politics, Ecologies, Genealogies." In S. Paulson, L.L. Gezon and M. Watts (Eds.), *Political Ecology across Spaces, Scales, and Social Groups* (pp. 17–37). Research, Center for International Forestry. "Khat Cultivation in Ethiopia Fuels Economy, Reduces Deforestation." http://blog.cifor.org/8059/khat-cultivation-in-ethiopia-fuels-economy-reduces-deforestation.

Rivera, J.H.V., Ortega-Huerta, M.A., Sarkar, S., and Rappole, J.H. 2012. "Modelling the Potential Winter Distribution of the Endangered Black-Capped Vireo (Vireo Atricapilla)." *Bird Conservation International*, 21(1): 92–106.

Robbins, P. 2004. *Political Ecology: A Critical Introduction*. Malden, MA: Blackwell.

Rocheleau, D., Thomas-Slayter, B.P., and Wangari, E. 1996. *Feminist Political Ecology: Global Issues and Local Experiences*. New York: Routledge.

Sanabria, H. 1993. *The Coca Boom and Rural Social Change in Bolivia*. Ann Arbor: University of Michigan Press.

Schmink, M. and Wood, C.H. 1987. "The Political Ecology of Amazonia." In P.D. Little, M.M. Horowitz, and E.A. Nyerges (Eds.), *Lands at Risk in the Third World: Local-Level Perspectives* (pp. 38–57). Boulder, CO: Westview Press.

Singer, M. 2005. *The Face of Social Suffering: Life History of a Street Drug Addict*. Long Grove, IL: Waveland Press.

Singer, M. 2008. *Drugs and Development: The Global Impact on Sustainable Growth and Human Rights*. Long Grove, IL: Waveland Press.

Singer, M. and Baer, H. 1995. *Critical Medical Anthropology (Critical Approaches in the Health Social Sciences)*. Baywood Publishing.

Singer, M. and Page, J.B. 2013. *Social Value of Drug Addicts: Uses of the Useless*. Walnut Creek, CA: Left Coast Press.

Singer, M., Tootle, W., and Messerschmidt, J. 2013. "Living in an Illegal Economy: The Small Lives That Create Big Bucks in the Global Drug Trade." *SAIS Review*, 33(1): 123–135.

Taussig, M. 1999. *Defacement: Public Secrecy and the Labor of the Negative*. Stanford, CA: Stanford University Press.

Tefera, H., Assefa, K., Hundera, F., Kefyalew, T., and Teferra, T. 2003. "Heritability and Genetic Advance in Recombinant Inbred Lines of Tef (Egragrotis Tef)." *Euphytica* 131(1): 91–96.

Tefera, T.L. and Start, D. 2010. "Market Incentives, Rural Livelihoods, and a Policy Dilemma" Expansion of Khat Production in Eastern Ethiopia Beyond the Tesfaye." In E. Gebissa (Ed.), *Taking the Place of Food: Khat in Ethiopia*. Trenton, NJ: Red Sea Press.

Thiengkamol, N. 2011. "Development of a Food Security Management Model." *Canadian Social Science*, 7(5): 162–166.

Varisco, D.M. 1997. "The Twin Twigs: Coffee and Qat in Yemen." *World & I*, 12(7): 216–228.

Wallerstein, I. 2004. "*World-Systems Analysis: An Introduction*." *Contemporary Political Theory*.

Ward, C. 1999. *Yemen: Cdr Building Block*. The World Bank.

Warfa, N., Klein, A., Bhui, K., Leavey, G., Craig, T., Stansfeld, S.A. 2007. "Khat Use and Mental Illness: A Critical Review." *Social Science and Medicine*, 65(2): 309–318.

Wedeen, L. 2008. *Peripheral Visions: Publics, Power, and Performance in Yemen*. Chicago: University of Chicago Press.

Weir, S. 1985. *Qat in Yemen: Consumption and Soical Change*. London: British Museum Publications Limited.

Whiteford, L. and Whiteford, S. (Eds.) 2005. *Globalization, Water, & Health: Resource Management in Times of Scarcity (School of American Research Advanced Seminar)*.: SAR Press.

Zimmerer, K.S. and Bassett, T.J. 2003. *Political Ecology: An Integrative Approach to Geography and Environment-Development Studies*. New York: Guilford Press.

CHAPTER 17

Reestablishing the Fundamental Bases for Environmental Health: Infrastructure and the Social Topographies of Surviving Seismic Disaster

Stephanie C. Kane

Introduction: Infrastructure, Social Topography, and Seismic Culture

Using seismic disaster as a lens, an ethnographic approach provides a perspective on how traditional-yet-dynamic forms of resilience are tied to historically and geologically active landscapes which are transfigured in globally standardized ways by urban infrastructure.[1] Focusing on systematic analysis of survivors' accounts in two adjacent coastal cities on February 27, 2010 ("27/2"), when an 8.8 magnitude (M) megaquake shook parts of central and southern Chile, this chapter develops an infrastructural approach to safety seeking that can be

A Companion to the Anthropology of Environmental Health, First Edition. Edited by Merrill Singer.

applied to urbanized coastlines in the Pacific Rim countries and beyond. In the process, it provides a unique angle on environmental health that highlights immediate health-seeking practices by ordinary people in extraordinary circumstances.

In coastal cities, seismic events extend from the first moments of a major earthquake through the subsequent hours until the danger of a tsunami has passed. Strong aftershocks may further extend a seismic event. In the immediacy of seismic events, inhabitants organize action by assessing the patterns of probable safety and danger that are inherent in local topography. Based on this observation, I define the *social topography of seismic events* as hybrid, socially organized landscapes of action that emerge in the timeframe of a seismic event to provide the basic, ready-made yet informal building blocks of emergency response. Social topographical knowledge is shared intergenerationally through narrative accounts, which, I argue, constitute basic elements of what Chileans call "seismic culture." Social topography is thus a kind of practical knowledge – a locally attuned, culturally salient method for navigating severely disrupted environments. As a survival mechanism, social topography relies on the improvisatory activation of historical and geographic knowledge to solve the simultaneous and uncanny problems of collapsed infrastructure.

Infrastructures mediate relationships between humans and the environment, providing the necessary conditions for health, health seeking, and health services. Bringing natural forms (water, energy, sewage, and waste) into the city and taking them out of the city, infrastructure urbanizes space, sustaining and expanding cities (Kaika and Swyngedouw 2000). Infrastructural networks delineate a city's three-dimensional ecological footprint: the length, breadth, and depth of the material conglomerations characteristic of each city's streets, towers, tunnels, and buildings will eventually remain as the most prominent human stamp in the earth's crust.[2] Infrastructures also enter into personal and cultural histories, shaping and mobilizing emotions and manifesting the sense of order that guides navigation through local worlds (Larkin 2013 drawing on Benjamin 1999). How and for whom cities, nations, and multinational entities build infrastructure, and how the plans are designed to fit and extend existing hierarchies of development are ethnographic questions (Kane 2012).

Although in popular and official parlance it continues to be common for earthquakes and tsunamis to be called *natural* disasters, anthropologists and other social scientists have established that disasters emerge in a complex way from interpenetrating social and environmental relations (Oliver Smith 1998), or, in the language of social and technology studies (STS), that disasters are coproduced by hierarchically organized assemblages of human groups, the habitats in which they live, and the technology-based infrastructures they build (Latour 1993). True, earthquakes of great magnitude begin deep under the earth's surface beyond the agency of humans. Tectonic plates push against each other, rupture the earth's crust, releasing energy into the water and causing long waves to rise up and radiate across the ocean basin (Raichlen 2013). Disaster does not become an existential fact or event, however, until the waves approach inhabited shorelines. Closest to the epicenter, the sociotechnical assemblages of humans, nature, and the built environment suddenly disassemble and reassemble in new, emergent configurations.

Infrastructures shape cities and their socioecological environments in inherently ambivalent and long-lasting ways. As Monstadt (2009: 1926) writes: "they can be seen both as a vital root cause of many environmental problems and resources shortages and as an important key to solving them." Seismic events dramatize this ambivalence, rupturing some infrastructures and putting additional pressure on others. Animated by seismic waves, earth and water move, meet, and break against the edges of cities. Modernized cities, especially container port cities, tend to have inflexible, hard edges. Infrastructures – either singly or combined, whether failed, functional, or threatening – and the people who operate and maintain them structure emergency encounters. Through a city's preparation and response, people can potentially exacerbate and/or mitigate the unfolding effects when gas lines break and fires start; when electrical systems fail or are shut down to prevent explosions; when buildings and roads collapse and water and sewage systems malfunction. People reorient. They grope in the dark and reach for their cell phones only to find that their functionality may be radically limited. Family members attempt to locate each other, check for wounded, gather if they can, evacuate if they must. Communication systems, interrupted by tilted towers, downed power lines, and lack of emergency generators, trigger cascading effects through the local and international media, health systems, and global financial systems. Food, water, and medicine become difficult to access because even simple technologies like cash registers in supermarkets and pharmacies are decoupled from the vast and complex systems upon which their operation depend. Infrastructural breakdowns trigger social order problems that are often beyond the capabilities of local first responders – the police, firefighters, coast guard, hospital and ambulance workers – who, along with their families, also face immediate danger and disorientation. Although it varies with person, responsibility, and situation, most local responders first make sure their families, the "internal front," are taken care of before they rush to, or continue with, their professional responsibilities.[3] But even then, their vehicles, tools, and facilities are often ruined, limiting their routine abilities to help or control others until outside assistance arrives.[4] In short, the earth's crust radically reorders the human condition in particular urbanized locales.

In Pacific Rim countries, seismic events have recurred throughout history and the response to them (unlike, for example, responses to nuclear disasters such as Chernobyl and Fukushima) is based on cultural advantages that have evolved through the centuries (Kreps 1998). These cultural advantages have predisposed governments to prioritize disaster prevention and preparation activities, leading to safer and more flexible infrastructures for homes, schools, hospitals, and, less frequently, jails. The nation of Chile is certainly at the forefront of these efforts (for overviews of the 2010 earthquake see Castaños and Lomnitz 2012; Humboldt State University 2010). But even in the most technologically advanced nations, state of the art anti-seismic technology is far from ubiquitous and always unequally distributed across neighborhoods.[5] Buildings and neighborhoods are engineered to different standards. Luxury apartment towers can afford prime locations sited on rock rather than landfill and built according to the most sophisticated anti-seismic designs and codes; they can sway even in response to strong tremors. And if the road is intact, their entrances provide access for emergency vehicles. In contrast, irregular housing sited in ravines or on hillsides without good, if any, vehicular access roads, or on sand which flows when seismically activated, are in situations that increase the potential hazard from building collapse and undermine evacuation and rescue attempts (see Figure 17.1). It is therefore unlikely that everyone can be equally served by police, fire trucks, and ambulances. Patterns of vulnerability tend to coincide with patterns of social and spatial marginality. Because they inhabit "ecologies of poverty," the poor are generally more vulnerable (Han 2010). Children, the elderly, prisoners, the infirm, and tourists may also find themselves marginal to the core social organizational patterns through which recovery is organized.[6]

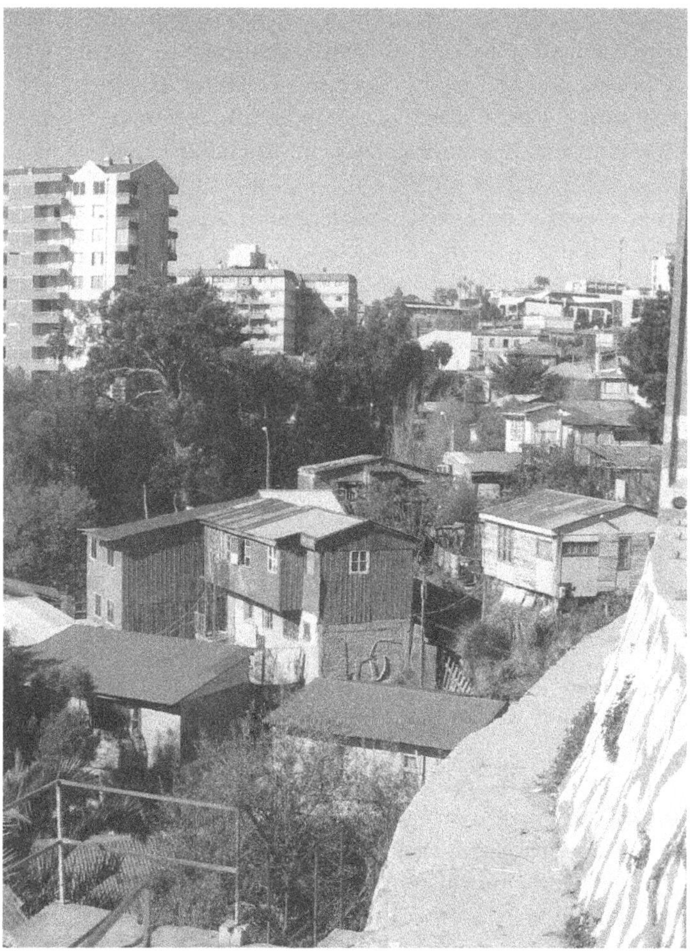

Figure 17.1 Differential patterns of architectural vulnerability have distinct implications in earthquakes and tsunamis.

In addition to governmental regulations and activities, cultural advantages are also transmitted through narratives based on the experiences of ordinary inhabitants. These narratives enhance survival by providing templates for self-organization in unpredictable and peculiar circumstances. They guide emergency action before trained first responders arrive to assist the wounded and endangered or where first responders are unlikely to arrive first. Although those at the bottom rungs of the social hierarchies tend to be more vulnerable to disaster, such narratives circulate across classes and neighborhoods. Wealthier neighborhoods will tend to fare better than poorer, but people do not stay where they sleep. They mix in public spaces, in plazas and thoroughfares, supermarkets and discothèques. In this sense, danger is always immanent in earthquake zones, for everybody. Localized effects of earthquakes and tsunamis are unpredictable, intersecting randomly with human activities. Scientists cannot discern the unfolding micro patterns of distributed seismic energy – that is, where, when, what a fault will do in the sea and on land. Rich or poor, in the immediacy of the seismic event one's fate is contingent on both chance and the availability and functioning of engineering codes, communication and energy technologies, emergency protocols, and backup systems in whatever location one happens to be – the techniques of stabilization developed in and maintained by government, family, and other civic institutions. To some extent, then, in the immediacy of seismic disaster, entrenched patterns of political economic division, along with the infrastructures that arise from and represent a material response to them, break down, causing systemic incoherence. Afterward, as recovery unfolds through time, the differential impact of social class on health will, along with normalcy, become entrenched once again, bringing political economic divisions more clearly into view. The degree to which class, race, and gendered identities structure emergency response will vary with the city and type of disaster. But here, I am concerned more generally with how city dwellers navigate through cities in the immediate timeframe of a seismic event; how they reestablish environmental health when the intertwining infrastructures, the elemental frameworks of their habitats and ordinary routines, are grievously disrupted.[7]

For the purpose of this analysis of action in disrupted habitats, it is useful to make a distinction between space and place. In the world of military and scientific experts in the Pacific Tsunami Warning Centers (PTWC), seismic data are continually mapped in cartographic space, and visually mediated through graphs tracking seismographic and oceanographic data and video feeds of coastal locales. Data recorded by measuring instruments, analyzed and mapped on to cartographic space by official protocols and communicated across the ocean basin, give governments some lead time in the organization of emergency warnings and preparations. The Pacific Basin, imagined as seismically active cartographic space, is a crucial, but nevertheless abstract, technological mediated arena where meaning is based on the interpretation of physical measurements defined by protocol as data. In the cultural logic of this technical space, reference points mark the location of places with specific seismic histories. But tsunami warnings cannot be issued for specific places, only entire coastlines. So although these reference points guide navy and coast guard commanders making large-scale decisions about how to organize emergency responses in particular places, they don't do much to help people who may already be in the throes of catastrophe.

Outside the PTWC domain of expertise, seismic culture attributes significance to *places*, not spaces. In contrast to spaces, places are socially constructed by people interacting with each other and with the material world (Tuan 1977; Lefebvre 1991). The everyday movements of people who find their ways through streets combine to shape the collective experience of cities in ways that have not necessarily been predicted on the abstract maps and drawings of planners and architects (De Certeau 1984). That places, identified socio-topographically and produced through language, discourse, and memory, acquire layered meanings is an important dimension of culture (Basso 1996; Gupta and Ferguson 1997; Low and Lawrence-Zuñiga 2003). In seismic culture, place occupies space in a peculiar way. In contrast to the assumptions of cartographic space, where the point indicating a locale is a fixed referent within a larger scale, embodied travel through a deconstructed seismic environment calls for frameworks of interpretation that do not rely upon assumptions regarding relatively fixed relationships between landscape, infrastructure, and health seeking or health services.

From the point of view of Chilean coastal inhabitants who must read radically altered landscapes during seismic events, it is not abstract space, but rather place, along with personal circumstances and timing, that shapes understanding of what survival entails. This mode of analyzing place can generally be applied to questions of environmental health; however, the specificities of seismic culture require that the commonsense assumption that there is a necessarily stable relation between space and place must be abandoned. As a neighborhood patriarch who lived through seismic events in Chile in 1960, 1970, 1985, and 2010, told me during an interview: "Everything starts falling in on itself and comes undone." Each person, he explains, must characterize the earth's natural movement based on their own experience. There is no universal risk scale. Proprioceptive predispositions toward usual, taken-for-granted aspects of stable ground in ordinary life are likely to fail. Historically informed common sense shifts toward the anticipation of *radical instability*. This shift motivates grandparents, parents, and teachers to teach children about how to evaluate danger immanent in different urban topographies and how to select from different modes of action so as to successfully negotiate the peculiarities of infrastructural collapse. That said, spatial reorientation is always socially organized – for, when a place suddenly becomes peculiar, it is established social relationships that provide the template for recovering stability. As the patriarch with four earthquakes in his life story says: "The first thing one thinks about is one's children – where are they, if they are near – then you just see what happens."[8]

The *habitus of emergency tradition* is encoded and transmitted through narrative performances of recalled perception, knowledge, and action (Bourdieu 1985; Scarry 2012). Narrated social topographies of encounter dramatize how the diverse members of human communities seek to limit physical and psychic hazards accompanying heaving ground and infrastructural collapse in urbanized landscapes. Ethnographic analysis of narrative reconstructions identifies micro strategies for reducing harm in the moments of danger and their immediate aftermath. In this analysis, oral texts are seen as basic elements of cultural transmission, a cross-culturally variable mode of seismic communication that could be considered a little-explored dimension of what Schoch-Spana *et al.* (2007) calls "civic infrastructure." The codes and capabilities for mitigating lethality are an essential component of cultural inheritance. Other things being equal, those who benefit from intergenerational traditions and institutional educational programs that inform emergency response are more likely to avoid injury and death.[9] In this sense, knowing how to enhance the probability of survival in a seismic event is the primary basis for reestablishing environmental health.

Studying Seismic Disaster

The ethnographic research project that I primarily draw on to develop the themes stressed in this chapter is comprised of personal, historical, and geoscience accounts collected in interviews and informal conversations with residents, first responders, and scientists.[10] My research assistant, Daniel Michler, and I asked local inhabitants to detail their experience and understanding of events on February 27, 2010 ("27/2"), when a megaquake shook parts of central and southern Chile. The Chile project extends my previous research on urban water ecology and infrastructure in Brazil and Argentina (Kane 2012). Research in Chile preceded two preliminary ethnographic projects about the 2007 earthquake and tsunami in Peru and periodic flash flooding in Singapore carried out in the summer of 2013. Together, these projects contribute to the development of a comparative research framework on water-related emergencies in cities. The themes developed in this chapter contribute to interdisciplinary theoretical and case-based scholarship on disaster studies, ethnography of infrastructure, and political ecology.

Fieldwork in Chile was carried out in two adjacent cities where the earthquake was strong but where there was no tsunami: in the port city and site of central navy command, Valparaíso, and in the adjacent, modern city of Viña del Mar. The core timeframe at issue begins with the first major quake at 3:34 a.m., followed by the first hours of reorientation. Medical emergencies reported by interlocutors in the context of describing events include drowning, crushing (e.g., by collapsed bridge, falling cornices), deaths from motor vehicle accidents, psychoses, anxiety, and a heart attack (due to a false alarm sent to a grandmother on Facebook). There were at least 521 deaths in Chile countrywide (Yamazaki and Cheung 2011). The disaster entailed the sudden, widespread loss of electricity, water, food, transportation, and phone and electronic communications, which delayed assistance to the places closest to the epicenter, and site of the tsunami, Talcahuano Bay and the city of Concepción (Castaños and Lomnitz 2012). Weaknesses in the communication infrastructure that had gone unnoticed for some time were revealed only in the moment of disaster, in part as a result of a phenomenon identified as "infrastructural drift" (Kane, Medina, and Michler 2015). In addition to face-to-face interviews, narrative accounts were collected in the context of participant observation and an open-ended Internet survey of geography students.[11] While narrative accounts of successful tactics of survival are often used as key examples in disaster preparedness education (e.g., for Chile, Hawaii, and Japan, see Atwater *et al.* 2009), this chapter presents a systematic analysis that identifies the place-based infrastructural dimensions of social topography and suggests how the findings in this one urbanized section of the Chilean coast can be generalized to other seismically active coastal cities. The narrative segments are thematically organized here to highlight the comparative potential of this communication mode during disasters.

How Social Topography and Seismic Culture Shape Emergency Response Narratives

Across Timescales and Cities: Valparaíso and Viña del Mar

The tectonic plate named Nazca is slowly grinding into and under the South American plate, moving through earthquake cycles over time. Eventually, the converging plates catch and release energy that punctuates the long rhythms of geological time. Like nuclear tests and atom bombs, volcanoes, tornadoes, bombings, and large lightning bolts, earthquakes register as significant events in the *longue durée* of recorded human history (Stein 2010: 72–74, 106). The tremors also interrupt individual life courses, cutting short everyday conversations in the Internet coffee shop on the corner. If the event is large, the energy pushes up the ocean into a tsunami and hurls it toward shore. In 1960, only one generation ago, Chile experienced the largest earthquake ever recorded in the world, 9.5 momentum magnitude (M). It was accompanied by a large tsunami in Valdivia, a city on the southern coast.[12] Despite considerable advances in seismic science, technology, and engineering, it is tricky to gauge where on the coast a tsunami will hit, how strong it will be, how far inland it will go and what human impacts it will have. Even for a singular locale such as Valparaíso, scientists cannot know *how* the depth of the bay will affect the wave, or even *if* depth will affect any particular wave, explains civil engineer Patricio Catalán Mondaca.[13] Officials must beware of sowing panic or crying wolf, and after the 2011 tsunami in Japan, when all their (officially accepted) predictions were smaller than the actual wave, it is clear that faulty prediction can undermine the best preparation.[14] Given the limitations of seismic science, Mondaca believes that ordinary inhabitants should use the historical and geological record to reorganize their thinking. It is always best to be prepared for the worst case. In practical terms, Mondaca advised the following: "If there is enough shaking that you cannot stand, or if shaking goes over 30 seconds, a tsunami is coming: Don't wait for a [tsunami] alarm."[15]

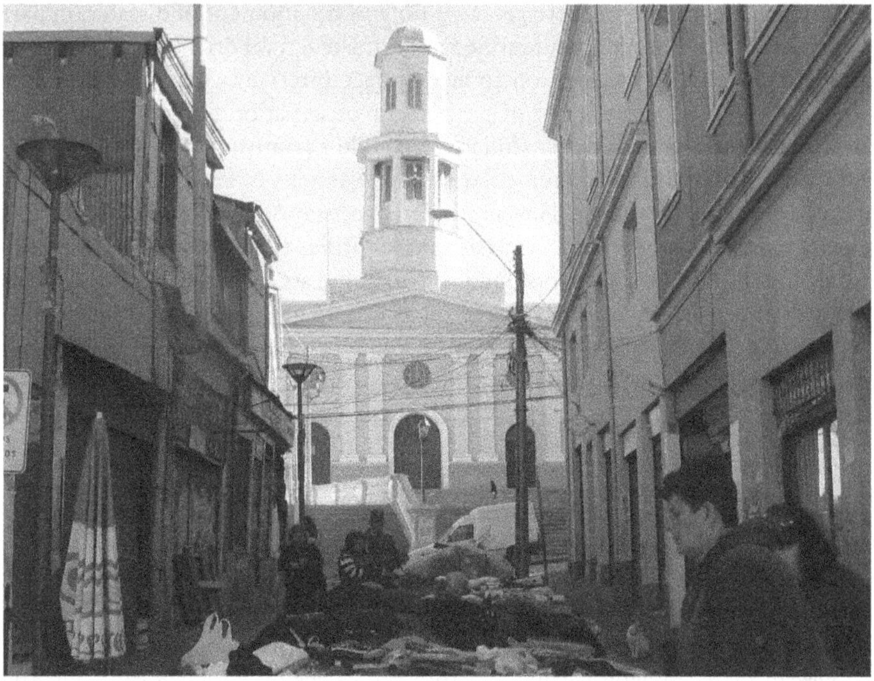

Figure 17.2 In 1730, a tsunami reached the level of La Matriz's steps. If a tsunami of that size occurred today, much of Valparaíso and all of Viña del Mar would be flooded.

Seeking to understand the geological record, geographer Marco Cisternas carefully digs through beds of buried sea grasses flattened and reoriented by the inland rush of past tsunamis.[16] This allows him to reach back to before the first written historical record, that is, before 1730, when the Spanish Chroniclers recorded a tsunami that lapped the steps of La Matriz church in Valparaíso (see Figure 17.2). Then a village, the church now sits on a small hill in the middle of the warren of the old port. To reach the church steps in 1730, the tsunami must have risen 10 meters. At 10 meters today, the part of the city that used to be an almond orchard, the Almendral (now also called the Plan), would be totally under water, as would be the whole city of Viña del Mar.

In the Plan: Before European colonization, mountain streams (*esteros*) crossed the surface of the coastal flats on their way to the sea. When the colonizers built the almond orchard in the flats not far from the La Matriz Church and the Customs House, streams still flowed across the surface. Eventually, however, the streams were covered over and the marshy areas between them were filled in. Today, the streams, the sand, and the fill lie hidden beneath the main avenues that structure the flow of inhabitants as they travel back and forth through the Plan, the city's business and government center (See Figure 17.3). Because they are flat and beside the ocean, both the Plan section of Valparaíso and the entire city Viña del Mar, built on similar terrain, are hazardous in earthquakes and tsunamis. Unlike undeveloped coastline, the hazard is intensified by the way the cities were created, that is, as a relatively inflexible built environment on top of

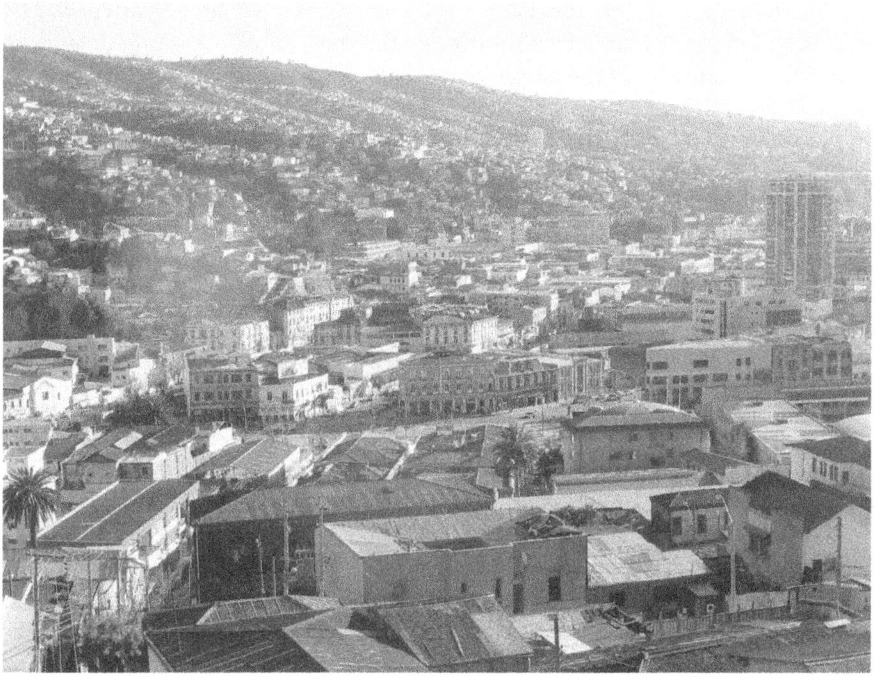

Figure 17.3 Under the avenues of the Plan, streams still flow from the mountains to the sea.

loose substrate that flows in concert with seismic waves. The earthquake hazard for occupants of Valparaíso's Plan is magnified by the adobe construction of its colonial buildings, the same architectural gems that led the city to be labeled a UNESCO World Heritage Site.

To avoid being swept away by a tsunami, people finding themselves in the Plan when a major earthquake strikes can run up into the hills that circle the city. In contrast, that mode of evacuation is not available to people in the modern city of Viña. There, where many of the buildings are engineered according to anti-seismic code – if the building does not collapse (and in 2010, some did) – most people know to evacuate vertically, that is, to stay in their building and go up to the fifth or sixth floor. If the building is strong, it can withstand the waves. Running to the closest hill could take half an hour, especially with all the rubble and other people and obstacles in the way. Taking the car is inadvisable because it will add to the havoc and not be able to traverse the rubble in the roads.

Generic Socio-topographical Narrative (Advice Mode)

Survival narratives, regularly shared among family members and in school education programs, focus on practical, social, and topographical guidelines for negotiating emergencies. The following two examples come from two people who live in Valparaíso. The first, a geographer (Augusto Guidi), a father of young children living in the Plan, speaks from his own life experience. The second, a geography student who lives in the hills, speaks as a granddaughter who respects and shares the advice of her elders:[17]

> Normally, people react based on their experience in the quakes of '71, '83, and now, 2010. Since one is a child, one knows what will happen. You leave the door open, stay away from windows, grab a flashlight, cut off the lights and the gas, know the difference between old buildings and new buildings, and move oneself to a low-risk region.[18]

In coastal cities, if a major earthquake is felt, "mov[ing] oneself to a low-risk region" generally implies that one should run to higher ground. But, as the next quote suggests, advice is far from homogeneous:

> People always say that you should run up to the hills but a better reaction is to think first. There can be an accident. If you run out into the street, you can get trampled; something can fall on your head. It's not a good idea to act out of panic and hysteria. My parents and grandparents always taught me: keep your shoes here, the oldest stays with the little children, stay calm, and think for yourself.

In everyday life, city dwellers overcome the problem of uncertainty by establishing and following routines. But when seismic events erase reference points, introduce cognitive problems, and make routines impossible, urban populations do not merely wait passively for the help of public authorities (Gilbert 1998: 97). On the contrary, citizens actively negotiate obstacles in their search for healthy environments. The above two quotes are examples of the condensed mode of general advice that circulates independently of specific events. Note that although the guidelines vary in regard to whether one should run or stay put, both examples are attuned to history (of buildings, infrastructure, and accidents) and a consideration along the vertical dimension of local topography. In the next section, I discuss narrative accounts that are tied to individual experience of unique infrastructural dilemmas that take place in the timeframe between earthquake, tsunami, and the immediate aftermath. Like the generalized advice, individual-experience based narrative transmissions are recounted to people across generations within families and friendship groups and between laypersons and professional researchers and journalists.

Coding Space and Infrastructure in Disaster Communication

One ethnographic thread runs across the scales of time and through the interpretive frameworks encountered in fieldwork on 2010 events: *successfully living through a major seismic event fundamentally depends upon topographical reorientation to the sudden overwhelming instabilities in the physical environment as they register sensually.* While Chileans ignore tremors that register at or below 3.0 M, not even defining them as earthquakes (and distinguishing them with the Spanish word *tremor*), a stronger quake (*temblor*) triggers conscious attention and assertive response. Chileans' perception of danger is precisely attuned to seismic scales. Their embodied skill is culturally specific. The personal experience narrative that follows suggests the implications of cross-cultural variation.

Luciana Alfaro Carrasco and Augusto Guidi (quoted above), a married couple who are both geographers, illustrated this phenomenon with this personal experience narrative. Carrasco told me the story as Guidi drove us to the University of Viña del Mar, where the ethnographic team would discuss our research and the students' experiences with her geography class:

> Some time ago, at a dinner gathering in Valparaíso, two visiting professors from Germany were sitting around a table enjoying dinner with Chilean friends and colleagues, when all of a sudden, they felt a tremor. The Germans leaped up from the table, ran to the archway connecting internal rooms. Stopping to catch their breath, they looked at each other, and then turned back to the table, where the Chileans continued to eat and drink as if nothing of import had happened. For their Chilean companions, quakes under 3 or 4 M are simply part of everyday life.

At the extreme end of the seismic scale, megaquakes are felt deeply in the body's muscular-skeletal interstices; they should upend ongoing interests, negotiations, and prior states of being. Lack of education can leave foreign visitors without the skills to translate this bodily perception into emergency action. That the perception of danger can be too weak is conveyed by stories of tourists transfixed by the vision of fish leaping wildly as the sea pulls away from the shore, not realizing how urgently they should be fleeing toward higher ground, away from the oncoming tsunami wave.[19]

Narrative reconstructions of seismic events are the vehicles for teaching emergency habitus. In them, socio-topographic conditions categorize the initial moment and set the parameters of possible escape. Within this categorization, the motif of infrastructure breakdown defines the character and extent of disaster. Narrated particulars contribute to the making of a kind of objective, publically shared knowledge. Depending on which infrastructures take center stage and what kind of networked interdependencies come into play, sociotechnical systems may present obstacles to, or support for, emergency action. The specific possibilities and consequences of breakdown in the seismic moment force new meanings for those involved. Whether or not infrastructure continues to function, the *uncanniness* accompanying the instabilities of socioenvironmental disruption adhere to it in memory. Another one of Carrasco's geography students shared this account:

> *We almost died on the road:* I was in Valparaíso on 27/2 but my family was in Concepción and Talcahuano [close to the epicenter, where the tsunami hit, although he could not have known that at the time]. I'd left work at 1:30 [a.m.] and was inside the house for about a half hour when the earthquake hit. Everything was broken up. At dawn, we went to the highway and started hitchhiking. There was nothing en route – no water, no motels. We slept in cars. At one point a car slowed down but went by without picking us up. *When we got a couple of miles down the road*, we saw a jeep on top of the car that had passed us. All the people inside were dead. It took us two days to get there. [Italics for emphasis added by author]

As told here, transport infrastructure sets up the conditions for unfolding *events*: the lack of vehicles, water, and housing made travel down the highway between the city and the hinterland difficult and strange. In addition, a highway accident serves as a rhetorical turning point in the plot of the narrative that would follow. Indeed, in many experiential accounts of seismic events, I find that the strain or collapse of infrastructure serves as a key image that indexes the extent and quality of material destruction and threats to well-being. Thus, the collapse of the *material* infrastructure in seismic events becomes the *narrative* infrastructure of emergency response communication. In the next narrative shared by another of Carrasco's students, infrastructure signals a significant change in awareness:

> It was holiday and we were in La Serena [a coastal town to the north]. There was only one night left to vacation. We had started dancing and felt a strong movement but our collective first reaction was: "Oh, I'm drunk." But one guy said, "*Temblor*!" But I still thought that I was just drunk. *When the lights went out, that's when we knew it was an earthquake.* It was only a 4 (M) there.

Crafted by inhabitants, narratives communicate both practical and emotional dimensions, the facts and the feelings, the instructions and the uncanny overtones of seismically active existence. The narratives emphasize that one's reorientation and search for safety in the midst of and immediately following a large quake calls for a practical consciousness, a mix of feeling and thought, a "structure of feeling" (Williams 1977: 132) that is tied to place and habitus through a layered composite of geological science, news, educational curricula, historical documents, and intergenerational oral narrative. And in 2010, when hand-held video recording devices were widely integrated into cell phone technology, a wealth of visual and auditory data was posted to YouTube to communicate the terrifying sounds of the breaking earth to the world. One usually expects stories that emerge repeatedly from structures of feeling to reinforce personal connections to place, to assert human dominance of landscapes, and, where dislocation has been experienced, to provide emotional continuity (Raffles 2002: 53–55). But in seismic culture, the repetition of the strategies, sensations, conditions, and logics arising in traumatic moments within disrupted social topographies necessitates more urgent readings of and decision making in landscapes.

As discussed, inhabitants key their evaluation of survival in the immediacy of hazard to infrastructural breakdown. However, as pointed out to me by another of Carrasco's geography students in Viña del Mar: "people are seismic sensors."[20] People too can function as infrastructure, transmitting information from the felt earth to their brain, and then sending their voice through communication infrastructure to the government agencies coordinating emergency response.[21] Inhabitants provide essential subjective data that combine in crucial ways with the seismic data inscribed by the seismometers in buoys that are distributed in the ocean by Chile and other member nations of the Pacific Tsunami Warning Center. The different registers of perception and evaluation distinguished by the Mercalli Scale, coding inhabitant perception, and the Richter scale, governing seismometer records and scientific analysis, combine to shape the circulating knowledge-in-process central to a national emergency response.

Both embodied and technically mediated perceptions of seismic and infrastructural changes on the earth's surface combine in the performance of emergency response. In support of Briggs's (2011) argument pertaining to an epidemiological arena of biosecurity, the modalities of disaster communication identified here indicate the weakness of top-down emergency models that rely on experts crafting and disseminating necessary knowledge to the public. The source of the most immediate and extensive knowledge is embodied in those affected by the strange geographical and infrastructural context.

In the Seismic Moment: "It all depends on where you are."[22]

When familiar places become strange and the structure of infrastructure breaks down, it takes a decisive journey through transformed landscapes to find relative environmental stability again. In these first moments, radios may or may not work, tsunami alerts may fail, an evacuation route may be blocked by a locked gate (all situations reported happening on 27/2). Although police and firefighters who happen to be on duty at the time surely participate in organizing emergency response, for most people, the initial phase of the journey out of chaos and danger is navigated according to traditional scripts: the familiar narrative recounting of conditions, decisions, and actions that people took to save lives become essential resources in moments of danger.

The cognitive map of city topography is sectioned by degrees of seismic hazard; in these differentiated spaces people map their social investments, emotions, and meanings (e.g., the neighborhood where home is and where family members might be at any given moment). The plot of emergency response narratives unfolds topographically: that is, they explicitly show how topographical orientation is accomplished in distinctive ways in the various spaces of the city and for what means and ends. Here I present narrative examples with contrasting topography: the first recounts 27/2 events in a neighborhood on a stable rocky outcrop high above the sea (Playa Ancha); a second pair takes place in the Plan, where colonial-era buildings and underground streams endanger inhabitants. These narratives emerge from and represent the kind of ordinary, theme-directed ethnographic conversations with people newly met in Valparaíso and in Viña del Mar. Although brief and serendipitous, the Playa Ancha story functions on three levels: (a) as a telling of the personal experience of 27/2 events, within which is embedded [in brackets] (b) seismic knowledge situated in a regional geography; and (c) advice to the ethnographic team (clearly newcomers who have not the slightest idea about how to survive an earthquake). To emphasize the kind of salient and generalizable narrative parameters that can be abstracted from the corpus we collected, I label the subsections.

Playa Ancha

Playa Ancha (on rocky outcrop high above the sea), neighbor:

1. *Serendipitous connection (set-up of our neighbor's narrative)*: The ethnographic team rented an apartment on the 27th floor of an apartment tower high above the

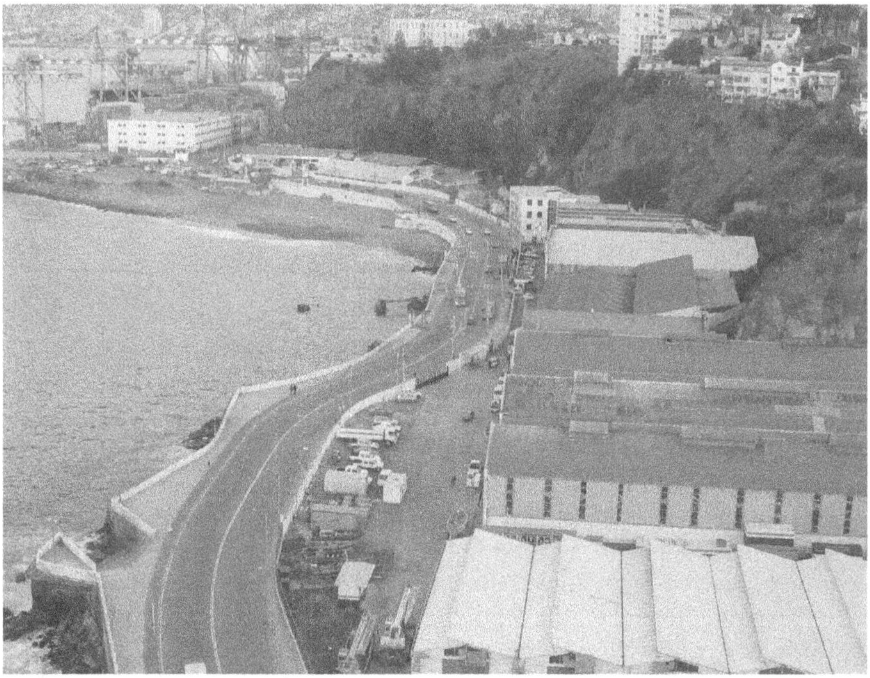

Figure 17.4 View of the coast road and container port in Valparaíso from an apartment tower in Playa Ancha.

ocean (see Figure 17.4). It was our first time trying to leave from the back of the building and we couldn't figure out how to get out of the locked parking lot. (In the event of a possible tsunami, one would take the back exit from the fourth floor, putting one partway up the hill, and avoid the main entrance in front, across the street from the sea wall.) That's when we met our neighbor, who I will call Amalia, the patriarch's daughter, who was bringing home groceries. Her gendered kinship story represents the kind of information conveyed in successful earthquake survival stories where people start at or close to home.[23]

2. *Enacting immediate safety moves*: First it was slow, then strong ... much underground noise, everything moving, glass breaking . . . loud and sonorous. I had my little son in hand and stood in the doorway ... [(Switching into advice mode): Always make sure to leave the door open because otherwise you could get locked inside ...] It was 3 in the morning, everyone was sleeping, the light was cut, telephone too. I dressed myself, looked for a flashlight, and pulled the car out. [(Switching into advice mode): Cars get flattened otherwise.] It was dangerous walking because everyone was running. [(Switching into advice mode): In the tower, you should stay well inside, away from windows, or well away from the building, which can fall.] So I went down the stairway, took the car out and waited for my parents to come. I realized when I got outside and looked around that the earthquake was really strong, that it was not just my perception. It was also really long compared to the one in the '80s.

3. *Seismic science (phenomenology)*: [(Switching into explanatory mode): When the shaking stops, one feels nothing for 1–2 minutes, 3–4 minutes. The shaking

movement can either be horizontal or vertical. Vertical is more dangerous. In 2010, it was horizontal. (She explains further about the Nazca plates.) In Papudo (Chile), there was a submarine volcano (which turned out to be a rumor).[24] Chile, like Japan, is in the most seismic region in the world. When there is shaking of 1, 2, or 3, we do not feel it. We only start to feel it at 3 or 4. We are so used to it.

4. *Topographic positions and relations*: In Playa Ancha we are on firm rock. Down under, in El Plan, where the central business district is, there is only sand and earth, landfill. The Plan shares characteristics with Mexico City, where a 5.0 quake destroyed much of the city because it is built on a lake and sand. At a certain grade, the earth liquefies like sand. [I keep pulling Amalia back from far and wide to her neighborhood account of 27/2]

5. *An infrastructural view with the gendered family at the center*: I was waiting for my parents … [SK: Had you called them?] No, I didn't call them. I knew they were coming. [SK: How?] My father stays very close (*muy apegado*). He is, above all, The Protector. [SK: What if you had a sister nearby?] Our brother lives in Viña. He called as soon as we got together, before communications were cut. Viña is far. [Here in Playa Ancha], we had no light, no water, no plumbing. [(Switching into advice mode: Most dangerous is the gas, which is in two forms: pipes, which can break and cause fires, and tanks, which can break …] We were without electricity for only one day. The water came back the day after that, as did the telephone (land line). But this varies greatly by sectors. In some sectors, they were without water for one month, without light or telephone as well. My mother and I missed the aftershock period (*tiempo de la replica*) because we went to Italy for my mother-in-law's funeral. But my father stayed behind. There is a film called *3:34* that shows the events of 27/2 from the point of view of families.[25] [In it, family members are caught in different socio-topographic conditions.]

6. *Reflections on psychological trauma*: One knows what to do, but it is still traumatic. People get really scared. One woman ran out of her house nude, she was so panicked. Living through an earthquake, it isn't written, it is personal. Every person lives through it in a different form … [(Switching to advice mode): When you feel a tremor, you remain calm. When it stops, go to the door.][26]

The Coastal Flats: El Plan (Almendral), Valparaíso

The ornate, multistoried public and private buildings of the European colonials are beautiful and hazardous. Many were broken on 27/2 and were still being repaired over a year later. When a major earthquake hits, people flee their homes and run to the hills, careful to stay in the middle of the jammed streets so as to avoid getting crushed by falling cornices and utility poles. Carrasco and Guidi were at home with their three young children in Almendral at 3:34 a.m. on 27/2. Their account emphasizes the importance of confronting instability with presence of mind:

Keep calm, follow the script, assess conditions and contingencies: Carrasco was in the front of the apartment when she felt the tremors. As the tremors grew stronger she held on to the baby with one arm and the new TV with the other. Meanwhile, Guidi was waiting in the back bedroom with their two daughters, the model of calm. As it turned out, they didn't have a lot of damage, but across the hall, the apartment was totaled. Though side by side, the apartments above street-level businesses were actually in adjoining buildings previously separated by an alleyway. They learned later why their neighbor's building fell and theirs was fine: when the owners joined the two spaces into one, they took out the supporting pillars in the middle, sacrificing building strength for commercial space.

Corruption can undo laws and codes in the most unintended and irresponsible ways, increasing the vulnerability of inhabitants in ways that, without knowing what really happened, is often attributed to the randomness of natural forces intersecting with the built environment.

Family emergency plans tend to work well when events are not complicated by dispersion. When everyone is at home, or at least in the same neighborhood, social reorganization is fairly straightforward. But often, families do not think about what will happen when its members are distributed across the urban landscape, at work, shopping, or at play. Two of Carrasco's students told us about what happened in a crowded disco in old colonial buildings, just about the worst kind of place to be in an earthquake. The first account is told in third person, the second, a more detailed account based on answering our questionnaire, is in the first person.[27] I have selected and reorganized the salient parts from the questionnaire and converted the second, longer account to a single narrative.

1. *Underground*: My friend was in Valpo, in a basement club, celebrating a promotion. Because it was below ground, when they felt the tremors, they panicked. It was terrible. There were only one or two escape routes, two small staircases, and the tremors were so strong, people ran in every direction. My friend hid under a table to protect herself from the people, so she wouldn't get stepped on.

2. *On the third floor*: I was not at home, having left work a short time before. I was in a discothèque, like the usual ones you find in Valparaíso. It was one of the emblematic architectural sites, an antique. I was on the third floor, in the grand dance salon, which was surrounded by columns. As soon as I felt the earthquake, I tried to go to a secure place and found myself near some of the columns. Most of the bottles and glasses had fallen from the bar and the floor was moving like a boat – not to mention there were more than 200 people in the place and everyone was running. The women were crying and pushing and one was always trying to calm them. I was hanging out with a large group and most of them were women. I got out of there immediately after the earthquake was over. What most occupied me was that right after the earthquake, there was a series of repeated aftershocks (*temblores*). *Upon leaving the place where I first found myself, I heard a kind of explosion: the whole region's energy was cut; the only lights came from cars in the streets. Once outside, one couldn't take the evacuation routes because one couldn't see anything. Only guessing where we were going, making sure we kept a distance from the buildings and away from streets where cornices were falling on top of cars and where we might have trampled those who had fallen there.* [Italics for emphasis added by author]

While this was happening, the idea that a tsunami could come never even entered my head. I was only thinking of the collective chaos that was occurring in the moment and trying to escape one way or another.

By way of contrast, one final mass-mediated account emphasizes the way that emergency habitus humanizes disaster preparedness:

Former dictator Augusto Pinochet moved the National Congress out of Santiago to a modernist building on the site of his family's home in the Plan. Minutes before Sebastián Piñera was about to be sworn in as the first right-wing president since Pinochet's fall, a series of strong aftershocks, up to 6.9 M, surprised the collection of Latin American presidents and other dignitaries present in the building. Although the reported Richter scale measure was just a shade under the 7.0 M level signaling the possibility of a tsunami, "Mr. Piñera refused to acknowledge the tremors during the ceremonies, continuing to smile and shake hands with world leaders even as the National Congress building in Valparaíso shook and television light stands swayed" (Barrionuevo 2010). Images of the event still circulating on the Internet all show the various presidents looking up toward the ceiling curiously. This case suggests the degree to which, despite wealth and power, those whose subjectivity has been shaped outside seismic culture can be made more vulnerable by officials (or multinational hotel chain managers) who decide not to err on the side of caution. Everyone should have been evacuated immediately. Had the visiting presidents been seismic culture insiders, they would have understood the assumed risks of remaining inside a building in the Plan at that moment. On the other hand, perhaps they would have assumed the risks to their persons in order to convey regional stability to the world.

Conclusion

Seismic culture provides an unusual angle by which to study the ways that local knowledge, encoded in oral narratives, enhances the abilities of ordinary citizens to reestablish the bases for environmental health.[28] First, although seismic and oceanographic sciences have made great strides in the study of earthquakes and tsunamis, on the scale of particular human localities, their abilities to decipher the exact spatiotemporal coordinates of impact are severely limited. As a result, in the timeframe of the seismic event, as defined here, traditional, place-based knowledge fills the gap. Without the intergenerational cultivation of dispositions and sensibilities that enable survival and promote resilience, inhabitants would not know how to get out of harm's way in suddenly disrupted, infrastructure-dense environments. Second, like Raffles (2002: 47) who shows how places are in the flow of becoming, and Nygren (1999), who studies multiple social actors who are differentially empowered to move through places, the study of seismic culture contributes to understanding the situated yet open-ended dynamics of local knowledge.

The narrative segments presented here convey and contrast social topographies of safety seeking on 27/2 in Valparaíso and Viña del Mar. Organized intergenerationally, in large part through family narrative, emergency habitus is an everyday dimension of civic infrastructure that travels into interpersonal communications and public education programs of every sort. There is no reason to believe that emergency habitus and its construction through narrative accounts is unique to the cities in which we did ethnographic research. They could be contrasted with like narratives collected in the Chilean hinterlands, for example, Iloca, a village situated in an estuary which, like other estuaries – where water runs over water – has a tendency to funnel seismic energy; or narratives could also be collected on offshore islands, like Juan Fernandez, where the earthquake was not felt and climbing a tree was the only escape from the tsunami.[29]

Indeed, it seems likely that all urbanized sections of the coastlines of Pacific Rim countries have characteristic socio-topographic narratives. I argue here that, as a genre, socio-topographic narratives of seismic culture penetrate cultural differences and operate as geomorphologically limited universals (e.g., everywhere in the Pacific Rim). Japan is an apt example of a technologically advanced nation in the same circle of subduction zones as Chile, which experienced a 9.0 M earthquake and tsunami along its northeast coast on March 23, 2011, little more than a year after Chile's 8.8 M. earthquake and tsunami. The "sawtooth" topography of the coastline increased the height and reach of the region's tsunamis that confronted inhabitants in locally distinctive ways. The water reached 127 feet above sea level in Aneyoshi in Iwate Prefecture (like being hit by a 13-story concrete wall if you are in its way). Because the villagers' ancestors carved four-foot-high stones marking the height of a historical tsunami, inhabitants knew to build their homes on higher ground, out of reach of the waves. In contrast, those who lived in Sendai's Wakabayashi ward, where the waves traveled five miles inland, ignored their ancestors' warnings and thousands of homes were lost (Birmingham and McNeill 2012: 38). I suggest that it is the power of narration that effectively carried the ancestral stone warnings in Aneyoshi and some distinctive lack in the cultivation of seismic culture, perhaps an overreliance on science and engineering, in Wakabayashi. The narratives that connect the generations to the material signs and stories of the past do not get reproduced in isolation, but rather they work in tandem with the most advanced technological systems (which often fail) and scientific knowledge, which tell us only so much. Each town and village practiced seismic culture in a different way. In Kamaishi, leaders heeded stories of the region's 1896 and 1933 quakes and tsunamis that killed thousands and brought in experts to give elementary and junior high school students emergency disaster lessons. When disaster struck on March 11, school microphone systems were knocked out. Students collectively decided to run to an evacuation site that they had learned about. There they met an elderly woman who had seen a cliff behind the evacuation site collapse. Convinced that a huge tsunami would come, she told them to run for higher ground. The older students helped the younger and when they turned back to look, they saw a massive wave engulfing the city (Birmingham and McNeill 2012: 38–39). Transmitted across generations, historical experience combined with state educational programs to give the youngsters the ability to save their own lives.

If systemically collected and analyzed on a wide scale, narrative accounts of survival could provide textual bridges between science-based, official communications, on the one hand, and the more topographically explicit, intergenerational, and popular forms of communication, on the other. This analysis suggests that the effectiveness of disaster communication could be improved by tailoring general seismic knowledge to locally situated, familiar socio-topographic patterns of hazard and safety. As a contribution to scholarly discussion, this chapter illuminates how people consciously engage with deeply embedded cultural dispositions and sensibilities – with emergency habitus – to make their way through infrastructural collapse to survive and reestablish environmental health in the context of sudden environmental change.

Postscript: The *Incendio* of 2014

As I was writing this chapter, a raging fire worked its way up the streambeds of Valparaíso, jumping from hill to hill. Fed by heavy winds and dry brush, the blaze was so enormous that the people in Santiago could see it 140 kilometers away. Fire trucks were stymied by the small winding roads or the lack of roads; when they did get to certain areas, they often faced a lack of operable water pumps. The houses of the hilltop neighborhoods had been legally regularized but remained infrastructure-poor and lacked emergency contingency plans (Gray 2014). With only the clothes on their backs and their children and pets in their arms, thousands ran *down or* across the hills to escape the flames threatening or consuming their homes then turned back to watch in horror from a safe distance.[30] The lesson of this disaster is that, even with the best preparation, the way that social topographies of disaster unfold depends on which and how natural forces and infrastructural shortcomings and breakdowns come into play. The fire disaster reversed the city's characteristic topographical orientation toward earthquake and tsunami evacuation. This strongly indicates that efforts to build effective and sustainable evacuation routes that connect different areas of the city should take into account the interactive patterns of infrastructural instabilities caused by earthquakes, tsunamis, fires, and wind.

ACKNOWLEDGMENTS

Thanks to Eden Medina and her grant from the Center for Applied Cybersecurity Research at Indiana University, Bloomington for funding ethnographic fieldwork in Chile. Special thanks to the people in Valparaíso and Viña del Mar who generously shared their knowledge and experience. Thanks to ethnographic team members Daniel M. Michler, field assistant and technology consultant, and C. Jason Dotson, videographer and editor.

NOTES

1 Although standardized, global technologies do not simply replicate unchanged in specific locales; rather, there is an assertion of, and resistance to, standards that connect landscapes and cities (e.g., Dunn 2005).

2 The nodes and tunnels of the human built environment are so prominent that paleontologists consider using them as markers of the Anthropocene (Williams *et al.* 2013).
3 Internal front is a coast guard term reported by Manuel Cofré Lizana, Captain of the Port. Interviews June 16 and 21, 2011.
4 Reported by Manuel Cofré Lizana, Captain of the Port. Interview June 21, 2011. See Kane *et al.*'s (2015) analysis of how Talcahuano Coast Guard's emergency response was severely limited by the 27/2 tsunami and not restored until the navy ship arrived three days later. See Sims (2010) for analysis of how the New Orleans police struggled to impose moral order without the benefit of communication networks and infrastructural circuits, including lockup facilities, in the floods accompanying Hurricane Katrina.
5 In Japan, which on a 1300-year average, has been hit by a tsunami every seven years, the seawalls protecting coastal cities vary greatly by height and configuration (Birmingham and McNeill 2012: 31, 50–51).
6 Cuban society, which organizes its community members to take special care of individuals who are members of these vulnerable groups, is known for its particularly effective modalities of evacuation in hurricanes (MEDICC Review 2005).
7 For an overview on social science and social studies of science approach to disrupted infrastructure, see Graham (2010).
8 Interview May 28, 2011.
9 Such traditions form the basis for what Chileans may label "instincts" (e.g., Meneses 2010 and Badal 2010, cited Massardo 2010).
10 The project was carried out in tandem with historian Eden Medina working in Santiago.
11 Fieldwork was carried out between May 20 and June 24, 2011 with the assistance of Daniel M. Michler, informatics consultant. We led a discussion with Professor Luciana Alfaro Carrasco's geography students at the University of Viña del Mar. We followed up this event with a class questionnaire administered via e-mail that elicited step-by-step events in the timeframe of the 27/2 earthquake.
12 At 9.5 M, the earthquake released more energy than the eruption of Krakatoa or the world's largest nuclear test, that is, equivalent to over 61 million tons of TNT (Atwater *et al.* 2009: 2–3; Stein 2010: 106).
13 Patricio Catalán Mondaca, professor of civil engineering at Universidad Tecnica Frederico Santa Maria. Interview June 10, 2011.
14 In 2009, seismologists of Japan's National Institute of Advanced Industrial Science and Technology (AIST) were ignored when they tried to warn officials that a massive earthquake that hit the Tohoku coastline in 869 should be considered in the regulation of the nuclear industry. And rather than rely on their own nation's seismic culture and history – especially the 1896 Meiji Sanriku tsunami – Japanese officials used the Valdivia, Chile, tsunami height as standard for sea wall specifications, thereby missing the opportunity to avoid at least some of the tragedies of 2011 (Birmingham and McNeill 2012: 37–39).
15 Interview June 10, 2011.
16 Marco Cisternas, Geógrafo docente de la Escuela de Ciencias del Mar de la Universidad Católica de Valparaíso. Interview, May 30, 2011. See also Cisternas (2005).
17 I include the names of people whom I interviewed as professionals or officials, but protect the privacy of students, neighbors, and others, leaving them unnamed.
18 Interview, May 28.
19 Interview June 10.
20 Reported in class discussion at Universidad del Viña del Mar, June 17.

21 In Chile, this agency is ONEMI. See the action diagram of emergency decision making in Kane, Medina, and Michler (2015).

22 Interview May 28.

23 Interview May 27.

24 See http://volcano.si.edu/world/vol_extra.cfm?name=Papudo

25 http://www.youtube.com/watch?v=sv5UXne10nU

26 The following day, when I interview Amalia's family in their home, her father clarifies: "In old houses like this, a chain embedded in the portals strengthens them, but in new construction, doorways have no chains and should not be considered safe."

27 The first story was reported in class discussion at Universidad del Viña del Mar, June 17. The second story is from the June 21 questionnaire, field notes pp. 84–86.

28 The place-based contributions of local knowledge to human understanding and action have been well established (Geertz 1983). No longer conceptualized by anthropologists as monolithic, culturally bounded, or necessarily rural, local knowledge, like scientific knowledge, is understood to be socially constructed. Inhabitants produce knowledge within powerful hierarchies that connect and divide their localities to and from the wider world (Nygren 1999).

29 Interview June 10.

30 For visual data on the fires of April 12–14, 2014, search YouTube using the term "Incendio Valparaíso."

REFERENCES

Atwater, B.F., *et al.* 2009. *Sobreviviendo a un Tsunami: Lecciones de Chile, Hawai y Japón.* Circular 1218. Department of the Interior and the US Geological Service.

Badal, I. 2010. "Intuición Salvó del Tsunami a Habitantes de un Pueblo del Chile." *Reuters América latina*, March 1.

Barrionuevo, A. 2010. "Aftershocks Jolt Chile as New Presidents is Sworn In." *New York Times*, March 11. http://www.nytimes.com/2010/03/12/world/americas/12chile.html?_r=0 (accessed December 8, 2015).

Basso, K. 1996. *Wisdom Sits in Places: Landscapes and Language Among the Apache.* Albuquerque: University of New Mexico Press.

Benjamin, W. 1999. *The Arcades Project.* Ed. R. Tiedemann. Cambridge, MA: Harvard University Press.

Birmingham, L. and McNeill, D. 2012. *Strong in the Rain: Surviving Japan's Earthquake, Tsunami, and Fukushima Nuclear Disaster.* New York: Palgrave Macmillan.

Bourdieu, P. 1985. *Outline of a Theory of Practice.* Cambridge: Cambridge University Press.

Briggs, C. 2011. "Communicating Biosecurity." *Medical Anthropology*, 30: 1, 6–29.

Castaños, H. and Lomnitz, C. 2012. *Earthquake Disasters in Latin America.* New York: Springer.

Cisternas, M. 2005. "Suelos Enterrados Revelan la Prehistoria Sísmica del Centro-Sur de Chile Durante lost Últimos Dos Milenios." *Revista de Geografía Norte Grande*, 33: 19–31.

De Certeau, M. 1984. *The Practice of Everyday Life.* Trans. S.R. Rendell. Berkeley, CA: University of California Press.

Dunn, E. 2005. "Standards and Person-Making in East Central Europe." In A. Ong and S.J. Collier (Eds.), *Global Assemblages: Technology, Politics, and Ethics as Anthropological Problems* (pp. 173–193). Malden, MA: Blackwell.

Geertz, C. 1983. *Local Knowledge: Further Essays in Interpretive Anthropology.* New York: Basic Books.

Gilbert, C. 1998. "Reply to Hewitt." In E.L. Quarantelli (Ed.), *What Is a Disaster? Perspectives on the Question* (pp. 95–98). New York: Routledge.

Graham, M. 1824/1835. "Of the Reality of the Rise of the Coast of Chile, 1822." *The American Journal of Science and Arts*, 28 (Art. IV): 236–247. https://www.ntu.ac.uk/hum/document_uploads/75932.pdf (accessed December 8, 2015).

Graham, S. 2010. "When Infrastructures Fail." In S. Graham (Ed.), *Disrupted Cities: When Infrastructure Fails* (pp. 1–26). New York: Routledge.

Gray, S. 2014. "El Incendio Es Resultado de una Completa Irresponsabilidad que Se Ha Ido Acumulando con El Paso de los Años." *El Mostrador*, April 14. http://www.elmostrador.cl/pais/2014/04/14/el-incendio-es-resultado-de-una-completa-irresponsabilidad-que-se-ha-ido-acumulando-con-el-paso-de-los-anos/ (accessed December 8, 2015).

Gupta, A. and Ferguson, J. (Eds.) 1997. *Culture, Power, Place: Explorations in Critical Anthropology*. Durham, NC: Duke University Press.

Han, C. 2010. "Earthquakes in Chile: Poverty and Social Diagnosis." *Latin American Studies Association Forum*, 41(3): 9.

Humboldt State University. 2010. *Preliminary Tsunami Survey Team Report, April 3.* http://www.eqclearinghouse.org/co/20100227-chile/wp-content/uploads/2010/04/dengler_itst_hsu_preliminary_team_report1.pdf (accessed December 8, 2015).

Kaika, M. and Swyngedouw, E. 2000. "Fetishizing the Modern City: The Phantasmagoria of Urban Technological Networks." *International Journal of Urban and Regional Research*, 24(1): 122–148.

Kane, S.C. 2012. *Where Rivers Meet the Sea: The Political Ecology of Water*. Philadelphia, PA: Temple University Press.

Kane, S.C., Medina, E., and Michler, D. 2015. "Infrastructural Drift in Seismic Cities: Chile, Pacific Rim, 27 February 2010. *Social Text*, 122: 71–92.

Kreps, G.A. 1998. "Disaster as Systemic Event and Social Catalyst." In E.L. Quarantelli (Ed.), *What Is a Disaster? Perspectives on the Question* (pp. 31–55). New York: Routledge.

Larkin, B. 2013. "The Politics and Poetics of Infrastructure." *Annual Review of Anthropology*, 42: 327–343.

Latour, B. 1993. *We Have Never Been Modern*. Cambridge, MA: Harvard University Press.

Levebvre, H. 1991. *The Production of Space*. Trans. D. Nicholson-Smith. Malden, MA: Blackwell.

Low, S.M. and Lawrence-Zuñiga, D. 2003. *The Anthropology of Space and Place: Locating Culture*. Malden, MA: Blackwell.

Massardo, J. 2010. "El Terremoto en Chile: Una Manifestaciónde la Naturalezque Deja el Desnudo al Funcionamiento del Sistema." In *El Terremoto Social del Bicentenario*, 159–179. Santiago del Chile: Bolsillo.

MEDICC. 2005. *In the Eye of the Storm: Disaster Management Lessons from Cuba*. MEDICC Review: Health and Medical News of Cuba. http://www.medicc.org/resources/documents/medicc-review-disaster-management.pdf (accessed December 8, 2015).

Meneses, A. 2010. "Valparaíso: Porteños a Los Cerros por Alerta de Tsunami." *La Nación*, March 11.

Monstadt, J. 2009. "Conceptualizing the Political Ecology of Urban Infrastructures: Insights from Technology and Urban Studies." *Environment and Planning*, 41(8): 1924–1942.

Nygren, A. 1999. "Local Knowledge in the Environment-Development Discourse: From Dichotomies to Situated Knowledges." *Critique of Anthropology*, 19: 267–288.

Oliver-Smith, A. 1998. "Global Changes and the Definition of Disaster." In E.L. Quarantelli (Ed.), *What Is a Disaster? Perspectives on the Question* (pp. 177–194). New York: Routledge.

Raffles, H. 2002. *In Amazonia: A Natural History.* Princeton, NJ: Princeton University Press.

Raichlen, F. 2013. *Waves.* Cambridge, MA: MIT Press.

Scarry, E. 2012. *Thinking in an Emergency.* New York: Norton.

Schoch-Spana, M., Franco, C., Nuzzo, J.B., and Usenza, C. 2007. "Community Engagement: Leadership Tool for Catastrophic Health Events. *Biosecurity and Bioterrorism: Biodefense Strategy, Practice, and Science*, 5(1): 8–25.

Sims, B. 2010. "Things Fall Apart: Disaster, Infrastructure, Order, and the New Orleans Police Department's Response to Hurricane Katrina." *Social Studies of Science*, 37(1): 111–118.

Stein, S. 2010. *Disaster Deferred: How New Science Is Changing Our View of Earthquake Hazards in the Midwest.* New York: Columbia University Press.

Tuan, Y.-F. 1977. *Space and Place: The Perspective of Experience.* Minneapolis: University of Minnesota Press.

Williams, Mark, Zalasiewicz, J.A., Waters, C.N., and Landing, E. (Eds.) 2013. "Is the Fossil Record of Complex Animal Behavior a Stratigraphical Analogue of the Anthropocene?" *Geological Society, London, Special Publications*, 395. 10.1144/SP395.8 (accessed December 8, 2015).

Williams, R. 1977. *Marxism and Literature.* New York: Oxford University Press.

Yamazaki, Y. and Cheung, K.F. 2011. "Shelf Resonance and Impact of Near-field Tsunami Generated by the 2010 Chile Earthquake." *Geophysical Research Letters*, 38: 1.

PART IV

Adverse Feedback Loops in Environmental Health

CHAPTER 18

Modifying Our Microbial Environment: From the Advent of Agriculture to the Age of Antibiotic Resistance

Kristin N. Harper,
Gabriela M. Sheets, and
George J. Armelagos

Introduction

Tens of thousands of years ago, modern humans left Africa and expanded their terrestrial range dramatically. As they colonized every continent but Antarctica, they adjusted to a vast array of new ecological niches, from mountain valleys to swamps to deserts. After millions of years of hunting and foraging, around 10,000 years ago some cultures began to practice agriculture, and population density increased as this new development spread. Settlements turned into cities, and cities turned into metropolises. Growing populations placed major demands upon the surrounding environment. Forests were chopped down and wetlands drained. As humans wrought these changes upon their external habitat, equally

A Companion to the Anthropology of Environmental Health, First Edition. Edited by Merrill Singer.

dramatic (but less visible) changes occurred to their internal environment. New exposures, changing diet, improved hygiene, and medical advances have resulted in dramatic shifts in the composition of the microbial partners of many populations. Here, we explore the trends that characterize humanity's last several million years of history through the lens of the epidemiologic transition model, investigating how modification of the environment has often resulted in unintended changes at the microscopic level.

The Epidemiologic Transition Theory

The epidemiologic transition theory was developed by Abdel Omran (1971) to explain the trends in infectious disease epidemiology he had identified in Western European nations. He divided history into three epidemiologic phases: (1) the Age of Pestilence and Famine; (2) the Age of Receding Pandemics; and (3) the Age of Degenerative and Man-made Diseases. In the first phase, infectious diseases were rife and, together with malnutrition, a source of high mortality. Life during this age conformed to Hobbes's description of life in a state of nature: nasty, brutish, and short. In the second phase, postindustrial advances in medicine, hygiene, and food production reduced infectious disease mortality. Finally, in the third phase, which peaked in the twentieth century, chronic diseases, such as diabetes and cardiovascular disease, replaced infectious diseases as important sources of mortality. Each phase in the model represents a dramatically different environment with its own disease ecology.

Other researchers have since refined Omran's original model. Assessment of paleopathological markers of health, such as linear enamel hypoplasia and cribra orbitalia, indicate that health was actually relatively good for much of human history. Markers of infection and nutritional deficiency did not increase until the advent of agriculture (Steckel and Rose 2002; Cohen and Armelagos 2013), a result of growing dependence on a small number of crops and the appearance of high-density settlements. Thus, Barrett *et al.* (1998) presented a new model, in which agriculture spurred the first epidemiologic transition, leading to Omran's Age of Pestilence and Famine. Other investigators, focusing on non-Western nations, have drawn attention to the fact that epidemiologic transitions proceed differently in different places. For example, a more rapid progression through the stages has characterized some countries in which the second transition arrived later (Mackenbach 1994). And some low-income countries are currently experiencing multiple transitions simultaneously, with an increasing chronic disease burden joining the still-substantial risk of death from infection or malnutrition. We presented an in-depth exploration of the nuances of the epidemiologic transition theory in Harper and Armelagos (2010).

More recently, we have broadened the model's traditional focus on pathogen exposure to include beneficial or commensal microorganisms (Harper and Armelagos 2013). Increasingly, we are coming to appreciate the role of the microbiome, or the "ecological community of commensal, symbiotic, and pathogenic microorganisms that literally share our body space," as a determinant of health (Lederberg and McCray 2001). Once developed, the genetic composition of our gut microflora is unique and quite stable through time, similar to a fingerprint (Schloissnig *et al.* 2013). Though the collection of microbes in our gut varies quite a bit from person to person, the assembly of species within each of us tends to carry out similar roles (Turnbaugh *et al.* 2009, Qin *et al.* 2010). A dysbiotic, or imbalanced, microbial community has been linked to a number of diseases, including obesity (Turnbaugh *et al.* 2009; Le Chatelier *et al.* 2013), diabetes (Qin *et al.* 2012; Karlsson *et al.* 2013), malnutrition (Smith *et al.* 2013), cancer (Kostic *et al.* 2012; Geng *et al.* 2013), inflammatory bowel disease (Qin *et al.* 2010), and a growing list of other ailments. We now know that microbes play pivotal roles in a diverse array of physiological activities, including metabolism, vitamin synthesis, and immunity (Kau *et al.* 2011).

Just as the human pathogen-scape has been transformed by the many physical and social changes we have wrought upon our environment, so has the broader human microbe-scape. We are just beginning to understand the potential health implications of these changes. A better understanding of humans' changing microbial environment will not only lead to a more complete picture of the historical interactions between humans and microbes but may contribute to important health interventions.

The First Epidemiologic Transition: Agriculture and the Microbiome

The transition from a foraging subsistence to an agriculture-based society was accompanied by dramatic changes in the microbiome. First, close proximity to newly domesticated animals resulted in an increase in cross-species transfer events, introducing novel microbes into human populations. A few examples of pathogens that appear to have originated in domesticated animals include measles (Furuse, Suzuki, and Oshitani 2010), rotavirus A (Martella *et al.* 2010; Ghosh and Kobayashi 2011), influenza, and *Trichinella spiralis* (Rosenthal *et al.* 2008). While these species of pathogen came to permanently reside in humans, many more microbes are continually passed back and forth between humans and the animals they live with, as is illustrated by current populations living in close contact with domesticated animals. Studies of the Amazonian Wayera, for example, suggest that *Candida albicans*, a commensal yeast species that is also an opportunistic pathogen, is transmitted between humans and their domesticated animals (Angebault *et al.* 2013). In addition, research on humans and cattle living near Lake Victoria in Uganda indicates that considerable microbial exchange occurs between the two species (Ellis *et al.* 2013). Finally, we are all familiar with the outbreaks of pathogens such as *E. coli* 0157 and *Salmonella* that can be traced back to feed animals.

In addition, agriculture reshaped the external environment in which practitioners lived. For example, anthropologist Frank Livingstone (1971) asserted that malaria became hyperendemic in West Africa only after slash-and-burn agriculture became common there. He had observed the mosquito that transmits malaria,

Anopheles gambiae, breeding in the man-made spaces created by this form of agriculture. His prediction that breeding spaces produced by agriculture were necessary to support the *A. gambiae* lifestyle, and thus malaria transmission, has largely been borne out by the research. One way that investigators have studied the history of *Plasmodium falciparum*, the protozoa that causes malaria, is by tracing the development of human genetic resistance to the parasite. Studies have shown that the more intense the reliance on slash-and-burn agriculture, the higher the prevalence of sickle cell trait (Wisenfeld 1967; Piel *et al.* 2010). In addition, the A polymorphism of the *G6PD* gene, which confers protection against malaria, is estimated to have arisen roughly 12,000–4000 YBP, consistent with the adoption of slash-and-burn agriculture (Tishkoff *et al.* 2001).

There are other examples of infections transmitted via the activity of farming, of course. Irrigation and dams are an efficient means of transmitting schistosomiasis, a parasitic worm infection that represents a major source of morbidity in many low-income countries (Brinkmann, Korte, and Schmidt-Ehry 1988; Talla *et al.* 1990). The parasite's eggs hatch in water contaminated with the feces of the infected; the larval form then penetrates a new victim's skin. It has also been hypothesized that the introduction of cattle into formerly forested areas may drive vampire bats to shift from feeding on forest animals to cattle – and, if cattle are not in sufficient supply, to nearby humans (Stoner-Duncan, Streicker, and Tedeschi 2014). Changes in cattle density in rural, forest communities may help explain the clusters of vampire bat–transmitted rabies that are becoming more frequent in South America.

Increasing population density also exposed agricultural societies to a novel set of microbes. In the Paleolithic, hominid populations were small and widely dispersed. Early agricultural villages were also relatively small. For example, settlements in the Iraqi foothills of the Zagros mountains are estimated to have had only about 150 residents (Braidwood and Braidwood 1950). By 4500 YBP, however, the population of Ur in Mesopotamia was 350,000 (Woolley 1965). With time, settlements grew even larger, and so did the opportunities for crowd diseases. Genetic analysis suggests that measles arose from the rinderpest virus, which infects cattle, around the eleventh to twelfth century YBP (Furuse, Suzuki, and Oshitani 2010), and it has been estimated that measles requires a population of at least 300,000 in order to maintain a transmission chain (Grenfell and Bolker 1998). Thus, a combination of proximity to domesticated animals and high-density settlements appears to have provided the conditions in which it could emerge. Similarly, analysis of existing smallpox viruses suggests that they diverged from a rodent virus 3000–4000 YBP, possibly in the Horn of Africa (Shchelkunov 2009; Babkin and Babkina 2012).

Finally, the transition from foraging to agriculture altered the diet of farmers and thus the composition of their microflora. It has been estimated that over the course of history, humans have used over 5000 plants as food sources (Reid and Miller 1989). However, by the late twentieth century, just three species – wheat, rice, and corn – accounted for roughly 70 percent of the calories and 55 percent of the proteins humans consumed (Reid and Miller 1989). Historically, communities that rely heavily on a few crops have often experienced nutritional deficiencies. A problem in and of itself, compromised nutrition can increase susceptibility to infections as well (Mensforth *et al.* 1978; Scrimshaw 2003, 2010; Cohen and Armelagos 2013), increasing the representation of pathogens in the microflora. In addition, diet is an important determinant of nonpathogenic species. For example, the consumption of proteins and animal fats favors higher levels of bacterial groups such as *Bacteroides*, while carbohydrates are associated with groups such as *Prevotella*, which can efficiently extract energy from grains (Wu *et al.* 2005).

Based on these trends, we might predict that the transition to agriculture would (a) decrease microbial diversity, (b) increase the proportion of *Prevotella* species in the gut, and (c) increase *Bifidobacteria* at later stages in the lifecycle, as these bacteria aid in the digestion of dairy products. Directly testing whether these predictions are correct has proved difficult, as only one ancient DNA (aDNA) study has investigated pre-agricultural remains. Adler *et al.* (2013) compared dental plaque from the Mesolithic, and from agricultural groups from the Neolithic, the Middle Ages, and the present day. They showed that the microbial composition of all post-agriculture groups formed a cluster distinct from Mesolithic samples, emphasizing the shift that took place in the dental microbiome. An alternative approach has been to investigate the microbiota of modern hunter-gatherers. A recent study identified significant differences between the gut microbiomes of the Hadza of Tanzania and rural African agriculturalists (Schnorr *et al.* 2014). The proportion of unclassified bacteria (33%) in the Hadza microbiome highlights the potential for biodiversity in this niche. In addition, unlike other human groups analyzed to date, a significant difference in the microflora of males and females was observed among the Hadza. It is believed this may be related to dietary differences stemming from the division of labor between the sexes in this population. The absence of *Bifidobacteria* in adult Hadza samples suggests that the discontinuation of dairy after infancy in this group eliminates these bacteria from the intestine. Finally, as predicted, a study found that the saliva microbiome of the Batwa Pygmies of Uganda, who only recently abandoned their hunter-gathering lifestyle, was significantly more diverse than that of agriculturalists in Sierra Leone and the Democratic Republic of Congo (Nasidze *et al.* 2011).

Other clues about microbial shifts characteristic of the first epidemiologic transition are emerging. Coprolites from an agricultural Mexican site (1400 YBP) were found to be rich in *Prevotella*, similar to modern agriculturalist samples from rural Malawi and the Venezuelan Amazon (Tito *et al.* 2012). The gut microbiome of Ötzi, the Tyrolean iceman, was also found to be similar to that of modern-day non-Western agriculturalists (Tito *et al.* 2012). This suggests considerable continuity between the gut microbiomes of ancient and modern non-Western agriculture communities. Recently, aDNA studies of coprolites have provided insight into the viral composition of the gut of our farming ancestors as well. Analysis of a fourteenth-century coprolite recovered from a site in Belgium revealed that the majority of viral genomes within belonged to bacteriophages (Appelt *et al.* 2014). Many of these carried metabolic genes that would enable their bacterial hosts to process fats and amino acids, indicating that the role of viruses in metabolism must not be overlooked.

Thus, the novel environment associated with agriculture in the first epidemiologic transition introduced new pathogens and provided a context in which they could reproduce. In addition, the composition of agriculturalists' microflora changed, as diets became increasingly dependent on carbohydrates and substantially less diverse.

The Second Epidemiologic Transition: A Short-lived Reprieve from Infections

In recent decades, improved hygiene and medical advances have afforded high-income nations the power to modify their microbial environments at will, although, as will be discussed, there have been unintended consequences. In these countries, morbidity and mortality related to infections have decreased dramatically as a result of these developments. These changes, along with improvements in nutrition, constitute the second epidemiologic transition. The period following the establishment of the germ theory was a magical time for many Western nations. In the United States, for example, the crude infectious disease mortality rate declined from 800/100,000 per year in 1900 to 59/100,000 in 1996 (Armstrong, Conn, and Pinner 1999). Once-fatal diseases, such as syphilis, went from killing roughly 11/100,000 people per year in 1900 to zero following the discovery of penicillin (ibid.). The same was true of vaccine-preventable diseases such as diphtheria, which once killed >40/100,000 people per year, pertussis (>10/100,000 per year), and measles (>10,100,000 per year; ibid.). Although deaths attributable to infection were declining even prior to the use of vaccines and antibiotics, due to improvements in living conditions (McKeown 1979), these discoveries helped put an end to the reign of many pathogens in the West.

Antibiotics seemed a dream come true: They revolutionized the treatment of infections by rapidly eliminating once life-threatening pathogens. In recent decades, however, appreciation of the structure and function of symbiotic microbiota coupled with surges in antibiotic-resistant pathogens have complicated the issue. Research indicates that weeks and even months after completing antibiotic treatment, the original microflora of the mouth have not been restored (Dethlefsen and Relman 2011; Lazarevic *et al.* 2013). Similarly, following short-term antibiotic treatment, the level of drug-resistant genes in the gut remains elevated for years (Löfmark *et al.* 2006; Jernberg *et al.* 2007; Jakobbson *et al.* 2010). Moreover, antibiotic treatment can lead to adverse feedback loops, in which one infection leads to another. For example, healthy individuals carry potentially pathogenic microbes such as *Escherichia coli*, yeast, *Staphylococcus aureus*, and *Clostridium difficile*. However, disturbances, such as antibiotic treatment, that alter the community composition of the gut can allow these microbes to proliferate, causing disease. Antibiotic treatment is a well-known risk factor for *C. difficile*, an infection that kills 14,000 Americans a year (CDC 2013). Disturbances in the gut microflora can also make people more susceptible to the introduction of pathogens; the infectious dose of *Salmonella*, that is, the number of bacteria required to establish infection, is 1000-fold lower for individuals on antibiotics (Reid and Greene 2013).

Hygiene also led to a change in the composition of the microbial communities of societies undergoing the second epidemiologic transition. Rural to urban migration, declining subsistence farming, and public health campaigns all influenced patterns of microbial exposure during early childhood. The hygiene hypothesis posits that these changes have had an unfortunate side effect. A reduction in early childhood exposure to pathogenic and/or commensal microbes may have caused alterations in the immune system that trigger susceptibility to allergy and other chronic diseases later in life (Strachan 1989; Yazdanbakhsh, Kremsner, and Ree 2002; Zuckerman and Armelagos 2014). This hypothesis is controversial and is continually being revised (Liu and Murphy 2003; Matricardi 2010; Cramer *et al.* 2012); currently, the role of early microbial exposures, both pathogenic and symbiotic, in specific later-life diseases is being investigated.

One outcome of such research is that we are learning more about the complex roles that a single species can play in the microbiome. The prevalence of *Helicobacter pylori* infection has decreased markedly in high-income countries in recent decades, due to antibiotic treatment and improved hygiene (Roosendaal *et al.* 1997; Fujisawa *et al.* 1999; Apostolopoulos *et al.* 2002). *H. pylori* causes gastric cancer (Graham *et al.* 1992; Fuccio *et al.* 2009), and its declining prevalence has resulted in a concomitant decline in gastric cancer incidence, as might be expected. At the same time, esophageal cancer rates have been increasing (Thrift and Whiteman 2012). It is now thought that in addition to causing gastric cancer, *H. pylori* may protect against acid reflux, and thus against Barrett's esophagus and esophageal cancer (Corley *et al.* 2008; Thrift *et al.* 2012). Thus, this single pathogen, which has infected humans since our origins in Africa, is both friend and foe. What seemed like a simple solution to preventing gastric cancer – eliminating *H. pylori* infection – has turned out to be more complicated than we imagined.

In summary, the second epidemiologic transition set the microbial stage for modern life in high-income countries. Modern urban environments transformed the way that a large proportion of the world's population lived. Deaths from pathogens declined with the advent of antibiotics, vaccines, and improved hygiene. However, the declining prevalence of certain pathogens, such as *H. pylori*, revealed their dual role, raising the possibility they may provide health benefits. In addition, environments that minimized microbe exposure, particularly in early childhood, may have altered the representation of important commensal microbes.

The Third Epidemiologic Transition: Chronic Diseases Meet Antibiotic-resistant Infections

While antibiotics offered an almost miraculous solution to bacterial infections, there was quickly reason to think that the respite they offered might be temporary. Mass production of penicillin began in the mid-1940s, and penicillin resistance quickly followed. In 1946, 14 percent of *S. aureus* strains isolated at Hammersmith Hospital in London were resistant to penicillin; two short years later, resistance had climbed to 59 percent (Barber and Rozwadowska-Dowzenko 1948). It appears that sources for antibiotic resistance genes were abundant long before penicillin was discovered; one recent study demonstrated that fourteenth-century European bacteriophage carried many antibiotic resistance genes – more, even, than have been found in modern stool samples (Appelt *et al.* 2014). Thus, perhaps it is not surprising that, post-antibiotic treatment, the number of antibiotic resistance genes in the gut is elevated for years (Löfmark *et al.* 2006; Jernberg *et al.* 2007; Jakobbson *et al.* 2010).

Hospital-associated microbial resistance has received extensive attention. In laboratories in England and Wales, penicillin resistance in *Streptococcus pneumoniae*, a major cause of pneumonia, increased 2.4 percentage points between 1990 and 1995; resistance to erythromycin increased 4.8 percentage points over the same time period (Johnson *et al.* 1996). In US hospitals, the proportion of methicillin-resistant *S. aureus* strains increased from 2.4 percent in 1975 to 29 percent in 1991 (Panlilio *et al.* 1992). While *S. aureus* infections represent an important public health problem in low-income countries as well, little is known about the frequency of resistance outside of high-income nations (Nickerson *et al.* 2009).

The prevalence of antibiotic-resistant bacteria also has increased in healthy individuals. A study of Nigerian students found that the prevalence of *E. coli* isolates resistant to tetracycline, ampicillin, chloramphenicol, and streptomycin increased from 9–35 percent in 1986 to 56–100 percent in 1998 (Okeke, Fayinka, and Lamikanra 2000). In a 2005 study of over 3000 children in Peru and Bolivia, over 90 percent of commensal *E. coli* strains were resistant to ampicillin, trimethoprim-sulfamethoxazole, and tetracycline; 90 percent exhibited a multidrug-resistant phenotype (Bartoloni *et al.* 2006). Though the residents of low-income countries are less likely to reap the benefits of the second epidemiologic transition, the carriage of resistant strains seems to be amplified in such populations. In one comparative study, nearly half the children studied in Boston (18 of 39) had no antibiotic-resistant *E. coli* strains, while all but 1 of 41 children from Caracas and all but 2 of 53 children from Qin Pu, China carried resistant strains (Lester *et al.* 1990). Resistance to five or more antibiotics was observed in 20 percent of Qin Pu strains and 6 percent of Caracas strains, but no Boston strains (ibid.).

As a result of the growing problem of antibiotic resistance, physicians are running out of options for treating patients with formerly treatable infections. Consider the case of extensively drug-resistant tuberculosis, or XDR-TB. Between 2000 and 2004, analysis of strains worldwide showed that roughly 20 percent of TB strains were multi-drug resistant (MDR) (CDC 2006). MDR-TB is a serious problem, but it pales in comparison to XDR-TB, which is resistant to the two most powerful anti-TB drugs, isoniazid and rifampicin, as well as fluroquinolones and at least one of the three injectable second-line drugs (amikacin, capreomycin, or kanamycin) (WHO 2012). This is problematic for a number of reasons. First, because the pathogen is resistant to most antibiotics, obtaining effective antibiotics is a challenge in many places in the world – especially places where XDR-TB is common. Moreover, the few drugs that do work are less effective and often have serious side effects. Finally, the cost of treating XDR-TB infections is extremely high. In the United States, the cost of hospitalizing one XDR-TB patient is estimated at almost $500,000, roughly twice the cost of treating an MDR-TB patient (LoBue, Sizemore, and Castro 2009). Of MDR-TB strains, 4 percent in the US, 19 percent in Latvia, and 15 percent in South Korea were XDR in a 2006 survey (CDC 2006). A person can develop XDR-TB via two routes: (a) insufficient treatment for TB, due to either medication noncompliance or ineffective antibiotics; or (b) by contracting XDR-TB directly from someone who has it. Unfortunately, it is estimated that only 3 percent of MDR-TB cases are currently being treated according to WHO standards (WHO 2009). This is not surprising when one considers the average treatment regimen: 13,664 pills and 244 shots over 28 months, which cause serious side effects in 33 percent of patients (Doucleff 2013). In a resource-poor environment, this type of treatment is often beyond reach. Thus, widespread treatment failure continues to create an environment conducive to the evolution of XDR-TB strains.

Interest in alternatives to antibiotics has been growing. For example, fecal transplants are gaining increasing acceptance as a first-line treatment for *C. difficile*. A recent randomized controlled trial had to be stopped early, after fecal transplants were shown to be a significantly more effective treatment, resolving 81 percent of infections versus 31 percent for vancomycin (van Nood *et al.* 2013). Similarly, transplantation of the gut microbiota from healthy, lean subjects improves insulin signaling in patients with metabolic syndrome (Vrieze *et al.* 2012). In addition, bacteriophage therapy, or treatment with viruses that target pathogenic bacteria, is receiving a new wave of attention. Popular in the Soviet Union in the early twentieth century, phage therapy became discredited in the West after early studies proved disappointing. As the problem of antibiotic resistance grows and the desire for more targeted therapies increases, however, more researchers have begun to investigate the potential of phage therapy. One recent study indicated that phage treatment was effective in treating chronic ear infections caused by antibiotic-resistant *Pseudomonas aeruginosa* (Wright *et al.* 2009). There has also been a case report of phage being used to treat a refractory urinary tract infection caused by *P. aeruginosa* (Khawaldeh *et al.* 2011), and animal experiments suggest that, someday, phage may also be used to treat *Pseudomonas* infections in cystic fibrosis patients (Morello *et al.* 2011). Finally, it has become clear that people are interested in using probiotics, or supplements that contain microorganisms with a perceived benefit, to alter the microbiome and improve health. In 2011, $770 million of probiotics were sold in the United States (Reddy 2012). Randomized controlled trials have shown that probiotics can help prevent acute diarrhea in children and adults (Sazawal *et al.* 2006), reduce infant gut inflammation and thus crying time (Savino *et al.* 2007), relieve IBS symptoms (Moayyedi *et al.* 2010), and treat atopic dermatitis (Michail *et al.* 2008). However, the optimal strains and doses for treatment remain unclear, and, not surprisingly, it appears that the treatment must be carefully matched to the disease targeted (Ritchie and Romanuk 2012). Moreover, commercially available preparations often do not contain the strains advertised at the levels described, and not all are effective at treating illness (Canani *et al.* 2007). For example, one study of European probiotics found that 10 of 24 preparations did not contain the amount of bacteria advertised (Toscano *et al.* 2013). In four of the preparations, no viable colonies of an advertised bacterial species were found (ibid.).

We are also coming to better understand the feedback loops governing the microbes that inhabit our body. As discussed, imbalances in the microbiome have been linked to a variety of diseases, including inflammatory diseases (Qin *et al.* 2010), metabolic conditions (Qin *et al.* 2012; Karlsson *et al.* 2013), and cancer (Kostic *et al.* 2012; Geng *et al.* 2013). Does this mean that the shifts cause the disease – or that the shifts result from the disease? In the case of obesity, animal experiments are starting to clarify some of these relationships, demonstrating causal relationships between our diet, the microbiome, and metabolism. When germ-free mice are inoculated with the microflora of obese mice, they gain more weight than those inoculated with the microflora of lean controls, even when both groups receive the same amount of food (Turnbaugh *et al.* 2006). This highlights the role of microbes in digestion and metabolism. In addition, two months of eating a Western diet transforms the composition of the mouse microbiome (Turnbaugh *et al.* 2008). Again, taking this acquired high-fat microbiome and transferring it to another mouse will cause that mouse to gain weight. Thus, diet drives changes in the microbiome that result in weight gain, and weight gain, in turn, increases caloric requirements, which influence diet. This represents a powerful positive feedback loop.

By contrast, negative feedback loops are thought to play an important role in stabilizing microflora composition and, perhaps, maximizing diversity. In negative feedback, an organism alters its own environment in a way that decreases its fitness, thus keeping its growth in check. One example of this type of feedback loop comes from the guts of infants; the higher redox potential of their gut facilitates the growth of facultative anaerobes such as *E. coli* and some *Lactobacillus* species early in development. These species reduce the amount of oxygen available, however, which favors their replacement by strict anaerobes, resulting in the maturation of the microbial composition of the gut (Stark and Lee 1982).

Along with antibiotic use and adult eating habits, early childrearing environments have changed dramatically in the third epidemiologic transition, interrupting the vertical inheritance of microbiota from parent to offspring. Although little is known about the transmission of microbes in the womb, the fetal microbiome is becoming a focus of study (Funkhouser and Bordenstein 2013). It has been shown that an infant's first postpartum bowel movement, which consists of amniotic fluid ingested in utero, contains an array of gut bacteria, and studies in mice demonstrate that *Enterococcus* strains ingested by a mother can be transmitted to her fetus in the womb (Jiménez *et al.* 2008). In addition, the composition of the placental microflora is linked to factors such as prenatal infections and preterm birth (Aagaard *et al.* 2014). Afterward, birth mode further contributes to the infant's initial exposure to maternal microbes. Across multiple body sites, babies delivered vaginally develop a microbiome that mirrors that found in their mother's vagina (Dominguez-Bello *et al.* 2010). In addition, the guts of vaginally delivered infants host *Bifidobacterium* strains seeded from their mothers' gut microflora (Makino *et al.* 2013). By contrast, babies delivered via C-section have a body microflora that resembles that found on their mother's skin (Dominguez-Bello *et al.* 2010). Strikingly, differences in the microflora linked to delivery mode are still evident in 7-year-old children (Penders *et al.* 2006).

After delivery, early feeding becomes a primary selector of infant bacteria, with breast milk or formula providing nutrients for the maintenance and growth of microbial communities (Blaut and Clavel 2007). The third epidemiologic transition witnessed widespread adoption of formula, which revolutionized infant feeding practices. In 2006, for example, only about 30 percent of 3-month-old babies in the United States were exclusively breastfed; by 6 months, this number fell to 10 percent (OECD 2009). The gut microbiome of breast-fed infants is typically high in *Bifidobacteria* and *Lactobacilli*. Formula-fed infants, by contrast, harbor a microbiome that is initially more diverse and complex, but less stable (Rautava *et al.* 2012). It is believed that these differences are related to the bioactive components of breast milk, which serves as a source of *Bifidobacteria* and *Lactobacilli* (Marques *et al.* 2010) and promotes the maintenance and growth of these beneficial bacteria via the oligosaccharides it contains (Chierici *et al.* 2003).

The functional importance of gut microbiome differences in infants is not yet well understood. It is known that children of normal weight have higher levels of fecal *Bifidobacteria* as infants than obese children do (Kalliomäki *et al.* 2008). While future research should clarify these issues, it is concerning to think that differences in C-section and breastfeeding rates by socioeconomic status and race (Forste, Weiss, and Lippincott 2001; Leeb *et al.* 2005; Amir and Donath 2008) may underlie health inequalities that begin as early as the delivery room. Such findings would further contribute to evidence that the foundation for the chronic health conditions that characterize the third epidemiologic transition, such as obesity and diabetes, is established quite early (Curhan *et al.* 1996; Boney *et al.* 2005; Pirkola *et al.* 2010; Laitinen *et al.* 2012). Moreover, C-section rates are skyrocketing in many low- and middle-income nations, accounting for 46 percent of births in Brazil and 42 percent in Iran and the Dominican Republic (Gibbons *et al.* 2010). The percentage of exclusively breastfed four-month-old babies is also extremely small in many low- and middle-income countries, including Chad (2%), Djibouti (2%), Suriname (3%), Gabon (7%), Burkina Faso (8%), Venezuela (7%), and Thailand (8%) (UNICEF 2009). Clearly, more research on the health effects of changes to the early dietary environment is needed.

Diet has also played a role in shaping the adult microbiome in the third epidemiologic transition. If the first and second epidemiologic transitions led to a decrease in the diversity of microbial communities, the Western diet appears to have led to an even greater narrowing of that diversity. Analysis of dental plaque samples indicates that phylogenetic diversity is significantly lower in modern samples than in Mesolithic or even Neolithic samples; moreover, the prevalence of cariogenic bacterial species, such as *Streptococcus mutans*, is higher in modern samples (Adler *et al.* 2013). Similarly, a number of studies have shown that the Western gut microbiome is less diverse than those found in non-Western agriculturalist populations in Dhaka, rural Malawi, and the Venezuelan Amazon (Yatsunenko *et al.* 2012; Lin *et al.* 2013). Comparisons of Western and non-Western agriculturalist populations also suggest that gut microbiomes resulting from high-fat, high-protein diets are enriched in *Bacteroides* species (Lin *et al.* 2013), although it remains unclear what effect this might have on health. Although there has been much interest in the association between specific gut microbes and obesity, as has been noted, it has been difficult to elucidate consistent trends. However, a study of obese and lean twins in the United States has shown decreased bacterial diversity in the feces of obese participants (Turnbaugh *et al.* 2009). Moreover, a decrease in gut bacterial richness is associated with metabolic dysfunction, including insulin resistance, as well as obesity (Le Chatelier *et al.* 2013).

In short, as the third epidemiologic transition unfolds in an environment where both antibiotics and infections are plentiful, there has been an increase in antibiotic resistance and rising interest in antibiotic alternatives that capitalize on our growing knowledge of the microbiome. In addition, we are gradually beginning to elucidate the complicated relationships between diet, microflora, and health outcomes. Changes to the early life environment, including birthing and nursing practices, have altered the establishment of the microflora. Meanwhile, the Western diet continues to influence the composition of the gut microbiome into adulthood. Finally, it is important to note that a number of other important disease trends, which we are not able to explore at length in this chapter, characterize the third epidemiologic transition. For example, novel zoonotic infections, emerging as humans increasingly encroach on animal habitat, have come to dominate the face of emerging infectious diseases (Jones *et al.* 2008; Zuckerman *et al.* 2014). Simultaneously, the process of globalization is allowing both novel and established pathogens to spread at heretofore unprecedented scales and rates (Barrett *et al.* 1998; Harper and Armelagos 2010). Nading (2014), for example, has documented the process by which the dengue virus quickly became entrenched in Nicaragua after the global trash trade reintroduced its mosquito vector, *Aedes aegypti*, into Central America. Singer (2010) has argued that the third epidemiologic transition is increasingly characterized by the syndemic interaction of infectious and other diseases, driven by processes such as globalization, global warming, and social factors such as poverty and discrimination. In the midst of this upheaval, many researchers hope to gain information that will allow us to modify the internal environment to optimize health, turning back the clock on some of the changes that have occurred as a result of epidemiologic transitions.

Conclusion

Emerging research on the microbiome is shifting how we view the role of microbes in our lives. Wide-scale environmental changes since the advent of agriculture have transformed the microbial ecology of the majority of the world's people.

The community structure of intestinal microbiomes in high-income countries is significantly less diverse than that of non-Western agriculturalists, and likely hunter-gatherers. Nascent understanding of the form and function of our microbial partners is broadening our concepts of health and disease. Although the human genome cannot keep pace with the rapid dietary, ecological, and technological changes occurring globally, it is possible that the human microbiome can. Many researchers anticipate that by learning more about our microbiomes, we can develop innovative and culturally appropriate health interventions. The narrowing in taxonomic diversity seen in Western populations has raised concerns. Some have questioned whether this reduced diversity could result in the loss of microbes that confer important health benefits (Lozupone *et al.* 2012). As the Western diet goes global, this loss of microbes may as well. Researchers have called for the preservation of microbial DNA from a range of environments (Fuerst and Hugenholtz 2000), and the human body should be one of the sites sampled.

The environmental changes that have resulted from humanity's success in expanding across the planet have created complicated feedback loops governing the composition of the microbes inside us. Some of the changes, such as the relative freedom of many high-income populations from epidemic infections such as smallpox and measles, are universally viewed as beneficial. Others, such as changes in the microflora that appear to predispose high-income populations to obesity and diabetes, act along complex, adverse feedback loops. As we learn more about the feedback mechanisms linking environment, microbes, and health outcomes, there are some glimmers of hope that knowledge of the microbiome may be used to modify diet and improve health. For example, studies show that by limiting carbohydrates or fat, we can induce statistically significant changes in the composition of our gut microflora (Ley *et al.* 2006). In fact, as soon as 24 hours after the initiation of a low-fat, high fiber diet, changes in the composition of the microbiome are evident (Wu *et al.* 2011). The species/gene-level changes that result are quite small compared to the differences observed between individuals. But is it possible they could be clinically significant? It seems so. When obese or overweight subjects ate an energy-restricted high-protein diet for 6 weeks, followed by a weight-maintenance diet for another 6 weeks, the diversity of genes in their microbes increased significantly and triglyceride levels improved (Cotillard *et al.* 2013). It should be noted that disparities in access to healthy foods may limit the utility of such interventions, even in high-income countries. The third epidemiologic transition is just beginning, and only time will tell which trends characterize it. With luck, our growing understanding of the microbiome will allow us to set in place negative feedback mechanisms, counteracting microbial alterations that began in the first epidemiologic transition and have compromised health.

ACKNOWLEDGMENTS

We dedicate this chapter to the memory of George J. Armelagos, a groundbreaking scholar and an even better friend.

REFERENCES

Aagaard, K., Ma, J., Antony, K.M., Ganu, R., Petrosino, J., and Versalovic, J. 2014. "The Placenta Harbors a Unique Microbiome." *Science Translation Medicine*, 6(237): 237–265.

Adler, C.J., Dobney, K., Weyrich, L.S., Kaidonis, J., Walker, A.W., Haak, W., Bradshaw, C.J.A., ... and Cooper, A. 2013. "Sequencing Ancient Calcified Dental Plaque Shows Changes in Oral Microbiota with Dietary Shifts of the Neolithic and Industrial Revolutions." *Nature Genetics*, 45: 450–455.

Amir, L.H. and Donath, S.M. 2008. "Socioeconomic status and Rates of Breastfeeding in Australia: Evidence from Three Recent National Health Surveys." *Medical Journal of Australia*, 189: 254–256.

Angebault, C., Djossou, F., Abélanet, S., Permal, E., Soltana, M.B., Diancourt, L., Bouchier, C. ... and Bougnoux, M.E. 2013. "*Candida albicans* Is Not Always the Preferential Yeast Colonising Humans: A Study amongst Wayampi Amerindians." *Journal of Infectious Diseases*, 208(10): 1705–1716.

Apostolopoulos, P., Vafiadis-Zouboulis, I., Tzivras, M., Kourtessas, D., Katsilambros, N.,and Archimandritis, A. 2002. "*Helicobacter pylori* (*H pylori*) Infection in Greece: The Changing Prevalence during a Ten-Year Period and Its Antigenic Profile." *BMC Gastroenterology*, 2: 11.

Appelt, S., Fancello, L., Le Bailly, M., Raoult, D., Drancourt, M., and Desnues, C. 2014. "Viruses in a 14th-century Coprolite." *Applied & Environmental Microbiology*, doi: 10.1128/AEM.03242-13.

Armstrong, G.L., Conn, L.A., and Pinner, R.W. 1999. "Trends in infectious Disease Mortality in the United States during the 20th Century." *JAMA*, 281: 61–66.

Babkin, I.V. and Babkina, I.N. 2012. "A Retrospective Study of the Orthopoxvirus Molecular Evolution." *Infection, Genetics and Evolution*, 12(8): 1597–1604.

Barber, M. and Rozwadowska-Dowzenko, M. 1948. "Infection by Penicillin-resistant Staphylococci." *Lancet*, 2: 641–644.

Barrett, R., Kuzawa, C.W., McDade, T., and Armelagos, G.J. 1998. "Emerging and Re-Emerging Infectious Diseases: The Third Epidemiological Transition." In W. Durham (Ed.), *Annual Review Anthropology* (pp. 247–271). Palo Alto, CA: Annual Reviews Inc.

Bartoloni, A., Palecchi, L., Benedetti, M., Fernandez, C., Vallejos, Y., Guzman, E., Villagran, A.L., Mantella, A., Lucchetti, C., Bartalesi, F., Strohmeyer, M., Bechini, A., Gamboa, H., Rodríguez, H., Falkenberg, T., Kronvall, G., Gotuzzo, E., Paradisi, F., and Rossolini, G.M. 2006. "Multidrug-resistant Commensal Escherichia coli in Children, Peru and Bolivia." *Emerging Infectious Diseases*, 12.

Blaut, M. and Clavel, T. 2007. "Metabolic Diversity of the Intestinal Microbiota: Implications for Health and Disease." *Journal of Nutrition*, 137: 751–755.

Boney, C.M., Verma, A., Tucker, R., and Vohr, B.R. 2005. "Metabolic Syndrome in Childhood: Association with Birth Weight, Maternal Obesity, and Gestational Diabetes Mellitus." *Pediatrics*, 115(3): 290–296.

Braidwood, R. and Braidwood, L. 1950. "Jarmo: A Village Early Farmers in Iraq." *Antiquity*, 24(96):189–195.

Brinkmann, U.K., Korte, R., and Schmidt-Ehry, B. 1988. "The Distribution and Spread of Schistosomiasis in Relation to Water Resources in Mali." *Tropical Medicine and Parasitology*, 39(2): 182–185.

Canani, R.B., Cirillo, P., Terrin, G.L., Cesarano, L., Spagnuolo, M.I., de Vincenzo, A., de Marco, G., Manguso, F., and Guarino, A. 2007. "Probiotics for Treatment of Acute Diarrhoea in Children: Randomised Clinical Trial of Five Different Preparations." *BMJ*, 335: 340.

CDC (Centers for Disease Control and Prevention). 2006. "Emergence of Mycobacterium Tuberculosis with Extensive Resistance to Second-Line Drugs – Worldwide 2000–2004." *MMWR Morbidity and Mortality Weekly Report*, 55(11): 301–305.

CDC (Centers for Disease Control and Prevention). 2013. "*Clostridium difficile* Infection." http://www.cdc.gov/hai/organisms/cdiff/cdiff_infect.html (accessed December 8, 2015).

Chierici, R.S., Fanaro, S., Saccomandi, D., and Vigi, V. 2003. "Advances in the Modulation of the Microbial Ecology of the Gut in Early Infancy." *Acta Paediatrica*, 92: 56–63.

Cohen, M.N. and Armelagos G.J. (Eds.) 2013. *Paleopathology at the Origins of Agriculture*. Gainesville, FL: University Press of Florida.

Corley, D.A., Kubo, A., Levin, T.R., Block, G., Habel, L., Zhao, W., Leighton, P. ... and Parsonnet, J. 2008. "*Helicobacter pylori* Infection and the Risk of Barrett's Oesophagus: A Community-based Study." *Gut*, 57: 727–733.

Cotillard, A., Kennedy, S.P., Kong, L.C., Prifti, E., Pons, N., Le Chatelier, E., Almeida, M. ..., and Erlich, S.D. 2013. "Dietary Intervention Impact on Gut Microbial Gene Richness." *Nature*, 500: 585–590.

Cramer, C., Link, E., Koletzko, S., Lehmann, I., Heinrich, J., Wichmann, H.E., Bauer, C.P. ..., and Krämer, U. 2012. "The Hygiene Hypothesis Does Not Apply to Atopic Eczema in Childhood." *New Trends in Allergy and Atopic Eczema*, 96: 15–23.

Curhan, G.C., Willett, W.C., Rimm, E.B., Spiegelman, D., Ascherio, A.L., and Stampfer, M.J. 1996. "Birth Weight and Adult Hyptertension, Diabetes Mellitus, and Obesity in US Men." *Circulation*, 94: 3246–3250.

Dethlefsen, L. and Relman, D.A. 2011. "Incomplete Recovery and Individualized Responses of the Human Distal Gut Microbiota to Repreated Antibiotic Perturbation." *PNAS*, 108(S1): 4554–4561.

Dominguez-Bello, M.G., Costello, E.K., Contreras, M., Magris, M., HIdalgo, G., Fierer, N., and Knight, R. 2010. "Delivery Mode Shapes the Acquisition and Structure of the Initial Microbiota across Multiple Habitats in Newborns." *PNAS*, 107(26): 11971–11975.

Doucleff, M. 2013. "What It Takes to Cure Drug-Resistant Tuberculosis." Accessed http://www.npr.org/blogs/health/2013/07/09/200387607/what-it-takes-to-cure-drug-resistant-tuberculosis (accessed December 8, 2015).

Ellis, R. J., Bruce, K.D., Jenkins, C., Stothard, J.R., Ajarova, L., Mugisha, L., and Viney, M.E. 2013. "Comparison of the Distal Gut Mcirobiota from People and Animals in Africa." *PLoS ONE*, 8(1): e54783.

Forste, R., Weiss, J., and Lippincott, E. 2001. "The Decision to Breastfeed in the United States: Does Race Matter?" *Pediatrics*, 108(2): 291–296.

Fuccio, L, Zagari, R.M., Eusebi, L.H., Laterza, L, Cennamo, V., Ceroni, L., Grilli, D., and Bazzoli, F. 2009. "Meta-analysis: Can *Helicobacter pylori* Eradication Treatment Reduce the Risk for Gastric Cancer?" *Annals of Internal Medicine*, 151(2): 121–128.

Fuerst, J.A. and Hugenholtz, P. 2000. "Microorganisms Should Be High on DNA Preservation List." *Science*, 290(5496): 1503.

Fujisawa, T., T Kumagai, T Akamatsu, K Kiyosawa, and Y Matsunaga. 1999. "Changes in Seroepidemiological Pattern of *Helicobacter pylori* and Hepatitis A virus over the Last 20 Years in Japan." *American Journal of Gastroenterology*, 94: 2094–2099.

Funkhouser, L.J. and Bordenstein, S.R. 2013. "Mom Knows Best: The Universality of Maternal Microbial Transmission." *PLoS Biology*, 11(8): e1001631.

Furuse, Y., Suzuki, A., and Oshitani, H. 2010. "Origin of Measles Virus: Divergence from Rinderpest Virus between the 11th and 12th Centuries." *Virology Journal*, 7: 52.

Geng, J., Fan, H., Tang, X., Zhai, H., and Zhang, Z. 2013. "Diversified Pattern of the Human Colorectal Cancer Microbiome." *Gut Pathogens*, 5: 2.

Ghosh, S. and Kobayashi, N. 2011. "Whole-genomic analysis of Rotavirus Strains: Current Status and Future Prospects." *Future Microbiology*, 6(9): 1049–1065.

Gibbons, L., Belizán, J.M., Lauer, J.A., Betrán, A.P., and Althabe, F. 2010. "The Global Numbers and Costs of Additionally Needed and Unnecessary Caesarean Sections Performed per Year: Overuse as a Barrier to Universal Coverage." In *World Health Report 2010 – Working Paper.*

Graham, D.Y., Lew, G.M., Klein, P.D., Evans, D.G., Evans, D.J., Saeed, Z.A., and Malaty, H.M. 1992. "Effect of Treatment of *Helicobacter pylori* Infection on the Long-Term Recurrence of Gastric or Duodenal Ulcer: A Randomized, Controlled Study." *Annals of Internal Medicine*, 116(9): 705–708.

Grenfell, B.T. and Bolker, B.M. 1998. "Cities and Villages: Infection Hierarchies in a Measles Metapopulation." *Ecology Letters*, 1(1): 63–70.

Harper, K.N. and Armelagos, G.J. 2010. "The Changing Disease-scape in the Third Epidemiological Transition." *International Journal of Environmental Research and Public Health*, 7: 675–697.

Harper, K.N. and Armelagos, G.J. 2013. "Genomics, the origins of Agriculture, and Our Changing Microbe-Scape: Time to Revisit Some Old Tales and Tell Some New Ones." *Yearbook of Physical Anthropology*, 152(S57): 135–152.

Jakobbson, H.E., Jernberg, C., Andersson, A.F., Sjölund-Karlsson, M., Jansson, J.K., and Engstrand, L. 2010. "Short-term Antibiotic Treatment Has Differing Long-Term Impacts on the Human Throat and Gut Microbiome." *PLoS ONE*, 5 (3): e9836.

Jernberg, C., Löfmark, S., Edlund, C., and Jansson, J.K. 2007. "Long-term Ecological Impacts of Antibiotic Administration on the Human Intestinal Microbiota." *ISME J*, 1(1): 56–66.

Jiménez, E., Marín, M.L., Martín, R., Odriozola, J.M., Olivares, M., Xaus, J., Fernández, L., and Rodríguez, J.M. 2008. "Is Meconimum from Healthy Newborns Actually Sterile?" *Research in Microbiology*, 159(3): 187–193.

Johnson, A.P., Speller, D.C.E., George, R.C., Warner, M., Domingue, G., and Efstratiou, A. 1996. "Prevalence of Antibiotic Resistance and Serotypes in Pneumococci in England and Wales: Results of Observational Surveys in 1990 and 1995." *BMJ*, 312: 1454.

Jones, K.E., Patel, N.G., Levy, M.A., Storeygard, A., Balk, D., Gittleman, J.L., and Daszak, P. 2008. "Global Trends in Emerging Infectious Diseases." *Nature*, 451: 990–993.

Kalliomäki, M., Collado, M.C., Salminen, S., and Isolauri, E. 2008. "Early Differences in Fecal Microbiota Composition in Children May Predict Overweight." *American Journal of Clinical Nutrition*, 87: 534–538.

Karlsson, F.H., Tremaroli, V., Nookaew, I., Bergström, G., CJ Behre, C.J, Fagerberg, B., Nielsen, J., and Bäckhed, F. 2013. "Gut Metagenome in European Women with Normal, Impaired and Diabetic Glucose Control." *Nature*, 498: 99–103.

Kau, A.L, Ahern, P.P., Griffin, N.W., Goodman, A.L., and Gordon, J.I. 2011. "Human Nutrition, the Gut Microbiome and the Immune System." *Nature*, 474(7351): 327–336.

Khawaldeh, A., Morales, S., Dillon, B., Alavidze, Z., Ginn, A.N., Thomas, L., Chapman, S.J. …, and Iredell, J.R. 2011. "Bacteriophage Therapy for Refractory *Pseudomonas aeruginosa* Urinary Tract Infection." *Journal of Medical Microbiology*, 60(11): 1697–1700.

Kostic, A.D., Gevers, D., Padamallu, C.S., Michaud, M., Duke, F., Earl, A.M., Ojesina, A.I. … and Meyerson, M. 2012. "Genomic Analysis Identifies Association of *Fusobacterium* with Colorectal Carcinoma." *Genome Research*, 22: 292–298.

Laitinen, J, Jääskeläinen, A., Hartikainen, A.L., Sovio, U., Vääräsmäki, M., Pouta, A, Kaakinen, M., and Järvelin, M.R. 2012. "Maternal Weight Gain during the First Half of Pregnancy and Offpsring Obesity at 16 Years: A Prospective Cohort Study." *BJOG*, 119: 716–723.

Lazarevic, V., Manzano, S., Gaïa, N., Girard, M., Whiteson, K., Hibbs, H., François, P., Gervaix, A., and Schrenzel, J. 2013. "Effects of Amoxicilin Treatment on the Salivary Microbiota in Children with Acute Otitis Media." *Clinical Microbiology and Infection*, 19(8): E335–342.

Le Chatelier, E., Nielsen, T., Qin, J., Prifti, E., Hildebrand, F., Falony, G., Almeida, M. …, and Pedersen, O. 2013. "Richness of Human Gut Microbiome Correlates with Metabolic Markers." *Nature*, 500: 541–546.

Lederberg, J. and McCray, A. 2001. "'Ome Sweet'Omics – A Genealogical Treasury of Words." *The Scientist*, 17(7).

Leeb, K., Baibergenova, A., Wen, E., Webster, G., and Zelmer, J. 2005. "Are There Socio-Economic Differences in Caesarean Section Rates in Canada?" *Healthcare Policy*, 1(1): 48–54.

Lester, S.C., Pla, M.P., Wang, F., Schael, I.P., Jiang, H., and O'Brien, T.F. 1990. "The carriage of Escherichia coli Resistant to Antimicrobial Agents by Healthy Children in Boston, in Caracas, Venezuela, and in Qin Pu, China." *New England Journal of Medicine*, 323(5): 285–289.

Ley, R.E., Turnbaugh, P.J., Klein, S., and Gordon, J.I. 2006. "Human gut Microbes Associated with Obesity." *Nature*, 444: 1022–1023.

Lin, A., Bik, E.M., Costello, E.K., Dethlefsen, L., Haque, R., Relman, D.A., and Singh, U. 2013. "Distinct distal Gut Microbiome Diversity and Composition in Healthy Children from Bangladesh and the United States." *PLoS ONE*, 8(1): e53838.

Liu, A.H. and Murphy, J.R. 2003. "Hygiene Hypothesis: Fact or Fiction?" *Journal of Allergy & Clinical Immunology*, 111(3): 471–478.

Livingstone, F.B. 1971. "Malaria and Human Polymorphisms." *Annual Review of Genetics*, 5: 33–64.

LoBue, P., Sizemore, C., and Castro, K.G. 2009. "Plant to Combat Extensively Drug-resistant Tuberculosis Recommendations of the Federal Tuberculosis Task Force." *MMWR*, 58 (RR03): 1–43.

Löfmark, S., Jernberg, C., Jansson, J.K., and Edlund, C. 2006. "Clindamycin-induced Enrichment and Long-term Persistence of Resistant *Bacteroides* spp. and Resistance Genes." *Journal of Antimicrobial Chemotherapy*, 58(6): 1160–1167.

Lozupone, C.A., Stombaugh, J.I., Gordon, J.I., Jansson, J.K., and Knight, R. 2012. "Diversity, Stability and Resilience of the Human Gut Microbiota." *Nature*, 489: 220–230.

Mackenbach, J.P. 1994. "The Epidemiological Transition Theory." *Journal of Epidemiology and Community Health*, 48: 329–331.

Makino, H., Kushiro, A., Ishikawa, E., Kubota, H., Gawad, A., Sakai, T., Oishi, K., Martin, R., and Ben-Amor, K. 2013. "Mother-to-Infant Transmission of Intestinal Bifidobacterail Strains Has an Impact on the Early Development of Vaginally Delivered Infants' Microbiota." *PLoS ONE*, 8(11): e78331.

Marques, T.M., Wall, R., Ross, R.P., Fitzgerald, G.F., Ryan, C.A., and Stanton, C. 2010. "Programming Infant Gut Microbiota: Influence of Dietary and Environmental Factors." *Current Opinion in Biotechnology*, 21(2): 149–156.

Martella, V., Bányai, K., Matthinjnssens, J., Buonavoglia, C., and Ciarlet, M. 2010. "Zoonotic Aspects of Rotaviruses." *Veterinary Microbiology*, 140(3–4): 246–255.

Matricardi, P.M. 2010. "Controversial Aspects of the 'Hygiene Hypothesis'." *Clinical & Experimental Immunology*, 160(1): 98–105.

McKeown, T. 1979. The Role of Medicine. *Dream, Mirage or Nemesis?* Oxford: Blackwell.

Mensforth, R.P., Lovejoy, C.O., Lallo, J.W., and Armelagos, G.J. 1978. "Part Two: The Role of Constitutional Factors, Diet, and Infectious Disease in the Etiology of Porotic Hyperostosis and Periosteal Reactions in Prehistoric Infants and Children." *Medical Anthropology*, 2(1): 1–59.

Michail, S.K,. Stolfi, A., Johnson, T., and Onady, G.M. 2008. "Efficacy of probiotics in the Treatment of Pediatric Atopic Dermatitis: A Meta-Analysis of Randomized Controlled Trials." *Annals of Allergy, Asthma & Immunology*, 101(5): 508–516.

Moayyedi, P., Ford, A.C., Talley, N.J., Cremonini, F., Foxx-Orenstein, A.E., Brandt, L.J., and Quigley, E.M.M. 2010. "The efficacy of Probiotics in the Treatment of Irritable Bowel Syndrome: A Systematic Review." *Gut*, 59: 325–332.

Morello, E., Saussereau, E., Maura, D., Huerre, M., Touqui, L., and Debarbieux, L. 2011. "Pulmonary Bacteriophage Therapy on *Pseudomonas aeruginosa* Cystic Fibrosis Strains: First Steps towards Treatment and Prevention." *PLoS ONE*, 6(2): e16963.

Nading, A.M. 2014. *Mosquito Trails: Ecology, Health, and the Politics of Entanglement*. Oakland, CA: University of California Press.

Nasidze, I., Li, J., Schroeder, R., Creasey, J.L., Li, M., and Stoneking, M. 2011. "High Diversity of the Saliva Microbiome in Batwa Pygmies." *PLoS ONE*, 6(8): e23352.

Nickerson, E.K., West, T.E., Day, N.P., and Peacock, S.J. 2009. "Staphyloccus aureus Disease and Drug Resistance in Resource-limited Countries in South and East Asia." *Lancet Infectious Disease*, 9(2): 130–135.

OECD. 2009. OECD Family Database: *Breastfeeding Rates*.

Okeke, I.N., Fayinka, S.T., and Lamikanra, A. 2000. "Antibiotic Resistance in Escherichia coli from Nigerian Students, 1986–1988." *Emergency Infectious Diseases*, 6(4): 393–396.

Omran, A.R. 1971. "The epidemiologic Transition: A Theory of the Epidemiology of Population Change." *Millbank Memorial Fund Quarterly*, 49(4): 509–538.

Panlilio, A.L., Culver, D.J., Gaynes, R.P., Banerjee, S., Henderson, T.S., Tolson, J.S., Martone, W.J., and NSISS. 1992. "Methicillin-resistant *Staphyloccus aureus* in US Hospitals, 1975–1991." *Infection Control and Hospital Epidemiology*, 13: 582–586.

Penders, J., Thijs, C., Vink, C., Stelma, F.F., Snijders, B., Kummeling, I., van den Brandt, P.A., and Stobberingh, E.E. 2006. "Factors Influencing the Composition of the Intestinal Microbiota in Early Infancy." *Pediatrics*, 118(2): 511–521.

Piel, F.B., Patil, A.P., Howes, R.E., Nyangiri, O.A., Gething, P.W., Williams, T.N., Weatherall, D.J., and Hay, S.I. 2010. "Global Distribution of the Sickle Cell Gene and Geographical Confirmation of the Malaria Hypothesis." *Nature Communications*, 1: 104.

Pirkola, J., Pouta, A., Bloigu, A., Hartikainen, A.L., Laitinen, J., Järvelin, M.R., and Vääräsmäki, M. 2010. "Risks of Overweight and Abdominal Obesity at Age 16 Years Associated with Prenatal Exposures to Maternal Prepregnancy Overweight and Gestational Diabetes Mellitus." *Diabetes Care*, 33: 1115–1121.

Qin, J., Li, R., Raes, J., Arumugam, M., Burgdorf, K.S., Manichanh, C., Nielsen, T. ..., and Wang, J. 2010. "A Human Gut Microbial Gene Catalogue Established by Metagenomic Sequencing." *Nature*, 464: 59–65.

Qin, J., Li, Y., Cai, Z., Li, S., Zhu, J., Zhang, F., Liang, S. ..., and Wang, J. 2012. "A Metagenome-wide Association Study of Gut Microbiota in Type 2 Diabetes." *Nature*, 490: 55–60.

Rautava, S., Luoto, R., Salminen, S., and Isolauri, E. 2012. "Microbial Contact during Pregnancy, Intestinal Colonization and Human Disease. " *Nature Reviews: Gastroenterology and Hepatology*, (10): 565–576.

Reddy, S. 2012. "Probiotics' Benefits May Be More Than a Gut Feeling." *Wall Street* Journal. http://online.wsj.com/news/articles/SB10001424127887324784404578143402702878118 (accessed December 8, 2015).

Reid, A. and Greene, S. 2013. *Human Microbiome FAQ.* Washington, DC: American Society for Microbiology.

Reid, W.V. and Miller, K.R. 1989. "Food Crops and Biodiversity. Keeping Options Alive: The Scientific Basis for the Conservation of Biodiversity." *World Resources Institute.* http://wwwwriorg/node/8584/.

Ritchie, M.L. and Romanuk, T.N. 2012. "A Meta-analysis of Probiotic Efficacy for Gastrointestinal Diseases." *PLOS ONE*, 7(4): e34938.

Roosendaal, R., Kuipers, E.J., Buitenwerf, J., van Uffelen, C., Meuwissen, S.G., van Kamp, G.J., and Vandenbroucke-Grauls, C.M. 1997. "*Helicobacter pylori* and the Birth Cohort Effect: Evidence of a Continuous Decrease of Infection Rates in Childhood." *American Journal of Gastroenterology*, 92(9): 1480–1482.

Rosenthal, B.M., LaRosa, G., Zarlenga, D., Dunams, D., Chunyu, Y., Mingyuan, L., and Pozio, E. 2008. "Human Dispersal of *Trichinella spiralis* in Domesticated Pigs." *Infection, Genetics and Evolution*, 8(6): 799–805.

Savino, F., Pelle, E., Palumeri, E., Oggero, R., and Miniero, R. 2007. "*Lactobacillus returi* (American Type Culture Collection Strain 55730) versus simethicone in the Treatment of Infantile Colic: A Prospective Randomized Study." *Pediatrics*, 119(1): e124–e130.

Sazawal, S., Hiremath, G., Dhingra, U., Malik, P., Deb, S., and Black, R.E. 2006. "Efficacy of probiotics in Prevention of Acute Diarrhoea: A Meta-Analysis of Masked, Randomised, Placebo-controlled Trials." *Lancet Infectious Disease*, 6(6): 374–382.

Schloissnig, S., Arumugam, M., Sunagawa, S., Mitreva, M., Tap, J., Zhu, A., Waller, A. … and Bork,P. 2013. "Genomic Variation Landscape of the Human Gut Microbiome." *Nature*, 493: 45–50.

Schnorr, S.L., Candela, M., Rampelli, S., Centanni, M., Consolandi, C., Basaglia, G., Turroni, S. … and Crittenden, A.N. 2014. "Gut Microbiome of the Hadza Hunter-Gatherers." *Nature Communications*, 5: 3654.

Scrimshaw, N.S. 2003. "Historical concepts of Interactions, Synergism and Antagonism between Nutrition and Infection." *Journal of Nutrition*, 133(1): 316–321.

Scrimshaw, N.S. 2010. "INCAP Studies of Nutrition and Infection." *Food Nutrition Bulletin*, 31(1): 54–67.

Shchelkunov, S.N. 2009. "How Long Ago Did Smallpox Virus Emerge?" *Archives of Virology*, 154: 1865–1871.

Singer, M. 2010. "Ecosyndemics: Global Warming and the Coming Plagues of the 21st Century." In A. Swedlund and A. Herring (Eds.), *Plagues and Epidemics: Infected Spaces Past and Present* (pp. 21–37). London: Berg.

Smith, M.I., Yatsunenko, T., Manary, M.J., Trehan, I., Mkakosya, R., Cheng, J., Kau, A.L. …, and Gordon, J.I. 2013. "Gut Microbiomes of Malawian Twin Pairs Discordant for Kwashiorkor." *Science*, 339: 548–554.

Stark, P.L. and Lee, A. 1982. "The Microbial Ecology of the Large Bowel of Breast-Fed and Formula-Fed Infants during the First Year of Life." *Journal of Medical Microbiology*, 15(2): 189–203.

Steckel, R.H. and Rose, J.C. (Eds.) 2002. *The Backbone of History: Health and Nutrition in the Western Hemisphere.* Cambridge: Cambridge University Press.

Stoner-Duncan, B., Streicker, D.G., and Tedeschi, C.M. 2014. "Vampire Bats and Rabies: Toward an Ecological Solution to a Public Health Problem." *PLos Neglected Tropical Diseases*, 8(6): e2867.

Strachan, D.P. 1989. "Hay Fever, Hygiene, and Household Size." *BMJ*, 299(6710): 1259–1260.

Talla, I., Kongs, A., Verle, P., Belot, J., Sarr, S., and Coll, A.M. 1990. "Outbreak of Intestinal Schistosomiasis in the Senegal River Basin." *Ann Soc Belge Med Trop*, 70: 173–180.

Thrift, A.P., Pandeya, N., Smith, K.J., Green, A.C., Hayward, N.K., Webb, P.M., and Whiteman, D.C. 2012. "*Helicobacter pylori* Infection and the risks of Barrett's

Oesophagus: A Population-based Case-Control Study." *International Journal of Cancer*, 130(10): 2407–2416.

Thrift, A.P., and Whiteman, D.C. 2012. "The Incidence of Esophageal Adenocarcinoma Continues to Rise: Analysis of Period and Birth Cohort Effects on Recent Trends." *Annales of Oncology*, 23(12): 3155–3162.

Tishkoff, S.A., Varkonyi, R., Cahinhinan, N., Abbes, S., Argyropoulos, G., Destro-Bisol, Drousiotou, A., ..., and Clark, A.G. 2001. "Haplotype diversity and Linkage Disequilibrium at Human G6PD: Recent Origin of Alleles That Confer Malarial Resistance." *Science*, 293(5529): 455–462.

Tito, R.Y., Knights, D., Metcalf, J., Obregon-Tito, A.J., Cleeland, L., Najar, F., Roe, B. ..., and Lewis. 2012. "Insights from Characterizing Extinct Human Hut Microbiomes." *PLoS ONE*, 7(12): e51146.

Toscano, M, de Vecchi, E., Rodighiero, V., and Drago, L. 2013. "Microbiological and Genetic Identification of Some Probiotics Proposed for Medical Use in 2011." *Journal of Chemotherapy*, 25(3): 156–161.

Turnbaugh, P.J., Ley, R.E., Mahowald, M.A., Magrini, V., Mardis, E.R., and Gordon, J.I. 2006. "An Obesity-associated Gut Microbiome with Increased Capacity for Energy Harvest." *Nature*, 444(7122): 1027–1131.

Turnbaugh, P.J., Backhed, F., Fulton, L., and Gordon, J.I. 2008. "Marked Alterations in the Distal Gut Microbiome Linked to Diet-induced Obesity." *Cell Host Microbe*, 3(4): 213–223.

Turnbaugh, P.J., Hamady, M., Yatsunenko, T., Cantarel, B.L., Duncan, A., Ley, R.E., Sogin, M.L., ... and Gordon, J.I. 2009. "A Core Gut Microbiome in Obese and Lean Twins." *Nature*, 457: 480–485.

UNICEF. 2009. *Infant and Young Child Feeding*. http://www.childinfo.org/breastfeeding_countrydata.php.

van Nood, E., Vrieze, A., Nieuwdorp, M., Fuentes, S., Zoetendal, E.G., de Vos, W.M., Visser, C.E. ...and Keller, J.J. 2013. "Duodenal Infusion of Donor Feces for Recurrent *Clostridium difficile*." *New England Journal of Medicine*, 368: 407–415.

Vrieze, A., van Nood, E., Holleman, F., Salojärvi, J., Kootte, R.S., Bartelsman, J.F., Dallinga-Thie, G.M. ..., and Nieuwdorp, M. 2012. "Transfer of Intestinal Microbiota from Lean Donors Increases Insulin Sensitivity in Individuals with Metabolic Syndrome." *Gastroenterology*, 143(4): 913–916.

WHO (World Health Organization). 2009. "M/XDR-TB: A Deadly, Infectious Disease That Knows No Borders." http://www.who.int/tb_beijingmeeting/mxdr_tb/en/ (accessed December 8, 2015).

WHO (World Health Organization). 2012. "Frequently Asked Questions – XDR-TB." http://www.who.int/tb/challenges/xdr/faqs/en/ (accessed December 8, 2015).

Wisenfeld, S.L. 1967. "Sickle-cell Trait in Human Biological and Cultural Evolution." *Science*, 157: 1134–1140.

Woolley, L. 1965. *Beginnings of Civilization, History of Mankind*. Vol. 1, Part II. New York/Toronto: The New American Library/Mentor Books.

Wright, A., Hawkins, C.H., Anggard, E.E., and Harper, D.R. 2009. "A Controlled Clinical Trial of a Therapeutic Bacteriophage Preparation in Chronic Otitis due to Antibiotic-Resistant *Pseudomonas aeruginosa*; A Preliminary Report of Efficacy." *Clinical Otolaryngology*, 34(4): 349–357.

Wu, G.D., Chen, J., Hoffmann, C., Bittinger, K., Chen, Y.Y., Keilbaugh, S.A., Bewtra, M. ..., and Lewis, J.D. 2011. "Linking Long-term Dietary Patterns with Gut Microbial Enterotypes." *Science*, 334: 105–108.

Wu, M.S., Lee, W.J., Wang, H.H., Huang, S.P., and Lin, J.T. 2005. "A Case-Control Study of Association of *Helicobacter pylori* Infection with Morbid Obesity in Taiwan." *Archives of International Medicine*, 165(13): 1552–1555.

Yatsunenko, T., Rey, F.E., Manary, M.J., Trehan, I., Dominguez-Bello, M.G., Contreras, M., Magris, M. …, and Gordon, J.I. 2012. "Human gut Microbiome Viewed across Age and Geography." *Nature*, 486: 222–228.

Yazdanbakhsh, M., Kremsner, P.G., and van Ree, R. 2002. "Allergy, Parasites, and the Hygiene Hypothesis." *Science*, 296(5567): 490–494.

Zuckerman, M.K. and Armelagos, G.J. 2014. "The Hygiene Hypothesis and the Second Epidemiological Transition." In M.K. Zuckerman (Ed.), *Modern Environments and Human Health: Revisiting the Second Epidemiologic Transition* (pp. 291–310). Hoboken, NJ: Wiley-Blackwell.

Zuckerman, M.K., Harper, K.N., Barrett, R., and Armelagos. G.J. 2014. "The Evolution of Disease: Anthropological Perspectives on Epidemiologic Transitions." *Global Health Action*, 7: 23303.

CHAPTER 19

China's Cancer Villages: Contested Evidence and the Politics of Pollution

Anna Lora-Wainwright and Ajiang Chen

Introduction

In February 2013, the Chinese government publicly acknowledged the existence of "cancer villages" (clusters of high cancer incidence typically correlated with pollution), feeding a controversy that started in 2001 with the first appearance of the term. An official document titled "Guard Against and Control Risks Presented by Chemicals to the Environment during the 12th Five-Year Plan (2011–2015)" (Ministry of Environment 2013) stated that the widespread production and consumption of harmful chemicals forbidden in many developed nations are still found in China: "Toxic chemicals have caused many environmental emergencies linked to water and air pollution. … There are even some serious cases of health and social problems like the emergence of *cancer villages* in individual regions" (Ministry of Environment 2013, emphasis added). As Wang Canfa, veteran Beijing-based lawyer and professor who defends pollution victims, pointed out, it was the first time the "cancer village" phrase had appeared in a ministry document (see BBC 2013). This official mention of the

A Companion to the Anthropology of Environmental Health, First Edition. Edited by Merrill Singer.

term triggered a spate of media reports both in China and abroad (see BBC 2013; Dewey 2013). A search for media articles containing "cancer village" in the keywords on CNKI (China National Knowledge Infrastructure, the main database of Chinese newspapers and academic publications) in July 2013 identified only 13 reports in 2012 and already 106 in the first half of 2013, with an additional 19 by November 10, 2013.[1]

In the ministry document, however, as in most of the media reports, the term "cancer village" remains undefined. Given long latency periods and multiple causality for several cancers, cancer villages are a contested field. Except for cases of acute poisoning and where there is a relatively clear understanding of health effects (as is the case for lead poisoning and for benzene, for instance) establishing causal links between exposure and health effects is complex for several reasons. Science on chemicals is unreliable by contemporary standards of scientific truth and there are no scientific studies for a large number of chemicals (Murphy 2006; Brown 2007; Steingraber 2010). Causation is also complex: exposure may take place over a long-term period, risk may be posed by a multiplicity of factors rather than single substances, incidence of chemical exposure is difficult to pinpoint, and symptoms may not fit a typical pattern. For these reasons, it is often difficult to determine causal paths between exposure to a particular contaminant and specific health effects. Scientific methods currently available are also inadequate. Laboratory tests on animals are short term, do not necessarily prove that a given element has the same effects on humans, and they do not take into account how exposure may interact with other factors. Epidemiology, by contrast, requires a long timeframe and is better at studying the interaction of a variety of factors in causing illness rather than singling them out (Tesh 2000).

This has important implications. First, as a consequence of such complex causality, many conditions which are attributed to environmental causes are "highly contested and the source of considerable confusion, anger and resentment" (Brown, Kroll-Smith, and Gunter 2000: 9). Second, although uncertainty associated with assessing causality is a genuine challenge even for those who want to attribute responsibility fairly, it may be exploited and maintained by industry-sponsored science (Murphy 2006). For example, evidence required to prove environmental health harm and gain compensation from liable companies or state agencies is typically defined very narrowly (Petryna 2002; Waldman 2009; Phillips 2012). "Toxic uncertainty," in other words, is rooted in uneven power relations and is a form of domination (Auyero and Swistun 2009). This is a phenomenon that Brown, Kroll-Smith, and Gunter term "organizational deceit," that is, privileging the well-being of organizations over human health (Brown, Kroll-Smith, and Gunter 2000: 10–12).

Those affected by pollution respond to politically sanctioned uncertainty in a variety of ways. They may mount opposition against it, in the form of protests, resort to the law and the media, lobby polluting companies, and demand government redress (Fortun 2001; Petryna 2002; Lerner 2005, 2010; Shevory 2007). Their actions may take a relatively NIMBY (not-in-my-backyard) form or be part of a more networked movement across different localities (Szasz 1994). They may form coalitions with scientific experts to challenge uncertainty and collect their own evidence of harm – for instance, by using alternative air pollution monitoring technology or by mapping health effects onto the physical presence of pollution. Such citizen-science alliances took shape in the Woburn (Massachusetts) childhood leukemia cluster (Brown and Mikklesen 1997) and in parts of Louisiana's "cancer alley" (Allen 2003; Lerner 2005; Singer 2011; Ottinger 2013). In these locations, and to varying degrees, citizens put forward a "popular epidemiology" (Brown 2007), an alternative way to prove the effects of environmental health threats by demonstrating concurrence of pollution with illness and holding industries and governments accountable (see also Balshem 1993). In doing so, these coalitions question the dominant epidemiological paradigm which emphasizes genetics and lifestyle and makes individuals responsible for their suffering. Elements in this complex spectrum of attitudes and responses – from various forms of opposition by affected communities to the denial of pollution by industries and local governments, or selected interventions – may be visible at different times in different localities, or they may coexist in the same site. This chapter examines some of these dynamics in the case of China's cancer villages.

Since the initial appearance of the term, cancer villages have been at the center of a controversy involving the national and international media, a range of government officials and state institutions, nongovernmental organizations (NGOs), natural and social scientists and the general public, particularly populations directly affected. Most often there is no conclusive scientific evidence to link village-size clusters of high cancer incidence epidemiologically to pollution.[2] If cancer refers to an individual bodily illness, cancer village delineates a shared social life, a space which is at once natural and social. Growing concern and unrest over pollution and its health effects mean that cancer villages are not only a medical phenomenon, but also a deeply social, cultural, and political one.[3]

Through a set of examples drawn from multi-sited fieldwork, we examine discourses and actions on the part of local residents, campaigners, polluting firms, local and higher government, the legal system, and the media. These elements form a complex web which shapes the evolving social, political, and scientific life of this concept, its implications, and the various effects its adoption has had on those living in the shadow of high cancer rates. The social and political life of cancer villages is molded by such interactions. In this chapter, we assess what knowledge is produced about pollution's effects on health by the different parties that are involved, what kinds of action it may convert into among local communities, and what responses it triggers on the part of local and higher levels of government. Different parties have different (though mutually shaping) paradigms for what constitutes a cancer village, and each has different aims and different outcomes. We then ask: How did a village first become seen as cancer village? How was this definition confirmed or contested? What were its effects on local strategies for seeking justice and on their relative success? In examining different cases, we show some commonalities but also differences in villages' ability to attract attention and obtain redress.

Developing an Understanding of Cancer Villages

Both authors have worked on pollution in rural China for almost a decade, and have carried out fieldwork in a range of severely polluted locations. As a foreign researcher, Lora-Wainwright was unable to carry out research in highly sensitive cancer villages which had generated significant controversy. Her research focused instead on sites which did not attract media attention and did not identify as cancer villages but were nevertheless affected by severe environmental degradation and health problems (see Lora-Wainwright 2013a, 2013b). She has conducted participant observation and semi-structured interviews with villagers in three sites since 2009. Her research in these polluted villages forms an important analytical background for understanding the sites where Ajiang Chen and his team conducted their research. Chen and his graduate students also faced considerable obstacles in accessing cancer villages, but were able to conduct extended research at six sites, through repeated visits. In each of these sites, they employed mixed research methods, including participant observation, questionnaires, and semi-structured interviews with villagers, the village doctor, village and township officials, representatives of the local industries, members of county environmental protection bureaus, and public health bureaus. They also conducted documentary research on each site and cross-checked lists of cancer deaths with the village doctor and where possible with the families of the deceased.

Here we only focus on three sites which attracted considerable attention: Huangmengying (pollution in the Huai basin, Henan, based on fieldwork in 2009 and 2011), Shangba (heavy metal extraction, Guangdong, based on fieldwork in 2010 and 2011), and Dongjing (Julong chemical industry, Jiangsu, studied by Chen's former student, Yajuan Luo, in 2007, 2008, 2009, and 2011).[4] We will also briefly refer to additional sites which provide valuable comparisons. Although pollution sources differ, these cases are comparable to the extent that in each of them the local population self-identified as living in a cancer village and sought redress for pollution. With assistance from Yajuan Luo, Lora-Wainwright also conducted an extensive content analysis on cancer village news reports and academic articles in Chinese which have appeared since 2001 and are listed in the CNKI database. This helped to provide additional information on some of the sites studied by Chen and his team and to contextualize them within the wider development of the label "cancer village" as a politico-semiotic paradigm.

The Appearance of "Cancer Villages" as a Politico-semiotic Paradigm

Media accounts of cancer villages have had perhaps the biggest and certainly the most visible impact on the development of the term. Reports over the past decades linked cancer villages first and foremost with the chemical industry, and secondly with paper factories, resource extraction and processing, downstream pollution (particularly from industry and mining), and heavy metals (caused by the above forms of pollution). The first article which contained the term cancer village was published in 2001 in the Chinese mining newspaper (Zhu 2001) about the village of Shangba (Guangdong). Some of the tropes mentioned in this initial piece are present in many of the future reports on cancer villages, and both authors found them to be prominent among villagers' evidence of pollution: changes in the color of the stream, livestock deaths, crop failures, high cancer rates, and men's inability to pass the physical test required to join the army. According to this article, tests on the stream water and on the soil revealed heavy metal content in excess of China's guidelines: lead in the soil exceeded by 44 times and cadmium by 12 times. In the list of deaths provided by village officials in 2001, 210 of 250 deaths were from cancer.

The number of media reports reached 12 in 2004 and 8 in 2005. An article in the state-run *China Daily*, headlined "Cancer Village in Spotlight," (quoted in Cody 2004) drew national attention, but officials ordered newspapers to stop covering the story. In the same year, an influential short documentary was aired on CCTV (China Central Television) titled "Rivers and Villages," which suggested pollution in the Huai River basin caused Huangmengying to become a "cancer village" (CCTV 2004). In subsequent years, report numbers remained relatively stable – between 3 and 11 per year – with a peak of 28 in 2011 (a third of them covering the case of chromium contamination in Qujing, Yunnan), a fall back to 13 in 2012, and the soaring peak of 106 in the first half of 2013. This sudden rise is first of all due to the official mention of cancer villages in the Ministry of Environment's document. Soon after this, the state-run news agency *Global Times* posted a "cancer village map" including 247 cases on their microblog (Wertime 2013), accompanied by a weeping emoticon and a caption referring to the Ministry of Environment document. This map, compiled by journalist Deng Fei and based on the cover story "cancer villages" for *Phoenix Weekly* (2009), had been circulating online for years (Doubleleaf 2009), but this was the first time that it had been posted by the state media. There were also additional reasons for the rise in reports. The 12th Five-Year Plan announced in late 2012 put emphasis on building an "ecological civilization," placing the environment in a position of unprecedented attention and therefore allowing more coverage of environmental issues. In March 2013, there were also two instances of extremely severe air pollution in Beijing, spurring a rise in media coverage. Finally, news items on the contamination of deep wells also heightened concerns about the effects of pollution.

The approaches taken in these reports are predictably diverse. A strong and recurrent theme is the critique of the high importance placed on GDP (gross domestic product) growth. Articles often contain lists of cancer victims, presented as evidence that cancer is the result of the proliferation of polluting enterprises promoted by the national emphasis on rapid economic development. In most cases, pollution is attributed to official corruption, which poses an obstacle to implementing environmental regulations. For instance, an article examining three cancer villages (in Shandong, Jiangsu, and Zhejiang) published as part of a series on water pollution documents how villagers' attempts at seeking redress failed due to insufficient evidence or through uncooperative officials bribed by polluting industries (Nanfang Dushi 2007a, 2007b). This emphasis became particularly prominent in 2008, 2009, and 2010 after the failure of attempts to measure "green GDP" (taking environmental losses into account when measuring GDP) and the publication of data from a project by the World Bank and China's State Environmental Protection Agency which showed that cancers associated with water pollution, such as liver and stomach cancer, are well above the world average (World Bank 2007), though it did not explicitly prove that those cancers were caused by water pollution.

Significantly however, many reports also promote a more balanced view of cancer villages and stress the remediation efforts underway. This is evident in articles about Huangmengying, in Shenqiu county, Henan province (CCTV 2004; Li 2004; Deng 2005), a village affected by pollution in the Huai River basin (the Huai is China's third largest and most polluted river), which became globally infamous because of its level of pollution. A 2004 news item on Huangmengying highlighted that the government had been making efforts to clean up the area since the 1990s and had now embarked on a new investigation and remediation program. This emphasis on attempts to clean up damaged areas was also present in a piece on Shangba (Yang and Fang 2005, later translated in English in Human Rights Forum 2007). This report portrayed a dire situation but also expressed some hope for the future given ongoing remediation efforts, particularly government investments in a water reservoir and investigation by scientific units as the basis for ecological remediation. Later articles on Shangba (Cao 2009; Cao 2013) continued to describe the achievements of remediation efforts and clean water programs funded by the province and city development commission which provided clean water for over 3000 villagers. The most recent piece on Shangba (Cao 2013) highlights that villagers and local officials alike are now keen to shed the label "cancer village" which has brought them so much bad publicity. These developments show a trend for media coverage becoming more mixed than it had been at first, and for highlighting government efforts to address the problem rather than simply pointing to its existence and urgency.

While few reports explicitly mention the word "evidence" (*zhengju*), this is at the core of many of the conflicts over recognition and redress. This tension is clear in news items on the infamous case of illegal dumping of waste leaching chromium into the soil in Qujing (Yunnan) in 2011. A villager complains: "our crops failed, our livestock died, and the environmental protection bureau says we have no evidence." The head of the county environmental testing unit defends their position: "the agricultural bureau needs to confirm that the crops failed, livestock death needs to be confirmed by the animal welfare department, they need to prove it is linked with the chemical industry" (Li 2011). Indeed, while initially news articles used the term "cancer village" to point the finger at polluting firms and complicit local governments, more recently some reports dispute the validity of the term (Chen 2013; Li 2011) and accuse villagers of using the law "unscientifically" (Duan 2007). Despite attempts to silence contestation with reference to science, recent levels of contestation (and the government's recent recognition of the existence of cancer villages) suggest that cancer villages are a social and political fact which cannot be dismissed with reference to narrow standards of evidence. Discourses around evidence are mobilized differently in different cases by villagers, campaigners, and local and higher authorities. The following section examines how such contention may develop, particularly among the population and government officials. The rest of this chapter looks at these differences through three examples.

Popular Epidemiology with Chinese Characteristics – The Struggle over Evidence

Initially popularized by the media, the term cancer village is frequently employed by those who identify their village as affected by high rates of cancer that they attribute to pollution. Residents engage in popular epidemiology (collaboration between laypersons and experts to establish a correlation between pollution and health effects, see Brown 2007) as influenced by Chinese cultural frames and collect what they regard as evidence of pollution and its link to cancer. In the United States, popular epidemiology often proceeds by creating local maps of pollution sources and illnesses. In China, villagers do not draw maps but instead, sometimes in collaboration with journalists, compile "name lists" of cancer victims to serve as "scientific evidence" about the extent of harm. The term cancer village and the lists compiled to support the term serve as "weapons of the weak" (Scott 1985), politically sensitive practices which serve to attract attention and demand redress where the local community has otherwise little or no power to do so. As these lists became a prominent feature of high-profile news coverage (such as the CCTV report on Huangmengying in 2004), they were adopted by other villages which sought to prove the detrimental effects of pollution on health. Chen and his team collected four name lists from their six research sites, and Lora-Wainwright found a similar list in one of her sites (a lead and zinc mining village) compiled in 2011 by locals in their attempt to demand compensation and a cleaner environment.

These lists face two major challenges. First, the scale at which their data is collected – typically villages of no more than 3000 people, sometimes much smaller – is too small epidemiologically to count as a valid sample (see Steingraber 2010), even if their data were accepted as accurate.[5] The conventions and scientific standards for confirming the existence of a cancer cluster are at odds with the level at which life is experienced. For instance, epidemiological studies require a long timeframe and a large sample, but cancer villages are by definition village-level entities. Villagers' terms of contention are dismissed by the standards of science. Second, their data cannot be validated by official data collected by the county-level Environmental Protection Bureau (EPB) or the Chinese Center for Disease Control and Prevention (CDC), because the lowest level at which statistics are aggregated is the township level, and therefore high rates in one village are diluted among many other villages where cancer rates are lower. Of course, in theory this does not negate the possibility that specific villages may have abnormally high rates, but it may be used by county governments to disprove villagers' claims by pointing to normal cancer rates at the county level.

One example illustrates this clearly. In Dingbang, a village of 192 some 100 km from Shanghai, cancer rates from 2000 to 2007 were four times the national average according to villagers (Cheng 2013). Villagers pointed to the metal furniture factory in particular (one among a total of 91 industries in the surrounding area) as a culprit. Waste water from the factory contains sulfuric acid and other pollutants. Though their scientific correlation with cancer rates is not clear, villagers were convinced this pollution was to blame for local cancers. According to villagers, staff from the local EPB had visited the metal factory once, but no information on pollution was released. The CDC is responsible for investigating cases of high incidence of serious illnesses, but this had not happened either. In 2010, CDC staff told Chen's team that in 1992 they began to establish a resource hub for recording illness data, but that abnormally high cancer incidence is not visible at the county level. The CDC is unable to assess illness rates at a micro scale, which is where villagers themselves experience it. As a consequence, villagers are trapped between their own village-level evidence and the scale at which the government operates.

Access to data is a serious obstacle to gaining recognition by the government and courts alike. In Dingbang as in many other places, villagers are not legally entitled to enter the factory or demand full records of a factory's emissions. Most often, villagers are unable to collect the necessary evidence to support their claims that pollution causes cancer. This evidence gap – between residents' understanding and what official records, scientific parameters, and the law allow them to prove – has potentially disparate effects:

1 In some cases, it undermines villagers' confidence in the effects of pollution. They may still believe they are victims of pollution, but become very aware of their powerlessness to prove it and, conversely, of the power of industry and local government to contest their claims. One villager in Baocun, a heavily polluted village surrounded by a large fertilizer plant where Lora-Wainwright carried out fieldwork in 2009, put this most clearly. She explained that when locals complained to the factory about pollution's effects on health, one member of staff sniggered "You go and find the evidence!" She reflected that such evidence was very difficult to gather, and therefore villagers were unable to prove their suspicions (Lora-Wainwright 2013b).
2 Limitations on villagers' ability to prove a causal connection between pollution and cancer also motivates them to reframe the ways in which they understand pollution and the demands they make to polluting firms and local governments. Particularly where there is little or no media coverage and where no charismatic, knowledgeable local leader emerges to champion villagers' concerns, initial demands for a cleaner environment and better health may turn into demands for financial compensation for losses incurred (Lora-Wainwright *et al.* 2012).
3 Conversely, in some cases villagers face the obstacles posed by limited data head on and make documenting pollution (rather than proving it has

particular health effects) their main focus. This is particularly likely when educated or well-connected figures live in the area and invest time and energy in collecting information and pressuring industries and governments into taking action (see Huangmengying's example).

4 When villagers try to prove that pollution caused particular damages (instead of only documenting its existence) and to pin responsibility on particular firms, the path is more complex. On this front, cancer villages are also similar to many other polluted villages across China in terms of the wider range of actions adopted to obtain redress. Villagers often first try to liaise directly with polluting firms; second, call on various levels of the government and organize petitions; third, contact the media, NGOs, and a range of "experts"; and finally, if they are still dissatisfied with the outcome, they may resort to lawsuits. While events do not always neatly follow this order and particular strategies (like petitions) may continue throughout, this gives a good indication of how activist strategies unfold. The choice of target and of complaint methods has a powerful effect on how villagers present the problem and what response they receive. Equally, levels of social cohesion influence the ways in which villagers understand the problem, the strategies they embrace to tackle it, and subsequent outcomes (see Shangba's example).

Government responses to villagers' complaints and to the media are as diverse as villagers' strategies, and vary depending on the level of government. At the lowest level of the village and its cadres, responses are sometimes supportive. As we will see in Shangba below, village officials supported petitions against the provincial mines, and even helped to organize them. Similarly in Dongjing, Party members in the village took part in petitioning. In Dingbang, a former township Party secretary who was from the village played a key role in lobbying for attention at higher levels, since he knew personally some of the township officials. Village officials, however, are not always supportive and they may become obstructive if the township puts pressure on them to maintain order. Village cadres in Dongjing explained that they were trapped between needing to maintain villagers' support and demands from the township to curb petitions given the township's reliance on tax revenue from the chemical plant. Sometimes village officials are themselves owners or managers of polluting enterprises, making them, predictably, less supportive of complaints.

At the level of the township and the county, responses to villagers' complaints are almost always negative, at least initially – both in terms of suppressing any resistance (as in Dongjing), refusing to carry out tests, or declaring that data collected by the CDC and EPB do not support villagers' allegations (as in Dingbang). When problems are exposed to higher government levels but there is no sustained media attention or successful campaign to request intervention from them, the common outcome is that pressure is placed back upon local governments to maintain social stability and deal with pollution. Given the financial pressures on township and county governments, they may opt for limited pollution monitoring and repression of local protests. In a few cases – where a media storm successfully attracts too much attention to the region for the status quo to continue undisturbed – pressure and funding from higher levels enable and require township and county governments to monitor pollution and to engage in remediation initiatives, as was the case in Shangba and Huangmengying. Even in such cases, however, the results are not entirely satisfactory for villagers and redress may only be partial.

Shangba: Media Storms, Choosing Targets, and the Importance of Cohesive Communities

Shangba is a village of 3400 residents located in a mountainous area of northern Guangdong province. Villagers have been severely affected by iron mining since it began there decades ago. The main mine is owned by the province, but villagers themselves also opened private mines following the start of economic reforms in the 1980s. Due to mining, local water and soil have become contaminated by heavy metals including lead, zinc, cadmium, and copper. Cadmium is a known human carcinogen and lead is regarded as a possible human carcinogen; therefore the scientific base for a correlation between pollution and cancer is strong. Villagers told Chen's team in 2010 that they started to complain about pollution in the 1970s. They initially became aware of pollution's effects because the water was smelly and "poisonous," prawns and fish died in great numbers, and their skin was irritated if it came into contact with water. Their case attracted the attention of the media, with the first report appearing in 2001 (Zhu 2001) and high-profile coverage in subsequent years (Yang and Fang 2005). These articles in turn attracted scientific and civil society interest to the area (ibid.). According to local records consulted by Chen's colleagues, there were 214 cancer deaths from 1986 to 2005 – that is, 315 people per 100,000 per year, more than twice the average cancer incidence in rural China of 112.57 per 100,000 per year. Attention by the media and researchers further convinced locals that pollution affected their health and provided them with scientific evidence to support their suspicions. However, as mining was carried out by both the provincial mine and by locals, attributing responsibility remained a contested issue.

The ways in which Shangba villagers tackled pollution is deeply influenced by the social texture of the village. Shangba villagers all shared the same surname, which endowed them with great cohesion and high organizational capacity. The ancestral hall is built near the village committee offices and because village cadres are part of the same kinship group, they are trusted and they are effective in coordinating villagers and organizing collective action. This enabled them to organize petitions from the 1980s onward, to attract media attention and to file lawsuits. They compiled lists of cancer victims, and these were used by the media as evidence of high cancer rates. As a result of citizens' efforts and media coverage, the provincial mine and provincial and municipal government offered 14 million yuan to build a reservoir and to connect tap water to all homes in Shangba.[6]

The choice of target and of complaint methods affects how villagers present the problem and what response they received. Shangba villagers' complaints were met with a mixed reception by the local government. The villagers' committee supported petitions which requested compensation from the provincial mine, but not from private mines. This taught villagers to target their complaints at the provincial mine rather than those in private ownership. This strategic approach, however, gave the provincial mine directors grounds to refuse complete responsibility for pollution, and villagers' requests for compensation and clean irrigation water remain unfulfilled. Shangba's case shows that even when evidence is relatively strong and there are high-profile media reports, results are mixed. Beyond the lack of complete remediation, Shangba's notorious reputation as a cancer village affected locals' ability to sell their produce in the market and men's ability to find wives. Though the label of "cancer village" had served to secure clean drinking water, during the latest visit by Chen's team, villagers and village officials alike were keen to shed it and embrace a different identity.

Dongjing: From Violent Protests to Petitioning and Lawsuits

Dongjing villagers followed a similar path of action though the results were partly different.[7] Dongjing is a village with over 2000 inhabitants in northern Jiangsu, a region which is historically underdeveloped as compared to southern Jiangsu. The local government therefore is keen to attract investors and prepared to cut environmental corners to do so. In 2000, the township government which presides over Dongjing made a deal with a chemical industry, Julong, which started to operate in Dongjing later that year. The main products are phloroglucinol and o-chlorophenol; both are organic compounds and derivatives of phenol, the first used in pharmaceutical production and the second in pesticide production, and neither is clearly correlated with increased rates of cancers. However, villagers held local pollution responsible for local cancers. Water tests which found chloride in excess of safe standards by 2000 times provided them with what they considered "iron evidence" of serious pollution.

Local residents told Luo during her fieldwork in 2007, 2008, 2009, and 2011 that they had agreed to having Julong in Dongjing because they had been told it would not cause pollution, but they soon realized that the industry had lied. They recalled that the air became smelly, thick, and unbearable, fish and prawn died, the water tasted strange and turned red. They did not dare eat their own food because it tasted of chemicals. Angered by the factory's behavior, in 2001 they surrounded it to stop production. As Julong ignored them, some began to damage the industry's chimney, some windows and waste water pipes. The police soon arrived and arrested several people and threatened they would not release them unless they promised not to protest again.

This experience taught villagers that direct confrontation tactics were not successful and that the township government was on the side of industry, not of villagers. Instead, they began to collect evidence of harm and pursued peaceful methods to complain. A key figure in this was Duan, a villager in his 60s with a rich life experience and some understanding of the law. Duan had not joined the protests. He made meticulous calculations about the losses incurred by villagers and collected records of cancer deaths between 2001 and 2005, according to which 83 villagers (out of 2115) developed cancer and 64 died. This is over five times higher than the average for rural areas. Most cases were digestive cancers (54), the highest being esophagus cancer (40). In 2008, one woman, whose home is adjacent to the factory and who lost three family members to cancer in three years, said, "We are a famous cancer village." Between 2002 and 2004 Duan, 10 village party members, and 20 villagers phoned the county EPB to report pollution and made countless petitions to the county government and to provincial levels but received no redress. This taught villagers that EPB staff at the county and city level also denied responsibility; they would inform the township before they carried out investigations, and allow the industry to temporarily comply with regulations during the EPB visit. Duan concluded that "officials protect each other."

Following a water contamination accident in March 2005, villagers led by Duan tried to contact the local media but the program was never aired because the township bribed journalists. Having lost faith in the local government and the media, Duan petitioned the central government. This attracted a journalist from Beijing (who did not accept any bribes despite vigorous attempts) who published an incriminating report in November 2005. Many journalists visited the area soon after, but eventually the media interest died down and villagers felt that the media too had failed to solve the problem. No government bureau intervened to control pollution. Villagers had initially put high hopes on higher levels of government to intervene. But this experience made them realize that when higher levels of government are alerted to local misconduct, they simply contact lower levels and tell them to sort it out. In other words, whether problems are solved ultimately depends on the local government. Yet local industry contributes a large share of local government revenue through taxation and through fines for pollution, therefore the local government is unlikely to regulate it too stringently.

As the next step, villagers decided to take the county EPB to court for not fulfilling its responsibility of controlling and investigating the level of firms' pollution as stipulated by law. A "barefoot lawyer" (a villager who taught himself law) from the neighboring town agreed to be their attorney. In March 2006, Duan and three others filed an administrative lawsuit demanding that the county EPB monitor Julong and ensure they abide by environmental protection. The county government responded by requiring Julong to stop production by May 31, 2006 and to move to the county ecological chemical park by the end of 2007. Villagers, however, were still not satisfied. Although Julong moved, it never compensated villagers for all the damage it caused in previous years.

Despite intimidation and offers of bribes by the town and county government, Duan and three others acted as representatives (attorneys) of 369 villagers and filed a civil lawsuit at the city people's court, demanding that Julong pay losses of 738,032 yuan (about US$118,000). The sum was based on detailed calculations about spiritual damages to relatives of cancer victims, and compensation for lost vegetables and for rice. However, the court required the villagers to present evidence of these losses and proof that they were caused by Julong, and on these grounds the villagers lost their case. Their appeal to the provincial court met with the same outcome. The verdict by the Supreme Court stated: "they could not provide proof that crops decrease, vegetables were inedible, and that fish and prawns died because of pollution. There was no proof of the extent, cost and range. They could not provide illness history for cancer cases and death certificates nor provide authenticated conclusion from relevant authorities" (Luo 2013).[8]

Because of legal parameters, villagers were unable to turn pollution's effects, which for them were a social fact, into a legal fact. In such circumstances, the law ultimately makes their suffering invisible, caught as they are in a double bind of being victims of pollution but unable to achieve recognition of their suffering (see Phillips 2012). This begs the question: if courts do not take into consideration the ability of villagers to compile the kind of data required, who or what are they protecting? Are they actually safeguarding justice? Although environmental litigation in China has grown in recent years (Stern 2013), it is little wonder that lawsuits are not villagers' first resort, and that they employ many more and diverse strategies. As in Shangba, results were mixed: the polluting company moved, but villagers failed to gain compensation for past losses. In Dongjing (unlike in Shangba or Huangmengying), there was a clear polluter, but villagers were unable to make it liable to pay compensation. Dongjing's case suggests that through persistence and laborious collection of evidence under the leadership of a skillful villager, villagers may be able to obtain some redress, but that obtaining compensation is a thorny and elusive business. Given these complexities, some campaigners focus instead on documenting the severity of pollution, rather than its effects on bodies and crops. The case of the Huai River basin is an example of this strategy.

Huangmengying and the Huai River Basin: Strong Civil Society and High-level Attention

The most striking example of the power of the media and civil society to affect cancer village cases is Huangmengying and the wider Huai River basin. The Huai River is naturally prone to flooding, and has been the object of several hydraulic projects since the 1950s. However, as industry boomed in the area with the advent of economic reforms in the 1980s, this system of reservoirs and canals aimed to prevent flooding and allow irrigation also spread polluted water in the surrounding area. For this reason, it is also difficult – if not impossible – to trace pollution to specific sources and industries. An accident in 1994 attracted the attention of the central government, which invested in a multi-billion pollution control project. However, similar accidents took place in 1995, 1999, and 2004, pointing to the inadequacies of the project and to continuing pollution.

Long before the State Council (China's cabinet) took notice, villagers already suspected a connection between cancer and water pollution and they were drilling wells as early as the 1980s to avoid having to drink from the river.

Newspaper photographer Daishan Huo played a key role in their efforts to obtain redress. A resident of Shenqiu county in Henan, home to China's largest cluster of cancer villages on the Huai River, Huo began to document local pollution in 1987, soon after local residents began to notice it. Huo turned to campaigning full time in 1998 and formed a group called "Guardians of the Huai River" in 2000. Since then, Huo and his group have trained hundreds of volunteers who now work in teams to regularly monitor the river and conduct water-testing, pushing companies to implement pollution-control measures. They have mounted 70 exhibitions in cities, universities, and villages; they have written letters exposing the illegal activities of local officials and factory owners; and they have raised awareness of local pollution through the media and conferences. They have installed deep-water wells and low-cost water filtration systems in local communities with support from government and private institutions and provided hundreds of cancer patients with medicines. They also have built cooperative relations with local authorities and industries, most prominently a local monosodium glutamate factory, one of China's largest MSG manufacturers and a major polluter. In recognition of these achievements, Mr. Huo won the prestigious Ramon Magsaysay Award in 2010.

These efforts attracted high-profile media attention, and major central government investigations and remediation projects. The report "Rivers and Villages" aired on CCTV in 2004 suggested that water pollution in the Huai basin had severe effects on public health. It stated: "According to the village committee's record of dead residents from 1990 to 2004, 204 people died during this period of 14 years .... 105 people died because of cancer, accounting for 51.5% of the deceased ... Obviously, cancer is prevalent here. Most people who died of cancer are about 50 years old. However, the youngest is only one year old." The village pond water was tested as part of the report and it was found to contain levels of chemical oxygen demand, ammonia, and of five other indicators in excess even of type 5 water, deemed unsuitable for any use.

Significantly, however, Huo's efforts focused on documenting the horrendous extent of local pollution rather than on proving that it caused cancer. Similarly, former journalist and Goldman Prize winner Ma Jun established the Institute of Public and Environmental Affairs (http://www.ipe.org.cn), which for several years has compiled online pollution maps to inform citizens about environmental hazards, demand transparency, and put pressure on polluters to clean up. More recently, a nonprofit group called the IT Engineers for Environmental Protection Association created Danger Maps (weixian ditu: http://www.epmap.org/ngo), an open platform which resorts to crowd-mapping and allows users and NGOs to upload their own pollution data. In both cases, maps do not include the minute level of detail that may be needed to map pollution sources in cancer villages (Danger Maps is still limited in its geographical scope), nor do they make claims to prove that pollution causes illness, but rather to show the extent, type, and location of pollution. Likewise, the "Guardians of the Huai River" avoided making a case for causal connections between cancer and pollution but focused instead on documenting its severity. Given the difficulties in proving such causal connections, the choice is no doubt a strategic one.

Local and central governments have taken actions to tackle pollution in the Huai River basin in a range of different ways, doubtlessly spurred not only by the gravity of the situation but also by the increasing pressure created by civil society. After the report on China's central television in 2004, the central government designed nation-wide and locally based programs for cancer prevention and treatment and it tasked the Center for Disease Control and Prevention with an investigation on cancer and water pollution in the Huai basin which would last for eight years. Gonghuan Yang, a Beijing-based professor of public health at the Chinese Academy of Medical Sciences who was deputy director of CDC at the time, was assigned to lead the project. Lack of data was an obstacle for Yang as it had been for villagers. Many of the area's rural residents were unregistered with health authorities and had never been to a hospital; village doctors had some statistics on the cancer death toll, but the figures were unreliable (Xie and Liu 2013). The findings of their study were published on June 28, 2013 in the *Atlas of the Water Environment and Digestive Cancer Mortality in the Huai River Basin*, a collection of 108 maps showing the severity of water pollution in the Huai River and its tributaries, and rates of digestive cancer deaths in the region. For the first time, they officially correlate high rates of cancer to pollution in the Huai River basin. Because the scale of the study is sufficiently large and aggregates data at the county rather than village level, it has statistical validity. Polluted water, the study suggests, may be directly blamed for several especially prevalent cancers of the gastrointestinal system in the area, including those that attack the esophagus, colon, and rectum.

Some campaigners in China have expressed hope that the newly published atlas could be used as evidence in future environmental public interest lawsuits aimed at winning compensation for victims of pollution (Wang 2013a, 2013b). The atlas, however, does not provide evidence to link specific pollutants or industries to health effects in particular villages. Indeed, it is typically the lack of this information which hinders villagers' and campaigners' efforts to obtain redress from polluters. The fact that pollution has multiple sources and that local flood control and irrigation systems spread it across wide areas further complicates attempts to pin down particular polluting firms for damage in specific sites. Nevertheless, the atlas has created the institutional momentum to close polluting factories in the area and to support further cleanup initiatives, even if it does not offer the evidence which would be required to deem specific polluters responsible for health effects and require that they compensate local populations.

This outcome suggests that high-profile attention is crucial in obtaining intervention, even when specific causal links between pollution and health may be unproven. By contrast, this remains a major hurdle for villagers who demand redress in areas which receive less attention by the central government and the media. And yet, even in areas like Huangmengying, which has been the focus of so much media and central government attention, results are mixed. Media reports and central government initiatives spurred action at the local level. During their fieldwork in Huangmengying, Chen's team found that the government built three deep wells in the village to supply clean drinking water to residents. These wells served an area with 40,000 people, including those outside the village. Shenqiu county authorities took action in 2005 by connecting village water supplies to 47 newly dug wells. Twenty villages with the highest cancer rates were among those benefiting. This was part of a wider initiative by the State Council to provide clean water to rural areas as stipulated in both the 10th and 11th Five-Year Plans (2001–2005 and 2006–2010). Typically this initiative would not have been applied to villages like Huangmengying because, according to regulations, pollution of drinking water should be resolved by the parties responsible for causing pollution. That it was applied successfully here is due to the notoriety of the site, which put pressure on the local government to solve the problem and secured higher government funding to do so, in the absence of evidence of liability for particular firms. All these efforts have improved the situation, but the Huai River is still far from clean (personal communication to Daishan Huo, November 12, 2013; Wang 2013b).

Conclusion

Discourses around cancer villages – among affected villagers, reporters, campaigners, polluters, and various agents of the state – and the types of actions they have triggered have changed dramatically over time. The year 2013 witnessed two major turning points: the first mention of the term in an official document and the publication of a government-sanctioned study which proves the existence of county-level clusters of high cancer incidence due to pollution. Citizens and the media have played a crucial role in making this happen by putting pressure on the government to recognize the existence of the problem and to take action. Cancer villages remain largely a sociopolitical rather than an established medical fact. When enough controversy surrounds a particular site, controversy itself becomes evidence of harm, or at least threatening enough to social stability (still the key principle for China's party-state) that the government opts to intervene. The relative scientific clarity of a link between cancer and local pollution does not seem to be, by itself, a strong explanatory principle for whether villages are able to attract attention or even resolution. In Dongjing and Dingbang the connection between local pollution and cancer rates remained scientifically tenuous, but both sites were able, respectively, to force the industry to close (Dongjing) and to require it to install water treatment equipment (Dingbang).

The government's official recognition of cancer villages and publication of Yang and Zhuang's atlas have not made the topic less contentious (see Barry 2012). On the contrary, the stark increase in reports is evidence of increased debate, which may result in residents of cancer villages making stronger efforts to reach out to government, media, and NGOs. The appearance of Danger Maps in 2013 is one example of this. The official recognition of the existence of cancer villages may serve as an opening for civil society forces concerned with the environment to raise their complaints or to legitimize their activities.

But they may also be part of an effort by the Chinese Communist Party to reclaim the terms of the debate on cancer villages and to silence further protests by suggesting that the government is already tackling this problem. The publication of the atlas may not help other polluted villages to make their case and attract attention. Indeed, it could be used as a standard against which other localities are measured, to stipulate that until a large, longitudinal, and in-depth study such as the one carried out in the Huai basin is done on other places, there is no proof of a correlation between cancer and pollution.

As any Chinese campaigner knows all too well, the line between what is acceptable or even praised by the government and what may result in severe repercussions is a blurred and shifting one. Crackdown on those "spreading rumors" online in 2013 may well extend to those who compile crowd-sourcing maps, if their claims are deemed to lack sufficient evidence. Yet, as we have shown, claims by courts, local governments, and industries that there is "insufficient science" to back allegations about cancer villages do not suffice to dispel anxiety around pollution's effects. Indeed, this may actually exacerbate anxiety, and add to it a deep sense of injustice. Their existence is something that the government has learnt it should recognize rather than deny.

The lesson for the anthropology of environmental health is that social, economic, political, and cultural contexts have crucial importance in influencing villagers' ability to turn cancer villages into social facts. While lack of scientific evidence may fail them in their attempts to gain compensation in court (as in Dongjing's case), it is far from the only determining factor of whether they gain redress. Which places gain attention, recognition, and redress clearly does not only depend on the severity of pollution, on the rates of cancer, or on the demonstrability of a link between them, but on how determined villagers and campaigners are, on the support and skills of local "elites" (like Daishan Huo) and the media, on what strategies they employ, and on their relationships with each other, with the polluters, and with the local state.

ACKNOWLEDGMENTS

Fieldwork for this project was supported by grants from China's National Social Science Funding Program on "Harmony between People and Water: Rural Research in the Tai Lake and the Huai River Basin" (07BSH036) and from the Social Science Research Council's China Environment and Health Initiative on "Public Understanding and Response Strategies to Environmental Health Risks: Research on Cancer Villages." A Leverhulme Trust Research Fellowship (RF-2012-260) and a writing residency at the Rockefeller Foundation Bellagio Center provided the time to complete the chapter. We thank Merrill Singer and Jennifer Holdaway for their comments on earlier drafts. Some of this work was presented at Glasgow University, at a workshop on "Infrastructures of Exposure" at the Centre for Research in the Arts, Social Sciences and Humanities in Cambridge University, and at a panel on "Global Cancer" at the Anthropological Association Annual Meeting in 2013. We benefited greatly from comments at these events.

NOTES

1 Confusingly, it seems that the database was revised between July and November 2013, so the search on November 10, 2013 returned only 68 reports until July, not 106 as in the original search.
2 A new, groundbreaking atlas of cancer and pollution in the Huai river basin is a notable exception (Yang and Zhang 2013), though its data are aggregated at the county rather than village level.
3 For an excellent English-language overview, see Liu (2010). See Deng (2009) for an influential report in the Hong Kong-based magazine *Phoenix Weekly*.
4 Given that these are high-profile cases, and are therefore easily identifiable, we use their real names. Some of the other examples mentioned briefly by contrast are anonymized to protect local informants.
5 We are grateful to Merrill Singer for pointing out that one of the cruel ironies is that everyone in a village of 500 could die of cancer and the scale of the data could be portrayed as too small to be meaningful.
6 By contrast, a neighboring village which also lacked clean water but where villagers did not share the same surname and lacked organizational capacity was unable to obtain clean water.
7 For a fuller description of this case, see Luo (2013).
8 According to Chinese law, in compensation lawsuits concerning environmental pollution, the polluter carries the burden of proof with respect to "demonstrating the lack of causal link between the polluter's actions and the harmful result. In practice, however, courts are still known to require plaintiffs to produce evidence sufficient to demonstrate causation. Given the difficulty of proving causation in environmental pollution cases, this reversal of burden of proof is often the critical determinant of outcome in environmental litigations" (Wang 2006: 209).

REFERENCES

Allen, B. 2003. *Uneasy Alchemy: Citizens and Experts in Louisiana's Chemical Corridor Disputes.* Cambridge: MIT Press.

Auyero, J. and Swistun, D. 2009. *Flammable: Environmental Suffering in an Argentine Shantytown.* Oxford: Oxford University Press.

Balshem, M. 1993. *Cancer in the Community.* Washington, DC: Smithsonian Institution.

Barry, A. 2012. "Political Situations: Knowledge Controversies in Transnational Governance." *Critical Policy Studies*, 6(3): 324–336.

BBC. 2013. "China Acknowledges 'Cancer Villages'." BBC News Online. http://www.bbc.co.uk/news/world-asia-china-21545868 (accessed December 9, 2015).

Brown, P. and Mikkelsen, E. 1997. *No Safe Place: Toxic Waste, Leukemia and Community Action.* Berkeley, CA: California University Press.

Brown, P., Kroll-Smith, S., and Gunter, V. 2000. "Knowledge, Citizens and Organisations. An Overview of Environments, Diseases and Social Conflicts." In S. Kroll-Smith, P. Brown, and V. Gunter (Eds.), *Illness and the Environment: A Reader in Contested Medicine* (pp. 9–25). New York: New York University Press.

Brown, P. 2007. *Toxic Exposures: Contested Illnesses and the Environmental Health Movement.* New York: Columbia University Press.

Cao, L. 2013. "'Cancer Village' Label Is Opposed by Villagers." *Xinhua Meiri Dianxun*, April 11.

Cao, W. 2009. "Shangba Villagers Drink Safe Water." *Shaoguan Ribao*, February 21.

CCTV (China Central Television). 2004. "Rivers and Villages." http://www/cctv/com/news/china/20040810/102281.html (accessed March 4, 2005).

Chen, A. 2013. "Inward and Outward Perspectives on Cancer Villages." In A. Chen, P. Cheng, and Y. Luo (Eds.), *Cancer Village Research: Understanding and Responding to Environmental Health Risks* (pp. 1–28). Beijing: Chinese Social Science Press.

Chen, J. 2013. "The Multiple Facets of 'Red Well Water.'" *Wenhui Bao*, April 11,.

Cheng, P. 2013. "A Rich 'Cancer Village.'" In A. Chen, P. Cheng, and Y. Luo (Eds.), *Cancer Village Research: Understanding and Responding to Environmental* Health (pp. 67–97). Beijing: Chinese Social Science Press.

Cody, E. 2004. "Chinese Newspapers Put Spotlight on Polluters." *Washington Post*, May 25. http://www.washingtonpost.com/wp-dyn/articles/A53012-2004May24.html# (accessed December 9, 2015).

Deng, F. 2009. "China's 100 Cancer Causing Places." *Phoenix Weekly*, no. 11, April 2009.

Deng, J. 2005. "Cancer Villages on the Banks of the Shaying River." *Zhongguo Shehui Bao*, May 19.

Dewey, C. 2013. "Chinese State Media Release a Map Showing the Spread of 'Cancer Villages.'" *Washington Post*, February 22. http://www.washingtonpost.com/blogs/worldviews/wp/2013/02/22/chinese-state-media-releases-a-map-showing-the-spread-of-cancer-villages/ (accessed December 9, 2015).

Double Leaf. 2009. "China Cancer Villages Map." Created May 7 and updated June 1, 2009. http://maps.google.com/maps/ms?hl=en&ie=UTF8&lr=lang_en&msa=0&msid=104340755978441088496.0004696l1a28a0d8a22dd&ll=34.098728,117.292099&spn=0.268943,0.4422&z=11 (accessed December 9, 2015).

Duan, J. 2007. "The Expression 'Cancer Village' Is Not Scientific: Workers in Science and Technology Have a Duty to Promote Environmental Health Science to the Public." *Dazhong Keiji Bao*, July 1.

Fortun, K. 2001. *Advocacy After Bhopal: Environmentalism, Disaster, New Global Orders.* Chicago: Chicago University Press.

Institute of Public and Environmental Affairs. No date. "Institute of Public and Environmental Affairs." http://www.ipe.org.cn.

IT Engineers for Environmental Protection Association. No date. "Danger Maps." http://www.epmap.org/ngo (accessed May 12, 2014).

Lerner, S. 2005. *Diamond: A Struggle for Environmental Justice in Louisiana's Chemical Corridor.* Cambridge, MA: MIT Press.

Lerner, S. 2010. *Sacrifice Zones: The Front Lines of Toxic Chemical Exposure in the United States.* Cambridge, MA: MIT Press.

Li, J. 2004. "Huai River Pollution Causes Several 'Cancer Villages.'" *Xinhua Meiri Dianxun*, June 29.

Liu, L. 2010. "Made in China: Cancer Villages." *Environment Magazine* (March–April) http://www.environmentmagazine.org/Archives/Back%20Issues/March-April%202010/made-in-china-full.html (accessed December 9, 2015).

Li, X. 2011. "'Chromium Crisis in Luliang, Yunnan." *Diyi Caijing Ribao*, August 24.

Lora-Wainwright, A. 2013a. "Plural Forms of Evidence and Uncertainty in Environmental Health: A Comparison of Two Chinese Cases." *Evidence and Policy*, 9(1): 49–64.

Lora-Wainwright, A. 2013b. "The Inadequate Life: Rural Industrial Pollution and Lay Epidemiology in China." In *Dying for Development: Illness and the Limits of Citizens' Agency in China*, special collection edited by A. Lora-Wainwright in *China Quarterly*, 214(June): 302–320.

Lora-Wainwright, A., Zhang, Y., Wu, Y., and Van Rooij, B. 2012. "Learning to Live with Pollution: The Making of Environmental Subjects in a Chinese Industrialised Village." *The China Journal*, 68 (July): 106–124.

Luo, Y. 2013. "'Cancer Village' in Subei." In A. Chen, P. Cheng, and Y. Luo (Eds.), *Cancer Village Research: Understanding and Responding to Environmental Health Risks* (pp. 29–66). Beijing: Chinese Social Science Press.

Ministry of Environment. 2013. "Guard Against and Control Risks Presented by Chemicals to the Environment During the 12th Five-Year Plan (2011–2015)." http://www.zhb.gov.cn/gkml/hbb/bwj/201302/W020130220539067366659.pdf (accessed March 10, 2013).

Murphy, M. 2006. *Sick Building Syndrome and the Problem of Uncertainty: Environmental Politics, Technoscience, and Women Workers.* Durham, NC: Duke University Press.

Nanfang Dushi. 2007a. "China's Water Crisis." *Nanfang Dushi*, November 2. http://www.nddaily.com/sszt/watercrisis/ (accessed November 21, 2007).

Nanfang Dushi. 2007b. "A Diary of Three Villages of Death." *Nanfang Dushi*, November 5. http://www.nddaily.com/A/html/2007-11/05/content_299441.htm (accessed November 21, 2007).

Ottinger, G. 2013. *Refining Expertise: How Responsible Engineers Subvert Environmental Justice Challenges.* New York: New York University Press.

Petryna, A. 2002. *Life Exposed: Biological Citizens after Chernobyl.* Princeton, NJ: Princeton University Press.

Phillips, T. 2012. "Repressive Authenticity in the Quest for Legitimacy: Surveillance and the Contested Illness Lawsuit." *Social Science and Medicine*, 75: 1762–1768.

Scott, J. 1985. *Weapons of the Weak: Everyday Forms of Peasant Resistance.* New Haven, CT: Yale University Press.

Shevory, T. 2007. *Toxic Burn: The Grassroots Struggle against the WTI incinerator.* Minneapolis, MN: Minnesota University Press.

Singer, M. 2011. "Down Cancer Alley: The Lived Experience of Health and Environmental Suffering in Louisiana's Chemical Corridor." *Medical Anthropology Quarterly*, 25(2): 141–163.

Steingraber, S. 2010. *Living Downstream: An Ecologist's Personal Investigation of Cancer and the Environment*, 2nd ed. Cambridge, MA: Da Capo Press.

Stern, R. 2013. *Environmental Litigation in China: A Study in Political Ambivalence.* Cambridge: Cambridge University Press.

Szasz, A. 1994. *Ecopopulism: Toxic Waste and the Movement for Environmental Justice.* Minneapolis, MN: University of Minnesota Press.

Tesh, S. 2000. *Uncertain Hazards: Environmental Activists and Scientific Proof.* Ithaca, NY: Cornell University Press.

Waldman, L. 2009. *The Politics of Asbestos: Understandings of Risk, Disease and Protest.* London: Earthscan.

Wang, A. 2006. "The Role of Law in Environmental Protection in China: Recent Developments." 8 *Vermont Journal of Environmental Law*, pp. 195–223.

Wang, Y. 2013a. "The Voice of the Polluted." *NewsChina*, vol. 062 (September). http://www.newschinamag.com/magazine/the-voice-of-the-polluted (accessed December 9, 2015).

Wang, Y. 2013b. "Death Maps." *News China* (October). http://www.newschinamag.com/magazine/death-maps (accessed December 9, 2015).

Wertime, D. 2013. "Chinese State Media Shares Powerful Map of 'Cancer Villages' Creeping Inland." *Tea Leaf Nation*, February 22. http://www.tealeafnation.com/2013/02/chinas-state-run-media-shares-powerful-map-of-cancer-villages-creeping-inland (accessed February 23, 2013).

World Bank. 2007. *The Cost of Pollution in China.* http://siteresources.worldbank.org/INTEAPREGTOPENVIRONMENT/Resources/China_Cost_of_Pollution.pdf (accessed December 9, 2015).

Xie, H. and Liu, H. 2013. "Sip of Death Plagues Cancer Villages." *Caixin*, October 15. Republished in *Chinafile*: http://www.chinafile.com/sip-death-plagues-river-villages.
Yang, C. and Fang, Q. 2005. "A Village of Death and Its Hopes for the Future." *Nanfang News Evening Edition*, November 18. www.southcn.com/news/dishi/shaoguan/ttxw/200511180238.htm (accessed December 9, 2015).
Yang, G. and Zhuang, D. 2013. *Atlas of the Water Environment and Digestive Cancer Mortality in the Huai River Basin*. Beijing: Zhongguo Ditu Chubanshe.
Zhu, H. 2001. "Mining Waste Water Harms a Village." *Chinese Mining Newspaper*, January 20.

CHAPTER 20

Mining and Its Health Consequences: From Matewan to Fracking

Elizabeth Cartwright

Thinking Into the Future: Eco-Risks of Extractive Mining Industries

I begin with two mining scenarios. They occur on opposite sides of the globe and they are different on many levels. What unites them is what unites all the ethnographic scenarios and illnesses that I include in this chapter – the occupation of mining. Extracting minerals from the earth comes at a high cost in human health and well-being. In each situation there is a cultural construction of risk. That risk is comprised of local notions of the dangers that surround mining combined with the current technologies used to perceive those dangers. These are combined with the ways in which groups of people try to legally, or otherwise, control and mitigate the damages caused by mining (Cartwright and Thomas 2000). Are the dangers inherent in mining worth the risk and what price are individuals and groups of individuals willing to pay in an increasingly industrialized world that so depends on the mining of many types of minerals? How does the risk taken by some benefit or damage the lives of others?

Scenario One: As the current Apple store advertisement enticingly describes it, the newest iPhone is one amazing little machine and it "feels great in your hand" (retrieved from Apple.com, February 23, 2014). What is it that makes

A Companion to the Anthropology of Environmental Health, First Edition. Edited by Merrill Singer.

that sleek little intelligent phone tick? Coltan. According to Hayes and Burge (2003), the mining of coltan in Central Africa occurs in areas near rivers where the soil is unstable and where accidents, many of them serious in nature, occur on a regular basis. Coltan is considered a conflict mineral because it is often mined under dangerous and illegal conditions and it is used to create profit for armed groups through theft, control of production at mine sites, taxation/ extortion, and trade in the Congo to finance military conflicts. As reported by the Costa Rican company Magma Coltan (a company that specializes in conflict-free mining of coltan in Costa Rica):

> As the demand for coltan capacitors for electronics has steadily increased over the last several years, more residents than ever of the Democratic Republic of Congo (DRC) have turned to the often dangerous and sometimes fatal practice of illegal mining. Why do so many people end up doing this backbreaking, lethal form of extracting ore? The reasons are often more complex than most people realize. While some are forced into service by guerilla warriors and tribal leaders embroiled in local wars, others choose to extract columbite-tantalite ore because of the impressive tantalum price on the open market ... [In the most common form of coltan mining] men, women and children mine by hand. They dig basins in or alongside streams by scraping away the mud and letting the stream's water rush in. They then swirl the water around, creating a minor whirlpool that washes away lighter debris while the ore settles to the bottom. (Magma Coltan 2012)

Working in coltan mining, especially in illegal mining operations, puts an individual at risk for the physical hazards of crushing injuries from rock falls, drowning in the streams, and the local social conditions of violence, malnutrition, lack of medical care, and all the other maladies associated with extreme poverty that create a maelstrom of suffering.

Scenario Two: It was the mid-1990s, and I was doing research in Sonora, Mexico. I had a particularly memorable discussion about mining and illness with a Mexican colleague of mine on a drive down to Cananea, Sonora. We were discussing workmen's compensation and she said that the miners in the nearby copper mines received their retirement benefits from the company based on the amount of lung damage from silicosis that they could medically document. Each year, the miners underwent lung function tests and were given a "percent of lung damaged" certificate. The more damaged their lungs, the higher their compensation packages would be upon retirement. Because their lung damage was cumulative, if they could stay on working in the mine for a longer period of time their retirement benefits would be higher. Many of them tried to stay on for as long as humanly possible. With each passing year their ability to breathe decreased as their retirement benefits concomitantly increased. It was, and likely still is, a tragic trade-off. (See Finn 1998 for an interesting comparison case.)

The health consequences of the mining industry that I will discuss in the following sections have some overlap with diseases and situations discussed in other chapters in this edited volume. Miners experience illnesses that come from air pollution, water pollution, contaminated food, and the myriad diseases of poverty. I am interested in pursuing the idea that the occupation of mining brings together a unique constellation of dangers that when taken in their totality are a huge burden of ill health for miners, their families, and their communities across the globe. Studying the effects of the mining industry on human health can be approached from many different levels of magnification; it is a matter of scale. While the health consequences of mining can be far-reaching, such as in the case of fracking (Cartwright 2013) and with "down-winders" (see Singer and Hodge, this volume), the miners and their families are the ones who most often experience the devastating health consequences of the processes of mining (Zhuang *et al.* 2009). As miners, they make their livelihoods from this occupation and they often view it as the best possible occupational opportunity available to them – something that is just as true in the western United States as it is in the remote regions of South America, China, Africa, and elsewhere. Mining salaries in the western US have skyrocketed in the last 10 years, making places like Wyoming and North Dakota attractive for individuals seeking employment. The same sort of economic decision making engaged in by the US miners may be leading the miners in the DRC to choose to enter the coltan mines. Despite the short-term gains of this kind of employment, mining is one of the most dangerous occupations in the world and it is one that often highlights the effects of class and lives lived in situations of structural and physical violence.

I use the term "eco-risk" to highlight how individuals and groups of individuals react to dangers that they perceive as coming from their environment. As I have defined the concept of eco-risk in past work (Cartwright 2013), it is the multilevel process of understanding and reacting to threats to our health and well-being that emanate from our environment. These environmental threats come in all sizes, from the molecular level that is impossible to perceive without the aid of technology, to the most blatant and overwhelming mountains of uranium tailings, deep black coal smoke, and earthquakes caused by fracking (Hand 2014). These dangers are both short term and long term and they are very difficult to escape, especially in the situation where your occupation (in this case mining) forces you into prolonged, unremitting contact with disease-producing elements in the environment. The concept of eco-risk highlights how the creation of an "accepted" risk is a process that is comprised of (a) cultural recognition of the dangers, (b) that recognition is predicated and instantiated based on the available technologies of perception (*pace* Foucault), and (c) the manner in which the particular risk is legitimized or disallowed via legal systems that enforce health and safety standards and/or legitimate claims of wrongdoing. I want to emphasize that the recognized dangers are enmeshed in the ways that the minerals being mined are valued both as commodities and as sources of pride, power, and aesthetics (Richardson and Weszkalnys 2014). The process of understanding local eco-risks is similar, if not on the same scale, as the cultural construction of medical risk described by my colleague Jan Thomas and myself (Cartwright and Thomas 2000).[1] Through keeping the focus here on the occupation of mining, I want to force the issue that there are, or should be, legal systems that can be brought to bear on infringements of existing health and safety standards. Legal systems also can be used as a tool to develop better health and safety standards in the future; and, importantly, legal systems can also provide a route to demand justice in the case of ongoing and past negligence.

The ethnographies produced by nonmedical anthropologists, such as those by Sawyer (2004), Kirsch (2008), and Li (2009), contain exceptional material about local notions of illness, curing, and the role of the mine-impacted environment on indigenous health and well-being; the boundaries between "cultural" and "medical" anthropology blur. Talking across subdisciplinary boundaries becomes crucial. A multidisciplinary approach implemented with ethnographic descriptions is an effective approach in documenting such things as chemical and physical exposures and hazards that occur in locales studied by anthropologists. Legal action against wanton polluting as well as medical attention for industrially produced health problems rest on precise documentation of exposures; this implies a way of doing anthropology that includes both broadly construed, culturally focused, meaning-centered descriptive work and the quantifiable work of our colleagues in the "hard sciences."

As we move to a more and more globalized economy, the effects of mining may be more widespread and more difficult to trace. There are old patterns of illnesses such as the ubiquitous "black lung" and concomitant high rates of ever-evolving HIV/AIDS and TB; there are new patterns of danger associated with small-scale artisanal mining for coltan (and gold), and there are new forms of "black lung" disease that are being documented in the eastern United States (Petsonk, Rose, and Cohen 2013). With the burgeoning economies in China, India, and other parts of the world, the scale of mining is growing explosively. There is a need for a critical medical anthropology of mining, mining labor, and the plethora of illnesses that are a result of exposure to the toxic substances and social environments created by the industry. As Kirsch (2008) points out, highlighting the logics behind local, oftentimes indigenous, responses to the toxicities of mining yields descriptions of new ways of envisioning "sustainable development"; the alternative to finding a new way to conceptualize our way forward is to keep reliving our past.

A Bit of Mining History: Nothing New Under the Sun ...

> By sunset on May 19, 1920, ten men lay dead in the coal mining town of Matewan, West Virginia, the result of a gun battle between striking coal miners and Baldwin Felts detectives hired by the Stone Mountain Coal Corporation. The Matewan Massacre, as it was later called, became one of the most famous events in West Virginia and Appalachian history. It was also a galvanizing point for the United Mine Workers of America (UMWA). (Lies 2009)

The 1920 massacre of miners agitating for union representation at Matewan, West Virginia resulted in further cementing the nascent worker's union (the UMWA) that was established in 1890 and that flourished under the 40-year leadership of John L. Lewis (1920–1960). The UMWA is still a major labor organizing force in the United States. The UMWA has successfully implemented mining safety standards and workers' compensation funds for its members in the US. It is respected industry-wide for the expertise it brings to bear on occupational hazards and labor disputes. For instance, the UMWA was called in to investigate the Upper Big Branch (UBB) mine disaster that occurred in West Virginia in 2010 that killed 29 miners. The UBB mine was not a unionized mine. The UMWA was brought in as an outside investigative agency; their investigation found that the health and safety regulations of the mine had been compromised at the expense of the workers. The final UMWA report on the Upper Big Branch mine disaster included a detailed letter of explanation to the families of the miners killed in that explosion. The letter was very clear that the Performance Coal Company was negligent.[2]

In the United States and other well-off countries, there are safety laws, such as those that were flaunted at the UBB mine, that have significantly decreased the number of fatal mining accidents over the last hundred years. The laws cannot rid this industry of all its inherent risks, even those that are considered to be preventable according to current safety standards. This is also a case of an industry whose safety is heavily dependent on continued upkeep and surveillance of the equipment being used in the extraction processes. When management changes, when economic fortunes wane, when any number of things happen that result in less oversight and less maintenance, the result quickly becomes lethal. For instance, in the UBB mine the gas accumulated because the ventilation system was not functioning correctly. Once the shovel hit the hard rock and caused sparks, gases were ignited and caused the fire which the sprinkler system should have been able to put out. The sprinkler heads had been removed and/or were not functioning. At that point, the fire became unstoppable. Miners knew of the problems but, because they needed the jobs and were not able to take their complaints to management for fear of retribution, they felt they were powerless to prevent the buildup of conditions that led to the disaster. Autopsies on the 29 victims showed the cause of death to be carbon monoxide poisoning for 19 individuals, trauma for the remaining 10 (Petsonk, Rose, and Cohen 2013).

An investigation into the deaths by the West Virginia State Medical Examiner and outside specialists that was included in the Governor's Special Investigation Report also revealed shocking physical evidence about the state of the miners' lung health, namely that 17 out of the 24 miners (72%) had coal worker's pneumoconiosis (CWP) and five of those had less than 10 years' experience working in the mine. This is a much more rapid progression of the disease than expected. Sixteen of the seventeen miners with CWP had started working after the modern dust limits were put in place in1969 (Petsonk, Rose, and Cohen 2013).

In the United States, approximately 28 times the number of miners die from CWP disease every year as die from mining accidents (McAteer 2011). Beginning in the year 2000, two different physicians began reporting to the International Labor Office (ILO) that they were seeing an increase in cases of CWP in underground miners in Appalachia and that the disease is beginning earlier in miners' working lives than in the past. This was the first up-tick in the prevalence of CWP since stricter safety standards were implemented in the Federal Coal Mine

Health and Safety Act of 1969 (Petsonk, Rose, and Cohen 2013). The change, while still not totally understood, is being attributed to working in "thinner layers" of mineral deposits where miners need to drill through more silica-containing rocks than they did in the past. Smaller mining operations with fewer safety measures may play a role as well. Cumulative dust exposure, masks that clog with the ever-finer dust created by more powerful drills, and long (12-hour) shifts that don't allow miners to clear out their lungs in fresh air are all probably part of the process producing more and earlier cases of CWP (Baxter *et al.* 2000: 682).

The UBB mine disaster was ultimately attributed to company negligence and greed, perhaps some of the more intractable aspects of this industry. In regions of the world where workers have less access to labor organizations, mining conditions are even more dangerous than they are in the United States, Canada, and the European Union. In South Africa, for example, the mining industry is widely recognized to be one of the most fatal in the world. With high rates of death in underground mines, poor living conditions for miners, and very high rates of communicable diseases such as HIV/AIDS and TB, miners and their families in southern Africa live and work in desperate situations (Stuckler *et al.* 2013). In the global sense, the concept of health disparities and class, structural vulnerability, and violence lend an important critical voice to workers' demands and demonstrations for reasonably safe working conditions (Cartwright 2011; Quesada, Kain, and Bourgois 2011; Pine 2013). Through keeping the focus on the occupation of mining, we intellectually group many disparate health problems and at the same time we force comparisons between regions of the world and between subfields of the industry. Collectively, the litany of environmental health impacts creates a conceptual tool that can be used to critique our currently unfettered trajectory of industrial development. Corporate and government-focused medical anthropological ethnographies of mining companies and national governments via a multi-sited approach like those used by Nordstrom (2007) could elucidate how decision making with respect to health decisions, such as the ratification of the International Labor Organization's Safety and Health in Mines Convention 176, plays out in the context of multinational mining companies. It is in the offices, far from the heat and dust and noise of the mines, where the power is held and where the decisions are made – in short, where livelihoods and lives are decided. The anthropological tool of ethnography can be used to incisively bring together the levels of the processes involved in mineral extraction, processing, transport, and refining and connect it to the health issues that emerge at each step in the production chain.

"The Importance of Time"

The human activity of mining both produces the energy that we need to power our carbon-based societies while it negatively affects our individual and collective health and well-being in profound ways. Anthropologists have studied mining communities in many places worldwide (Ballard and Banks 2003;

Kirsch 2008; Welker 2009; Carrasco 2011; Rolston 2013). As Kirsch notes, anthropologists are particularly situated to see the inherent contradictions that the activity of mining brings to light in the way that we choose to live and exploit our environment:

> The US Environmental Protection Agency identified mining as the nation's leading source of toxic pollution for the last 9 years. Pollution from a single mining project can affect hundreds of square miles and acid mine drainage can render environments inhospitable to organic life for centuries. Yet despite the indisputable evidence of the environmental damage caused by mining, for the last decade the industry has aggressively promoted the corporate oxymoron of sustainable mining. (Kirsch 2010: 88)

There is nothing sustainable about mining; the jobs aren't sustainable as they last just until the deposit is extracted (at least with existing technology and in light of prevailing market prices); the benefits aren't sustainable as they are predicated on a way of life that is too consumptive for our planet; the technologies aren't sustainable as they pollute water and air, create deforestation, cause loss of topsoil, loss of land, and diminished sea productivity that will stretch in the far future. And, with reference to the concerns of medical anthropology, the well-being of the people who work in the mines is not sustainable as they endure a myriad of threats to their health, both physical and mental.

Time is a critical component to consider when thinking through the effects of mining on health. Much of what is mined is dangerous when it is extracted and it remains that way for hundreds if not thousands of years. Mining practices are still with us from the past. A recent article in the *New York Times* described the present-day situation for Navajos living near abandoned mines situated on their homelands:

> In this dusty corner of the Navajo reservation, where seven generations of families have been raised among the arroyos and mesas, Bertha Nez is facing the prospect of having to leave her land forever. The uranium pollution is so bad that it is unsafe for people to live here long term, environmental officials say. Although the uranium mines that once pocked the hillsides were shut down decades ago, mounds of toxic waste are still piled atop the dirt, raising concerns about radioactive dust and runoff. And as cleanup efforts continue, Ms. Nez and dozens of other residents of the Red Water Pond Road community, who have already had to leave their homes at least twice since 2007 because of the contamination, are now facing a more permanent relocation. Although their village represents only a small sliver of the larger Navajo nation, home to nearly 300,000 people, they are bearing the brunt of the environmental problems …
>
> "Our umbilical cords are buried here, our children's umbilical cords are buried here. It's like a homing device," said Tony Hood, 64, who once worked in the mines and is now a Navajo interpreter for the Indian Medical Center in Gallup. "This is our connection to Mother Earth. We were born here. We will come back here eventually." (Frosch 2014, see Singer and Hodge, this volume)

Navajos living and working near the uranium mines have increased rates of lung cancer, COPD, pulmonary fibrosis, and anxiety and depression (Dawson and

Madsen 2011; Singer and Hodge, this volume). The following section discusses a plethora of health problems that emanate from mining. As in the case of the uranium tailings on the Navajo reservation, the toxic remains from mines can create health consequences far into the future; the safe disposal of what we currently understand to be toxic materials can falter over time; and what we think is safe now maybe be discovered to be toxic in the future.

Health Consequences of Mining: A Brief Overview

While it is beyond the scope of this chapter to go into the vast detailed literature that describes the health problems most often faced by miners, their families, and their surrounding communities, I will briefly describe the main health issues in order to flesh out the scope of what environmental health-oriented medical anthropologists *could* study in the future. I will then include some ethnographic excerpts that best illustrate the situations. Much work remains to be done on this topic. Medical anthropology has barely scratched the surface of what matters for millions of mine workers and their families.

Physical Hazards

The many hazards of mining have been documented in occupational health journals (Donoghue 2004); medical anthropology's task is to undertake the study of the social and cultural meanings and contexts of these hazards. I start this discussion with a focus on the physical hazards of mining.

> Physical hazards of mining include: traumatic injuries from rock falls, fires, explosions, falls from heights, entrapments and electrocutions. There is the danger of flooding that can occur both inside and outside of the mine. There is the noise that comes from drilling, blasting, cutting, ventilation and ore processing all resulting in hearing loss when not controlled. Radon exposure and solar UV exposures come from working in above surface mines. There are increased heat and humidity that lead to serious exhaustion and whole body vibration, hand and arm vibration that lead to skeletal pain and disability. (Donoghue 2004: 283–284)

Rolston's (2013) ethnographic work on open-pit coal mining in Wyoming gives a visceral perspective on what it is like to be in the huge mine equipment that is used in large-scale extractive processes. The walls of earth, carved hundreds of meters deep through differently hard and soft layers, are a constant danger in the pits. The large shovels, draglines, and haul trucks shake workers' bodies, creating stresses to joints and organs. The vibrations from the explosions, sounds of the equipment, and sounds of falling rocks on the roof of the vehicles all contribute to a less than healthy workplace. Rolston describes what it is like for a woman to operate the heavy equipment in the open-pit mines in Wyoming:

> By the end of decades of work at a mine, Jo had operated almost every single piece of machinery and trained new hires. Convinced that the Caterpillar equipment was "designed for men and male body types," she explained, "women are longer in the

legs, men in the waist. You have to lean forward when you're operating a blade, and they didn't design the seat for a woman." Nicole also combated sex-specific adjustments. She vividly remembered her first attempts operating the scrapers: "I got on there and I did the best job I knew … It was scary, I mean, because you get up on your side, yeah, and you got your tires off the ground and you're kind of rooting and rolling around and stuff, and it was nerve wracking. And I got to where I loved it, but I hurt when I got off of it." An older crewmember warned her to be careful, telling her that he did not want to appear sexist, but that "your kidneys aren't attached the same way mine are. Mine are tucked in a little tighter and yours are out a little bit. I don't want you to spend that much time in there, jiggling, and your kidneys break loose." His concern reinforced her own. "I enjoy it but I don't want to be on it much anymore," she said. "I do hurt, and it's just not … a good piece of equipment. But I love it and I'm good at it, and I would love to get on it every once in a while." She eventually started operating dozers but found that as with most of the equipment, "you just get beat up." That specific wording – getting "beat up" by the equipment – was pervasive throughout the basin. (Rolston 2013: 586)

The mechanical harms that come from noise, heat, and vibration can have profound impacts on the health of individuals. Hearing loss, deafness, tinnitus, and vertigo can be debilitating as can hand/arm vibration (from drills) and whole-body vibration from driving heavy equipment (Baxter *et al.* 2000). The ramifications of hearing problems, carpal-tunnel syndrome, low-back pain, and so on play into the other chronic health problems that come from working in these large-scale, highly mechanized mines. Driving heavy equipment is taxing in many ways, but it is not hard physical labor – indeed it is very sedentary, resulting in a workforce that is increasingly overweight and obese with concomitant high rates of diabetes, heart disease, and other associated problems (Rolston 2013).

Chemical Hazards

The next group of hazards is classified as "chemical," but includes diseases as different as "black lung" disease and the mental health problems that come from mercury poisoning.

Chemical hazards in mining start with the ubiquitous silicosis and silico-tuberculosis that comes from the additional damage that occurs in the lungs when one has TB and silicosis, like the majority of the miners do in places such as South Africa. Chronic obstructive pulmonary disease comes from prolonged exposures to silica as does lung cancer. Beyond the silica itself is the coal dust that causes "black lung"/pneumoconiosis and COPD. Asbestos-related diseases, while largely controlled in places like the US, continue to occur in much of the world. Exposures to diesel particulates cause lung cancer as do the arsenic that comes from copper smelting and nickel that comes from nickel refineries. Many chemicals, during the metallurgical processing, increase one's risk of lung cancer and nasal cancer. Mercury exposures that lead to an array of psychological pathologies are a serious issue in gold mining, especially in areas of the world where processing is not controlled. (Donoghue 2004)

The health effects of chemical exposures are always dependent on which chemical or chemicals one is dealing with and in what form that chemical is in when one is exposed to it, as well as the dose (quantity of chemical taken into the body), the duration of the exposure, the route (inhalation, ingestion, dermal, etc.), and the age and the health of the person. Assessing these variables is an area that is clearly ripe for transdisciplinary work. An example of chemical hazards exemplifying the multilevel eco-risks in mining are the kinds of dangers coming from small-scale, artisanal gold mining. This kind of mining is highly dangerous and mostly unregulated. It occurs where there are gold deposits deemed too small or too remote to be profitably mined by large mining companies. Mercury is used in the extractive processing that is often carried out in small buildings near residential areas:

> About 20% of the world's gold is produced by the artisanal and small-scale gold mining sector. This sector is also responsible for the largest releases of mercury to the environment of any sector globally. A major source of air pollution from mercury, artisanal and small-scale gold mining releases approximately 400 metric tons of airborne elemental mercury each year. Located in over 55 countries, small scale gold buying and refining facilities (commonly referred to as "Gold Shops") are an important part of this production process, and are a major cause of air pollution from mercury. The burning of mercury-gold amalgam in these Gold Shops can have serious health effects both locally and globally. (EPA n.d.)

A recent article in the journal the *Lancet* describes one such mining community in South America:

> The airborne mercury in Segovia (Colombia) emanates from scores of small gold mills, locally known as *entables*, where gold-flecked rocks from nearby mines are pulverized in rolling steel drums containing mercury, which forms an easily retrieved amalgam with gold. Once the mercury-gold amalgam is removed from the drums, it is heated in small furnaces that vaporize the mercury, producing semi-pure gold while disseminating a powerful airborne neurotoxin into the city's air. These health-threatening gold production practices, which were pioneered centuries ago but long-abandoned by large-scale gold companies, are used by an estimated 200,000 artisanal miners in Colombia, and as many as 13 million others in 70 nations worldwide. (Webster 2012: 1379)

As described by Webster (2012), the process of artisanal gold mining in this area not only creates an environment full of mercury which can cause changes in mentation, anxiety, depression, muscle tremors, kidney failure, respiratory failure, and death, but additionally, the Colombian case discussed here is characterized by high levels of interpersonal violence, robberies, extortion, and paramilitary oppression due to the increased cash flows in the context of an ongoing civil war of 60 years plus duration. China, India, South Africa, and many other nations similarly use these outdated and dangerous methods to mine for gold, creating deadly community health situations especially for those directly involved with the burning off of the mercury during processing.

Gold mining, like other heavy metal ore and coal mining, also creates a phenomenon called acid mine drainage. Mining exposes pyrite, a very common mineral. When mining operations are finished, water seeps back into contact with the now-exposed pyrite and causes a reaction that results in the creation of sulfuric acid, which in turn can dissolve any heavy metals left in the rock walls, slag pits, tailing piles, etc. This produces serious water pollution with many minerals and arsenic. According to the trade journal *Mining Weekly*'s May 8, 2009 issue, acid mine drainage is the "single most significant threat to South Africa's environment." This widespread source of water pollution contributes to the overall ill health associated with mining communities in the present and will continue to produce these chemical hazards long into the future unless large-scale, costly remediation is undertaken (Johnson and Hallberg 2005).

Another example of the ramifications of chemical exposures is that of coal mine dust lung disease (CMDLD). CMDLD includes the spectrum of diseases that result from prolonged exposure to dust in coal mines; these include CWP, silicosis, mixed-dust pneumonconiosis and dust-related diffuse fibrosis, and chronic obstructive pulmonary disease (COPD). CMDLD is often found occurring in the presence of various pathogens (TB, HIV etc.), resulting in increased severity of all the diseases precisely because of the fact that they are coexisting and interactive, thus creating a perfect syndemic storm (Singer 2009):

> Miners have significantly elevated risks of pulmonary disease, arising from cumulative exposure to toxins inside the mines. Silica dust inhalation causes silicosis, an occupational lung disease leading to scarring of the lungs. About one-quarter of miners had silicosis in 2008, roughly the same prevalence recorded in the early 1900s ... Silicosis increases risks of lung cancer by two-fold ... and lung TB by four-fold ... Silica dust increases the risk of TB in a dose-response relationship, even without the development of silicosis. Because of these pulmonary hazards, workers in South Africa's gold mining industry have among the highest incidences of TB in the world, of between 3,000 and 7,000 cases per 100,000 population per year, compared with global incidence of 128 per 100,000 population per year and rates in South Africa of about 920 per 100,000 per year. (Stuckler *et al.* 2013: 640–641)

Coal mine dust lung disease (CMDLD) can be analyzed through the lens of the concept "eco-risk." The first part of the equation of an eco-risk is to see the pathology within a three-dimensional space of contagion. Starting from the interior physiological processes of disease transmission and pathophysiological states, there are the cellular levels. In the case of silicosis, thin silica fibers in the coal dust wend their way into the distal cellular structures of the lung causing fibrosis (excess connective tissue), that leads to emphysema, lung cancer, obstructive lung disease, and silicosis. Other fibrotic changes also occur from other substances in the coal dust. With CMDLD tuberculosis risk increases concomitantly as silicosis increases, and the presence of silicosis and HIV on tuberculosis is "multiplicative" in that each condition is exponentially worsened by the coexistence of the other conditions. Smoking additionally compounds pathological manifestations of all of these diseases (Chen *et al.* 2012) and poor nutrition and obesity exacerbate the symptoms of decreased cardiopulmonary functioning, leading to increased rates of heart failure and death (Petsonk, Rose, and Cohen 2013). Assessing the source of the risk to health all of a sudden becomes a process of choosing between many different culprits. Diagnosis of these diseases is predicated on access to imaging technologies. Without the process of diagnostic imagery the danger remains unnamed and as such is not subject to proper treatment and compensation via labor unions, health insurance, and other sources of aid. Depending on the occupational laws of the mining region, compensation may or may not be within the reach of the affected miners.

TB on top of silicosis on top of lung cancer on top of HIV/AIDS on top of malnutrition – the buildup of pathologies becomes staggering. What is normal? How do we make judgments regarding physiology when the textbooks on physiology were written using healthy people and singly occurring pathologies (see Singer 2009)? Local biologies of miners that are culturally informed, and locally produced understandings of what is normal (pace Lock 1993), reflect the reality that half or more of the working miners already have changes in their breathing by the time they are in their 30s and 40s or worse, *even in the United States.* A different kind of "normal" emerges. People's expectations change; they live their lives through a different kind of filter that includes expecting to be breathless at the top of a flight of stairs, expecting to have that telltale grey tinge to the skin, expecting to die by the age of 40.

As local biologies change, integrating the different forms our bodies can assume, then the "danger" becomes locally defined and the eco-risk is dealt with in local ways. US lawsuits seeking damages for black lung are rarely settled in favor of the miner seeking compensation. In a recent report from the Center for Public Integrity, it was stated that about 85 percent of cases are denied during the first trial (Hamby 2014). Even though some cases are approved in appeals, many cases are subsequently re-appealed and won by coal industry lawyers. X-rays are read and reread by "experts" on both sides, each side giving the opposite diagnosis (Hamby 2014). Cases last for years and decades without resolution. Lawyers for the miners cannot be paid until the cases are settled and therefore many lawyers won't take black lung cases. Miners try to represent themselves and often are not successful. The technologies of perception are fallible, as are those who interpret them; the "Black Lung Benefits Law" originally passed in 1969 has been modified to more stringent standards, but even those standards are proving not rigorous enough to prevent this disease from developing (Hamby 2014).

Psychosocial Hazards

In this section I want to highlight the violences present in mining communities, both those that are obvious and expected and also those that may not be so apparent. Caxaj and colleagues (2014) describe a mining company's impact on a Mam Mayan community, San Miguel Ixtahuacan, Guatemala. Her descriptive research illustrates a community divided along the lines of who supports the mining company and who doesn't. The money, jobs, and social power that come from working for the mines benefit a minority of the community, leaving the rest of the population disenfranchised and terrorized:

> Many reported that the community had been safe and peaceful before the arrival of mining operations. With the arrival of the company, however, participants reported experiences of more overt targeting and control exerted through local militias that they believed to be hired or paid for by Goldcorp. Adding to this militarized environment was an increased ownership of guns in the community, particularly among mine workers seeking to protect their earnings outside of a banking system. Participants recounted experiences of being followed and monitored, as well as threats, intimidation, kidnappings, torture, witnessing the murder of loved ones and being victims of attempted murder. Threats and intimidation were often delivered via cell phone messages, drunken yelling outside of individuals' homes, in person, or hand-delivered notes. (Caxaj *et al.* 2014: 53)

Increased violence and interpersonal strife often accompanies mining operations, as do full-fledged violent protests (Sawyer 2004). In their work in South Africa, Campbell and her colleagues detail the complexities of the structural violence of a mining town filled with miners far from home, large numbers of sex workers, and exceptionally high rates of HIV/AIDS, TB, and silicosis (Campbell and Williams 1999; Campbell 2003). The psychosocial hazards that come from hard work, low pay, being far from home, and working under very dangerous conditions create a complexly pathological situation for these gold miners (Campbell and Cornish 2011).

In a more recent study, Steele (2013) describes the migration of men to work in the South African gold mines 10 years after Campbell and her team did their initial work. Steele paints a picture where interpersonal violence is still ubiquitous:

> this large-scale movement of men without their wives and girlfriends is fueling demand for sex workers in mining communities ... Criminal gangs, realizing the profits to be made from the sex industry around mines, have turned to forcing, coercing, or deceiving women and girls into sexual slavery ...There is little data on the scope of this exploitation, but accounts suggest that some women are exposed to violence, abuse, and rape at the hands of gangs and, sometimes, even at the hands of boyfriends who sell these women and girls to their mine co-workers. (Steele 2013: 666)

Conditions among miners in Africa of forced labor, debt bondage, slavery, pornography, and sex work have been condemned by the US Department of State in its annual *Trafficking in Persons Report* (2012). This report goes on to document forced labor of young children in many countries across Africa and other countries. A recent editorial published in the *Lancet*, based on information from Human Rights Watch, included this interview:

> I was hungry and in need of money so I decided to go there," said 13-year-old Rahim, just one of thousands of children facing hazardous conditions and long-term illness working in Tanzania's small-scale gold mines. Toxic Toil, a report

> published on August 28 by Human Rights Watch (HRW), describes children as young as 8 years old living in poverty turning to mining to make money for basic necessities for themselves and their families. The children have no knowledge of the health risks they will be exposed to. During interviews of more than 200 children while visiting 11 mining sites, HRW found that young girls were sexually exploited and at risk of contracting sexually transmitted diseases. School attendance was poor and alternative employment opportunities lacking, making the mines one way to earn a living. (Lancet 2013: 834)

The webs of socialities that link miners to their jobs and to their communities are reflective of past ways of life and contemporary constellations of needs and desires. These webs are also those that link and bind the bodies of miners, their families, and the larger community into contact with toxic chemical exposures as well as toxic social milieus.

Eco-risks of Mining: The Medical Anthropology of an Occupation

A recent story on National Public Radio highlights another side of the mining issue:

> Girls in clunky roller skates whizz past their coach. They're sweaty, rowdy, and covered in tattoos. Gillette's roller derby team proudly represents coal country, as does their name. "We're called the Coal Miner's Daughters, number one because Loretta Lynn rocks!" Katie Buffington, president of the team, explained. "Number two because coal is the main source of income in the area. And we really wanted to get back to our roots, where we come from." And yes, there are actual coal miners' daughters on the team. And others, like Buffington are coal miners themselves. "Coal is so deeply rooted in the community that you really can't go anywhere without meeting a coal miner's daughter, at roller derby or not," Buffington said. Maybe that's because one out of every hundred Wyoming residents works in the coal industry. And the state produces a whopping 40% of the nation's coal. So, despite concern over climate change, competitive natural gas prices, and greater availability of renewables, Wyoming's coal industry lives on. (Paterson 2014)

Miners and their families are often proud, stoic and deeply immersed in the culture of mining. The occupation carries connotations of history and family ties that can span generations. The monetary value of minerals reinforces the value of the work and creates a lens through which mining-caused illness are made sense of. Richardson and Weszkalnys argue for an understanding of the meaning of minerals that simultaneously takes into account the geophysical spaces where they are found, and the cultural and technological aspects of their use: "that natural resources are inherently *distributed things* whose essence or character is to be located neither exclusively in their biophysical properties nor in webs of socio-cultural meaning. By 'distributed,' we refer to both the spatial and temporal extensions of specific resources, and their material and ontological dispersion." (2014: 8).

The materiality of the disease-producing aspects of mining takes one even deeper into the realm of, as Richardson and Weszkalnys call it, this particular "resource environment." The resource environments that I've been describing become interiorized as the polluted dust, air, and water from the mines seep into the distal regions of the lungs, the blood, and the brain. As in the process of fracking, where water is forced under pressure into the cracks and crevices of the earth with little regard as to where it might end up and with little thought as to the ramifications of the creation of deep unnatural mixtures and pressures, so, too, in other settings, the silica, the mercury, the asbestos, and the uranium enter into the deep recesses of the human body causing cellular havoc and corporeal breakdown now and into the future.

How will the "Coal Miners' Daughters" live their lives into the coming decades and centuries in rural Wyoming? How will they experience and appraise their repetitive motion injuries from driving heavy equipment? How will they understand and act upon the risks that they perceive of the neurological, oncological, and psychological illnesses that will come from the increasingly polluted aquifers, the increasingly polluted air that they breathe, and the social problems associated with lots of extra spending money and lots of drugs and alcohol? How will their bosses and their companies respond to worker demands as the mining workforce ages and the boom and bust economics of mining play out once again across the short grass prairies cum national treasure houses of natural resources? As this chapter has illustrated, there are myriad states of ill health that accompany the occupation of mining. Given mining's continued importance in our industrialized world and its complexities, both physical and social, there remains much to be done in understanding how it impacts local realities and cultures across the globe.

NOTES

1 We described how medical risks are culturally constructed through three basic components: locally recognized dangers, perceived through (in this case biomedical) technologies that are adjudicated and instantiated through a legal (in this case malpractice) system.

2 Letter from the United Mine Workers of America:

October 25, 2011

To the workers at the Upper Big Branch mine and the families of the victims of the explosion:

The 29 miners who died in the Upper Big Branch mine on April 5, 2010, did not go to work that day with the expectation that it was the last day of their lives. They kissed their wives and children goodbye and drove the twisting roads of Raleigh County, W. Va., to make their way to the mine. Once there, they got into their work clothes, joked around with their buddies, then made ready to go to work. They perhaps knew something about the serious safety problems at the mine. Everyone who worked there knew something was off. But they didn't know just how bad it was, and anyway they figured there was nothing they could do about it. After all, fixing the mine's problems was the responsibility of management, under the oversight of the federal and state safety and health agencies. The workers were right. But they were also, tragically, let down by the very people who were supposed to be keeping them safe. And because of that, those 29 husbands, fathers, brothers, sons and grandsons never came home.

There were many factors that led to this disaster. But there is only one source for all of them: A rogue corporation, acting without real regard for mine safety and health law and regulations, that established a physical working environment that can only be described as a bomb waiting to go off. And that same company established a working environment where, operating through subterfuge, fear and intimidation, management prevented any opportunity for the workers to know the full range of dangerous conditions in the mine, or to effectively protest them even if they did know.

Federal and West Virginia mine safety and health law is very clear: It was the responsibility of the mine's operator, Performance Coal Company, and its parent company, Massey Energy, to operate the mine in a safe and healthy manner in compliance with laws and regulations. That did not happen at UBB. Indeed, the UMWA's investigation reveals that well-established safety and health laws were deliberately flouted at UBB, even after the federal and/or state agencies cited the operator multiple times for breaking the law. The only conclusion that can be drawn is that Massey simply did not care if it broke the law. The safety of its employees was not worthy of its concern.

The only thing that mattered was getting the coal out.

This attitude was not a creation solely of management at the UBB mine. Far from it. This was a company-wide practice, fomented and directed by those at the highest corporate levels. The UBB mine was not unique in its manner of operation – other Massey Energy mines were similar. It is unconscionable, in the 21st Century, for a mine to be operated in the manner that UBB was. (United Mine Workers of America 2011)

REFERENCES

Ballard, C. and Banks, G. 2003. "Resource Wars: The Anthropology of Mining." *Annual Review of Anthropology*, 32(1): 287–313. doi: 10.1146/annurev.anthro.32.061002.093116.

Baxter, P.J., Adams, P.H., Aw, T.C., Cockcroft, A., and Harrington, J.M (Eds.) 2000. *Hunters Diseases of Occupations.* London: Arnold.

Campbell, C. 2003. "Letting Them Die" *Why HIV/AIDS Prevention Programmes Fail.* Bloomington, IN: Indiana University Press.

Campbell, C. and Cornish, F. 2011. "How Can Community Health Programmes Build Enabling Environments for Transformative Communication? Experiences From India and South Africa." *AIDS and Behavior*, 16(4): 847–857. doi:10.1007/s10461-011-9966-2.

Campbell, C. and Williams, B. 1999. "Beyond the Biomedical and Behavioural: Towards an Integrated Approach to HIV Prevention in the Southern African Mining Industry." *Social Science & Medicine*, 48 (April): 1625–1639.

Carrasco, A. 2011. "One World, Many Ethics: the Politics of Mining and Indigenous Peoples in Atacama, Chile." Doctoral dissertation, University of Arizona.

Cartwright, E. 2011. "Immigrant Dreams: Legal Pathologies and Structural Vulnerabilities Along the Immigration Continuum." *Medical Anthropology*, 30(5): 475–495. doi: 10.1080/01459740.2011.577044.

Cartwright, E. 2013. "Eco-Risk and the Case of Fracking." In S. Strauss, S. Rupp, and T. Love (Eds.), *Cultures of Energy* (pp. 201–212). Walnut Creek, CA: Left Coast Press.

Cartwright, E. and Thomas, J. 2000. "Risk, Technology and Malpractice in Maternity Care in the United States, Sweden, Canada and the Netherlands." In R. DeVries,

E. van Teijlingen, and S. Wrede (Eds.), *Birth by Design* (pp. 218–228). New York: Routledge.

Caxaj, C.S., Berman, H., Varcoe, C., Ray, S.L., and Restoulec, J.-P. 2014. "Gold Mining on Mayan-Mam Territory: Social Unravelling, Discord and Distress in the Western Highlands of Guatemala." *Social Science & Medicine*, 111(C): 50–57. doi: 10.1016/j.socscimed.2014.03.036.

Chen, W., Liu, Y., Wang, H., Hnizdo, E., Sun, Y., Su, L., Zhang, X. *et al.* 2012. "Long-Term Exposure to Silica Dust and Risk of Total and Cause-Specific Mortality in Chinese Workers: A Cohort Study." Edited by Naftali Kaminski. *PLoS Medicine* 9(4): e1001206. doi: 10.1371/journal.pmed.1001206.

Dawson, S.E. and Madsen, G.E. 2011. "Psychosocial and Health Impacts of Uranium Mining and Milling on Navajo Lands." *Health Physics*, 101(5): 618–625. doi: 10.1097/HP.0b013e3182243a7a.

Donoghue, A M. 2004. "Occupational Health Hazards in Mining: An Overview." *Occupational Medicine*, 54(5): 283–289. doi: 10.1093/occmed/kqh072.

EPA (Environmental Protection Agency). n.d. "Reducing Mercury Pollution from Artisanal and Small-scale Gold Mining." http://www.epa.gov/international-cooperation/reducing-mercury-pollution-artisanal-and-small-scale-gold-mining (accessed December 9, 2015).

Finn, J.L. 1998. *Tracing the Veins: of Copper, Culture, and Community From Butte to Chuquicamata.* Berkeley, CA: University of California Press.

Frosch, D. 2014. "Amid Toxic Waste, A Navajo Village Could Lose Its Land." *New York Times February* 19, 2014.

Hamby, C. 2014. "Breathless and Burdened." *Center for Public Integrity.*

Hand, E. 2014. "Injection Wells Blamed in Oklahoma Earthquakes." *Science*, 345(6192): 13–14.

Hayes, K. and Burge, R. 2003. *Coltan Mining in the Democratic Republic of Congo: Flora and Fauna International Conservation Reports.*

Johnson, D.B. and Hallberg, K.B. 2005. "Acid Mine Drainage Remediation Options: A Review." *Science of the Total Environment*, 338(1–2): 3–14. doi: 10.1016/j.scitotenv.2004.09.002.

Kirsch, S. 2008. "Social Relations and the Green Critique of Capitalism in Melanesia." *American Anthropologist*, 110(3): 288–298. doi: 10.1111/j.1548-1433.2008.00039.x.

Kirsch, S. 2010. "Sustainable Mining." *Dialectical Anthropology*, 34: 87–93.

Lancet, The. 2013. "Child Labour: the High Cost of Gold." *The Lancet*, 382(9895): 834. doi: 10.1016/S0140-6736(13)61845-0.

Li, F. 2009. "Documenting Accountability: Environmental Impact Assessment in a Peruvian Mining Project." *PoLAR: Political and Legal Anthropology Review*, 32(2): 218–236. doi: 10.1111/j.1555-2934.2009.01042.x.

Lies, E. 2009. "Matewan Before the Massacre: Politics, Coal, and the Roots of Conflict in a West Virginia Mining Community (Review)." *The Oral History Review*, 36(2): 294–296.

Lock, M. 1993. *Encounters With Aging: Mythologies of Menopause in Japan and North America.* Berkeley, CA: University of California Press.

Magma Coltan. 2012. "Life of African Miners Is One of Suffering." http://www.magmacoltan.com/announcements/life-of-african-coltan-miners-is-one-of-suffering?A=SearchResult&SearchID=8681251&ObjectID=91172&ObjectType=7 (accessed December 9, 2015).

McAteer, J.D. 2011. *Upper Big Branch: the April 5, 2010,* Explosion*: A Failure of Basic Coal Mine Safety Practices. Report to the Governor.*

Nordstrom, C. 2007. *Global Outlaws: Crime, Money, and Power in the Contemporary World.* Berkeley, CA: University of California Press.

Paterson, L. 2014. "*In Wyoming Coal Culture Runs Deep.*" Wyoming Public Media, National Public Radio.

Petsonk, E.L., Cecile R., and Cohen, R. 2013. "Coal Mine Dust Lung Disease. New Lessons From Old Exposure." *American Journal of Respiratory and Critical Care Medicine*, 187(11): 1178–1185. doi: 10.1164/rccm.201301-0042CI.

Pine, A. 2013. "Revolution as a Care Plan: Ethnography, Nursing and Somatic Solidarity in Honduras." *Social Science & Medicine*, 99: 143–152. doi: 10.1016/j.socscimed.2013.05.028.

Quesada, J., Hart, L.K., and Bourgois, P. 2011. "Structural Vulnerability and Health: Latino Migrant Laborers in the United States." *Medical Anthropology* (July), 1–26. doi: 10.1080/01459740.2011.576725.

Richardson, T. and Weszkalnys, G. 2014. "Introduction: Resource Materialities." *Anthropological Quarterly*, 87(1): 5–30. doi: 10.1353/anq.2014.0007.

Rolston, J.S. 2013. "The Politics of Pits and the Materiality of Mine Labor: Making Natural Resources in the American West." *American Anthropologist*, 115(4): 582–594. doi: 10.1111/aman.12050.

Sawyer, S. 2004. *Crude Chronicles: Indigenous Politics, Multinational Oil, and Neoliberalism in Ecuador.* Durham, NC: Duke University Press.

Singer, M. 2009. *Introduction to Syndemics: A Critical Systems Approach to Public and Community Health.* San Francisco, CA: Jossey-Bass.

Steele, S. 2013. "Human Trafficking, Labor Brokering, and Mining in Southern Africa: Responding to a Decentralized and Hidden Public Health Disaster." *International Journal of Health Services*, 43(4): 665–680. doi: 10.2190/HS.43.4.e.

Stuckler, D., Steele, S., Lurie, M., and Basu, S. 2013. "Introduction: 'Dying for Gold': the Effects of Mineral Mining on HIV, Tuberculosis, Silicosis, and Occupational Diseases in Southern Africa." *International Journal of Health Services*, 43(4): 639–649. doi: 10.2190/HS.43.4.c.

United Mine Workers of America. 2011. "Industrial Homicide: Report on the Upper Big Branch Mine Disaster," October, pp. 1–154.

US Department of State. 2012. *Trafficking in Persons Report 2012.* http://www.state.gov/documents/organization/192587.pdf (accessed December 9, 2015).

Webster, P.C. 2012. "Not All That Glitters: Mercury Poisoning in Colombia." *The Lancet*, 379(9824): 1379–80. doi: 10.1016/S0140-6736(12)60582-0.

Welker, M.A. 2009. "Corporate Security Begins in the Community": Mining, the Corporate Social Responsibility Industry, and Environmental Advocacy in Indonesia." *Cultural Anthropology*, 24(1): 142–179. doi: 10.1111/j.1548-1360.2009.00029.x.

Zhuang, P., McBride, M.B., Xia, H., Li, N., and Li, Z. 2009. "Health Risk From Heavy Metals via Consumption of Food Crops in the Vicinity of Dabaoshan Mine, South China." *Science of the Total Environment*, 407(5): 1551–1561. doi: 10.1016/j.scitotenv.2008.10.061.

PART V

Pluralea Interactions and Ecosyndemics in a Changing World

CHAPTER 21 Pluralea Interactions and the Remaking of the Environment in Environmental Health

Merrill Singer

Introduction: Rethinking Environment Health

The field of environmental health is tied historically to the emergence of industrialization and its effects on human well-being. In 1831, Charles Thackrah, through his experience treating worker health issues in England, connected the growth of industrial factories to rising rates of "painful disease and premature disablement or death" (Simon 1897: 125). In the United States, focus on the health consequences of industrialization awaited the turn of the twentieth century. In 1908, reflecting on her experience-based apprehensions about the health of industrial workers, physician-activist Alice Hamilton initiated ground-breaking studies of the dangerous properties of industrial metals and chemical compounds. Her first book (1925) on the topic provided an eye-opening introduction to industrial toxicology. Over time, concern about the environmental impacts of industrialization beyond the factory had a growing impact on our conception of the environment. A critical moment in this expanded focus on environment was the publication over 50 years ago of Rachel Carson's classic *Silent Spring* (1962), which examined the adverse ecosystem effects of DDT and the potential role of DDT in cancer and birth defects in humans.

A Companion to the Anthropology of Environmental Health, First Edition. Edited by Merrill Singer.

Our understanding of the environment as a dynamic system was advanced by the work of Ernst Haeckel, who in 1855 defined the term "ecology" as the study of the relationship of organisms with their environmental contexts (as contrasted with laboratory studies). In this, Haeckel was strongly influenced by Darwin's discussion of the mutual relations of organisms (Stauffer 1957). Wrote Darwin, "Let it be borne in mind how infinitely complex and close-fitting are the mutual relations of all organic beings to each other and to their physical conditions of life" (1859: 69). The biological concept of ecology shares with the anthropological concept of ethnography a recognition of the fundamental importance of the physical setting as a shaping force rather than merely a background or locational reference. In anthropology, specific emphasis on human societies in their natural contexts was consolidated in the mid-1950s under the rubric of "cultural ecology" (Steward 1972). Central to Steward's cultural ecological project was the explanation of cultural variation in terms of adaptation to specific local environmental conditions. Of lesser concern were the issues of environmental change and the role of humans in this process. In 1956, however, the Wenner-Gren Foundation for Anthropological Studies sponsored a major conference on ecology that drew focused attention to human impact on the environments of Earth (Thomas 1956). This issue became increasingly prominent in anthropology when ecological and cultural ecological approaches were integrated with the study of political economy to form the field of political ecology (Wolf 1972), leading to recognition that "human activities can modify physical and biological events, sometimes many miles away (e.g., deforestation contributing to flooding downstream) or many years later (e.g., the introduction of a new seed or animal, or the substitution of one form of architecture for another, less safe, one)" (Wisner *et al.* 2003: 7).

Introduction of the term "Anthropocene" early in the twenty-first century marked a critical moment in the growing awareness of how extensively humans change ecological systems. The name Anthropocene was proposed for the contemporary era of Earth's history and the significant impact of human behavior in shaping planetary climate and environments (Crutzen and Stoermer 2000). In the Anthropocene, environmental health becomes an ever more significant shaper of human well-being, health experience, and health behavior. In the view of Crutzen, the origin of the Anthropocene can be traced to the latter part of the eighteenth century, based on the analyses of air trapped in polar ice that revealed growing global concentrations of carbon dioxide and methane. This date coincides with James Watt's invention of the steam engine in 1784 and the world-changing advent of the Industrial Revolution. Realization of the extent of our impact on the planet increased significantly after World War II when the human population doubled, soaring from three billion in 1950 to six billion in 2000, and the scale of industrial production, consumerism (which more accurately might be called hyper-consumption), and globalism accelerated rapidly. Today, Earth "is being anthroposized at high speed" (Crutzen and Schwägerl 2011). The Anthropocene is characterized by active and multidimensional global human interaction with the rest of nature based on the ongoing "interrelatedness of human actions and biogeophysical processes" (Dearing 2007: 27), an interaction that has significant health implications. Most notably, human release of greenhouse gases is now established as the primary driver of global warming, a process that is significantly reshaping ecological systems and producing multiple challenges to the health of humans and other species. In fact, health is being put at risk in the contemporary moment by multiple anthropogenic environmental degradations including polluting of air and water, clearing of forests, release of toxic chemicals, degradation and loss of top soil, depopulation of ocean fish stocks, and much more. Moreover, there is occurrence of ecocrisis interaction (Singer 2009). Rather than being stand-alone threats to human well-being, adverse anthropogenic effects on the environment act in tandem to magnify their overall health threat. I argue here that this interaction and enhanced effect of multiple adverse ecological changes, termed "pluralea," must become a growing concern in a world with rising temperatures and consequential climatic events.

The term "pluralea," constructed from the Latin words *plur*, meaning "many" and *alea*, meaning "hazards," labels the growing number of health-related interactions that transpire across the full array of environmental degradations in our increasingly human-dominated and human-restructured environment. As Rosenzweig (2008), observes, "Separating the influence of human-caused temperature increases from natural climate variations or other confounding factors, such as land-use changes or pollution is a real challenge." Nonetheless, the tendency in environmental studies has been to seek single-cause understandings based on the separation and independent analysis of selected health risks in the "natural" and built world around us. In the assessment of Spratt and Sutton (2008: xi), however, climate change comprises only the exposed "tip of [a far] broader global sustainability iceberg" that includes numerous other environmental disruptions that are not only coterminous but are "converging rapidly in a manner not previously experienced."

In this light, health has come to be recognized as an ecologically mediated state that is heavily influenced by human activities that produce varied intentional and unintentional changes in the environment, and increasingly so since the beginning of the Industrial Revolution. This chapter argues that climate change is not occurring in isolation but is adversely magnifying a wide range of other health-related ecocrises produced by human activity. Specifically, in this chapter I examine the origins and features of pluraleal interactions, the ways in which they are reconstituting the ecosystems of human and other species' habitats, and the implications for human health and social well-being.

Defining Pluralea

Central to the pluralea perspective is the development of an understanding of the pathways and mechanisms through which two or more ecocrises interact to produce synergistic and enhanced environmental and human health impacts. What is of importance about pluralea is not just the number of environmental health risks we have created but the ways their interactions magnify their overall adverse effects (Rees 2003). The dominant outlook on contemporary ecocrises, reflecting a siloed (one problem at a time) approach, produces fragmented and often competing mitigation responses. The pluraleal perspective, by contrast, seeks to assess pathways of interaction and consequences in light of the entwined nature of ecosystems.

The pluraleal approach stems from recognition that Earth, as a complex interlinked planetary ecological system, has limits and that human technologies today have the capacity to overtax "planetary boundaries" and "trigger abrupt or irreversible environmental changes that would be deleterious or even catastrophic for human beings" (Rockström *et al.* 2009). The term "planetary boundaries" draws attention to the biophysical processes that shape the self-regulating capacity of the planet and to the existence of immutable thresholds and tipping points, the crossing of which, for prolonged periods, can set in motion nonlinear changes that jeopardize "the safe operating space for humanity" on Earth (Rockström *et al.* 2009). Ecocrises interactions, because of their multiplying effects, constitute mounting threats to planetary boundaries and hence to the health of our species and that of the many other inhabitants of Earth. Consequently, the pluraleal perspective is based on a view of humans and their cultures as being within and not separate from nature as well as an assessment of the ways that a productivist ethic of endless economic expansion and social injustice is environmentally expressed and experienced and can push ecological systems beyond the coping capacity of species, including our own. As living systems, human and otherwise, we face a form of destruction from within, a set of circumstances that "can be called, without hyperbole, threatened apocalypse" (Foster, Clark, and York 2010: 109).

I examine these issues below by way of three case studies of anthropogenic-impacted environmental changes – air pollution, superstorms, and coral reef loss – that have significant pluraleal components and multiple health-related consequences,

Case Study 1: Health and the Air We Breathe

The first pluraleal case discussed here involves the interaction between anthropogenic air pollution and global warming in the exacerbation of respiratory and cardiovascular disease around the world. The Global Burden of Disease report indicates that 3.1 million people die and 22 percent of disability-adjusted life years (DALY) are lost because of atmospheric particulate air pollution, including finely divided solids and liquids such as dust, fly ash, soot, smoke, aerosols, fumes, mists, and condensing vapors that are suspended in the air for extended periods of time (Lim *et al.* 2012). Most of the particulate matter that pollutes the air we breathe is generated from various human activities, including the burning of fossil fuels by vehicles and industrial manufacture, agricultural operations, combustion of wood (e.g., fireplaces), construction and demolition activities, and entrainment of road dust into the air. Other sources of particulate matter are windblown dust and wildfires (both of which are impacted by human activities). Additional toxic anthropogenic air pollutants, including carbon monoxide (CO), nitrogen dioxide (NO_2), and ozone (O_3), also are contributing to a rise in health risks around the world.

Intensification of these airborne pollutants has contributed to notable increases in the reported frequency of a range of respiratory symptoms and diseases like asthma, especially among poorer and disadvantaged populations in both developed and developing nations. The World Health Organization (WHO 2008) estimates that 300 million people currently suffer with asthma, and approximately a quarter of a million people, mostly living in low- and lower-middle income countries, die of this disease each year. This represents one of every 250 deaths in the world annually. Asthma, a disease named after the Greek word for panting, ranked as the 25th leading cause of disability-adjusted life years lost in 2001. The number of DALYs that annually are lost to this respiratory disease worldwide is estimated to be 15 million, a level that is on par with diabetes and cirrhosis (Masoli *et al.* 2004). Growth in asthma rates is occurring worldwide, especially among the urban poor (Laurent *et al.* 2008). Even in settings where treatment is reasonably available, "poorly controlled asthma continues to be reported in developed and developing countries" alike (Hanania 2009: 2). The United Nation's Global Initiative for Asthmas (2009: 3) stresses that in Africa, Latin America, and sectors of Asia, "the global burden of asthma is continuing to rise." Focusing on asthma and other respiratory conditions in West Africa, Gbadero *et al.* (1995: 739) note:

> With the inevitable atmospheric pollution from increasing urbanisation and industrialisation, paediatric asthma morbidity in the tropics may approach the current "epidemic" proportions of the western world. Acute respiratory infections currently constitute a research priority area worldwide, and justifiably so in the third world where mortality related to acute respiratory infections continues to soar.

Likewise, in Tijuana, Mexico, following the passage of NAFTA (North American Free Trade Agreement), numerous foreign-owned factories (*maquiladoras*) sprang up along the US/Mexico border, resulting in an increase in industrial air pollution and, "a dramatic rise in the incidence of childhood asthma" (Schwartz 2004: 215).

A growing literature indicates that respiratory health has deteriorated in recent decades "because of interaction between heavier pollen loads and increased air pollution; thunderstorms and extreme precipitation events; worsening heat-related ground-level ozone pollution; increased ambient air pollution from natural and anthropogenic sources; and air pollution related to wildfires" (Shea *et al.* 2008: 445). This conclusion is supported by the findings of high-resolution climate/air pollution computer modeling (Noyes *et al.* 2008).

In the case of asthma, there is growing evidence that a synergistic interaction that is helping to drive increases in the disease involves growth in the annual loads of environmental allergens like ragweed – a change that has been tied to global warming and its impacts on the timing of plant pollen production and release – and the presence of respiratory pathogens. One feature of global warming in some locations is the early arrival of spring and late departure of fall, combined with increases in precipitation (Ziska *et al.* 2011). In combination with historically high levels of carbon dioxide in the air, these environmental conditions promote pollen manufacture by trees and plants as well facilitate mold and other fungal growth and the discharge into the air of allergy-triggering spores.

To assess the interaction between allergens and pathogens in the onset of asthma attacks, Murray and colleagues (2006) enrolled children ages 3–17 admitted to hospital with an acute asthma flare-up into a case control study. Index cases were matched with two control groups: outpatients with stable asthma and patients with nonrespiratory conditions. Participants were tested for allergic sensitivity to various allergens and tested for various nasal pathogens. Findings showed that case group participants were at a significantly higher risk of having been both exposed and sensitive to allergens and of having a higher respiratory pathogen loads than the control groups. The presence of both risk factors was found to increase the risk of hospital admission by almost 20-fold. These researchers (Murray *et al.* 2006: 381–382) concluded that their findings "indicate that there appears to be a combined rather than an individual effect of natural virus infection and real life allergen exposure in allergic asthmatic children in inducing asthma exacerbations."

Beyond respiratory health, deteriorating air quality in some locations is contributing to cardiovascular problems. In a recent study in Chile (Franck, Leitte, and Suppan 2014), for example, researchers acquired data on a range of air quality measures for particulate matter, CO, NO_2, and O_3 levels for the years 2004–2007 from seven weather monitoring stations around the city of Santiago de Chile. They compared these data with health ministry records on the number of hospital admissions during the target period for heart problems. The researchers employed a lagged analysis that allowed them to determine the specific impact that varying levels of pollution had on hospital admission rates, with inclusion of both immediate effects and those that occurred over several subsequent days. They found that as levels of CO, NO_2, and particulate matter increased so did hospital admissions for cardiovascular disease, and that hospital admission upswings lasted one to two days past peak pollution levels. In a parallel study, Cesaroni *et al.* (2014) examined the heart effects of long-term exposure to various airborne pollutants, including 2.5 and 10 size particulate matter (PM), soot, and NO as well as traffic exposures in 11 European cohorts. These researchers assessed acute coronary events (i.e., myocardial infarction and unstable angina) per fixed increments of the measured pollutants with adjustment for sociodemographic and lifestyle risk factors (e.g., smoking). They found that a 5 $\mu g/m^3$ increase in estimated annual mean PM2.5 was associated with a 13 percent increased risk of coronary events while a 10 $\mu g/m^3$ increase in estimated annual mean PM10 was associated with a 12 percent increased risk of coronary events. Long-term exposure to particulate matter, they concluded, is directly linked to incidence of adverse coronary events.

The specific pluraleal linkages that have been identified among global warming, air pollution, and respiratory and cardiovascular health include: (1) the deleterious effects of toxins produced by motor vehicles, industrial power plants, and industrial chemicals as a result of expanded environmental discharge and increasing planetary temperatures; (2) forest fires that produce ever greater quantities of hazardous particulate matter, carbon monoxide, and polyaromatic hydrocarbons as a result of global warming and drier environmental conditions; (3) noxious mold exposures facilitated by changes in precipitation patterns, farmland restructuring, drought, and more frequent flooding and water intrusion in buildings as a result of climate change; and (4) expansions in both the range and quantity of pollen produced by global climate change (Ontario Lung Association 2008). Moreover, because the human respiratory system is a primary site where diverse environmental threats to health cluster, intermingle, and multiply their adverse impacts (e.g., diesel fuel droplets with bacteria, allergens with infectious agents), there is a set of ecosyndemic threats to health that also are being ushered in by the contemporary pluraleal interaction of air pollution and global warming (Singer 2013).

Case Study 2: Superstorms: The Example of Hurricane Sandy

What has been called Superstorm Sandy, which broke 16 historical storm-tide records along the east coast of the United States, is exemplary of a health-threatening pluralea that may be representative of the increasingly erratic and turmoil-causing weather to come because of the ocean-warming and other effects of climate change. Sandy began as a hurricane that devastated parts of the Caribbean during the busy 2012 hurricane season, the likes of which (in terms of hurricane size and impact) are being predicted by climate scientists to become more frequent. As summarized by Jeff Masters, director of meteorology at Weather Underground, a commercial online weather service, "the predictions for the future are pretty solid. As you warm up the oceans, you will tend to make the strongest storms stronger" (quoted on PBS Newshour 2013). Adds Kevin Trenberth, a climate scientist at the National Center for Atmospheric Research: "sea temperatures are higher by over a degree Fahrenheit or so on a global basis because of global warming, because of human influences. And going along with that, the air in the atmosphere is warmer and moister. And that's what fuels all of these storms" (quoted on PBS Newshour 2013).

Ultimately, Sandy became the largest Atlantic hurricane on record (by diameter) and the deadliest (with 286 fatalities), as well as the most destructive storm in the region in 2012, with winds spanning an area of 1100 miles. Sandy damaged or destroyed at least 650,000 homes and caused approximately $70 billion in losses, the second-costliest hurricane in US history after Hurricane Katrina, which struck the United States only eight years earlier. The storm made landfall on the US mainland near Atlantic City, New Jersey as a post-tropical cyclone with hurricane-force winds estimated to be about 80 mph (NOAA [National Oceanic and Atmospheric Administration] 2013a). All told, it impacted 24 states, especially New Jersey and New York, but had effects as far west as Wisconsin. Sandy caused ocean water levels to rise along the entire east coast. The greatest storm surges and maximum inundation, which reached record levels, occurred in New Jersey, New York, and Connecticut. These states experienced catastrophic, record-shattering water levels.

In New York City, a 13-foot flood surge saturated streets, tunnels, and subway lines, cutting power in and around the city. Homes were cracked open and gutted by the storm's intensity, and family possessions and cars were washed away. Hospitals lost power just as they were receiving emergency storm victims. More than 1000 patients had to be evacuated from New York City hospitals. Thousands of elderly with chronic conditions were trapped without power for days on the upper floors of high-rise buildings. Raw sewage spilled into homes when a sewage plant flooded. Individuals like Anthony Narh, a 58-year-old Ghanaian immigrant who worked at Empire Parking in the heart of Tribeca's evacuation zone, drowned when tons of water rushed into the basement parking garage. Frank Suber, who was on Broad St. when the storm surge hit, was washed through a revolving door into a commercial building, where he drowned. Others died from flooding, collapsing structures and trees, and electrocution. In Breezy Point in Queens, damaged electrical lines caused a massive blaze. In all, over 100 fires were attributed to Sandy (Otis 2013). Additionally, Sandy raised apprehensions about safety conditions in nuclear power plants in the storm zone, leading the Nuclear Regulatory Commission to shut down three facilities.

In light of ocean rise caused by global warming of approximately one foot over the last 100 years along the New Jersey coast and the fact that the Atlantic Ocean is now about 2 degrees warmer than a century ago, the notable extent of the flooding is believed to have been directly influenced by global warming (Sweet *et al.* 2013). According to the National Oceanic and Atmospheric Administration (NOAA) (2013b),

> climate-change related increases in sea level have nearly doubled today's annual probability of a Sandy-level flood recurrence as compared to 1950. Ongoing natural and human-induced forcing of sea level ensures that Sandy-level inundation events will occur more frequently in the future from storms with less intensity and lower storm surge than Sandy.

Similarly, in a *Washington Post* editorial (2013), Kevin Trenberth, senior scientist at the National Center for Atmospheric Research, and Michael Oppenheimer, a climate scientist at Princeton University, asserted with reference to Sandy, "Had the storm surge not been riding on higher seas, there would have been less flooding and less damage. Warmer air also allows storms such as Sandy to hold more moisture and dump more rainfall, exacerbating flooding" (Oppenheimer and Trenberth 2013). Indeed Oppenheimer and colleagues predicted 8 months before Sandy hit that because of global warming New York was highly vulnerable to extreme hurricane-surge flooding (Cooper, Beevers, and Oppenheimer, 2008). His research team projects 100-year surge flooding in New York City to occur every 3–20 years and 500-year flooding of the city every 25–240 years by the end of the twenty-first century (Lin *et al.* 2012).

That Sandy turned inland along the Atlantic Coast and not out to sea, as has historically been the case with such storms, also has been attributed to the influence of climate change, with specific reference to the impact of planetary warming on the northern hemisphere jet stream. This stream of rapidly moving air flowing west to east, caused by a combination of the rotation of Earth on its axis and atmospheric heating, is a primary determinant of weather patterns in North America as it transports air masses and creates clashing zones that generate storm formations. As noted in the Fifth Assessment Report of the Intergovernmental Panel on Climate Change (IPCC 2013: 2–5), global warming has caused air circulation features to move "poleward since the 1970s, involving a widening of the tropical belt, a poleward shift of storm tracks and jet streams, and a contraction of the northern polar vortex." While factors influencing the jet stream are complex, there is evidence that as the Arctic warms faster than the tropics, a lessening of the temperature gradient between the equator and the North Pole slows down the jet stream. As this occurs, it increases the probability of extreme weather events, a process known as Arctic amplification (Francis and Vavrus 2012).

Additionally, Sandy merged with an Arctic front that some climate scientists attribute to global climate change. This robust high-pressure body of cold air, hovering over Newfoundland, blocked Sandy from taking the usual path out to sea. As a result, rather than dissipating over the ocean, the full destructive potential of the storm was forced inland. Notably, a feature of the anthropogenic warming of Earth has been a pattern of increasing record highs in temperature and a decreasing number of record lows over North America. These conditions may be related to the warming of the Arctic, which, in turn, is changing wind patterns in the northern hemisphere (Betts 2012).

Adding to the impact of Sandy was the anthropogenic elimination of wetlands and sand dune areas and their replacement by concrete in places like Staten Island, which experienced some of the most severe flooding. During Sandy, shore towns that had retained their dunes suffered less damage than those without dunes. Similarly, wetlands and marshes have been found to slow down fast-moving currents, dissipating the energy in water as it floods over grasses, roots, and other materials, generating friction. While Sandy would have been a devastating storm even if these natural barriers had not been eliminated by development, their absence contributed to Sandy's noted destructiveness and creation of flood conditions (Freed 2013).

In sum, Sandy was a pluraleal event that united several climatic and environmental factors influenced by anthropogenic global climate and other human restructuring of the environment. The potential health risks of a superstorm like Sandy are several. Immediate risks from flooding are evident in the morbidity and mortality statistics produced by the storm. Moreover, flooding in urban settings like New York City with its extensive subway system can displace rat populations (which at least equal the number of people in the city) and the diseases they carry, including leptospirosis, hantavirus pulmonary syndrome, typhus, enteritis salmonellosis, and plague. One possible consequence of such a shift is greater contact with humans as rats flee flooded areas and settle into new, drier locations. Beyond rat bites and ectoparasites as sources of human infection, rodent feces and urine can spread hantavirus (Schmaljohn and Hjelle 1997).

At the same time, loss of power and a significant upswing in the use of home generators led to a significant increase in reported carbon monoxide exposures (Chen *et al.* 2013). Crowding of displaced residents in emergency shelters created a risk for post-storm outbreaks of infectious diseases. In the post-storm period, which struck during flu season, New York City witnessed a massive increase in visits to health care facilities for influenza-like illnesses, especially among young children. Additionally, post hurricane assessment showed that legionellosis, a bacterial disease that can cause pneumonia, was statistically significantly associated with increased occurrence in flooded/impacted areas (Green *et al.* 2013). Standing pools of water produced by the storm constituted another source of infectious disease risk caused by Sandy. Of most concern in urban areas is the bacterium *Escherichia coli*. Found normally in the lower intestine, where it plays a role in digestion, it can be toxic if it enters the stomach. Floods that carry raw sewage into densely populated areas can be a source of infection with this microbe. Cases of vibrio bacterial infections, which enter the body through open cuts (and were reported after Hurricane Katrina), present another infectious disease threat of hurricanes. Finally, floods produce damp environments that promote the growth of humidity-loving fungi, some of which can be quite harmful to humans. While not all of these infectious disease threats were realized with Sandy, the increased frequency of major multifaceted climate events predicted by climate scientists as a result of global warming, coupled with other environmental degradations and increasing population densities along coastlines worldwide, appear likely to cause a stormier future endured by more storm-stressed people tenuously supported by overtaxed infrastructures.

Case Study 3: Coral Life and Human Well-being at Risk

The final pluraleal case involves the multiple ways human activities are contributing to the loss of coral reefs around the planet and the consequences for various populations of this loss. One of the most biologically diverse habitats in the world, coral reefs constitute a dispersed ecosystem (often ecologically tied to mangroves and seagrass stands) found especially in tropical waters throughout the world (although deep-water corals are found in nontropical settings). Situated on the interface between land and sea, it is estimated that warm-water reefs cover approximately 600,000 km^2, somewhat more than a third of which occur in near-surface shallow waters adjacent to the coastline of over 100 countries (Spalding, Green, and Ravilious 2001). The most extensive shallow reef habitats, of particular importance to human populations, are found in the South Pacific, followed by Southeast Asia (especially Indonesia and the Philippines), the Indian Ocean, the Middle East, the Caribbean, and the Atlantic.

The coral reefs of the world are not in good condition. An analysis by the World Resources Institute and 25 other research organizations (Burke *et al.* 2002) concludes that currently three-quarters of the world's coral reefs are at risk and that by 2050 virtually all such systems will be in danger. Already, the Great Barrier Reef in Australia has lost more than half of its coral cover since

1985, with two-thirds of this loss occurring since 1998 (De'ath *et al.* 2012). The consequences of coral reef loss for countries in what has been called the Coral Triangle (Indonesia, Malaysia, Papua New Guinea, the Philippines, Solomon Islands, and Timor-Leste), as well as in the Caribbean and elsewhere, that depend for food on the fish and other animals attracted by coral reefs are projected to be severe.

It is estimated that 275 million people around the world live near (within 30 km of) coral reefs and many people in these areas depend on reefs for their livelihood (Burke *et al.* 2012). NOAA (2012) reports that fish that live on and near coral reefs are a keystone food source for over a billion people worldwide. In Southeast Asia, for example, 350 million people live within 50 km of the coast and the communities they inhabit are heavily dependent on marine and coastal resources. While reef fisheries in this region generate US$2.4 billion annually (Burke *et al.* 2002), coral food sources are particularly important for small-scale fisher families dwelling in rural areas, many of whom depend on coral species both as a primary source of food and as income. Overall, it is estimated that most of the 30 million small-scale fishers in the developing world rely at least to some degree on coral reefs, with 25 percent of all marine fish caught coming from coral reef sites (Jameson, McManus, and Spalding 1995). This pattern is seen clearly in the Philippines, where most of the population dwells in coastal areas that are bordered by the third largest reef area linked to a single nation. In the Philippines, more than one million small-scale fishers depend directly on coral reefs for sustenance and revenue and reefs are the primary source of most of the protein in many people's diets, as more than 50 percent of animal protein in the Philippines is derived from marine fisheries and aquaculture (United Nations Environment Program World Conservation Monitoring Center 2006). Beyond direct primary producers, it is estimated that at least 20 million people in the world are involved in small-scale fish processing and marketing (McGoodwin 2001). While reefs constitutes constitute the primary resource for millions of people, for many others they serve as a safety net reserve that enables them to survive periods of extreme hardship, such as climate-related droughts. Thus, small-scale farmers sometimes are forced by weather conditions or other crises to turn to reefs for crucial survival resources.

Two-thirds of countries with reefs are developing nations, including about one-quarter of the least developed countries in the world (United Nations Development Program 2002). In these settings, a significant number of people who are dependent on near-shore reefs live in poverty. The presence of coral reefs provides vital opportunities for the poor, including the young, the old, and women, sociodemographic groups that often have the least access to means of livelihood. The reefs allow them to harvest food on foot and by hand, or with the use of cheap and locally available technologies. Among female-headed households and those headed by widows, which frequently are among the poorest and most marginalized of households in poor communities, accessible reef resources constitute a critical lifeline under the bleakest of conditions.

The largest proportion of people living on less than 1 US$ a day in the world is found in sub-Saharan Africa, followed by South Asia, Latin America and the

Caribbean, East Asia, and the Pacific, areas characterized by large coral reefs. Of these areas, reefs are especially important in the lives of the poor of East Africa and Southeast Asia. In Mozambique, for example, the sixth poorest country in the world, reefs are found on the northern coast of Cabo Delgado. The province is one of the poorest in a country with one of the lowest Human Development Indices globally (Spalding *et al.* 2001). Other expressions of poverty include a high illiteracy rate (75%), a high infant mortality rate (174.4 per 1000 live births), a high proportion of low birth weight (highest in the country), and a life expectancy of only 37.9 years (Cabo Delgado Biodiversity and Tourism Project 2006). While a radio is one of the first purchases made by a household with disposable income, the vast majority of families in the province do not own one. Fishing traditionally has been the main economic activity for those living along the coast and on islands of the province, supplemented by cassava and other farming. Fishing methods are simple, with access to the reefs gained by using unmotorized dugouts, outrigger canoes, and dhows. Because of poverty, however, boats and nets are rare and fishers in some coastal villages can barely provide enough fish to ensure subsistence. This is especially the case during February and March, the lean period for fishery stocks. Mollusks and crustaceans also are taken, primarily by women in the intertidal zone, for family consumption, while sea cucumbers are harvested and dried and sold to commercial traders (although overharvesting has significantly degraded this resource). Poor households tend to have higher dependence on intertidal bivalve resources, which are reported to be progressively declining (Wilson, Muchave, and Garrett 2003). Were the reefs to die off, reef-dependent communities would face starvation. Increasing levels of child malnutrition amongst coastal communities in the Philippines, for example, has been linked to declining fishery production associated with degraded reef resources (McAllister 1988).

Research carried out in India and Mozambique (International Institute for Environment and Development 2003) has identified some of the reasons reefs constitute a vital resource for the poor as well as some of the reasons this means of livelihood is at increasing risk. Generally coastal areas, locations where different ecosystems meet and interact, tend to be characterized by multiple resource opportunities and intensified productivity, a feature that has been called the "edge effect" (Levin 2009). Assessment project findings, however, indicate that coral reefs differ from many other coastal resources used by the poor because they cannot easily be occupied or alienated from public access by the rich. The shallow and complex physical structure of reefs and their noted high level of biodiversity do not lend themselves readily to intensive exploitation or to increasing economies of scale. As a result, they tend to remain open areas accessible to the poor even when other nearby coastal resources are privatized by social elites. Moreover, coastal areas may be highly vulnerable to storms and flooding, making them challenging places to live. Because of these conditions, they may be avoided by wealthier classes and as a result become locations where the poor can establish households. Coral reefs also have been found to play a role in the way some people are able to cope with structural violence such as the impact of structural adjustment policies and the displacement of people from prior livelihoods in government employment. For example, on the south Pacific island of Niue, elimination of government-sector jobs in response to structural adjustment produced an increase in fishing pressure on reefs, as laid-off government workers took up fishing as a means of survival (Pasisi 1995).

Despite the open nature of reefs, the lure of tourist spending has begun to change patterns of access, as have some conservation efforts. Coral reef zones have seen huge increases in tourism development in recent years, with many millions of people now visiting reefs for recreational purposes. In the Caribbean, for example, 20 million people visit coastal areas annually and coral reefs attract 60 percent of the world's scuba-diving tours (International Coral Reef Initiative 2002). As a result, large areas of reef are being claimed by emergent profit-driven tourist industries in a number of countries and poor and displaced families are being blocked from access.

Increased tourism also has been linked to coral degradation. Research by Canty (2008) on the island of Utila, Honduras is illustrative. The approximately 9000 residents of Utila traditionally relied on offshore work and fishing as a means of livelihood. Since the 1980s, low-budget dive tourism has significantly expanded and today the local economy is based primarily on the dive industry, with cruise ships and backpackers making the island a desired travelers' destination. Divers interviewed by Canty reported noticeable declines in marine life in recent years, including some local keystone species. Also noted was damage to corals through contact or inappropriate use of anchors or diver behavior. The steadily increasing popularity of diving and the increasing accessibility of recreational diving to previously remote areas has generated concerns about diver effect on coral, with poor diver etiquette, inexperience at controlling buoyancy, improperly secured gear, photography flashes, and blasts from fin kicks being important diver-induced damage to reef structures (Fishman 1991).

Beyond the impacts of immediate harvesters and tourists, propelled by a growing demand from the restaurant and hotel industries, a global market for reef species like grouper has developed, making reefs a significant site of resource extraction and foreign exchange (Hughes *et al.* 2003). In the Philippines, this extraction, with a focus on the Hong Kong and Chinese markets, has contributed to overfishing, and the decline or collapse of some reef fisheries (Fabinyi and Dalabajan 2011). Reef fisheries are also often tied to other forms of fishing, as they are used as a place for catching bait fish used in hooking highly desired fish foods like tuna, which themselves depend on reef species as part of their food source (Whittingham, Campbell, and Townsley 2003). In the Maldives, for example, 25 percent of the workforce is employed in fishing, predominantly tuna fishing, an industry that is dependent on reefs to attract target fish and for live bait supplies (Zuhair 1998). Moreover, there is a global market for hobby reef fish and a sizeable percentage of fish and marine invertebrates in the aquarium trade are taken from coral areas and shipped, primarily, to wealthy countries in Europe and North America. Additionally, large numbers of corals, shells, starfish, puffer fish, seahorses, and other reef species are taken for sales in the curio trade (United National Environmental Program 2006).

Adding to their importance to human communities, coral reefs are a vital barrier that protects coast lands and islands from erosion, storm surges, flooding, and salinization of crop lands and fresh water sources (Wilkinson 2006). Reefs function as coastal buffers by absorbing most of the force produced by ocean waves. When reefs are damaged or destroyed, their absence results in increased damage to coastal communities from both normal wave action and violent storms. Reefs also protect other ecosystems that contain vital resources, such as mangroves and seagrass meadows.

Finally, reefs have emerged as a source of new medicines, and their degradation puts this health-resource aspect of coral areas at risk. Marine organisms found on reefs often contain pharmaceutically active compounds, many of which have not been investigated. Already, reef inhabitants have been used as the source of both an HIV treatment and a painkiller and active research is investigating reef species as a source of cancer drugs (Millennium Ecosystem Assessment 2005).

As suggested above, the anthropogenic threat to coral reefs has several sources. Climate change, by raising the temperature of the oceans, is leading to coral bleaching, which is a stress response to rising ocean temperatures (Donner *et al.* 2005). For example, reef systems in Mozambique were particularly badly affected by the major El Niño bleaching event of 1998 (Samoilys *et al.* 2011). It is estimated that 16 percent of the coral reefs distributed across the world died during this warm ocean event, especially reefs in the Indian Ocean and Western Pacific (Wilkinson and Souter 2008). As the ocean waters around reefs heat up, zooxanthellae, the tiny algal organisms that provide coral reefs with their brilliant colors and much of the energy for coral growth, emigrate or are expelled by their hosts in massive numbers, killing themselves and bleaching the coral they leave behind. Migration is driven by the heat-propelled production of toxic compounds in coral algae that are transferred to the host coral. Bleached coral is highly susceptible to death due to disease and starvation. This occurred in 2005 in the Caribbean, which contains about 10 percent of the world's reefs, when rising temperatures produced one of the warmest years on record and resulted in corals being bathed in abnormally warm waters for 4 to 6 months. During this episode, the greatest coral death was recorded in the US Virgin Islands, which lost about 51 percent of its reefs due to bleaching and subsequent diseases. The 2005 coral die-off "followed a long, slow decline in the status of Caribbean coral reefs … especially during the last 50 years," with coral reefs of the Caribbean losing "up to 80% of their coral cover during this time" due to diverse anthropogenic activity (Wilkinson and Souter 2008: 7).

Additionally, greenhouse gas emissions are increasing the dissolved carbon dioxide composition of the ocean, altering ocean chemistry (making it more acidic), resulting in a slowing of coral growth and a weakening of coral structures. Since the Industrial Revolution, oceans have absorbed at least a quarter of the carbon dioxide released by human activity. While this has somewhat slowed overall global warming, it has increased ocean acidification, sometimes referred to as "the other CO^2 problem" (Doney *et al.* 2009), by 30 percent over the last 150 years. Existing research suggests that ocean acidification "may be proceeding at a rate that is 100 times faster and with a magnitude that is 3 times greater than anything experienced on the planet in the last 21 million years" (Wilkinson and Souter 2008: 12). Carbon dioxide dissolution is known to directly alter the carbonate chemistry of seawater and reduce the availability of ions required by marine life to form shells and coral structures. Various studies have documented the sensitivity of marine organisms including coral to pH changes at the level they are now occurring in the oceans. One response to disruption caused by changing external CO_2 levels in tropical corals is a reduction in growth likely tied to the increased energy needed to sustain the proper acid balance that sustains normal metabolic activity. Acid-base imbalance in corals can result in metabolic suppression, reduced protein synthesis, and reduction in long-term fitness (Pandolfi *et al.* 2011). Recent research with corals has shown that ocean acidification may begin to impair the calcification process when acid-base and ion regulatory systems are unable to maintain homeostasis in the calcifying cells (Kaniewska *et al.* 2012).

In many environments, corals compete for space with seaweed. Seaweed grows much faster than coral, giving it a potential competitive advantage. Humans, however, have helped to tip this balance strongly in favor of seaweed in many locales through various environmental changes such the over-extraction of the fish and other herbivores that keep seaweed under control. Overfishing may contribute to algal growth as the absence of herbivorous fish results in the proliferation of green filamentous algae on dead coral. This transition may be followed by the settlement of brown frondose algae and the transformation of a previous reef area into an algae-dominated zone (McClanahan 1997). This shift can be facilitated by the inability of a reef to recover from damage caused by a severe storm of the sort increasingly produced in coral zone areas by global warming. Algae has been found be more resilient to weather and other disturbances than corals and consequently may be more stable once it is established (McManus *et al.* 2000). Reef researchers in Mozambique, for example, note that

> low densities of reef fishes is of concern and indicates that fishing pressure may be relatively high. Further, with such a high proportion of [coral genus] *Acropora* on these reefs, their vulnerability to future bleaching from sea surface temperature increases is likely to be high. It is therefore crucial that other stresses such as overfishing are minimised to maximise the ability of these reefs to recover from a future bleaching event. (Samoilys *et al.* 2011: iv)

Notably, fishing pressure on places like the northern reefs of Mozambique is expected to increase in coming years as the national government builds infrastructure in Pemba, the province capital. Limited electricity in parts of the province in the past limited the making of ice and the ability to store fish, which controlled the scale of reef fish harvesting. Extension of the electric grid has begun to eliminate this control. Other local threats to northern Mozambique reefs include growing levels of immigration, construction of improved access to wider markets and technology, and the initiation of exploratory efforts for oil and gas extraction (Hill *et al.* 2009). All of these developments are likely to contribute to increased demand for reef fish foods, overfishing, algal growth, and resulting reef loss.

Moreover, the release into the oceans of human sewage, urban runoff, industrial effluents, fertilizer-rich farm runoff, and other organic pollutants rich in nitrogen or phosphorus provides nutrients for rapid seaweed and algal growth, to the disadvantage of corals. Especially important in this anthropogenic eutrophication process are rivers, loaded with organic pollutants that empty into oceans. This pattern is noted throughout the Caribbean where there has been a shift from coral-dominated reefs toward macroalgal domination (Idjadi *et al.* 2006).

The interaction of climate change with ocean acidification, sewage dumping, pollutant release, overfishing, and dive tourist disturbance in the demise of coral reefs affirms the significance of pluraleal interactions as a growing risk factor in a time of global climate change. Given the critical importance of coral reefs as a source of food, other resources, and income for millions of people, especially the poorest people in low-income countries in several parts of the world, degradation and loss of reefs presents a major threat to food security and to global human health and well-being.

Conclusion

The World Health Organization (2014) promotes a definition of environmental health that encompasses "all the physical, chemical and biological factors external to a person." While this international body does not emphasize the importance of the interactions that occur among environmental threats to health, it does recognize, for example, that many of the major environmental sources of human mortality in the world, such as diarrheal diseases, malnutrition, malaria, and dengue, that are enhanced by various anthropocentric factors (e.g., polluted water, deforestation, urbanization, land use pattern), "are highly climate-sensitive and are expected to worsen as the climate changes" (World Health Organization 2013). While this is a useful start, the approach of the World Health Organization, as well as that of other environmental health institutions, tends to direct focus toward individual environmental threats to health and associated outcomes. A pluraleal approach, by contrast, is centrally concerned with the ways that environmental risks intersect and how their adverse health effects are multiplied through interaction. As emphasized in all three of the case studies, climate change is a significant interactive and amplifying contributor to worsening environmental health globally. Thus, rising planetary temperatures magnify the respiratory and cardiovascular damage caused by air pollution; worsen the food security impacts of overfishing, toxic ocean dumping, ocean acidification, and tourist pressure on coral reefs. In interaction with the intentional removal of natural barriers like wetlands and seagrass (but mangroves and coral reefs as well), climate change intensifies storms, flooding, and related health risks like waterborne diseases and exposure to fungal spores. By drawing attention to multiple interacting anthropogenic ecological crises and to the fact that because of human activities we have entered an era of novel environmental conditions on Earth, a pluraleal approach facilitates a rethinking of the concept of environmental health that promotes the development of holistic models and multidimensional, multisectorial responses appropriate to the complexities of contemporary life.

ACKNOWLEDGMENTS

I thank Pamela I. Erickson for her comments on an earlier draft of this chapter.

REFERENCES

Betts, A. 2012. "Extreme Weather and Climate." *Rutland Herald*. http://alanbetts.com/workspace/uploads/feature-2012nov11-extremeweather-and-1352669502.pdf. (accessed December 11, 2015).

Burke, L., Reytar, K., Spalding, M., and Perry, A. 2012. *Reefs at Risk Revisited in the Coral Triangle*. Washington, DC: World Resources Institute.

Cabo Delgado Biodiversity and Tourism Project. 2006. *Management Plan*. Pemba, Mozambique: Cabo Delgado Biodiversity and Tourism LDA.

Canty, S. 2008. "Positive and Negative Impacts of Dive Tourism: The Case Study of Utila, Honduras." *Master's thesis*, Lund University Centre for Sustainability Studies, Sweden.

Carson, R. 1962. *Silent Spring*. Boston: Houghton Mifflin.

Cesaroni, G., Fortastiere, F., Stafoggia, M., Andersen, Z., Badaloni, C., Beelen, R., *et al.* 2014. "Long-term Exposure to Ambient Air Pollution and Incidence of Acute Coronary Events: Prospective Cohort Study and Meta-analysis in 11 European Cohorts from the ESCAPE Project." *British Medical Journal*, 348: f7412.

Chen, B., Shawn, L., Connors, N., Wheeler, K., Williams, N., Hoffman, R., *et al.* 2013. "Carbon Monoxide Exposures in New York City following Hurricane Sandy in 2012." *Clinical Toxicology*, 51(9): 879–885.

Cooper, M., Beevers, M., and Oppenheimer, M. 2008. "The Potential Impacts of Sea Level Rise on the Coastal Region of New Jersey, USA." *Climate Change*, 90: 475–492.

Crutzen, P. and Schwägerl, C. 2011. "Living in the Anthropocene: Toward a New Global Ethos." *Yale Environment* 360. http://e360.yale.edu/feature/living_in_the_anthropocene_toward_a_new_global_ethos/2363/ (accessed December 11, 2015).

Crutzen, P. and Stoermer, E. 2000. "The Anthropocene." *Global Change Newsletter*, 41: 17–18.

Darwin, C. 1859. *On the Origin of Species by Means of Natural Selection, or the preservation of favoured races in the struggle for life*. London: Watts.

De'ath, G., Fabricius, K., Sweatman, H., and Poutinen, M. 2012. "The 27-year Decline of Coral Cover on the Great Barrier Reef and Its Causes." *Proceedings of the National Academy of Sciences*. doi: 10.1073/pnas.1208909109.

Dearing, J. 2007. "Human–Environment Interactions: Learning from the Past." In R. Constanza, L. Graumlich, and W. Steffen (Eds.), *Sustainability or Collapse: An Integrated History and Future of People on Earth* (pp. 19–38.) Cambridge, MA: Massachusetts Institute of Technology.

Doney, S., Faby, V., Feely, R., and Kleypas, J. 2009. "Ocean Acidification: The Other CO2 Problem." *Annual Review of Marine Science*, 1: 169–192.

Donner, S., Skirving, W., Little, C., Oppenheimer, M., and Hoegh-Guldberg, O. 2005. "Global Assessment of Coral Bleaching and Required Rates of Adaptation under Climate Change." *Global Change Biology*, 11: 2251–2265.

Fabinyi, M. and Dalabajan, D. 2011. "Policy and Practice in the Life Reef Fish for Food Trade: A Case Study from Palawan, Philippines." *Marine Policy*, 35: 371–378.

Fishman, D. 1991. "Loving the Reef to Death." *Sea Frontiers*, 37: 14–18.

Foster, J.B., Clark, B., and York, R 2010. *The Ecological Rift: Capitalism's War on the Earth*. New York: Monthly Review Press.

Francis, J. and Vavrus, S. 2012. "Evidence Linking Artic Amplification to Extreme Weather in Mid-latitudes." *Geophysical Research Letters*, 39: L06801.

Franck, U., Leitte, A., and Suppan, P. 2014. "Multiple Exposures to Airborne Pollutants and Hospital Admissions due to Diseases of the Circulatory System in Santiago de Chile." *Science of the Total Environment*, 468/9(15): 746–756.

Freed, A. 2013. "Global Cities Need Natural Defenses." Nature Conservancy. http://blog.nature.org/conservancy/2013/05/30/global-cities-need-natural-defenses/ (accessed December 11, 2015).

Gbadero, D., Johnson, A.-W., Aderele, W., and Olaleye, D. 1995. "Microbial Inciters of Acute Asthma in Urban Nigerian Children." *Thorax*, 50: 739–745.

Global Initiative for Asthma. 2009. *Global Strategy for Asthma Management and Prevention*. Vienna: World Health Organization.

Greene, S., Wilson, E., Konty, K., and Fine, A. 2013. "Assessment of Reportable Disease Incidence after Hurricane Sandy, New York City, 2012." *Disaster Medicine and Public Health Preparedness*, 7(5): 513–521.

Hamilton, A. 1925. *Industrial Poisons in the United States*. New York: Macmillan.

Hanania, N. 2009. "Asthma Control: A New Perspective on the Management of Asthma." *Current Opinion in Pulmonary Medicine*, 15(1): 1–3.

Hill, N., Davidson, J., Sivla, I., Mucave, S., Muaves L., Guissamulo, A., Debney, A., and Garnier, J. 2009. "Coral and Reef Fish in the Northern Quirimbas Archipelago, Mozambique – A First Assessment." *Western Indian Ocean Journal of Marine Science*, 8(1): 113–125.

Hughes, T., Baird, A., Bellwood, D., Card, M., Connolly, S., Folke, C., Grosberg, R., … and Roughgarden, J. 2003. "Climate Change, Human Impacts, and the Resilience of Coral Reefs." *Science*, 301: 929–933.

Idjadi, J., Lee, S., Bruno, J., Precht, W., Allen-Requa, L., and Edmunds, P. 2006." Rapid Phase-Shift Reversal on a Jamaican Coral Reef." *Coral Reefs*, 25: 209–211.

International Coral Reef Initiative. 2002. *Deciding on Priorities to Protect and Manage the World's Coral Reefs*. Townsville, Australia: International Coral Reef Initiative.

International Institute for Environment and Development. 2003. *Reef Livelihoods Assessment (RLA) Project: Global Overview of Reef Dependent Livelihoods and the Poor*. London: IIED.

IPCC (Intergovernmental Panel on Climate Change). 2013. Working Group I Contribution to the IPCC Fifth Assessment Report. *Climate Change 2013: The Physical Science Basis*. Stockholm.

Jameson, S., McManus, J., and Spalding, M. 1995. State of the Reefs: Regional and *Global Perspectives*. Background Paper, Executive Secretariat, International Coral Reef Initiative. Washington, DC: US National Oceanic and Atmospheric Administration.

Kaniewska, P., Campbell, P., Kline, D., Rodriguez-Lanetty, M., Miller, D., Dove, S., and Hoegh-Guldberg, O. 2012. "Major Cellular and Physiological Impacts of Ocean Acidification on a Reef Building Coral." *PLoS ONE*, 7: e34659.

Laurent, O., Filleul, L., Havard, S., Deguen, S., Declercq, C., and Bard, D. 2008. "Asthma Attacks and Deprivation: Gradients in Use of Mobile Emergency Medical Services." *Journal of Epidemiology & Community Health*, 62(11): 1014–1016.

Levin, S. 2009. *The Princeton Guide to Ecology*. Princeton, NJ: Princeton University Press.

Lim, S., Vos, T., Flaxman, A., Danei, G., Shibuya, K., Adair-Rohani, H., *et al.* 2012. "A Comparative Risk Assessment of Burden of Disease and Injury Attributable to Risk Factor Clusters in 21 Regions, 1990–2010: A Systematic Analysis for the Global Burden of Disease Study 2010. *Lancet*, 380(9859): 2224–2260.

Lin, N., Emanuel, K., Oppenheimer, M., and Vanmarcke, E. 2012. "Physically Based Assessment of Hurricane Surge Threat under Climate Change." *Nature Climate Change*, 2: 462–467.

Masoli, M., Fabian, D., Holt, S., and Beasley, R. 2004. *Global Burden of Asthma*. Wellington, New Zealand: Medical Research Institute of New Zealand.

McAllister, D. 1988. "Environmental, Economic and Social Costs of Coral Reef Destruction in the Philippines." *Galaxea*, 7: 161–178.

McClanahan, T. 1997. "Primary Succession of Coral-Reef Algae: Differing Patterns on Fished Versus Unfished Reefs." Journal of Experimental Marine Biology and Ecolecology, 218: 77–102.

McClanahan, T., Glaesel, H., Rubens, J., and Kiambo, R. 1998. "The Effects of Traditional Fisheries Management on Fisheries Yield and the Coral Reef Ecosystem of Southern Kenya." *Oceanographic Literature Review*, 45: 561–562.

McGoodwin, J. 2001. *Understanding the Cultures of Fishing Communities: A Key to Fisheries Management and Food Security*. Rome: United Nations Food and Agricultural Organization, Fisheries Technical Paper No. 401.

McManus, J., Meñez, L., Kesner-Reyes, K., Vergara, S., and Ablan, M. 2000. "Coral Reef Fishing and Coral-Algal Phase Shifts: Implications for Global Reef Status." *Journal of Marine Science*, 57: 573–578.

Millennium Ecosystem Assessment. 2005. *Ecosystems and Human Well-being: Synthesis*. Washington, DC: Island Press.

Murray, C., Poletti, G., Kebadze, T., Morris, J., Woodcock, A., Johnston, S., and Custovic, A. 2006. "Study of Modifiable Risk Factors for Asthma Exacerbations: Virus Infection and Allergen Exposure Increase the Risk of Asthma Hospital Admissions in Children." *Thorax*, 61: 376–382.

NOAA (National Oceanic and Atmospheric Administration). 2012. "Fisheries." http://coralreef.noaa.gov/aboutcorals/values/fisheries/ (accessed December 11, 2015).

NOAA (National Oceanic and Atmospheric Administration). 2013a. *Hurricane/Post-Tropical Cyclone Sandy. October 22–29, 2012*. Silver Springs, MD: National Weather Service.

NOAA (National Oceanic and Atmospheric Administration). 2013b. "New Analyses Find Evidence of Human-Caused Climate Change in Half of the 12 Extreme Weather and Climate Events Analyzed from 2012." http://www.noaanews.noaa.gov/stories2013/20130905-extremeweatherandclimateevents.html (accessed December 11, 2015).

Noyes, P., McElwee, M., Miller, H., Clark, B., Van Tiem, L., Walcott, K. Erwin, K., and Levin, E. 2008. "The Toxicology of Climate Change: Environmental Contaminants in a Warming World." *Environment International*, 35(6): 971–986.

Ontario Lung Association. 2008. "The Connections between Climate Change, Air Quality and Respiratory Health." http://www.lung.ca/protect-protegez/pollution-pollution/outdoor-exterior/climate-climatique_e.php (accessed January 26, 2014).

Oppenheimer, M. and Trenberth, K. 2013. "Climate Science Tells Us the Alarm Bells Are Ringing." *Washington Post*, Opinion section, June 7. http://www.washingtonpost.com/opinions/climate-science-tells-us-the-alarm-bells-are-ringing/2013/06/07/ca81cb84-cef6-11e2-8845-d970ccb04497_story.html (accessed December 11, 2015).

Otis, G. 2013. "Hurricane Sandy, One Year Later: Tracing the Superstorm's Path from Inception to Destruction." *Daily News*, October 20. http://www.nydailynews.com/new-york/hurricane-sandy/sandy-1-year-storm-winds-article-1.1495677 (accessed December 11, 2015).

Pandolfi, J., Connolly, S., Marshall, D., and Cohen, A. 2011. "Projecting Coral Reef Futures under Global Warming and Ocean Acidification." *Science*, 333: 418–422.

Pasisi, B. 1995. *Country statement – Niue Island.* South Pacific Commission and Forum Fisheries Agency Workshop on the Management of South Pacific Inshore Fisheries 1: 117–121.

PBA Newshour. 2013. "Why the Strongest Storms Are Getting Stronger." http://www.pbs.org/newshour/bb/climate-change-july-dec13-storms2_11-12/ (accessed December 11, 2015).

Rees, M. 2003. *Our Final Hour: A Scientist's Warning: How Terror, Error, and Environmental Disaster Threaten Humankind's Future in This Century – On Earth and Beyond.* New York: Basic Books.

Rockström, J., Steffen, W., Noone, K., Persson, A., Chapin, F., Lambin, E., *et al.* 2009. "Planetary Boundaries: Exploring the Safe Operating Space for Humanity." *Ecology and Society*, 14(2): 32.

Rosenzweig, C. 2008. "Warming Climate is Changing Life on Global Scale." Goddard Institute for Space Studies, NASA. http://www.giss.nasa.gov/research/briefs/rosenzweig_02/ (accessed December 12, 2015).

Rozenzweig, C., Solecki, W., Hammer, S.A., and Mehrotra, S. (Eds.) 2011. *Climate Change and Cities: First Assessment Report of the Urban Climate Change Research Network.* Cambridge: Cambridge University Press.

Samoilys, M., Ndagala, J., Macharia, D., da Silva, I., Mucave, S., and Obura, D. 2011. *A Rapid Assessment of Coral Reefs at Metundo Island, Cabo Delgado, Northern Mozambique.* Mombasa: CORDIO East Africa.

Schmaljohn, C. and Hjelle, B. 1997. "Hantaviruses: A Global Disease Problem." *Emerging Infectious Diseases*, 3(2): 96–104.

Schwartz, N. 2004. "Childhood Asthma on the Northern Mexico Border." *Medical Anthropology Quarterly*, 18(2): 214–229.

Shea, K., Truckner, R., Weber, R., and Peden, D. 2008. "Climate Change and Allergenic Disease." *Journal of Allergy and Clinical Immunology*, 122(3): 443–453.

Simon, J. 1897. *English Sanitary Institutions.* London: Smith, Elder and Co.

Singer, M. 2009. "Beyond Global Warming: Interacting Ecocrises and the Critical Anthropology of Health." *Anthropology Quarterly*, 82(3): 795–820.

Singer, M. 2013. "Respiratory Health and Ecosyndemics in a Time of Global Warming." *Health Sociology Review*, 21(1): 98–111.

Spalding, M., Green, E., and Ravilious, C. 2001. *World Atlas of Coral Reefs.* UNEP World Conservation Monitoring Centre. Berkeley, CA: University of California Press.

Spratt, D. and Sutton, P. 2008. *Climate Code Red: The Case for a Sustainability Emergency.* Melbourne: Friends of the Earth Australia.

Steward, J. 1972 (original 1955). *Theory of Culture Change: The Methodology of Multilinear Evolution.* Champaign, IL: University of Illinois Press.

Stauffer, R. 1957. "Haeckel, Darwin and Ecology." *Quarterly Review of Biology*, 32(2): 138–144.

Sweet, W., Zervas, C., Gill, S., and Park, J. 2013. "Hurricane Sandy Inundation Probabilities Today and Tomorrow." In "Explaining Extreme Events of 2012 from a Climate Perspective." Supplement to the Bulletin of the *American Meteorological Society*, 04(8): 17–19.

Thomas, W. 1956. *Man's Role in Changing the Face of the Earth.* Chicago, IL: University of Chicago Press.

United Nations Development Program. 2002. *Human Development Report.* Geneva: UNDP.

United Nations Environment Program World Conservation Monitoring Center. 2006. *In the Front Line: Shoreline Protection and Other Ecosystem Services from Mangroves and Coral Reefs.* Cambridge, UK: WNEP-WCMC.

Whittingham, E., Campbell, J., and Townsley, P. 2003. *Poverty and Reefs.* Vol. 1: *A Global Overview.* London: Intergovernment Oceanographic Commission of UNESCO.

WHO (World Health Organization). 2008. "Air Quality and Health." http://www.who.int/mediacentre/factsheets/fs313/en/index.html (accessed December 11, 2015).

WHO (World Health Organization). 2013. "Climate Change and Health." Fact Sheet No. 266. http://www.who.int/mediacentre/factsheets/fs266/en/index.html (accessed December 11, 2015).

WHO (World Health Organization). 2014. "Environmental Health." http://www.who.int/topics/environmental_health/en/ (accessed December 11, 2015).

Wilkinson, C. 2006. "Status of Coral Reefs of the World: Summary of Threats and Remedial Action." In I. Côté and J. Reynolds (Eds.), *Coral Reef Conservation* (pp. 3–39). Cambridge. Cambridge University Press.

Wilkinson, C. and Souter, D. 2008. *Status of Caribbean Coral Reefs After Bleaching and the Hurricanes of 2005.* Townsville, Australia: Global Coral Reef Monitoring Network and Reef Rainforest Research Centre.

Wilson, J., Muchave, P., and Garrett, A. 2003. "A Case Study from Mozambique." In E. Whittingham, J. Campell, and P. Townsley (Eds.), *Poverty and Reefs: Case Studies* (pp. 73–111). Paris: DFIC-IMM-IOC/UNESCO.

Wisner, B., Blaikie, P., Cannon, T., and Davis, I. 2003. *At Risk: Natural Hazards, People's Vulnerability and Disasters.* New York: Psychology Press.

Wolf, E. 1972. "Ownership and Political Ecology." *Anthropological Quarterly*, 45(3): 201–205.

Ziska, L., Knowlton, K., Rogers, C., Dalan, D., Tierney, N., Elder, M., *et al.* 2011. "Recent Warming by Latitude Associated with Increased Length of Ragweed Pollen Season in Central North America. *Proceedings of the National Academy of Sciences*, 108(10): 4248–4251.

Zuhair, M. 1998. "Conservation by Local Communities in the Maldives." In B. Taneja (Ed.), *Communities and Conservation: Natural Resource Management in South and Central Asia* (pp. 102–116). New Delhi, India: Sage.

CHAPTER 22

Private Cars as Environmental Health Hazards: The Critical Need for Public Transit in the Era of Climate Change

Hans A. Baer

Introduction

Motor vehicles with their internal combustion engines embody the social structural contradictions of the capitalist world system. The world now has an estimated 700 to 800 million cars, and this number continues to grow rapidly as certain developing countries – particularly China and India but certainly others – imitate developed societies in their adoption of a culture of automobility. Sperling and Gordon (2010: 4) project that there will be over 2 billion motor vehicles, at least half of them cars, by 2020 while the International Monetary Fund projects the presence of some 3 billion cars in the world by 2050 given the current pace of car production (Richter 2010: 118). The latter projection may be unlikely given the impact of climate change over the course of the next several decades, which is likely to have grave effects on the global economy and life as we more or less know it in the current era. Part and parcel of these impacts, motor vehicles have affected and will continue to affect patterns of consumption, settlement, traffic congestion, mass transportation, social relations, the environment, and environmental health. They

A Companion to the Anthropology of Environmental Health, First Edition. Edited by Merrill Singer.

constitute a major contributor not only to air and noise pollution but also to greenhouse gas emissions and ultimately to climate change as well as fatalities, injuries, stress, social isolation, and obesity.

The private automobile constitutes the ultimate commodity for many people around the world, indeed a *killer commodity* and a *death machine*, around which numerous other industries operate, including the oil, accessory parts, highway construction, insurance, and even health care industries. As Matthew Paterson (2007: 92) astutely observes, "[a]cross a wide range of political/economic discourses the car has been seen to play a fundamental role in the promotion of economic growth in the twentieth century [as well as the twentieth-first century], and thus in the reproduction of capitalism as a system." The state has served as a staunch ally of automobile companies by facilitating road construction, allowing the systematic neglect and downplaying of public transportation, fiscal policies which essentially privilege the car over other forms of transportation, and rescue of the car industry from economic collapse (Paterson 2007: 115).

Adopting a critical medical anthropological perspective, this chapter examines four environmental health hazards of private cars: (1) air pollution, (2) greenhouse emissions, (3) auto accidents that result in injuries and fatalities, and (4) mental health consequences. Cars also contribute to the restructuring of food production as valuable farmland is converted from the production of food to the production of biofuels, thus depriving an increasing number of people of subsistence necessary for sustenance, nutrition, and health. In the conclusion of this chapter I examine the pressing need for structural change to reduce the considerable adverse impacts of automobility. Ultimately, for the sake of both the ecological and the human body, it is imperative that humanity rethink the sustainability and value of the private car.

The Private Car as a Manifestation of Global Culture of Automobility

James Flink (1988: viii) contends that the rise of the automobile industry and a massive network of roads are "central to the history of the advanced capitalist countries, and explains an especially large part of the history of the American people." Although Europeans invented the internal combustion engine, the United States assumed the lead in car production by the early twentieth century. Sociologist John Urry (2004: 25–26) delineates six key aspects of *automobility*. In his view, cars are:

- "the quintessential *manufactured object* produced by the leading industrial sectors and the iconic firms within 20th-century capitalism" and, one might add, early 21st-century capitalism;
- "the major item of *individual consumption* after housing which provides its owner/user through its sign-values (such as speed, security, safety, sexual desire, career success, freedom, family, masculinity)";

- "an extraordinarily powerful *complex* constituted through technical and social interlinkages with other industries";
- "the predominant global form of 'quasi-private' *mobility* that subordinates other mobilities of walking, cycling, travelling by rail and so on," and which defines work and recreation;
- "the dominant *culture* that sustains major discourses of what constitutes the good life;" and
- "the single most important cause of *environmental resource-use*" which serves as a major source of pollution, carbon dioxide emissions, health problems, as well as an indirect contributor to warfare, particularly in efforts to ensure oil supplies.

The production and consumption of cars became a major component of Fordism as a corporate vision of mechanized production coupled with the mass consumption of standardized products. Henry Ford systematically embarked upon a campaign to socialize his and other workers into core American values, which included the purchase of one of his automobiles at a purportedly affordable price. In reality, people were induced to sacrifice other needs and desires in order save up the money to purchase a Model T Ford. In the case of Ford's workers, the raising of wages to $5 a day resulted in a rigid discipline mechanism:

> The $5-a-day rate was about half pay and half bonus. The bonus came with character requirements and was enforced by the Socialization Organization. This was a committee that would visit the employees' homes to ensure that they were doing things the "American way." They were supposed to avoid social ills such as gambling and drinking. They were to learn English, and many (primarily the recent immigrants) had to attend classes to become "Americanized." Women were not eligible for the bonus unless they were single and supporting the family. Also, men were not eligible if their wives worked outside the home. (Worstall 2012)

In their classic community study of Middletown (Muncie, Indiana) during the 1920s, Robert and Helen Lynd (1929: 950) reported that the "make of one's car is rivalling the looks of one's place as an evidence of one's belonging among members of the 'business class.'" Fordism, however, propelled the automobile from its status as a luxury commodity into a mass commodity. Lynd and Lynd stated that despite the Depression, by the mid-1930s the car had become an essential object for the Middletown worker, for whom "it gives the status which his job increasingly denies, and, more than any other facility to which he has access, it symbolizes living, having a good time, that things that keeps you working" (Lynd and Lynd 1937: 245). Particularly in the wake of World War II, it had become commonplace for the vast majority of American families to own an automobile, a pattern that Ford had set in motion. Private motor vehicles, perhaps more than any other consumer item, exemplify the culture of consumption par excellence. In describing the economic situation in US society during the 1970s, Paul Sweezy (1973: 7) contended that the "private interests which cluster around and are directly or indirectly dependent upon the automobile for their prosperity are quantitatively far more numerous and wealthy than those similarly related to any other commodity or complex of commodities in the U.S. economy."

In both developed and developing countries, the car has come to be viewed by many people as a necessity rather than a luxury, one which often traps them into a complex web which functions as anthropologist Daniel Miller (2001: 2) describes as a "villain that has separated us from world and threatens to take over as we come to serve it more than it serves us." In a similar vein, Lenora Bohren (2009: 370) posits the car as a form of cultural adaptation that became highly maladaptive in that it "has caused many unintended consequences to the environment." She notes that the "car also brought on problems of intense resource and energy use and environmental degradation" (Bohren 2009: 372).

For city dwellers seeking relief from the hectic pace of urban life, the car and even the camper or recreational vehicle offer an escape to imagined idyllic locations. In reality, most trailer parks in North America, Europe, and Australia are flooded with urbanites who are parked closely to each other while they watch TV, drink, and cook over a camp stove brought from the city. Automobile companies in their advertisements often depict cars in natural, remote settings, such as mountain tops, canyon lands, and secluded beaches. As Nickolas Low *et al.* (2005: 234) indicate, "Nature, like sex, sells cars! And yet nothing despoils nature like cars!"

However, slick advertisements ultimately cannot effectively stimulate car sales during periods of economic downturn. For instance, the global financial crisis that erupted in 2008 resulted in a downturn in automobile sales, with a 30 percent reduction in late 2008 over the previous year (Barbier 2010: 79). General Motors (GM) and Chrysler declared bankruptcy in the United States with GM receiving a US government bailout. The US government spent taxpayer money to rescue the automobile industry without requiring CEOs to lower their overinflated salaries, the companies to guarantee jobs for auto workers, or even the industry to shift much of its production from cars to public transportation infrastructure. Indeed, tax dollars were used in some cases to provide company executives with bonuses.

While the United States undoubtedly represents the leading example of the culture of automobility, the private car constitutes a component, and often a leading component, of societies around the world, particularly developed countries, such as Germany, the United Kingdom, Italy, Japan, Canada, and Australia, but increasingly developing countries, particularly China, India, and Brazil. In Australia, war bonds posters urged people to save for a post-World War II car (Davison 2004: 3) and the Holden station wagon became in the late 1950s a "mobile embodiment of a middle-class suburb family life" (Davison 2004: 21). Although Canberra, the national capital, has grown to a sprawling city of some 375,000 people with an elaborate road system consisting of concentric circles, roundabouts, and a bus system vastly superior to most US cities of roughly the same size, politicians, city planners, and a substantial number of residents postpone the inevitable day of reckoning in terms of increasing traffic congestion by arguing that a light-rail system would be prohibitively expensive.

In recent decades, automobile firms have been searching for new markets in the developing world and, with the collapse of the Soviet bloc, in Eastern

Europe. As Schaefer *et al.* (2009: 3) observe, "[s]ince about 80 percent of the world population lives in the developing countries, the largest wave of motorization is yet to come." Car production in South Korea jumped from 20,000 a year in the early 1980s to 2.4 million in 2000 (Dicken 2003: 359). Thailand has evolved into the "car capital" of Southeast Asia with many major foreign automobile companies having manufacturing facilities there due to cheaper labor costs than in developed societies.

These operations are dwarfed by a burgeoning car manufacturing sector in China and India. The Chinese car industry consists of state companies as well as a number of joint operations between these companies and foreign companies, including Volkswagen, Toyota, Nissan, Honda, Hyundai, and General Motors (Dicken 2003: 396–397). According to Sachs (2008: 76), "China's annual production is now soaring, up to around 7 million in the year 2000." Various studies project that China will have approximately 200 million cars by 2020 and nearly 400 million cars by 2030 on the road (Montgomery 2010: 37). Whereas vehicle sales dropped 50 percent in the United States and 40 percent in other countries as a whole in 2009 in the midst of the global financial crisis, China overtook the United States during that year as the largest domestic market for cars in the world and became General Motor's largest market (Achoff 2011: 134).

Whereas in 1951 India had an estimated 300,000 cars, this number had increased to about 85 million by 2005 (Shiva 2008: 52). Tata launched the mini-car Nano in India in 2008 as an alleged "people's car'." It plans to market the Nano in Southeast Asia, Latin America, and Africa (Montgomery 2010: 37). General Motors, Honda, Volkswagon, and other companies plan to build new factories in India and Fiat, Nissan, and Renault are forming partnerships with Indian car manufacturers (Shiva 2008: 50).

Cities around the world vary considerably in their utilization of cars for transportation. For instance, car or motorcycle utilization runs from 16 percent in Hong Kong, to 39 percent in Berlin, to 51 percent in Madrid, to 76 percent in Melbourne, to 88 percent in Chicago (Gilbert and Perl 2010). In China, car ownership varies widely from area to area: "In Beijing, there were 108 cars per 1,000 residents in 2004, 72 percent were privately owned. In Gansu, Guizhou, and Jiangxi provinces, there were fewer than 5 per 1,000, and only 42 percent of these cars were privately owned" (Gilbert and Peel 2010: 74). Even in Singapore, which reportedly has an excellent public transportation system, many affluent people are being seduced by the culture of automobility. In this densely populated and compact city-state of only 274 square miles,

> Mileage per vehicle is very high: the average car in Singapore travelled 21,100 km in 2006, double the figure for 1980 and virtually identical to the 21,317 km reported for Los Angeles … The number of Singapore residents rose by 6 per cent in the five years to 2007, but the number of cars jumped 19 per cent, traffic entering Singapore's CBD grew by 14 per cent and CBD traffic speeds fell by up to 30 percent. (Mees 2010: 45)

Not only in Singapore but throughout much of Southeast Asia, South Asia, and East Asia, cities are increasingly characterized by traffic congestion in which motor vehicles make their way across large cities such as Bangkok, Jakarta, Beijing, Shanghai, Mexico City, and São Paulo in a long series of starts and stops. In short, urban areas around the world find themselves, to a greater or lesser degree, literally choked by private motor vehicles of one sort or another – in terms of air pollution, noise, greenhouse gas emissions, and congestion – a situation that severely counteracts many of the redeeming aspects of urban life, such as cultural diversity and cosmopolitanism.

Environmental Health Hazards of Private Cars

Along with industrial pollution, motor vehicles have transformed many cities around the world into environmental disaster areas accompanied by a wide array of health problems. Along with their environmental impacts, motor vehicles have had major impacts on not only patterns of consumption but also energy utilization, settlement patterns, social relations, public policy, and congestion, all of which in one way or another affect health. Woodcock and Aldred highlight the complex linkages between car-based transportation and public health:

> The burning of fossil fuel, oil, produces the kinetic energy that kills 1.2 million people and injures 50 million on the roads each year. Urban pollution for motor vehicles is responsible for hundreds of thousands of deaths per year, while noise pollution is implicated in cardiovascular disease, and inhibits cognitive development. The obesity epidemic is linked to the shift from human powered to fossil fuel power transportation, which contributes to an imbalance between energy expenditure and energy consumption. Major roads can sever communities by barring local access, communication and social integration, with implications for social capital. These harms and benefits are unequally distributed. (Woodcock and Aldred 2008: 3)

Indeed, car-related injuries, deaths, and diseases are ultimately disproportionally inflicted by the affluent upon the poor.

While the role of motor vehicles in transmitting infectious disease remains a thinly studied topic, Gewald, Luning, and van Walraven (2009) maintain that the advent of the motor vehicle has been a mixed blessing for Africans. Whereas, on the one hand, it has improved access to inoculation campaigns, primary health care, hospitals, and medical extension work, on the other hand:

> these vehicles have, at the same time, become the main vectors for the spread of disease and the speed of transfer of viruses from forest enclaves to cities, and vice versa, along roads transecting the continent has increased markedly. The most notable has, of course, been the rapid and devastating spread of HIV/AIDS. (Gewald, Luning, and van Walraven 2009: 8)

Air Pollution from Motor Vehicles

Along with industrial pollution, motor vehicles have contributed to air pollution in cities around the world, particularly those in developing countries. Mage and Zali (1992: viii) report: "Exposure to high levels of motor vehicle pollutants occurs essentially in three situations: (a) while inside vehicles (from immediately surrounding traffic); (b) while working in, or walking alongside congested areas, and (c) through residence in urban neighborhoods with high motor vehicle traffic pollution (and or ozone), in urban areas downwind from the city center." Of the estimated 4.4 million tons of human-generated pollutants emitted into the air of Mexico City in 1989, 76 percent were produced by motor vehicles (Freund and Martin 1993: 67). Indeed, Bohren (2009: 374) views the growth of the car culture as an important force in making Mexico City the "most populated and polluted city in the world." In contrast, of the 3.5 million tons of human-created pollutants emitted into the air of Los Angeles – the most polluted city in the United States – in 1985, 63 percent were created by motor vehicles.

Motor vehicles emissions consist of sulfur oxides, nitrogen oxides, carbon monoxide, hydrocarbon, volatile organic compounds, toxic metals, lead particles and particulate matter, carbon dioxide, which contribute to acid rain, climate change, and cardiovascular, pulmonary, and respiratory ailments. Bongardt *et al.* (2013: 38) report that "[e]xposure to such emissions can lead to increased blood pressure, liver/kidney damage, impairment of fertility, comas, convulsions, an, in the worse cases, death." One of the major by-products of gasoline exhaust is benzopyrene, a carcinogenic chemical that is suspended in urban air. Lead constitutes one of the most dangerous pollutants emanating from motor vehicles. According to Rob Bowdon, "When released into the atmosphere, even in relatively small quantities, it can cause lead poisoning in humans. The effects of lead poisoning can include headaches, stomach pains, tremors and in severe cases even death. Lead is especially harmful to young children as it affects the development of the brain" (Bowdon 2004: 16).

Although lead has been gradually removed from motor vehicle fuel in developed countries since the 1970s, it is still present in fuel in many developing countries. The high levels of carbon monoxide coming primarily from motor vehicle emissions in congested areas "can lead to levels of 3% carboxhhemoglobin (COHB) which produce adverse cardiovascular and neurobehavioral effects and seriously aggravate the condition of individuals with ischemic heart disease" (Mage and Zali 1992: vii). Another motor vehicle emission gas, nitrogen dioxide, produces a brownish-red haze and can contribute to respiratory problems, particularly in asthmatics and young children.

The American Lung Association estimated that in 1985 motor vehicle pollution contributed to some 120,000 deaths in the United States (Freund and Martin 1993: 29). Sixty percent of the residents of Calcutta, India, were found to have pollution-related respiratory problems (Freund and Martin 1993: 67). Chakraborty conducted an epidemiological study of the distribution of cancer and respiratory risks from exposure to motor vehicular pollutants in the Tampa Bay Metropolitan Statistical Area (MSA) that found African Americans and Hispanic Americans were at a greater risk than were European Americans in the area, even after controlling for socioeconomic status, because the former tend to reside near major thoroughfares. Furthermore, "densely populated neighbourhoods in the more urbanized parts of the MSA are more likely to experience higher traffic volumes and are thus exposed to greater health risks from vehicular emissions" (Chakraborty 2009: 690). Ironically, people of low socioeconomic status who do not even own cars are among those at greatest risk for traffic-related air pollution, again because they tend to live relatively close to major thoroughfares.

While, as Black (2006: 262) observes, it is difficult to precisely determine how much of air pollution is attributable to motor vehicles, he reports, based on research undertaken in the Los Angeles area: "Transportation sources account for some 60 to 90 percent of all air pollution in Los Angeles County and three adjacent counties," and that in California, "all forms of air pollution cause some nine thousand premature deaths, nine thousand hospitalizations, 1.7 million cases of respiratory illness, 1.3 million school absences, and 2.8 million lost days, according to the state's Air Resources Board."

While developing countries generally have few cars per 1000 population, "each vehicle is likely to emit more air pollutants per mile than the vehicles in developed nations due to a lack of or less stringent emission controls, and/or poor quality," particularly adversely impacting upon informal workers, such as street vendors and hawkers, who are more prevalent in developing countries (Flachsbart 1992: 106). Ray and Lahiri identify three significant sources of air pollution in Indian cities:

- emissions from motor vehicles due to combustion and evaporation of automotive fuels;
- emissions from industrial units and construction of buildings and infrastructure in and around cities; and
- emissions from domestic sources. (Ray and Lahiri 2010: 167)

While it is difficult to determine precisely the health consequences of each of these sources of air pollution, they note that, "of these, the contribution vehicular source is increasing over the years" whereas "emissions from industrial and domestic sources are declining because coal-based industries are increasingly using cleaner fuel, highly polluting industrial units are being shifted outside the city areas, and liquefied petroleum gas (LPG), a relatively cleaner fuel, is replacing coal and biomass as the cooking fuel in urban households" (Ray and Lahiri 2010: 167–168). Ray and Lahiri (2010: 169) report that the number of motor vehicles in India has increased by a factor of 29, from 1.9 million in 1971 to 55.0 million in 2001, over the course of three decades. In a similar vein, the number of motor vehicles in Brazil doubled during the period 1999–2009, reaching some 59 million vehicles in 2009 and resulting in increased levels of atmospheric air pollution through the release of carbon monoxide and other harmful particulates which give rise to various respiratory problems and allergies (Assis and Silva 2012: 2169).

Greenhouse Gas Emissions from Cars

In that they emit greenhouse gases, particularly carbon dioxide and nitrous oxide, as well a black carbon, motor vehicles are a major contributor to climate change and its various health impacts. The Environmental Defense Fund (2007) provides the following sobering statistics on motor vehicles and their contribution to greenhouse gas emissions in the United States alone:

- 30 percent of the world's automobiles are situated in the United States.
- There are 232 million registered vehicles.
- US cars and light trucks traveled 2.7 trillion miles in 2004.
- The average US car consumes 600 gallons of gasoline per year.
    - The average US car emits 12,000 pounds of CO_2 each year (for a total of 2784 trillion pounds of CO_2/year).
    - The United States accounts for 45 percent of the world's automotive CO_2 emissions.

Aside from the amount of CO_2 that cars emit, the CO_2 emissions "required to produce the energy to make the car in the first place as well as the energy to make and maintain the roads and to extract the fuel and raw materials that go into the car's tank, tires, and body" also contribute to emissions (Robbins, Hintz, and Moore 2010: 136).

Transportation emissions account for 29 percent of US greenhouse gas emissions of global greenhouse gas emissions (US Department of Transportation 2010: 2–5). In the case of the US transportation emissions, 58.7 percent come from light duty vehicles (passenger cars, SUVs, and pickup trucks), 19.2 percent from freight trucks, 0.6 percent from buses, 8.2 percent from domestic flights, and 3.4 percent from international flights (US Department of Transportation 2010: 2–7). Ribeiro *et al.* (2007) report that about one-quarter of world energy-related greenhouse gas emissions can be attributed to transportation and nearly 85 percent of transportation-related greenhouse gas emissions is caused by land modes of transportation. NASA (National Aeronautics and Space Administration) reports:

> Cars, buses, and trucks release pollutants and greenhouse gases that promote warming, while emitting few aerosols that counteract it. In contrast, the industrial and power sectors release many of the same gases – with a larger contribution to radiative forcing – but they also emit sulfates and other aerosols that cause cooling by reflecting light and altering clouds. (Quoted in Shahan 2010: 1)

Cities and countries vary greatly in terms of CO_2 emissions. Whereas the transportation-produced CO_2 in the New York metropolitan area totaled 3378 kilograms per capita in 1990, it was 5193 kilograms in the Houston area (Newman and Kenworthy 1999: 120). By contrast, Toronto has 46 percent less CO_2 per capita production than the average US city, largely due to an extensive public transportation system. While the catalytic converter "effectively breaks down the various nitrous oxides that contribute to smog and local air pollution ... it creates nitrous oxide, benign in smog creation but 3000 times more potent than carbon dioxide as a greenhouse gas" (Porter 1999: 81).

Car Accidents in the Form of Injuries and Fatalities

Motor vehicles are a major source of injuries around the world. According to Urry (2007: 118), "[c]rashs are a normal and predictable outcome of the car system although they are typically referred to as 'accidents', aberrations rather than 'normal' features of what Beckmann [2001] terms the 'auto-risk society'." Forman, Watchko, and Sequi-Gomez (2011) refer to deaths and wounds from automobile collisions as an "overlooked epidemic" deserving of medical anthropological study. Indeed, automobiles' very hazardous nature began to be apparent very early in their history. Brian Ladd reports:

> In 1906–07, over 90 percent of the two thousand cars registered in Berlin were involved in accidents. Too often the victims were pedestrians. Most were poor and anonymous, but not all: in 1914 two members of the German parliament were run down on a Berlin street. Already a member of the Prussian parliament had complained that "there is hardly a person in Berlin who has not been on the verge of being run over." (Ladd 2008: 73)

Whereas some 260,000 Britons were killed as a result of World War II between 1939 and the 1945, by 1984 more Britons – 287,000 – had died in road accidents over a 75-year period (Hamer 1987: 141).

Automobile accidents reportedly result in more than 1.24 million deaths per year worldwide and an estimated 20 million to 50 million injuries, of which 91 percent occur in low- and middle-income or developing countries where safety standards are not as developed as in high-income or developed countries (WHO 2013). Road traffic accidents are projected to increase from 1.3 million in 2004 to 2.4 million in 2030 due to the anticipated increase in number of motor vehicles world-wide (Lynch and Smith 2005). Urry (2007: 207) boldly asserts that the "freedom to drive is the freedom to die." In a similar vein, Woodcock and Aldred (2008: 5) propose that the term "motorized violence" is a more appropriate designation for what generally are termed "road accidents" for a phenomenon that in essence has become "socially naturalised" and for which "justice systems in many countries impose minimal penalties upon drivers causing death or serious injury." They also assert that the "threat of violence is embodied through obesity, diabetes, and cardiovascular disease," ailments that in large part are a consequence of diminished active travel that contributes to the obesity epidemic (Woodcock and Aldred 2012: 6). In other words, heavy reliance on cars as a mode of transportation contributes to less exercise through walking and cycling and thus to obesity and various diseases.

Referring to the United States, David Blanke observes:

> The most painful and direct cost of mass automobility is the toll in human lives. Between 1899 and 2003, nearly 3.2 million Americans died as a result of auto accidents. In 2001, motor vehicles were the single leading cause of death for Americans between ages four and thirty-four, and the eighth leading cause of all leading cause of death for all ages. (Blanke 2007: 3)

Indeed, Blanke provides interesting historical evidence comparing the fatality rates for selected infectious diseases with those emanating from motor vehicle accidents between 1910 and 1940 in the United States, as shown in Table 22.1.

While public health measures and medical treatment have, during the course of the early twentieth century, contributed to declining mortality rates from

Table 22.1 Fatality rate for selected infectious diseases and motor vehicle-related accidents, 1910–1940, per 100,000 population in the United States.

Year	*Syphilis*	*Tuberculosis*	*Whooping cough*	*Typhoid*	*Motor vehicle accidents*
1910	13.5	153.8	11.6	22.5	1.8
1920	16.5	113.1	12.5	7.6	10.3
1930	15.7	71.1	4.8	4.8	26.7
1940	14.4	45.9	2.2	1.1	26.2

Source: Adapted from Blanke (2007: 99).

infectious diseases, the growing utilization of motor vehicles during the same time period contributed to a rising mortality rate from their use. An epidemiological study by Sovacool (2010) revealed that in the United States in 2008, 36,710 deaths resulted from automobile fatalities while another 65,638 deaths resulted from particulate-matter pollution, much of it due to motor vehicle exhaust fumes. A German study reported that nearly one in twelve heart attacks are linked to motor vehicle traffic, although the researchers were uncertain whether stress or air pollution was the main cause (Pallarito 2008).

While working-class people are probably more apt to die as the result of automobile accidents, Mitika Brottman (2001: xv) asserts that the "car crash is the archetypal means of *celebrity death*":

> From motorcade and gold-plated Rolls to tour bus and stretch limousine, celebrities are particularly fond of their automobiles. Nothing makes a better tabloid headline than the celebrity car crash, especially if it involves drugs, alcohol, excessive speed, violence, or passengers who shouldn't have been there. Nothing ends a tale of beauty, wealth, and potential better than blood on the tracks.

R.J. Smeed (1949), a British statistician and road-safety expert, concluded (based upon research done in 20 developed countries) that the number of motor fatalities on the road rise up to a certain point, but then the fatality rates begin to drop and even the absolute number of fatalities drops. This is because with rising fatalities governments begin passing regulations that promote safety, such as the requirement to wear seat belts and restrictions on the amount of alcohol that a driver may consume, and so may make drivers more cautious in their road behavior (Vanderbilt 2008: 231). Siem Oppe (1991: 410) maintains that Smeed formulated his generalization at a time when automobile traffic was still on the rise, but that in some developed countries, particularly Japan, the "development of traffic volume is already reaching its point of saturation." Furthermore, it is not clear whether Smeed's generalization applies to developing societies, many of which have just begun to increase in traffic volume as more – and more particularly middle-class people – adopt private cars.

The motor vehicle accident rate appears to be the highest in developing countries, which have more recently acquired large numbers of cars and other motor vehicles compared with developed countries. This is illustrated in Table 22.2,

Table 22.2 Comparison of road fatalities and homicide rates.

	Mortality rate per 100,000 persons		
	Homicide	*Road crash*	*Ratio*
North America	6.5	14.8	2.3
Europe	1.0	11.0	11.0
Africa	22.2	28.3	1.3
Latin America	27.5	16.2	0.6
Southeast Asia	5.8	18.6	3.2
France	0.7	12.1	17.3
Japan	0.6	7.4	12.3
China	1.8	19.0	10.6
Canada	1.4	9.3	6.6
USA	6.9	15.0	2.2
Sweden	1.2	2.6	2.2
Mexico	15.9	11.8	0.7
Russia	21.6	9.7	0.4
Colombia	61.6	24.2	0.4

Source: Adapted from Gilbert and Perl (2010: 215).

which compares road fatalities and homicide rates for selected regions and countries around the world. A simple comparison of the United States and Canada with regard to mortality rates of both homicide and road crashes reveals that the United States on both counts is a more violent society than its neighbor to the north which has gun control laws and apparently somewhat safer drivers and/or driving regulations. Although the United States with its minimal gun control laws is commonly viewed as a violent society, more of this violence is perpetrated by motor vehicles than weapons.

Mortality rates in developing societies tend to exceed those in developed societies. According to Vanderbilt (2008: 231–232), "In China, one sees things … like bicycles traveling on restricted highways, scooter drivers carrying several children without helmets, and drivers stopping on the highway to urinate – but presumably, a number of years down the road, these things will largely be only memories." Hopefully so, but driver safety regulations will not eradicate the pollution and greenhouse gases emitted by motor vehicles in a country with a rapidly growing number of motor vehicles. While China has 2 percent of the world's cars, it has 15 percent of the world's traffic fatalities (Kingsley and Urry 2009). Wang and Dalal (2012) conducted an epidemiological study which examined road traffic injuries in the city of Shanghai. Of 1205 individuals who were involved in a total of 568 traffic accidents, 2 percent died, 43 percent sustained mild injuries, 7 percent received severe injuries, and 48 percent suffered no injuries. Wang and Dalal report: "The majority of the victims were passengers, motorcyclists and pedestrians. Road accidents mainly occurred at night between 19–20 p.m. [*sic* – should be 7–8 p.m.] being peak hours, and most deaths occurred at 3–5 a.m." (Wang and Dalal 2012: 79).

Traffic congestion in large cities in developing countries tends to be worse than it is in developed societies, in part due to poor public transportation systems. In contrast to developed societies where cars constitute the primary private mode of transportation, towns and cities in developing countries teem with motor scooters, motorcycles, and mopeds because they generally are considerably less expensive than cars (Metz 2008). Each car in Bangkok, for example, reportedly spends an average equivalent of 44 days per annum in traffic jams (Banister 2005). Furthermore, excessive lead levels, largely due to more motor vehicles, contribute to 200,000–400,000 cases of hypertension resulting from the stress associated with the frustration of sitting in congestion, and some 400 deaths a year in Bangkok.

Motor vehicles also pose hazards for pedestrians and cyclists. Motor vehicle driving, particularly under congested conditions, also induces stress and contributes to medical complications such as lumbar disk herniation, or motorist's spine, and contributes to a sedentary lifestyle. Truck drivers in particular suffer a high rate of back injuries. City bus drivers around the world experience a great deal of stress, particularly during peak hours. Reportedly, "[m]edical ailments send more than half of them into early retirement" (Vanderbilt 2008: 141).

In developed countries and probably in developing countries, motor vehicle fatalities on rural roads are considerably higher relative to population than in urban areas. In the case of the United States, "rural areas, as defined by traffic safety analysts, contain 23 percent of the national population but witness 56 percent of fatal crashes" (Meyer 2013: 94). Anthropologist Judith Barker (1999) presents a revealing case study of road traffic crashes on Niue Island in the South Pacific. She asserts:

> Most Pacific (e.g., Solomon Islands, Papua New Guinea, Western Samoa) exhibit road traffic crash (RTC) fatality rates consonant with low motorization but high with respect to total number of vehicles in country: that is, the death rate from RTCs is high with respect to the total number of vehicles in the country … By these measures, Niue is a Pacific nation with a high level of motorization and considerable societal costs from RTC. (Barker 1999: 214)

Barker gathered her data over 12 months in 1982–1983 when Niue had a population of some 2500 people, with most Niueans having opted to migrate to New Zealand (where they hold citizenship). In comparison to most Pacific states, Niue had a relatively high material standard of living because more than 80 percent of the population was employed in the service sector or in government or received remittances from expatriate relatives in New Zealand (but less so today as 90 percent of Niueans reside in New Zealand). These factors allowed many Niueans to own motor vehicles of one sort or other. Many young men and women drove motorcycles, which were hazardous to drive due to the fact that the major roads consisted of only two lanes and the road surface often was rough. Young men in particular mixed motorcycle riding with drinking and competition for young women. Barker estimates that nearly half of all RTC on

Niue in 1982–1983 were alcohol related. She observes: "In 1982, some 11.2% of all adult male hospital admissions were the result of RTCs, matching some of the highest RTC admission rates in the world" (Barker 1999: 228). Thus, while we generally associate traffic accidents and fatalities with urban life, the Niuean case indicates that even in a supposedly idyllic remote setting in the South Pacific motor vehicles have had adverse impacts.

Mental Health Consequences of Cars

Automobile transportation discourages social interaction which – at least sometimes – occurs in the process of taking public transport. It leads to social isolation, in that most motorists, especially in advanced capitalist societies, drive alone. As Wolf so aptly observes, "The car society reproduces an elementary phenomenon of the capitalist mode of production: the depersonalization and reification of human relationships. The alienation of the producers (wage earners) in the labour process is reproduced in the organisation of transport" (Wolf 1996: 192).

With the decline of public transportation, especially in the United States, mothers in particular function as chauffeurs for their children as they transport them to various activities in sprawling suburbs. Generations of children in developed societies have internalized car dependence and have been prevented from developing social connections with fellow students who walk to school, often in groups or at least in pairs. In contrast to 1969, when slightly over 40 percent of American children walked or cycled to school, by 2001 only about 15 percent of students were walking to school, a likely factor in increased childhood obesity (US Department of Transportation 2008). Moreover, traffic noise reportedly contributes to both physical and mental health problems, including disrupted sleep patterns, hearing damage, anxiety, and even depression (Rylander 1992; Engler and Mugyenyi 2011). Bongardt *et al.* (2013: 38) report that "[n]oise and vibration from transport contributes to sleep disturbance, which in turn can lead to increased blood pressure and heart attacks."

Low-income people, who already suffer from the injuries of class both materially and psychically, often find themselves further marginalized without access to adequate transportation in cities where an increasing number of jobs are located in outer suburb areas. Kay maintains: "The car culture has thus become an engine of inequality, raising high the barriers of race and class. Transportation that is difficult at best, non-existent at worse, darkens their lives in myriad ways and adds to the financial and social inequality they suffer" (Kay 1997: 38).

Conversely, many cities in developing societies are coming to resemble the majority of North American cities, characterized by a spatial separation between residences and work sites. Furthermore, "Shopping and leisure activities are undertaken in out-of-town areas. High fuel prices limit social exchange and work opportunities; many suburbs are run-down and develop into places of uncoordinated social unrest" (Bongardt *et al.* 2013: 41).

Elderly people with impaired vision often continue to drive because the automobile is necessary to maintaining social connections with friends and family scattered about urban areas. Finally, various studies have indicated that automobile drivers, particularly in conditions where traffic congestion is moderate to light, may exhibit "road rage" because they feel frustrated by their inability to reach their destinations quickly (Smith 2002). As Urry comments, "With 'road rage' emotions of aggression, competition and speed come to the fore although automobility is always polysemic, encouraging one to be careful and civilized *and* to enjoy speed, danger and excitement" (Urry 2007: 128).

Challenges and Alternatives to the Private Car

Referring to the society with the greatest number of cars in the world, Bohren (2009: 377) correctly argues that the car as a "symbol of the American ethos of individualism, personal freedom, and mobility, shaped twentieth-century America." In recognizing the maladaptive nature of the car in the twenty-first century, she asserts that "[c]hange is needed in the human sociocultural practices that have accompanied the adaptation to the car in order to reduce its contribution to global climate change" (Bohren 2009: 378). In his book *Ecotopia*, Ernest Callenbach (1975: 35) describes a fictional place situated in northern California, Oregon, and Washington State that has transcended cars. Aside from the question of whether such a place could exist in the modern world, as Peter Newman (2009: 108) observes, "The biggest challenge in an age of radical resource-efficiency requirements will be a way to build fast rail systems for the scattered car-dependent cities." At the present time, a powerful motor vehicle-highway lobby consisting of the automobile industry, oil companies, trucking companies, and road clubs poses a formidable barrier to the development of effective public transportation, especially in most American urban areas, but also in countries such as Australia. In the case of the United States, as Taebel and Cornehls (1977: 75) observe,

> [C]orporate administrators and technicians, particularly those of the auto industry, have long moved free in and out of the federal government, thus blurring the line between governmental interests and those of private business concerns. Nowhere is this mutuality of interests more clearly understood or more staunchly promoted than among the leaders of the auto corporations themselves.

Despite the existence of massive corporate support for the ongoing use of motor vehicles, there have been some counterhegemonic efforts to resist the automobilization of society by emphasizing the need for people to rely on other forms of transportation. Peter Newman and Christy Newman report:

> recent data from US and Australian cities that car use per person has been going down since 2004, and that public transport has been dramatically increasing. The first assessments of this suggest that something structural is happening, that younger people in particular are coming back into cities rather than choosing car dependence. Indeed car ownership among teenagers in the United States has dropped from fifteen million to ten million. Is it possible that a change in car culture is underway? (Newman and Newman 2012: 360)

Environmentalists and other social activists began to challenge the pollution, health hazards, traffic congestion, urban sprawl, and fragmentation of social life resulting from motor vehicles and highways in the 1960s and 1970s, a period of social ferment on many fronts around the world (Golten and Allen 1977). According to Ladd,

> Anti-freeway activists joined lovers of city life, conservationists (soon to be much more numerous and known as environmentalists), urban politicians, and a growing number of transportation planners in promoting a revival of mass transit during the 1960s. The car, they believed, was reaching the limits of its usefulness, even in the suburbs. (Ladd 2008: 133)

More recently, the SUV (sports utility vehicle), or what in Australia is generally simply called a four-wheel drive, "has become lightning rod for critics of American patterns of consumption and inefficiency" (Vandenheiden 2006: 24). The anti-SUV movement includes groups such as the Friends of the Earth, Earth on Empty, and the Evangelical Environmental Movement. Kay (1997: 286) asserts "that disposing the car from its domination over the earth is a radical, even revolutionary move" and argues that those who participate in this still burgeoning "countercultural rescue movement" must act as "promobility advocates: pro-walking, pro-cycling, pro-transit."

Newman and Kenworthy (1999: 144–189) propose five policies for overcoming automobility dependency: (1) traffic calming in which speed plateaus, neck-downs, and other strategies are employed to slow down traffic in order to make streets safer, particularly for pedestrians, cyclists, shoppers, and residents; (2) the construction of quality transit systems as well as cycling and walking paths; (3) the development of "urban villages" or multimodal centers with mixed, dense land use; (4) growth management to counter the urban sprawl; and (5) and increasing taxes on motor vehicle transportation.

Modern cities have evolved following, in large part, the dictates of capital with its need for manufacturing, financial, commercial, distribution, and communication centers, as well as state bureaucracies. In cities where significant public transportation infrastructure exists but has not been developed and upgraded sufficiently to discourage car use, the growing proliferation of cars also reduces the efficiency of road-based forms of public transportation. In Melbourne, for example, buses and trams are slowed greatly by congestion caused by cars. Fortunately, a few Melbourne trams operate as light-rail conveyances in some motor vehicle-free stretches between the city or central business district and various suburbs.

In addition to having a detrimental impact on the environment, cars are very expensive modes of transportation. Newman and Jennings (2008: 45) report, "Cities that are car dependent spend between 15 and 20 percent of their wealth just on getting around, whereas transit-oriented cities spend only 5 to 8 percent of the wealth on transport." Consequently, Register (2001) maintains that cities should be designed for people, not cars. Furthermore, he proposes the notion of *pedestrian cities* in which people will not need cars and will be able to walk, cycle, or take public transportation to get around. In this light, Groningen, a city of some 170,000 people in the Netherlands, removed the roads in its central business district in 1992 and adopted various policies that promote cycling (Korten 2001: 256). Unfortunately, most of the efforts to make cities greener have benefited the affluent much more than poor and working-class people.

A new urbanism that seeks to make cities more liveable and environmentally sustainable has emerged around the world and has begun to permeate urban planning. Various cities around the world, including Singapore, Hong Kong, Zurich, Copenhagen, Freiburg (Germany), Vancouver, Toronto, and Boston, are encouraging residents to rely on available forms of public transportation, including trains, trams, and buses. While the United States remains a highly car-dependent country, there are some signs that public transit has started to exhibit a modest upswing. Lane reports:

> Conventional bus service has been improved in many cities, and new modes of transit such as express bus and light rail have enhanced this serviceability and image of transit operations. Data from the American Public Transportation Association ... indicates that mass transit has been increasing in aggregate counts of unlinked passenger trips in the United States since the mid-1990s, while VMT [vehicular motor transportation] seems to have slowed to a halt and, since 2007, actually decreased. (Lane 2013: 110)

While most US cities constitute a "sea of auto-dependent sprawl," in contrast to most European cities that have efficient and highly utilized public transit systems, it is important to note that the "few American cities, such as New York, San Francisco, Chicago, or Boston, that have good public transportation systems and accompanying density have per-capita fuel/energy consumption and GHG emission that are not only lower than other parts of the United States, but in some cases lower than those in Europe" (Dutka 2013: 128). In these US cities, people tend to live in more compact living quarters and rely less on cars as a form transportation than in other US cities. Conversely, some European cities, such as Madrid, appear to have embraced some of the suburban sprawl characteristic of most large US cities.

A global movement to make inner cities car free has emerged in recent years. Sustainable transportation would entail many other measures, such as limiting the use of cars as much as possible, making them smaller and more energy efficient, and even banning four-wheel drives except in special circumstances (such as in the outback and rugged mountainous areas) and drastically limiting air travel. Electric cars are often offered as a more environmentally sustainable form of transportation. This might be the case if they derive their power from renewable sources of energy, but not necessarily if they derive their energy from coal-fired power plants. Furthermore, electric cars will not solve congestion problems and the need to build and maintain roads, which requires an enormous amount of concrete, the manufacture of which produces CO_2 emissions. While shifting from cars to public transit – such as intercity and suburban trains and trams or light-rail systems – would serve to diminish greenhouse gas emissions, these modes of transportation are not a panacea. While there is much discussion about high-speed passenger rail substituting for cars or plane travel, according to Todorovich and Burgess 2013: 145), various studies indicate that the "direct benefits from high-speed rail in terms of overall energy and emissions may be modest." Additionally,

> these analyses also neglect the indirect impacts in terms of land-use and city-entering, which may be large and are difficult to measure and attribute. It is our view that these indirect benefits may be more important than any direct reduction in energy utilization as passengers choose high-speed rail over alternative travel modes. (Todorovich and Burgess 2013: 145)

Much thought is being given to the best form of public transportation, such as train, tram, or bus, in urban areas, depending on the situation. Furthermore, there is the issue of connecting small towns and rural areas with cities. In Europe, many villages are relatively well connected to urban areas, but this is not generally the case in North America and Australasia. Thus, given that public transportation is often infrequent or even nonexistent, most people have become dependent on cars to connect them with commercial centers, family, friends, and acquaintances. Diana Young (2001) observes that the motor vehicle appears to be the most significant Western consumer item for the Anangu people in the South Australian outback: in their remote community it has multiple purposes, including providing relatives lifts to shop and work, picking up the mail, and paying bills, and constitutes an essential component of fulfilling social obligations. Likewise, the car or the pickup truck serves a similar purpose for Native Americans living on remote reservations, as any visitor to such communities will observe. Measures will need to be taken to connect rural communities to urban communities and to provide public transportation, perhaps in the form of regularly scheduled mini-buses in rural areas. Furthermore, it would be possible to reinstate the passenger rail services that serviced rural communities in both North America and Australia at a time in the past when their respective populations were considerably less than today.

For a variety of reasons, including poor scheduling or limited routes, buses are frequently underutilized. For example, as a frequent public transit user in Melbourne I have found that while trains and trams are well used, often requiring some passengers traveling at peak hours to stand, buses which serve to connect train and tram lines often are greatly underutilized. According to Paul Mees (2010: 38), "A bus with half a dozen passengers will be no more efficient, in greenhouse terms, than if the passengers travelled in cars at average occupancies." Conversely, various Latin American cities, such as Curitiba in Brazil, have created rapid, low-cost high-frequency bus systems that utilize bus-only lanes and feeder buses that link with the larger bus network (Metz 2008).

Many cities – including Canberra, the Australian national capital – also are increasing provisions for cycling and walking, as forms of active transport. Copenhagen has created bicycle right of ways and has fostered an ethos of respect for cyclists. Xia *et al.* (2013) maintain that active transport has pronounced health benefits. For instance, public transport usage could increase physical activity per day by 8–33 minutes. Regular cycling also has clear-cut health benefits but is an activity which varies considerably between urban areas around the world, ranging from less than 3 percent total of travel trips in some cities in the UK, USA, and Australia to over 30 percent of trips to work or school in the Netherlands and Denmark and 28 percent in Germany. Schiermonnikog, a national park off the northwest coast of the Netherlands, does not allow visitors to drive their private automobiles onto the island, thus meaning that "[c]yclists, local buses, taxis, pedestrians and the occasional car of one of the island's inhabitants share the streets without any problems" (Peters 2006: 128). In terms of countries, Switzerland, admittedly a small country, has the most extensive public transportation system in the world, one that connects urban and rural areas, including steep mountainous terrain. Zurich reintroduced trams "at a time when they were disappearing from many German cities, and new stretches of railway were laid when services were closing down in many other countries" (Welzer 2012: 113). Whereas the average person in EU countries makes 14.7 train trips a year, the average Swiss makes 47 train trips a year.

While cycling trips tend to decline with increasing age, 12 percent of Danes between ages 70 and 74 make such trips on a regular basis. Morabia and his colleagues (2010) conducted an experiment in which 18 people who commuted by car to Queens College in New York shifted to commuting for the next five days by public transportation. They found that "[c]ommuting by public transportation rather than by car increased energy expenditure (+124 kcal/day; P-.001) equivalent to the loss of 1 pound of body fat per 6 weeks" (Morabia *et al.* 2010: 2388). In another study, Maizlish and his colleagues (2013) increased median daily walking and cycling from 4 to 22 minutes, reduced the burden of cardiovascular and diabetes by 14 percent, and decreased greenhouse gas emissions by 14 percent, but ironically increased the traffic injury burden by 39 percent because of inadequate protection from moving motor vehicles. Dutka (2013: 138) reports that while the car-dependent United States as a whole has the highest obesity rate world-wide, Washington, DC, which is characterized by a high use of public transit, biking, and walking trips. exhibits the "third lowest obesity rate in the nation." Ironically, half of all driving trips in the United States are "within a 20-minute bicycle ride (3 miles or less), and a quarter of overall trips are within a 20-minute walk (1 mile or less)" (Mills 2013: 178). Promotion in American schools and media of walking and cycling for short trips has the potential to diminish the obesity epidemic in the United States, not to speak of other countries.

Conclusion

In light of the significant environmental health costs, sustainability challenges, and social damage wrought by private motor vehicles, it is evident that human societies need to move to less impactful means of transportation. In the long run, the contradictions associated with automobility, including those that impact the environment and health, can only be adequately addressed through the creation of an alternative world system, one premised upon meeting human social needs and creating a sustainable environment, including achieving a safe climate. In the short run, however, challenges to the hegemony of the private car, both collective and individual, constitute examples of what Andre Gorz (1973) calls "non-reformist reforms," which challenge existing power relations and pave the way for the more revolutionary changes in the larger society necessary for a more socially just and environmentally sustainable world. An example of a collective non-reformist reform would be the expansion of existing urban public transit systems and intercity passenger train systems, and an example of an individual non-reformist reform would be restricting or even eliminating one's driving. Fortunately, challenges to the hegemony of the private motor vehicle are coming from many quarters, including environmentalists, public transportation advocates, radical cyclists belonging to Critical Mass who ride through busy streets in order to express their opposition to a car-oriented society, progressive politicians, and even academics.

Following Freund and Martin (1993: 60), a political ecological approach to addressing the health consequences of automobility requires "changing the social and physical environment (e.g., building safer highways), producing safer cars, and making many alternative ways of traveling available to drivers." However, even the construction of safer highways and production of safer cars will not be enough because the health benefits will be far greater in moving away from an infrastructure that perpetuates motor vehicle utilization. In this transition, cities will have to be redesigned to accommodate emergency and delivery vehicles and special vehicles to transport disabled people. Furthermore, the development of green cities will have to be part and parcel of achieving social equality and will give ordinary people more options in their choices of where to live.

Despite its many health deficits, the culture of automobility is alive and well and increasingly spreading to developing countries and contributing to the creation of a dystopian world. These developments have prompted Ladd (2008: 179) to observe that the "grave crisis of civilization that some pessimists predict (whether precipitated by fuel shortages, global warming, or the collapse of urban order) may, in fact, if it arrives, be the only way to get people out of their cars – if it actually does so." In the long run, the contradictions associated with automobility, including those associated with the environment and health, can only be adequately addressed through the creation of a democratic ecosocialist world system, a system based upon meeting human social needs and creating a sustainable environmental and safe climate (Baer, Singer, and Susser 2013). Indeed, Herman Rosenfeld (2009), a member of the Canadian Socialist Project and the Greater Toronto Workers' Assembly, advocates a comprehensive socialist approach to the search for solutions to the economic and environmental crises generated by the North American automobile industry. He maintains that the private welfare state needs to be replaced by a set of strengthened, democratically administered, universal public programs; the banking and finance sector should be nationalized and socialized and operated by democratic bodies; auto production and trade should be regulated; and that much of the productive capacity presently used to manufacture cars should be redirected to produce other goods and services, including those presumably related to public transportation. Rosenfeld (2009) also notes that efforts to address climate change and the environmental crisis in general would require a shift to smaller vehicles reliant on nonfossil fuels; a strong emphasis on public transportation; the development of alternative sources of fuel and energy; and the creation of new ways of working and living. He believes that communities must be restructured to defend the right of workers to decent jobs and direct control over the production process.

In capitalist societies, "time is money," and this dictates rapid movement between places. Conversely, in a more leisurely paced world based on ecosocialist principles, people might find slower train travel – although faster than presently exists in most parts of North America and Australia – to be a time to slow down by reading, chatting with fellow passengers, enjoying the passing countryside, reflecting, and even sleeping. A more sustainable form of vacationing or holidaying would entail trips much closer to home – by train or bus, if possible – rather than to distant places either by plane or car. The global economic, ecological, and climate crises that are by the by-products of a capitalist world system require that we reexamine much of what we do in terms of work and leisure, what we eat and consume in general, in what sort of dwellings we reside, and how we move about our planet. The "simpler way" that eco-anarchist Ted Trainer (2011) has been advocating for years in his various writings strikes me as highly compatible with the goals of a healthier democratic ecosocialism delineated in the medical anthropology textbook that Merrill Singer, Ida Susser, and I have coauthored (Baer, Singer, and Susser 2013). From an ecosocialist perspective, Magdoff and Foster argue:

> An economic system that is democratic, reasonably egalitarian, and able to set limits on consumption will undoubtedly mean that people will live at a significantly lower level of consumption than what is sometimes referred to in a wealthy country as the "middle class" lifestyle (which has never been universalized even in those societies). A simpler way of life, although "poorer" in gadgets and ultra-larger luxury homes, can be richer culturally and in reconnecting with other people and nature, with people working the shorter hours needed to provide life's essentials. (Magdoff and Foster 2010: 26)

In addition to rejecting a high level of material consumption in general, a simpler way would also entail disposal or minimization of the use of private motor vehicles and reliance on alternative modes of transportation, including simple walking and cycling. Many of us, particularly those of us in the developed world, would do both humanity and other life forms on the planet a favor if we, as Katarine Alvord (2000) advises, divorce our cars.

REFERENCES

Achoff, N.M. 2011. "A Tale of Two Crises: Labour, Capital and Restructuring in the US Auto Industry." In L. Panitch, G., Albo, and V. Chibber (Eds.), *Socialist Register 2012 – The Crisis and the Left* (pp. 125–148). London: Merlin Press.

Alvord, K. 2000. *Divorce Your Car!: Ending the Love Affair with the Automobile.* Gabriola, BC: New Society Publishers.

Assis, U. Wasconcelos de, and Wasconcelos Silva, G. 2012. "VLT: A Sustainable Solution to Urban Mobility, in Joao Pessoa-BP." *Work*, 41: 2169–2174.

Baer, H.A., Singer, M., and Susser, I. 2013. *Medical Anthropology and the World System: A Critical Perspective*. Westport, CT: Praeger.

Banister, D. 2005. *Unsustainable Transport: City Transport in the New Century*. London: Routledge.

Barbier, E.B. 2010. *A Global Green New Deal: Rethinking the Economic Recovery*. Cambridge: Cambridge University Press.

Barker, J.C. 1999. "Road Warriors: Driving Behaviors on a Polynesian Island." In R.A. Hahn (Ed.), *Anthropology in Public Health: Bridging Differences in Culture and Society*. New York: Oxford University Press.

Beckmann, J. 2001. "*Risky Mobility: The Filtering of Automobility's Unintended Consequences*." Doctoral dissertation, University of Copenhagen.

Black, E. 2006. *Internal Combustion: How Corporations and Governments Addicted the World to Oil and Derailed the Alternatives*. New York: St. Martin's Press.

Blanke, D. 2007. *Hell on Wheels: The Promise and Peril of America's Car Culture, 1900–1940*. Lawrence: University Press of Kansas.

Bohren, L. 2009. "Car Culture and Decision-Making: Choice and Climate Change." In *Anthropology & Climate Change: From Encounters to Actions* (pp. 370–379). Walnut Creek, CA: Left Coast Press.

Bongardt, D., Creutzig, F., Hueging, H., Sakamoto, K., Bakker, S., Gota, S., and Boehler-Baedeker, S. 2013. *Low-Carbon Land Transport: Policy Handbook*. London: Earthscan Routledge.

Bowdon, R. 2004. *Transportation: Our Impact on the Planet*. Lewis, UK: White-Thomson.

Brottman, M. 2001. Introduction. In M. Brottman (Ed.), *Car Crash Culture* (pp. xi–xliii). New York: Palgrave.

Callenbach, E. 1975. *Ecotopia: The Notebooks and Reports of William Weston*. New York: Bantam Books.

Chakraborty, J. 2009. "Automobiles, Air Toxics, and Adverse Health Risks: Environmental Inequities in Tampa Bay, Florida." *Annals of the Association of American Geographers*, 99: 674–697.

Davison, G. 2004. *Car Wars: How the Car Won Our Hearts and Conquered Our Cities*. Sydney: Allen & Unwin.

Dicken, P. 2003. *Global Shift: Reshaping the Global Economic Map in the 21st Century*, 4th ed. New York: Guilford.

Dutka, P. 2013. "Taking the Car Out of the Carbon: Mass Transit and Emission Avoidance." In J.L. Renne and B. Fields (Eds.), *Transport Beyond Oil: Policy Choices for a Multimodal Future* (pp. 126–140). Washington, DC: Island Press.

Engler, Y. and Mugyenyi, B. 2011. *Stop Signs: Cars and Capitalism*. Vancouver, BC: RED Publishing.

Environmental Defense Fund. 2007. "Cars by the Numbers: Statistics on Automobiles and Their Global Warming Contribution." http://sustainablog.org/2008/08/environmental-defense-fund-transportation-by-the-numbers/ (accessed December 16, 2015).

Flachsbart, P.G. 1992. "Human Exposure to Motor Vehicle Air Pollution." In D. Mage and O. Zali (Eds.), *Motor Vehicle Air Pollution: Public Health Impact and Control Measures* (pp. 85–106). Geneva: World Health Organization and Geneva Department of Public Health.

Flink, J.J. 1988. *The Automobile Age*. Cambridge, MA: MIT Press.

Forman, J.L., Watchko, A.Y., and Sequi-Gomez, M. 2011. "Death and Injury from Automobile Collisions: An Overlooked Epidemic." *Medical Anthropology*, 30: 241–246.

Freund, P.S. and Martin, G. 1993. *The Ecology of the Automobile.* Montreal: Black Rose Books.

Gewald, J.-B., Luning, S., and van Walraven, K. 2009. "Motor Vehicles and People in Africa: An Introduction." In J.-B. Gewald, S. Luning, and K. van Walraven (Eds.), *The Speed of Change: Motor Vehicles and People in Africa, 1890–2000* (pp. 1–18). Leiden, The Netherlands: Brill.

Gilbert, R. and Perl, A. 2010. *Transport Revolutions: Moving People and Freight Without Oil.* London: Earthscan.

Golten, T.E. and Allen, B.R. (Eds.) 1977. *The End of the Road: A Citizen's Guide to Transportation Problem Solving.* Washington, DC: National Wildlife Federation.

Gorz, A. 1973. *Socialism and Revolution.* Garden City, NY: Anchor.

Hamer, M. 1987. *Wheels within Wheels: A Study of the Road Lobby.* London: Routledge & Kegan Paul.

Kay, J.H.. 1997. *Asphalt Nation: How the Automobile Took Over America and How We Can Take It Back.* New York: Crown.

Kingsley, D. and Urry, J. 2009. *After the Car.* London: Polity.

Korten, D. 2001. *When Corporations Rule the World*, 2nd ed. San Francisco, CA: Kumerian Press.

Ladd, B. 2008. *Autophobia: Love and Hate in the Automotive Age.* Chicago, IL: University of Chicago Press.

Lane, B. 2013. "Public Transportation as a Solution to Oil Dependence." In J.L. Renne and B. Fields (Eds.), *Transport Beyond Oil: Policy Choices for a Multimodal Future* (pp. 107–125). Washington, DC: Island Press.

Low, N., Gleeson, B., Green, R., and Radovic, D. 2005. *The Greencity: Sustainable Homes, Sustainable Suburbs.* Sydney: University of New South Wales Press.

Lynch, J. and Smith, G.D. 2005. "A Life Course Approach to Chronic Disease Epidemiology." *Annual Review of Public Health*, 26: 1–35.

Lynd, R.S. and Lynd, H.M. 1929. *Middletown: A Study in American Culture.* London: Constable.

Lynd, R.S. and Lynd, H.M. 1937. *Middletown in Transition: A Study in Cultural Conflict.* New York: Harcourt, Brace.

Magdoff, F. and Foster, J.B. 2010. "What Every Environmentalist Needs Know about Capitalism." *Monthly Review*, 61(10): 1–30.

Mage, D. and Zali, O. 1992. "Executive Summary." In D. Mage and O. (Eds.), *Motor Vehicle Air Pollution: Public Health Impact and Control Measures* (pp. vii–ix). Geneva: World Health Organization and Geneva Department of Public Health.

Maizlish, N. et al. 2013. "Health Cobenefits and Transportation-related Reductions in Greenhouse Gas Emissions in the San Francisco Bay Area." *American Journal of Public Health*, published online ahead of print, February 14.

Mees, P. 2010. *Transport for Suburbia: Beyond the Automobile.* London: Earthscan.

Metz, D. 2008. *The Limits to Travel: How Far Will You Go?* London: Earthscan.

Meyer, W.B. 2013. *The Environmental Advantages of Cities: Countering Commonsense Antiurbanism.* Cambridge, MA: MIT Press.

Miller, D. 2001. "Driven Societies." In D. Miller (Ed.), *Car Cultures* (pp. 1–33). Oxford: Berg.

Mills, K. 2013. "Health, Oil-free Transportation: The Role of Walking and Bicycling in Reducing Oil Dependence." In J.L. Renne and B. Fields (Eds.), *Transport Beyond Oil: Policy Choices for a Multimodal Future* (pp. 178–187). Washington, DC: Island Press.

Montgomery, S.L. 2010. *The Powers That Be: Global Energy for the Twenty-First Century and Beyond.* Chicago, IL: University of Chicago Press.

Morabia, A. et al. 2010. "Potential Health Impact of Switching from Car to Public Transportation when Commuting to Work." *American Journal of Public Health*, 100(12): 2388–2391.

Newman, P. 2009. "Transport Opportunities: Towards a Resilient City." In J. O'Brien (Ed.), *Opportunities Beyond Carbon: Looking for a Sustainable World* (pp. 98–115). Melbourne: Melbourne University Press.

Newman, P. and Kenworthy, J. 1999. *Sustainability and Cities: Overcoming Automobile Dependency*. Washington, DC: Island Press.

Newman, P. and Jennings, I. 2008. *Cities as Sustainable Ecosystems: Principles and Practices*. Washington, DC: Island Press.

Newman, P. and Newman, C. 2012. "Car." In P. Beilharz and T. Hogan, (Eds.), *Sociology: Antipodean Perspectives* (pp. 358–363). Sydney: Oxford University Press.

Oppe, S. 1991. "The Development of Traffic and Traffic Safety in Six Developed Societies." *Accident Analysis and Prevention*, 23: 401–412.

Pallarito, K. 2008. "Heavy Traffic Can Be Heart Breaking." MedicineNet.com. http://www.medicinenet.com/script/main/art.asp?articlekey=94566 (accessed December 16, 2015).

Paterson, M. 2007. *Automobile Politics: Ecology and Cultural Political Economy*. Cambridge: Cambridge University Press.

Peters, P.F. 2006. *Time, Innovation and Mobilities: Travel in Technological Cultures*. London: Routledge.

Porter, R.C. 1999. *Economics at the Wheel: The Cost and Drivers*. San Diego, CA: Academic Press.

Ray, M.N. and Lahiri, T. 2010. "Health Effects of Urban Air Pollution in India." In B.R. Gurjar, L.T. Molina, and C.S.P. Ojhas (Eds.), *Air Pollution: Health and Environmental Impacts* (pp. 165–201). Boca Raton, FL: CRC Press.

Register, R. 2001. *Ecocities: Building Cities in Balance with Nature*. Berkeley, CA: Berkeley Hills Books.

Ribeiro, K.S., Kobayashi, S., Beuthe, M., Gasca, J., Greene, D., Lee, D.S., Muromachi, Y., …, and Zhou, P.J. 2007. "Transport and Its Infrastructure." *In Climate Change 2007. Mitigation*. Contribution of Working Group III to the Fourth Assessment Report of the Intergovernmental Panel on Climate Change, edited by B. Metz, O.R. Davidson, P.R. Bosch, R. Dave, L.A. Meyer (pp. 323–385). Cambridge: Cambridge University Press.

Richter, B. 2010. *Beyond Smoke and Mirrors: Climate Change and Energy in the 21st Century*. Cambridge: Cambridge University Press.

Robbins, P., Hintz, J., and Moore, S.A. 2010. *Environment and Society*. Malden, MA: Wiley-Blackwell.

Rosenfeld, H. 2009. "*The North American Auto Industry in Crisis*." Monthly Review, June, pp. 18–36.

Rylander, R. 1992. "Effects on Humans of Environmental Noise Particularly from Road Traffic." In D. Mage and O. Zali, (Eds.), *Motor Vehicle Pollution: Public Health Impact and Control Measures* (pp. 63–83). Geneva: World Health Organization and Geneva Department of Public Health.

Sachs, J. 2008. *Common Wealth: Economics for a Crowded Planet*. New York: Allen Lane.

Schaefer, A, Heywood, J.B., Jacoby, H.D., and Waitz, I.A. 2009. *Transportation in a Climate-Constrained World*. Cambridge, MA: MIT Press.

Shahan, Z. 2010. "NASA Says: Automobiles Largest Net Climate Change Culprit." *Scientific American*, February 24.

Shiva, V. 2008. *Soil Not Oil: Environmental Justice in an Age of Climate Crisis*. Boston, MA: South End Press.

Smeed, R.J. 1949. "Some Statistical Aspects of Road Safety Research." *Journal of the Royal Statistical Society A*, 112(1): 1–34.

Smith, E.O. 2002. *When Culture and Biology Collide: Why We Are Stressed, Depressed, and Self-Obsessed*. New Brunswick, NJ: Rutgers University Press.

Sovacool, B.K. 2010. "A Transition to Plug-in Hybrid Electric Vehicles (phevs): Why Public Health Professionals Must Care." *Journal of Epidemiology and Community Health*, 64: 185–187.

Sperling, D and Gordon, D. 2010. *Two Billion Cars: Driving Toward Sustainability*. New York: Oxford University Press.

Sweezy, P. 1973. "Cars and Cities." *Monthly Review*, 24(11): 1–18.

Taebel, D.A. and Cornehls, J.V. 1977. *The Political Economy of Urban Transportation*. Port Washington, NY: Kennikat Press.

Todorovich, P. and Burgess, E. 2013. "High-speed Rail and Reducing Oil Dependence." In J.L. Renne and B. Fields (Eds.), *Transport Beyond Oil: Policy Choices for a Multimodal Future* (pp. 141–160.) Washington, DC: Island Press.

Trainer, T. 2011. *The Transition to a Sustainable and Just World*. Canterbury, New South Wales: Environbook.

Urry, J. 2004. "The 'System' of Automobility." *Theory, Culture & Society*, 21(4/5): 25–39.

Urry, J. 2007. *Mobilities*. London: Polity.

US Department of Transportation. 2008. "Travel to School: The Distance Factor." *National Household Travel Survey Brief*, January, http://nhts.ornl.gov/briefs/Travel%20To%20School.pdf (accessed December 11, 2015).

US Department of Transportation. 2010. Transportation's Role in Reducing U.S. Greenhouse Gas Emissions, Vol. 1: Synthesis Report. April.

Vanderbilt, T. 2008. *Traffic: Why We Drive the Way We Do (and What It Says about Us)*. London: Penguin.

Vanderheiden, S. 2006. "Assessing the Case against the SUV." *Environmental Politics*, 15: 23–40.

Wang, S.-M. and Dalal, K. 2012. "Road Traffic Injuries in Shanghai, China." *HealthMED*, 6(1): 74–80.

Welzer, H. 2012. *Climate Wars: Why People Will Be Killed in the Twenty-First Century*. Trans. P. Camiller. London: Polity.

WHO (World Health Organization). 2013. *Global Status Report on Road Safety*. Geneva: WHO.

Wolf, W. 1996. *Car Mania: A Critical History of Transport*. Trans. G. Fagan. London: Pluto Press.

Woodcock, J. and Aldred, R. 2008. "Cars, Corporations and Commodities: Consequences for the Social Determinants of Health." *Emerging Themes in Epidemiology*, 5(4): 1–11.

Worstall, T. 2012. "The Story of Henry Ford's $5 a Day Wages: It's Not What You Think." Forbes, March 4, http://www.forbes.com/sites/timworstall/2012/03/04/the-story-of-henry-fords-5-a-day-wages-its-not-what-you-think/ (accessed December 11, 2015).

Xia, T., Zhange, Y., Crabb, S., and Shah, P. 2013. "Cobenefits of Replacing Car Trips with Alternative Transportation: A Review of Evidence and Methodological Issues." *Journal of Environmental and Public Health*, 797312. doi: 10.1155/2013/797312 DOI:10.1155%2F2013%2F797312#pmc_ext .

Young, D. 2001. "The Life and Death of Cars: Private Vehicles on the Pitjantjatjara Lands, South Australia." In D. Miller (Ed.), *Culture Cultures* (pp. 35–57). Oxford: Berg.

CHAPTER 23 Health and the Anthropocene: Mounting Concern about Tick-borne Disease Interactions

Nicola Bulled and Merrill Singer

Linking Ticks, Human Health, and Anthropogenic Change

Environmental health is shaped by a multiplicity of factors, but critical, multidimensional approaches are needed to untangle immediate and ultimate causal factors. Even tiny components of the environment can have huge impacts on human health. Ticks, and the pathogenic species they transmit, relatively miniscule organisms, constitute one of the growing environmental threats faced by our species in a world we are changing, intentionally and unintentionally, domestically and globally, with telling consequence.

The fossil record suggests that ticks, hematophagous or blood-feeding ectoparasites, originated 65–146 million years ago, and hence have been present throughout human history. However, whatever their historic impact on human health at various points in the past, they have begun to play a growing role in human disease in recent years (Fuente 2003). Globally, ticks of varied species transmit a remarkably wide array of pathogens, including bacteria, spirochetes,

A Companion to the Anthropology of Environmental Health, First Edition. Edited by Merrill Singer.

rickettsiae, protozoa, viruses, and nematodes (Mayer 2010). Some tick-borne disease (TBD) outbreaks produce high case-mortality rates or long-term morbidity and considerable human suffering, and have become the sources of great alarm among populations who reside in endemic areas. For example, an outbreak of Brazilian spotted fever (Rocky Mountain spotted fever) in Minas Gerais State, Brazil between the years 2000 and 2008 had a case-fatality rate of 40.2 percent (53 of 132 cases died) (Amâncio *et al.* 2011). Other TBDs, including Crimean-Congo hemorrhagic fever and Kyasanur forest disease, have case-fatality rates that rival or exceed many of the most severe nontick-borne infectious human diseases (Hoogstraal 1979; Swanepoel *et al.* 1988; Nichter 1992; Pattnaik 2006). In parts of Europe and the United States, Lyme disease and other TBDs are the most extensive and medically significant of all vector-borne infectious diseases shaping human health (Randolph 2010; Levi *et al.* 2012).

The expansion in the impact of TBDs on human health over the past three decades is a result both of increases in the recognized number of human diseases transmitted by ticks (Paddock and Telford 2011) and the widening geographic range of the tick vectors. Novel disease-causing tick-borne microorganisms continue to be discovered. In 2014, for example, a new TBD was identified following the death of a man in Bourbon County, Kansas. Dubbed Bourbon virus, it is believed to have only been discovered now because of the introduction of new diagnostic techniques that allow earlier isolation and identification of viral species. While the man had symptoms suggestive of a TBD, including high fever, severe headache, muscle aches, and nausea, his condition was unresponsive to standard TBA treatment. Pathological analysis of his body revealed the previously unknown virus. Bourbon virus has been genetically linked to the family of RNA viruses known as Orthomyxoviruses, a group that includes animal and human influenza viruses (Hawkinson 2014). Similarly in 2012, the Heartland virus was identified and since then eight cases of infection with it have been confirmed in Missouri and Tennessee. With both Bourbon and Heartland virus infection anorexia is a distinctive symptom. Notably, other new studies have linked tick bites to unexpected outcomes, such as the onset of allergic reactions following the ingestion of red meat (Commins and Platt-Mills 2013; Platts-Mills and Commins 2013).

The adaptive versatility of ticks, allowing them to expand into new territories and survive despite changes in climate and environment, has earned them the nickname of the "Swiss Army knife of disease vectors" (Olson and Patz 2011). While the dispersal of TBDs has been uneven geographically – going up in some places and not others – "increases in the scope and magnitude of tick-borne infections have occurred worldwide" (Paddock and Telford 2011: 221). In the closing decades of the twentieth century and opening decades of the twenty-first, tick-borne disease epidemics have broken out in several countries around the world (Paddock and Telford 2011).

Despite the significant global health consequences of TBDs, our knowledge and understanding of them remains incomplete (Goodman, Dennis, and Sonenshine 2005; National Academy of Medicine 2011: 7). One such gap involves an understanding of TBD comorbidity and the health effects of suffering multiple TBDs, which is a notable possibility given that there are at least 12 known TBDs and that ticks can harbor several pathogens (simultaneously and/or in the same locality) (Reis *et al.* 2011). In relation to this, the home ranges of tick species are in flux, resulting in altered disease patterns and mounting geographic overlap. The state of Indiana, for example, home to the dog tick (*Dermacentor variablis*), vector of Rocky Mountain spotted fever, is facing the intrusion of the black-legged tick (*Ixodes scapulris*), vector of Lyme disease and other TBDs, from the north, and the lone star tick (*Amblyomma americanum*), vector of human ehrlichiosis, from the south. In the southern United States, there are rising concerns over the emergence of rickettsioses and the increased recognition of *Rickettsia amblyommii* as a suspected etiological agent of human disease (Apperson *et al.* 2008). The proceedings of a 2008 regional workshop to assess research and outreach needs in integrated management to reduce the incidence of TBDs in the southern United States concluded that concerns regarding increases and alterations in disease patterns and their impact are warranted given "key knowledge gaps that presently block progress towards more effective management of TBDs of public health importance" (Harkin 2009; CDC 2008a, 2008b).

The changing distribution of tick species and of TBDs reflects the significant and ever mounting human impact on the environment globally and regionally, a reflection of changing biopolitics and varied human behavioral patterns across time and space. The magnitude of the climatic and bioenvironmental changes wrought by humans on Earth prompted Dutch atmospheric chemist Paul Crutzen and ecologist Eugene Stoermer (2000) to suggest that the most recent segment of the geographic age of Earth in which we now live, more broadly known as the Holocence – an era that began roughly 12,000 years ago at the end of the last Ice Age – should be retitled the Anthropocene (Age of People). The term, new to geochronology, unites two Greek root words: *anthropo-* meaning "human" and *-cene* meaning "new." Crutzen and Stoermer argue that for the last 150 years, since the rise of the Industrial Revolution, human activities have had the most significant impacts on the biogeological environments of Earth and its climate. The Anthropocene, in short, is a "biogeochemical era of our own making" (Revkin 2008). Already, the human biomass is 100 times greater than any other large animal species that ever lived on Earth, dinosaurs included, according to calculations carried out by Edward O. Wilson (Kolbert 2011).

In the Crutzen/Stoermer view, the start of the Anthropocene can be dated to the latter part of the eighteenth century: analyses of air trapped in polar ice reveal a growing global concentration of carbon dioxide and methane gases as well as other related signs of a durable human imprint registered in the geological record. Human reshaping of the planet took a sizeable jump (known as the Great Acceleration) after World War II, when the human population doubled, going from three billion in 1950 to six billion in 50 years, and the scale of industrial production, consumerism, and globalism accelerated rapidly. These social changes, each dramatic in their own right but collectively sweeping in character, led to the accumulation of gases from coal and other fossil fuel burning as well as other technological developments like cement production for construction, a massive use of nitrogen fertilizers and other agricultural chemicals, and related technology-based expansions in production and the release of the by-products of manufacture into the environment (Steffen, Crutzen, and McNeill 2007). Today, Earth "is being anthroposized at high speed" (Crutzen and Schwägerl 2011). One unintended, indeed unforeseen, consequence has been a spread of tick species to new (climatically and geographically changed and now more hospitable) areas where they encounter growing numbers of humans in close proximity and therefore there is a resulting increase in TBDs of various kinds.

In this chapter, we examine the effects of the Anthropocene in several of its components in increasing the clustering and syndemic interaction of tick-borne diseases and their consequent mounting contribution to the global disease burden. The chapter is organized into two major sections suggested by the syndemics model of disease. The first addresses tick behavior, tick-mediated infections, and the pathways of tick-mediated syndemics as influenced by human altered physical environments. The second, framed by syndemics theory, engages a range of social and anthropogenic environmental factors at both the regional and global levels that are contributing to increased human–tick encounters. In this chapter we seek to promote an enhanced understanding of the global health importance of TBD syndemics within the anthropology of infectious diseases, given their worldwide distribution, growing importance in global health, and capacity to reveal fundamental ways in which human beings are "not simply agents of environmental change … [but] are also objects of that change" (Nash 2006: 7).

The Application of the Syndemics Model to TBDs

The analytic concept *syndemics* was introduced into medical anthropology in the early 1990s and has since diffused across a number of health-related disciplines, especially epidemiology but also nursing and medicine. A syndemic is the clustering of two or more adversely interacting diseases or other health conditions within a population (Singer 2009: xiii), a biological process that is promoted by social and environmental conditions. The related theoretical frameworks of critical medical anthropology and political ecology that gave rise to a focus on syndemics view increased disease burdens within specific populations as involving biosocial and political economic processes operating at several levels. In the case of infectious diseases transmitted by ticks, these perspectives strive to understand the nature of the relationship between what historian William McNeill (1976; also see Scheper-Hughes 1992) refers to as *microparasitism* (the pathogens and vectors, and their animal hosts that are the proximate causes of infection) and *macroparasitism* (structures of human social relations and resulting social conditions), which are seen as the distal but fundamental causes of infectious disease.

In all of the syndemics studied to date, involving both infectious and noninfectious diseases (e.g., Singer and Clair 2003; Freudenberg *et al.* 2006; Littleton and Park 2009; Singer 2011; Mendenhall 2012; Marshall 2013; Marsters 2013;

Bulled, Singer, and Dillingham 2014), social inequality, marginality, poverty, and other forms of political and economic oppression have played a critical role in both promoting the clustering of diseases and facilitating disease interactions. In the case of the SAVA syndemic, for example, either poverty and/or social discrimination promote drug use, which, in turn, facilitates the spread of HIV disease and interpersonal violence or, alternatively, discrimination and violence promote drug abuse and HIV risk (Singer 1996; Stall *et al.* 2003). Syndemics, in other words, have been closely linked with adverse social conditions and the physical and emotional traumas of marginalization and structural violence. More broadly, the biosocial link that underlies syndemics involves social structures and processes that shape the environments of human occupation and create exposures and vulnerabilities in populations.

As TBDs are especially common in wealthy suburban residential areas and outdoor recreation spaces, the application of syndemic theory may raise questions. As has been argued in the syndemics literature (Singer 2009), conditions of social injustice or structural violence typically play central roles, not only in causing the concentration of diseases in specific populations that allows interaction, but also in the weakening of bodies, the degrading of immune capacity, the failing of social support systems, and the disruption and inaccessibility of health care, factors that facilitate the development of syndemic interactions. It is argued here, however, that subaltern status and oppressive conditions are not the only direct and indirect political and economic factors that can promote the kinds of deleterious disease interface characteristic of syndemics. In addition, human reshaping of environments can also create the kinds of exposures and vulnerabilities that lead to novel disease–disease and other biosocial interactions, a pattern referred to as *ecosyndemics*. In the case of tick-borne syndemics, three broad ecosocial factors warrant particular attention: global climate change as a consequence of human action; collapses and disruptions of social systems as a result of political rearrangements and economic inequalities and their impacts on human behaviors and standards of living; and the development of residential and activity class boundaries and distinctions. These elements are discussed in relation to how they influence tick activities, tick exposures, and tick-borne disease interactions.

Ticks in Human Health

We begin our examination with a focus on ticks as vectors of disease, including factors in TBD clustering and indications of syndemic interaction. The assessment of ticks, their life cycles, feeding habits, hosts, and associated diseases offered here is limited, but aims to provide a foundation for a clearer understanding of the growing impact of TBDs in the Anthropocene.

Ticks and Tick-borne Disease

Ticks have been implicated as a source of disease for over a hundred years. Ricketts (1991) recognized the role of ticks as vectors of human disease in 1909 with his descriptions of the transmission of Rocky Mountain spotted fever by the wood tick (*D. andersoni*). In 1912, a Swedish dermatologist first reported characteristic skin lesions near Ixodes tick bites, which were termed erythema chronicum migrans (Afzelius 1921). In the 1920s, Garin and Bujadoux described a patient with meningoencephalitis, painful sensory radiculitis, and erythema migrans following a tick bite, and postulated the symptoms were due to a spirochetal infection. By the mid-1930s, neurologic manifestations of Ixodes tick bites were recognized (see Bransfield 2007). About a decade later, Bannwarth (1941, 1944) described several cases of chronic lymphocytic meningitis and polyradiculoneuritis, some of which were accompanied by red skin lesions. In 1975, an important milestone in tick-related health research was achieved when Steere and colleagues isolated cases of erythema migrans rashes in a group of children with juvenile rheumatoid arthritis living in Old Lyme, Connecticut (Steere, Malawista, Hardin *et al.* 1977; Steere, Malawista, Snydman *et al.* 1977). Seven years later, a spirochete (*Borrelia burgdorferi*) was isolated from Ixodes ticks by Burgdorfer and colleagues (Burgdorfer *et al.* 1982). This is currently accepted as the pathogen that is the immediate cause of Lyme disease. Globally, tens of thousands of new Lyme disease cases are reported every year, distributed across several continents.

During the last 30 years, the recognized number of distinct and epidemiologically important TBDs globally has increased considerably. Table 23.1 shows the estimated distribution of TBDs by geographic region. Since 1984, over 10 newly recognized spotted fever rickettsioses have been identified (Raoult, Broqui, and Roux 1996; Parola, Paddock, and Raoult 2005; Paddock *et al.* 2008; Shapiro *et al.* 2010). By 1998, the United States had a total of five recognized tick-borne infections, with Lyme disease, human anaplasmosis, and human monocytic ehrlichiosis being added to the list of previously identified TBDs (Rocky Mountain spotted fever and tularemia). Incidence rates of Lyme disease in the United States have ranged from a low of 19,804 in 2004 to a high of 29,959 (plus an additional 8000 probable cases) in 2009 (CDC 2012). Between 2000 and 2008, the annual reported incidence of Rocky Mountain spotted fever in the United States also increased dramatically, from 1.7 to 9.4 cases per million persons (Openshaw *et al.* 2010). From 2000 to 2007, the incidence of human anaplosmosis and human monocytic ehrlichiosis also grew, going from 0.80 to 3.0, and 1.4 to 3.0 cases per million population, respectively (Dahlgren *et al.* 2011).

TBD epidemics have been reported globally including tick-borne encephalitis in Central and Eastern Europe (Randolph 2008), Kyasanur forest disease in Karnataka state in India (Pattnaik 2006), Crimean-Congo hemorrhagic fever in northern Turkey and the southwestern regions of the Russian Federation (Maltezou *et al.* 2010), and Rocky Mountain spotted fever in Arizona and Baja California (Bustamente Moreno and Pon Méndez 2010; McQuiston *et al.* 2010). Several recent reports have indicated a widening spread of specific tick species in geographic areas that were not considered previously infected with these ticks, suggesting an expansion of possible TBD epidemic and endemic areas (e.g., Jaaskelainen *et al.* 2006; Nijhof *et al.* 2007; Gray *et al.* 2009; Jaenson *et al.* 2012).

Table 23.1 Incidence and geographic distribution of major tick-mediated infections by level of severity.

Disease severity	*Geographic region*
Very common (>10,000 new cases each year)	
Lyme disease	Holarctic
Common (1000–10,000 new cases each year)	
Tick-borne encephalitis	Holarctic
Tick-borne relapsing fever	Tropical Africa Western United States
Tick-borne spotted fever group rickettsioses	Global
Ehrlichiosis and anaplasmosis	Global
Masters' disease	Eastern, central, and south-central United States
Crimean-Congo hemorrhagic fever	Southern Europe Western and central Russian Federation North Asia Africa
Moderately common (100–1000 new cases each year)	
Colorado tick fever and other other coltivirus infections	Western United States Central Europe
Babesiosis	Northeastern United States Europe
Omsk hemorrhagic fever	Eastern Russia and Siberia
Tick-borne tularemia	Eastern and central United States Central Europe Russian Federation
Kyasanur forest disease	Karnataka and adjacent states in India Saudi Arabia
Rare (sporadic cases)	
Powassan/deer tick virus	Canada Northeastern and north-central United States

Source: Modified from Paddock and Telford (2011).

The distribution of tick-borne pathogens and risk of disease is believed to be closely linked with the life cycle of the tick, feeding habits, and the distribution and density of small-mammal species that act as pathogen reservoirs, a patterning increasingly influenced by human activity. For example, while *I. scapularis* ticks are widely distributed in the northeast and upper Midwest, the lack of human Lyme disease in the southern United States may be the result of distinct feeding habits in this region. In the south, immature *I. scapularis* ticks commonly feed on lizards (Oliver, Cummins, and Joiner 1993), which are incompetent as reservoir species for *B. bugdorferi* (Spielman *et al.* 1985; Lane and Quistad 1998), and adult ticks do not commonly bite humans.

Both host availability and climate influence the geographic placement of ticks and related TBDs. Table 23.2 presents a list of the major tick species, their geographic distribution, hosts, and the diseases they transmit to hosts. At least

Table 23.2 Major tick species, their primary hosts and associated diseases.

Tick species	*Geographic distribution*	*Host*	*Transmitted diseases*
Soft-bodied (Argasidae)			
Argas			
A. persicus	World	Poultry	Fowl spirochaetosis
A. reflexus	Europe	Pigeons, humans	*B. anserine*
A. polonicus		Pigeons	
Ornithodoros			
O. coriaceus	North America	Domesticated pigs	African swine fever virus (ASFV)
O. turicata			
O. puertoricensis			
O. parkeri	Sub-Saharan Africa	Domesticated pigs, warthogs	
O. savignyi	Europe		
O. moubata		Domesticated pigs	
O. erraticus			
O. marocanus			
Hard-bodied (Ixodidae)			
Ixodes			
I. scapularis (deer tick), *I. pacificus*	North America	Lizards, birds, mammals, humans	Lyme borreliosis, TBE, anaplasmosis, babesiosis, *B. microti*, *B. venatorum*, tularaemia, louping ill virus
I. ricinus	Europe, western Asia, North Africa	Lizards, birds, mammals, humans	
I. persulcatus	Northeastern Europe, North Asia	Lizards, birds, mammals, humans	
Haemaphysalis			
Ha. punctata	Europe, Asia	Livestock, cattle, horses, deer, cats, dogs, hares	Tick-borne encephalitis virus (TBEV), Bhanja virus, Crimean-Congo hemorrhagic fever virus (CCHFV), *Listeria monocytogenes*, *Brucella abortus*, tick paralysis
Ha. concinna	North Africa		
Ha. inermis			
Ha. sulcata			
Hyalomma			
Hy. Marginatum	Southern Europe, central and southern Asia, Middle East, most of Africa	Livestock, camels, rodents	CCHFV, Babesia caballi, *T. equi*, tropical theileriosis, *C. burnetii*
Hy. Anatolicum			
Hy. Excavatum			
Hy. Scupense			

Table 23.2 (*Continued*)

Tick species	*Geographic distribution*	*Host*	*Transmitted diseases*
Amblyomma			
Am. variegtum *Am. hebraeum* *Am. variegatum*	Sub-Saharan Africa, Caribbean	Livestock, humans	African tick bite fever
Am. maculatum *Am. americanum* (lone-star tick)	North America		Rocky Mountain spotted fever, tularaemia, Q fever, Lyme disease, tick paralysis, monocytic ehrlichiosis
Rhipicephalus			
Rh. Bursa *Rh. Anulatus* *Rh. Microplus* (cattle tick)	Africa	Domestic pigs and ruminants, horses, carnivorous mammals, rodents	Mediterranean spotted fever and other rickettsioses, Q fever, monocytic ehrlichiosis, canine babesiosis, hepatozoonosis, Nairobi sheep disease, East coast fever
Rh. Sanguineus (brown dog tick)	Worldwide	Domestic dog, wild and domestic animals, humans	
Dermacentor			
D. marginatus *D. reticulates*	Europe	Large mammals, dogs, hares, hedgehogs	*C. burnetii*, *R. conori*, *R. slovaca*, *R. sibirica sibirica*, *F. tularensis*
D. reticulates	Europe, Central Asia	Humans, rodents, birds	Babesia ssp., *T. equi*, *A. ovis*, *R. conori*, *R. raoultii*, *F. tularensis*, *D. reticulates*
D. andersoni (wood tick)	North America	Large domestic and wild mammals, cattle, horses, sheep, goats, pigs, small rodents, birds	Rocky Mountain spotted fever

Source: Modified from Farkas *et al.* (2012).

900 tick species exist today, inhabiting every continent (Dennis and Piesman 2005; Keirans and Durden 2005; Benoit *et al.* 2007). Morphologically, ticks are grouped into three families: (1) Nutalliellidae, with a single species; (2) Argasidae, soft-bodied organisms, with 186 species; and (3) Ixodidae, hard-bodied organisms, with 720 species (Barker and Murrell 2008). From the standpoint of human disease, hard-bodied ticks are of primary importance and the focus of our discussion below. Hard-bodied ticks are found throughout the world, with some species expanding their current ranges. For example, *I. scapularis* may have spread (or re-spread) to much of the eastern United States following reforestation and the subsequent resurgence of white-tailed deer populations within the past 30 years (Spielman *et al.* 1985; Healy 1989; Wilson 1998).

Among the hard-bodied ticks (Ixodidae), the largest genus, Ixodes, is widely distributed throughout the world. Ixodes ticks serve as primary vectors for Lyme disease, ehrlichiosis (human anaplasmosis and human monocytic erhlichiosis), babesiosis, tularemia, and tick-borne encephalopathy (Keirans and Durden 2005). In many regions Ixodes ticks are found beyond the areas of endeminicity of the pathogens they are known to transmit. A review of distribution records in the United States demonstrated the established existence of *I. scapularis* (deer tick) or *I. pacificus* (Western blacklegged tick) in 34 percent of counties, including much of the country east of the Great Plains and the West Coast (Dennis *et al.* 1998). However, only a limited proportion of US counties (2%) accounted for the majority (78%) of nationally reported Lyme disease cases in 1995 (CDC 1996). In 2011, 96 percent of Lyme disease cases were reported from just 13 US states, primarily those in the northeast and upper Midwest (CDC 2013). As mentioned above, this pattern is not well understood, but is believed to be related to tick habitat needs, feeding behavior, presence of tick predators, and host–reservoir dynamics.

The biological and behavioral characteristics of ticks make them ideal vectors of human pathogenic agents. Their hardiness and longevity enables them to survive long periods of unfavorable environmental conditions. The tick life cycle involves four stages of development – egg, larva, nymph, and adult – which generally take two years to process through. During each phase after hatching, the tick takes one blood meal. They feed slowly, allowing sufficient time for pathogen acquisition and transmission. For hard-bodied ticks, and males of some species, each blood meal typically requires 3–5 days to complete. One or more pathogens can be ingested from an infected host during an individual feeding session by tick larvae, nymphs, and adults. Additional pathogens also can be acquired during subsequent blood meals at later life stage. Moreover, transstadial transmission of disease pathogens, which allows pathogen interaction among agents acquired during two different feedings, perhaps on different hosts, occurs across the ticks' life stages. Finally, transovarial transmission (the transfer of pathogens to succeeding generations) allows nymphs and adult ticks of some species to emerge from molting having already been infected during a previous developmental stage and able to transmit disease to susceptible hosts. There are, therefore, multiple opportunities through which ticks can acquire a single or multiple interacting pathogens: during a single blood meal or passed along through subsequent life stages.

The wide range of possible hosts and the tendency to feed on several hosts throughout their life cycle further promotes opportunities for ticks to both acquire and transmit pathogens. Host preferences vary among species, at different developmental stages, seasonally, and relative to climate and environmental conditions (Dennis and Piesman 2005). Some tick species are host-specific, while others feed on several species. Host-specific ticks are less likely to bite humans. Species with nonspecific feeding habits draw blood from both animal species (reservoirs for tick-borne pathogens) and humans (to whom they transmit disease). Despite nonspecific feeding patterns, ticks tend to parasitize only a small fraction of the host population. Ticks stimulate other ticks to feed on the same host by releasing tick-specific pheromones, a phenomenon known as overdispersal (Norval, Hancock, and Yunker 1989). Overdispersal may promote disease coinfections in hosts as each additional tick bite increases the likelihood of coinfection in the host and pathogen transmission among cofeeding ticks (Ginsberg 2008). Finally, ticks have a high reproductive potential, ensuring large population densities and a high frequency of host–vector contact. All of these factors are potential facilitators of tick-borne disease syndemics.

Tick-borne Disease Syndemics

A growing number of studies indicate the occurrence of adverse syndemic interactions among tick-borne pathogens/diseases (Singer and Bulled in press). Existing research further suggests that there are pathogen-to-pathogen interactions in ticks involving both microbial facilitation and interspecies competition (Gotelli 2000). Facilitative and syncretic microbial interactions could increase human health risk if the acquisition, establishment, virulence, or maintenance of an infection caused by one microbial agent is promoted by another pathogen or multidirectional enhancements occur for two or more comorbid diseases (Ginsberg 2008). Conversely, competitive interactions might prevent the establishment or maintenance of multiple pathogens, decreasing the likelihood of coinfections arising from a single tick bite. Such competitive interactions suggest the possible occurrence of a countersyndemic (Singer 2009), where coinfection and interaction lowers the burden of disease in a population below the sum effects of the individual diseases agents involved (Ginsburg 2008; Singer 2010). In these cases, the presence of one pathogen and its biochemical or other actions within a host control or limit the virulence or reproduction of a coterminous pathogen. For example, countersyndemic outcomes have been described for malaria and certain helminth infections (Boel *et al.* 2010; Singer 2010). The continuum of potential interactions among comorbid diseases is displayed in Figure 23.1.

Table 23.3 presents an overview of major tick-borne diseases (both human and animal) showing the lowest and the highest observed pathogen prevalence,

Countersyndemics	Comorbid noninteraction or uneventful interaction	Syndemics

Figure 23.1 Continuum of consequential interactions among comorbid diseases.

Table 23.3 Prevalence of coinfections of Ixodes ticks with *Borrelia burgdorferi*, *Anaplasma phagocytophilum*, and *Babesia microti/divergens* by species and geographic region. *Indicates range over multiple studies.

Region	*Ixodes species*	*% Infection with:*			*% Coinfection with:*	
		B. burgdorferi	*A. phagocytophilum*	*B. microti or B. divergens*	*Two pathogens*	*Three pathogens*
North America						
California*	*I. pacificus*	3.8–6.7	3.2–7.2		1.0–1.3	
Maine	*I. scapularis*	22.3	2.8	0.8	1.0	0
Massachusetts*	*I. scapularis*	27.3–36.0	11.0	9.0–23.0	4.0–10.9	0
New Jersey*	*I. scapularis*	33.6–50.3	1.0–17.0	5.0–8.4	2.7–10	0
New York*	*I. scapularis*	26.0–66.0	21–53		5–28.2	5
Pennsylvania	*I. scapularis*	41.2	17.8		3.5	
Wisconsin	*I. scapularis*	11.2	7.9		2.2	
Europe						
Bulgaria	*I. ricinus*	32.1	33.9		13.4	
France	*I. ricinus*	3.3		20.6	2.1	1
Germany*	*I. ricinus*	8.6–37.4	0–6.5		0–9.1	1.3
Italy	*I. ricinus*	19.8	24.4		8.1	
The Netherlands	*I. ricinus*	13.0	28.9		3.3	
Poland*	*I. ricinus*	5.5–42.1	0-29.7	4.2–19.3	0–5.4	0–1.1
Russia	*I. persulcatus*	29.9	1.0	0.9	1.2	0
Slovakia	*I. ricinus*	45.0	20.0		7.5	
Switzerland	*I. ricinus*	40.0	0		0	
Asia						
China*	*I. persulcatus*	13.6–37.3	3.0–4.9		0.5	

Source: Modified from Swanson *et al.* (2006).

including coinfection, from separate studies from around the world. As indicated in Table 23.3, numerous studies have identified the prevalence of multiple human pathogens among ticks. These studies generally involve a small number of collected ticks and the identification of pathogens using polymerase chain reaction (PCR) analysis of DNA (see e.g., Schouls *et al.* 1999; Adelson *et al.* 2004; Swanson *et al.* 2006). Methods of tick collection, sample size, specimen preparation, DNA extraction, and selection of primers vary among studies. While it is difficult to compare findings given the considerable differences in methodology, collectively this research confirms that ticks can host multiple pathogen species at a single time.

The highest prevalence of dually infected ticks appears in regions where Lyme disease is endemic. In North America, evidence of coinfection with multiple disease-causing human pathogens has been demonstrated for Ixodes ticks samples from select geographic areas of California, Wisconsin, and the northeast (Swanson *et al.* 2006; Tokarz *et al.* 2010; Schulze *et al.* 2013). In Europe, the highest reported prevalence of dual pathogens in *I. ricinus* ticks occurs in Bulgaria (13%) (Christova *et al.* 2001), Poland (2–11%) (Stanczak *et al.* 2004; Siński 2009), and Germany (2.8–9.1%) (Schicht, Schnieder, and Strube 2012). Dual infections in *I. persulcatus* ticks have been reported in Russia and China (Alekseev, Semenov, and Dubinina 2003; Cao *et al.* 2003). Investigations of a cluster of spotted fever rickettsiosis cases in a family of three in southern France revealed that *Rh. sanguineus* ticks found in the family's home were coinfected with *Ri. conorii* and *Ri. massiliae* (Renvoisé *et al.* 2012).

Triple coinfection does not appear common among Ixodes ticks, although a limited number of studies have detected coinfection with three pathogens in *I. ricinus* ticks. A study conducted in France found the simultaneous presence of *Bartonella spp.*, *B. burgdorferi*, and *Babesia spp.* in *I. ricinus* ticks in which 7.6 percent of the ticks registered dual infection, and 1 percent were characterized by triple coinfection (Halos *et al.* 2005). A study of ticks in the northern German city of Hanover revealed triple infection with *Rickettsia spp.*, *B. burgdorferi*, and *A. phagocytophilum* in 1.3 percent of *I. ricinus* ticks (Schicht *et al.* 2012). A study in northwestern Poland similarly demonstrated a 1 percent prevalence of a triple infection of *B. burgdorferi*, *B. microti*, and *A. phagocytophilum* (Skotarczak *et al.* 2003). Examination of *I. persulcatus* in Russia identified triple infection with two tick species of Borrelia and Ehrlichia (Dubinina and Alekseev 1999). In addition, there is evidence of *Babesia microti* infection in multi-infected *I. persulcatus* ticks in Russia (Alekseev *et al.* 2003). Examination of *I. scapularis* ticks in New York detected polymicrobial infections in 30 percent of tested specimens and triple infections in 5 percent (Tokarz *et al.* 2010). Quadruple infection in ticks has been described in China (Sun *et al.* 2007) and New York (Tokarz *et al.* 2010).

Additionally, in coinfected ticks, pathogens can "potentially influence transmission of other pathogens in the tick by virtue of their effects on tick behavior and survival" (Ginsburg 2008: 30). Ginsberg (2008) suggests that patterns of pathogens in ticks include numerous cases of higher or lower levels of coinfection than would be expected due to chance alone. While the majority of these cases can be explained on the basis of vertebrate host associations, some studies demonstrate antagonistic interactions, while others potential mutualisms between pathogens within ticks. Transmission dynamics, though, likely depend on initial conditions. For example, when the number of tick bites is relatively low (i.e., human bites), changes of pathogen prevalence in ticks are predicted to have a commensurate effect on pathogen transmission. By contrast, when the number of tick bites is high (i.e., animal bites), changes in pathogen prevalence in ticks have relatively little effect on levels of disease transmission (Ginsberg 2008). In other words, an important issue in tick-borne syndemic research concerns the impacts of dual or multi-infection on the tick vector and not just impacts on the human host (Adelson *et al.* 2004; Václav *et al.* 2011).

Given the coexistence of two or more disease agents in Ixodes ticks, humans may become coinfected with several tick-borne pathogens with a single bite (Swanson *et al.* 2006). However, the risk of human coinfection differs by geographic location and depends on the density of ticks, tick hosts, and prevalence of pathogens within the local tick populations. The epidemiology and natural history of TBD coinfections in humans are not fully understood, with most data collected from studies of patients with suspected or confirmed Lyme disease from limited regions of endemicity within the United States and Europe (Swanson *et al.* 2006). Cross-sectional seroprevalence studies have found biomarkers of dual infection in 9–26 percent of patients with a tick-borne infection (Belongia 2002). However, these studies often fail to distinguish between simultaneous and sequential infections, an issue that may impact disease interaction. Nevertheless, a growing number of studies offer molecular and serological evidence of coinfection, adding to seroprevalence data. For example, serologic confirmation of concurrent babesiosis and Lyme disease was first reported in 1983 in an asplenic male from Shelter Island, New York (Grunwaldt, Barbour, and Benach 1983).

Animal models provide some clues as to the immunologic effects and pathogenesis of coinfections. For instance, a time-series study of field voles with recently cleared *A. phagocytophilum* infections showed increased susceptibility to *B. microti*; those with ongoing infections showed decreased susceptibility (Telfer *et al.* 2010). Conversely, new and chronic *B. microti* infections increased the risk of *A. phagocytophilum* infection. These observations suggest that immune-mediated mechanisms might not only increase susceptibility to additional infections, they may also prolong and increase the severity of infections. These animal models suggest that infection with *B. microti* and *A. phagocytophilum* explain variation in infection risk in addition to factors related to exposure risk, host condition, and tick modulation of the host immune response (Wikel, Ramachandra, and Bergman 1994).

Animal models also provide evidence that simultaneous infection with *B. burgdorferi* and *A. phagocytophilum* increases disease severity. Coinfection appears to modulate the host immune response increasing pathogen loads in blood and tissues, resulting in more severe Lyme disease associated arthritis than Lyme disease alone (Zeidner *et al.* 2000; Thomas *et al.* 2001; Holden *et al.* 2005). Coinfection increases the number of CD4 cells and drives cytokine release toward a T helper 1 lymphocyte response with increases in interleukin-4 and decreases in interleukin-2 levels (Zeidner *et al.* 2000, mouse model). A study in mice found increased levels of both pathogens resulting in diminished interleukin-12, gamma interferon, and tumor necrosis factor, and increased levels of interleukin-6 increasing pathogen burden (Thomas *et al.* 2001). In a similar study, spirochete numbers were found to increase in some mouse tissues while Anaplasma numbers remained constant (Holden *et al.* 2005). Antibody responses decreased for *A. phagocytophilum*, but not for *B. burgdorferi*. Researchers postulated that *A. phagocytophilum* appears to functionally impair neutrophils, limiting the host's immune system to mount an early defense against *B. burgdorferi* infection.

Coinfection with *B. burgdorferi* and *B. microti* has also been demonstrated to have immunologic effects in animal models (Moro *et al.* 2002). However, the results are not consistent across studies. While one study suggests increases in T helper 1 lymphocytes (Moro *et al.* 2002), another suggests that in dual infections *B. burgdorferi* and *B. microti* appear to follow an independent course (Coleman *et al.* 2005).

No human experiments have been conducted to assess the immunologic effects of coinfections. Consequently, uncertainties regarding implications of these animal models for the pathogenesis and immunologic effects of coinfections in humans remain. However, as Thomas and colleagues (2001: 3369) observed, research on TBD coinfection in mice

> may have implications for human Lyme disease … In particular, the increase in joint inflammation in the murine studies suggests that coinfection may influence the severity of human Lyme arthritis. Epidemiological studies have previously suggested that concurrent Lyme disease and babesiosis … result in increased Lyme disease severity, providing one clinically relevant example of this phenomenon … Our present murine studies now suggest that *B. burgdorferi* and the agent of HGE [human granulocytic ehrlichiosis] transmission and pathogenicity increase during coinfection, and this may be one explanation [for] differences in the severity of disease.

In humans, case reports of coinfections with tick-borne encephalitis (TBE) virus and *B. burgdorferi* globally are limited as the dual infection likely only occurs in a restricted number of geographic regions. These case reports and retrospective studies do not provide adequate evidence to suggest that multiple disease agents interact leading to more severe disease than a single infection of either TBE or *B. burgdorferi* alone. However, 12 patients in Slovakia with diagnosed dual infections were found to suffer increased rates of the central nervous system disorder neuroborreliosis (Lyme disease), possibly due to prior damage to the blood/brain barrier caused by the TBE virus (Cimperman *et al.* 1998).

The incidence of parasite coinfection appears highest among persons with Lyme disease. In areas where Lyme disease is endemic, between 4 and 45 percent of Lyme disease patients are coinfected with either human anaplasmosis or babesisiosis (Swanson *et al.* 2006). In the eastern United States, Lyme disease and babesiosis account for about 80 percent of coinfections (Belongia 2002). Numerous studies have confirmed that seroprevalence of *B. microti* is highest among persons with prior or active Lyme disease (Benach *et al.* 1985; Krause *et al.* 1991; Magnarelli *et al.* 1998; Wang *et al.* 2000). In a retrospective study in New York and Massachusetts from 1978 to 1984, approximately 50 percent of patients with confirmed babesiosis had antibodies to *B. burgdorferi* (Benach *et al.* 1985). Moreover, a study on Nantucket Island found that over a quarter of residents testing seropositive for Lyme disease also had serologic evidence of prior *B. microti* infection (Wang *et al.* 2000). Coinfection with Lyme disease and human anaplasmosis (*A. phagocytophilum*) is also relatively common. In the Great Lakes and northeastern US.regions, seropositivity for both pathogens has been found to range from less than 3 percent to 26 percent of tested patients (Swanson *et al.* 2006).

In Europe, evidence of potential coinfection with Lyme disease and human anaplasmosis pathogens has been demonstrated in Belgium, the Czech Republic, Germany, Italy, Norway, Poland, Slovenia, Switzerland, Sweden, and the United Kingdom (see Swanson *et al.* 2006). Coinfection prevalence of Lyme disease and human anaplasmosis in European countries ranges from 3.2 percent to 17 percent. In Central Europe and large parts of Asia, Lyme disease and TBE are the most important diseases transmitted by ticks. Coinfection with TBE virus and Borelia bacteria in humans is rare, but has been documented in a limited number of cases since 1986 (Kristoferitsch, Stanek, and Kunz 1986; Bröker 2012).

The single most important risk factor for babesial infection is a diagnosis of Lyme disease (*Boriella burgdorferi*) (Hu *et al.* 1996). According to an important study conducted on Block Island by Krause and colleagues (1996), ticks that carry both Lyme disease and babesiosis are very likely (as much as 95% of the time) to make the individuals they bite sick immediately and for a long period of time. Altered, more diverse and intensified symptoms, including fever, chills, sweats, headaches, fatigue, and nausea, are some of the experiential effects of interactions among TBDs in humans (Krause *et al.* 1996; Krause *et al.* 2002). Persistent symptoms appear to be more associated with coinfection than with isolated infections, with over half of Lyme disease/babesiosis coinfected patients reporting at least one symptom (mostly extreme fatigue) for over 3 months (Krause *et al.* 1996). Similarly, patients diagnosed with both Lyme disease and human anaplasmosis report more severe or persistent symptoms with significantly more chills, sweats, headaches, joint pain, and sore throats than patients with Lyme disease alone (Pancholi *et al.* 1995; Nadelman *et al.* 1997; Krause *et al.* 2002). In addition, anemia, decrease in blood platelets, and influenza-like symptoms, which are uncommon among patients with Lyme disease alone, occur during coinfection with Babesia or human anaplosmosis (Belongia *et al.* 1999; Krause *et al.* 2002; Gutman, Kotton, and Kratz 2003). In a study of patients with chronic fatigue syndrome, the severity of systemic signs and symptoms was directly related to the presence of multiple chronic coinfections, including babesiosis (Nicolson, Gan, and Haier 2005).

Longer duration of illness as a consequence of concurrent infection may often be attributable either to the direct effects of disease interaction or to a delay in diagnosis and treatment. This is a particular problem for Lyme disease/babesiosis coinfections. Babesiosis alone is not easily recognizable, as symptoms are either absent or low-grade. In addition, initial symptoms of Lyme disease can overlap with symptoms of babesiosis and disguise dual infection. Unless physicians are alerted to look for both, a diagnosis with Lyme disease can mask the presence of babesiosis. In a study in Wisconsin and Minnesota, of 60 patients diagnosed with Lyme disease, babesiosis, or human granulocytic ehrlichiosis that involved immunoserologic testing for coinfection, researchers found that suffering multiple TBDs explained "the variable manifestations" and unexpected clinical responses sometimes seen in patients diagnosed with one of these diseases (Mitchell, Reed, and Hofkes 1996: 726). Persons coinfected with *B. burgdoferi* and *B. microti*, however, do not appear to be at heightened risk for Lyme disease complications or greater disease burden (Krause *et al.* 1996; Krause *et al.* 2002; Wang *et al.* 2000). In a study of patients with Lyme disease, coinfected patients experienced more symptoms and more persistent episodes of disease than patients with babesial infection alone (Krause *et al.* 1996). Specifically, coinfected patients experienced fatigue, headache, sweats, chills, anorexia, emotional lability, nausea, conjunctivitis, and splenomegaly more frequently than those with Lyme disease alone. Half of coinfected patients were symptomatic for three months or longer as compared to four percent of patients with Lyme disease alone. These conflicting accounts suggest a greater understanding of pathogenic interactions and their impact on the immune system is needed.

There are limited data suggesting that dual infection between *A. phagocytophilum* and *B. microti* occurs (Swanson *et al.* 2006). Studies of rates of prevalence of dual infection in the United States have found ranges between less than 2 percent and less than 7 percent of patients suffering tick-borne illnesses (Magnarelli *et al.* 1998; Krause *et al.* 2002). Evidence of triple coinfection is rarer still, with the majority of studies reporting none to 2 percent of patients with a tick-associated illness demonstrating laboratory evidence of infection with *B. microti*, *A. phagocytophilum*, and *B. burgdorferi* (Swanson *et al.* 2006). In a study conducted in New England between 1997 and 2000, of 310 patients presenting during the summer months with Lyme-related conditions, 24 percent had dual coinfections and 3 percent had triple coinfections (Lyme disease, human anaplasmosis, and babesiosis) (Krause *et al.* 2002). Over half of the patients were diagnosed with acute Lyme disease; 45 percent of these patients demonstrated simultaneous evidence of coinfection with *B. microti* or *A. phagocytophilum*, suggesting that interactions between pathogens may affect the severity of disease.

As with other infections, it appears that the simultaneous coinfection or sequential active infection with human tick-borne pathogens has the potential to modulate transmission dynamics and influence disease severity (Singer 2010). These syndemic impacts, including alternations in the efficiency of transmission (Thompson *et al.* 2001), complicate disease diagnosis due to symptom overlap

(Belongia *et al.* 1999), confuse treatment protocols, and increase disease duration and severity. While there remain many unanswered questions about the pathogenesis, immunological effects, and clinical expressions of tick-borne syndemic interactions, and despite the shortcomings of existing studies, regional differences in species, and challenges of variability in the sociodemographic and prior health status of patients, it is now clear that some human studies and several animal models "demonstrate a potential for immunologic synergy and more severe outcomes" in polyinfected individuals (Belongia 2002: 271).

Syndemic Understanding of Increasing TBD Burden

The existing and growing potential for TBD syndemics is driven by environmental changes that, in turn, are promoted by political and economic forces operating at both global and regional scales. At the global level, anthropogenic climate change is emerging as an increasingly impactful force in the spread of TBDs.

Climate Change and Tick Distribution and Exposure

Assessing the impact of climate change on TBD syndemics is complicated by the diverse ecology and multistage/multihost developmental processes of tick vectors (Randolph 2004; Estrada-Peña 2009). Moreover, debates have developed among researchers about the significance of climate change in shifting patterns of TBDs distribution globally (e.g., Sumilo *et al.* 2007; Randoph 2009). Nevertheless, given what is known of tick biology and observations of their shifting geographic distributions, it appears that climate change is influencing tick behavior in such a way that TBDs are occurring in areas where previously they had not.

Tick activity (i.e., feeding patterns and even speed of maturation) differs dramatically by season and life stage. For example, hard-bodied larval *I. scapularis* ticks often show peaks in activity during early and late summer. However, if they did not feed in the fall, the adult *I. scapularis* ticks are active again during the spring months (Wilson and Spielman 1985; Neitzel, Jarnefeld, and Sjogren 1993). By contrast, the nymph stage is most active from late spring through mid-summer. As climates change, the activity levels of ticks similarly accommodate, with more activity in warmer climates and less in colder areas. As such, higher environmental temperatures increase development rates among tick larvae, nymphs, and adults, although the effect is mediated by stage of development, location, tick species, and host accessibility. Conversely, in cold temperatures and low humidity host seeking (referred to as questing) is known to decrease (Randolph 2004), and overall tick survival is reduced (Schulze *et al.* 2013). Thus, as Olson and Patz (2011: 272) have observed, "the literature consistently shows warmer temperatures increase tick abundance." Early spring and milder winters, climate change expressions seen in areas like the northeastern United States and Sweden, among other areas, are positively associated with tick abundance and Lyme disease incidence (Lindgren, Tälleklint, and Polfeldt 2000).

Research by Solveig Jore (2013; Jore *et al.* 2011) in Norway affirms this association beyond Lyme disease. Jore examined the relationship between the distribution of infected ticks and microclimatic conditions at seven data collection points along the southern coast of Norway. She reports that the degree of humidity in the air has a substantial impact on the ability of the tick-borne encephalitis virus to survive and reproduce in the *I. ricinus* tick and then be transmitted to humans in areas of the country where they previously were absent. As a result of climate change, as well as access to host animals like deer and changing human and livestock demography (e.g., the number of farms with ruminants), Jore found that the *I. ricinus* tick has been spreading over an ever wider geographic range and at higher altitudes in mountainous regions in Norway. The studies found that it is critical to examine local seasonal fluctuations in climatic variables, including seasonal weather extremes, and not just average climate changes as climatic conditions can have a decisive impact on the capacity of ticks to spread disease. Other research supports Jore's view that "Areas that are likely to experience increased or prolonged seasonal tick activity are … those located at the current extremes of the current range of distribution, areas where climate change will be felt most acutely" (Munderloh and Kurtti 2011: A148).

As ticks alter or expand their geographic areas, they not only overlap with other tick and host species, but also with other TBDs. Consequently, multiple pathogen infected ticks are becoming both more common and more likely. Coinfections are likely to become more common as tick species expand their geographic ranges, and with changing climate conditions also alter their activity levels. Consequently, previously uncommon occurrences of coinfections may become the norm.

While there are numerous confounding factors, from land cover and land use patterns to regional vicissitudes in the configurations of impacts of a warming planet, anthropogenic climate change appears to be contributing to the wider distribution of ticks and to increased exposure to tick-borne disease in humans. The engine driving climate change is a global industrial economy fed by the burning of fossil fuels and the voluminous emission of greenhouse gases like carbon dioxide (which has now reached 400 parts per million in the atmosphere, the highest level since the Pleistocene). Central to this economy is a focus on profit making, continual economic expansion, and a treadmill of production and consumption (Baer and Singer 2014). This productivist ethic underlying the capitalist worldview exerts "a negative impact on the environment on a much broader and profounder scale than any previous social system" (Baer and Singer 2009: 23). Of note in this regard is what Faber (2009) refers to as the "polluter-industrial complex," the group of powerful multinational energy, agribusiness, mining, manufacturing, and utility corporations that produce great quantities of greenhouse gases and vigorously oppose environmental regulations.

One of the core practices of the capitalism world economic system that puts it on a collision course with environmental sustainability is the transformation of everything in the natural world into commodities for sale on the market. Commodification, a process Chernomas and Hudson (2009) refer to as the privatization of nature and the empowerment of the capitalist class at the expense of the collective good, organizes the capitalist orientation toward the environment, beginning with the demarcation of elements of nature that can be assigned a market value. Under capitalism, stresses Foster (1994), the "cash nexus" has emerged as the preeminent link between human beings and the world they inhabit. With the development of the capitalist division of nature, components of the natural world are reduced to a common denominator – their exchange value. The hazardous waste products of manufacturing and other economic activities are not treated as costs but as externalities that can be released at will into the environment. This orientation toward the natural world drives greenhouse gas emission in the midst of growing scientific knowledge about the human contribution to global warming and resulting environmental changes, like those that facilitate the spread of tick species.

Global warming, in short, is not simply anthropogenic in origin; it has been driven historically by a particular mode of production and its associated patterns of consumption, including production in ostensive noncapitalist countries like China, which has been dubbed "the world factory" because it is the largest exporter in the world and because it produces numerous commodities for consumption by the West; environmental degradation; and hierarchical social organization. Climate change is therefore of relevance to the understanding of the biosocial aspects of TBD syndemics for two interrelated reasons. On the "bio" side, climate change has the potential to impact tick vectors and the microbial agents they transmit in ways that increase vector activity, host–vector interactions, and disease overlaps thereby promoting syndemic interaction and health consequence. On the "social" side, the dominant force in contemporary climate change is human activity, including socioeconomic interest-driven commitment to fossil fuel use and resulting greenhouse gas emissions.

Regional Ecosocial Changes and Increasing Tick Exposures

Unlike climate change, which more significantly influences the activities of ticks, changing ecosocial interactions alter human behaviors that influence exposure to disease-bearing tick vectors. In what follows we offer two regional examples of altered ecosocial interactions that increase human exposures to ticks and consequently disease risk. The first falls more obviously in line with syndemic theory, as we suggest that growing socioeconomic inequalities, particularly in the former Soviet countries of Latvia, Lithuania, and Estonia, has pushed impoverished communities to engage in subsistence agriculture and food foraging in forested areas inhabited by ticks. The second example explores the rise of Lyme and related TBD in the US context where it is not marginalized communities who suffer the greatest disease burden, but rather relatively affluent suburban residents or individuals with sufficient income to engage in outdoor recreation. While this example does not fit into the classic definition of a syndemic whereby social injustice or structural violence influences the clustering of disease, as suggested earlier, we expand the syndemic perspective here and argue that environmental mediated class boundaries and distinctions have perpetuated deleterious disease outcomes in certain (though not necessarily marginalized) social groups.

Collapse and Disruptions of Ecosocial Systems

Socially, the capitalist world system is organized around stark social inequalities including the unequal distribution of produced wealth. The considerable inequality that exists within the capitalist world system among nations, regions of the world, social classes, and ethnic/cultural groups is not a consequence of chance or a weakness of the system; it is, as Stevenson (1982: 368) indicates, "the direct and inevitable result of the 'normal' operations of the capitalist mode-of-production." While the extent of this disparity has varied over time, it has consistently grown wider since the 1970s, a period generally characterized by stagnated worker salaries, rising productivity, growing corporate class wealth, and significant increases in greenhouse gas emissions. These are not independent elements but are intrinsically linked as features of the modern capitalist accumulation process.

In addition to human/environment changes at the global scale, various sociopolitical disruptions of the environment at the regional scale also reflect the importance of social factors in the emergence of TBD syndemics. This can be seen in the case of the Baltic countries of Latvia, Lithuania, and Estonia. During the early 1990s, this region experienced explosive increases in the incidence of TBDs of as much as 22 percent in one year, especially in tick-borne encephalitis and Lyme disease. The same pattern occurred in Poland.

One explanation that has been proposed for this significant and sudden jump in tick-associated disease burden is the collapse of the Soviet Union, the return of capitalism, and the resulting social breakdowns in post-Soviet and Eastern bloc states that followed (Randolph 2001). In the Baltic nations, in the years after the collapse, there was a steep economic decline with an average loss in GDP (gross domestic product) of 53 percent (Scott 2000). During this period, there was a measurable rise in social inequality, involving increases in wealth for some and enhanced poverty for many others. As a result, people began turning to small-scale farming as a means of survival (Oxenstierna 2002). There was also an increase in the gathering of wild foods to supplement people's diets. Foraging is most common during the spring and summer months when ticks are most active. Public surveys conducted in all three of the Baltic nations revealed that the "Collection of nature products for self-consumption (berries, mushrooms, hunting, fishing) is more common among households in Estonia and Lithuania (51% and 49%) than in Latvia (35%). In Latvia and Lithuania such activities are most common in the lower income groups" (Aasland and Tyldum 2000: 8). Part and parcel of this shift was the movement of people and their domesticated animals and livestock into tick-infected fields and forested areas.

Very few people in studies of Baltic households report that they are prosperous. Half of the households in Latvia and Lithuania and one-third in Estonia identified as either poor or on the verge of poverty (Aasland and Tyldum 2000: 10). The need to rely on foraged foods and the raising of livestock on family and forest plots is especially great in households with unemployed adults as only a small minority of the unemployed in these countries receive unemployment benefits. More broadly, the governments of Baltic countries have been unable to provide social safety nets for the poor (Scott 2000). At the same time, among the minority that grew wealthier with the introduction of market economies, there was an uptake in outdoor recreational and leisure activities, as practiced in the West, that led more affluent people to increased entry into tick-populated areas.

The unexpected increase in TBDs following the breakup of the Soviet Union suggests the importance of both anthropogenic ecological disruptions and social upheavals generally as human drivers of TBD distribution and incidence. For example, the impacts of war on human/environment relations have been identified as a factor in some TBD outbreaks (Paddock and Telford 2011: 228):

> During World War II, following the occupation of Crimea by Axis forces, there was abandonment of agricultural lands and diminished hunting of European hares (*Lepus europaeus*) because of combat activities. When Soviet troops reoccupied the Crimean steppes in 1944, pastures and farms had become overgrown by weeds, and hares had become extremely abundant and were heavily infected with Hyalomma ticks. The combination of these factors is believed to have contributed to an epidemic of CCHF [Crimean-Congo hemorrhagic fever] among military personnel during 1944–1945, involving especially signalmen and surveyors, who frequented brushy areas.

In Turkey, the jump in diagnosed cases of CCHF from 20 in 2002/2003 to 1300 in 2008 has also been attributed to human involvement in habitat fragmentation. Important in this regard are farming activities that penetrate forests and leave standing small patches of plant undergrowth between cultivated areas and nearby urban spaces. "This unprecedented increase in habitat fragmentation," stress Estrada-Pena and colleagues (2010: 1201), "leads to greater contact between tick and reservoir, and therefore to a virus amplification cycle."

These examples affirm the role played by changing relations among people and people's relations with the environment in the ultimate origins of TBDs as threats to human health. Such cases reveal the degree to which social relations find expression in human relations with the environment as well as the unexpected health consequences of environmental disruption.

Class Boundaries and Distinctions

The third aspect of the social dimension of TBD syndemics involves the class relations that comprise a historic cultural construction of and interaction with nature that has helped to place more affluent people and ticks in increasingly closer encounters. It has been noted that "one of the most characteristic features of modern society is that the level of environmental concern is high and generalized" (Berenguer, Corraliza, and Martin 2005: 128). Contemporary environmentalism in Western culture can be viewed as involving such diverse components as conservationism, outdoor recreation and adventurism, Earth Day celebrations, organic farming, vegetarianism, back-to-nature ideologies, and green politics. These activities are generally practiced by the higher socioeconomic classes, who can afford higher priced organic produce and have time for vacation or recreation in the outdoors. Indeed, environmentalism in the United States began as a campaign by members of the privileged classes to preserve areas for their personal outdoor amusement and recreation. Affirming the elite nature of these groups, Silverira (2004: 504) points out, was the fact that "Working class individuals and ethnic minorities were generally excluded from conservation and preservation organizations."

The roots of American environmentalism lie in the work and legacy of John Muir, long honored as a ranking member of the pantheon of conservation prophets (Gore 1995; National Park Service, 2003). Muir's achievement was the popularization of a profoundly novel attitude in American land use that developed into a new American, and increasingly global, environmentalist narrative. Central to this narrative, as embodied in the activities of the Sierra Club, which Muir cofounded, is the dual idea that nature should be both protected and enjoyed. Thus, Muir successfully lobbied Congress to establish sites like Yosemite National Park where people could "experience nature" through participatory engagement but in which nature could be protected from the harms of prolonged human presence.

Despite his love of nature, Muir's perceptions of the indigenous peoples he encountered in untamed spaces were consistent with the cultural biases of the Christian perceptions of his day. Though he recognized Native Americans' comparatively low impact on the environment and their mistreatment by the dominant society, Muir believed that the indigenous people of Yosemite were not capable of appreciating the beauty of the environment and thus they had "no right place in the landscape" (Muir 1894: 93). Such attitudes, which Jacoby (2006: 3) refers to as part of the "elite discourse about conservation," rationalized the removal of Native Americans from the areas that were designated as national parks and made available through an array of exclusionary practices for recreational use and transcendent experience by the dominant population. "Whites only" signs were a common feature in the early years of the national park system (Dowie 2009).

Such attitudes have persisted into contemporary times. Public opinion research consistently shows a higher level of support for conservation in communities of color, yet it was noted in a Pyramid Communications assessment for the Nature Conservancy (2005) that, "Historically, white middle and upper class Americans have constituted the strongest base for conservation and environmental organizations." The Center for Diversity and the Environment (2007) reports that 33 percent of environmental organizations in the United States lack a person of color on their respective staffs, while only 9 percent of the board members of natural resource organizations are people of color in a country in which over one-third of the population reports a nonwhite ethnic identity.

A central element of the environmentalist narrative within and beyond environmental organizations is a negative appraisal of urban life. As bluntly phrased by Tarlock (1993: 466), "Environmentalists see cities as parasites on the landscape. This view reflects an Arcadian preference which [contrasts] the unnatural city to the natural environment." This depiction of the city, fully expressed in Odum's (1983) classic environmental text, *Basic Ecology*, had a discernible impact on post-World War II urban planning and residential aspiration. Inherent in white retreat from the city and the whole suburbanization drive during this era was a threefold view that: (a) urban areas were crowded, congested, confining, and polluted; (b) the city was populated by menacing poor people and people of color (who were also seen in some cases as a form of pollution); and (c) suburbia offered open spaces where people could live closer to "nature." A cultural theme that resonated with this population shift was the idea that "the good life" consisted of owning a home of one's own surrounded by a grassy yard and trees at some distance from the urban workplace.

The creation of affluent suburbs involved residential invasions of environments like broad-leaf forest woodlands, where wildlife tick hosts, including deer and mice, were abundant. Residential penetrations of this sort have contributed to habitat fragmentation involving the creation of small forest patches broken by housing developments, an environmental pattern that has been found to be associated with higher densities of infected nymphal ticks in some studies (Allan, Keesing, and Ostfeld 2003). This pattern occurred in the United States but also, on a more modest scale, in Europe (Randolph 2001). In addition to residential relocation, fueled by the broader environmentalist alignment, there has emerged a cultural emphasis on outdoor recreation that has further increased the opportunities for human/tick exposure. In the United States in 2011, for example, The Outdoor Foundation (2012: 1–2) reports that "Nearly half of the … population enjoyed various forms of outdoor recreation. That equates to a total of 141.1 million Americans, millions more participants than 2010 … In 2011, outdoor participants made 11.5 billion outings – that is 1.4 billion more outings than 2010."

This discussion suggests that the social origins of TBD syndemics involve diverse factors, including both global and regional social dynamics, shifting population/environment relationships, geographically expressed class and ethnic relationships, changing environments, and resulting fluctuations in the ecologies of tick vectors. In addition to having complex social structural causes, as discussed below, TBD syndemics reflect intricate patterns of species interaction at several levels (humans and other host animals, tick vectors, and tick-borne pathogens) within varying local contingencies.

Conclusion

In this chapter, we argue that the existence of tick-borne disease syndemics are of global health significance because of the continued identification of tick-borne pathogens, increasing geographic diffusion of ticks caused by ongoing anthropogenic environmental/climate changes, and shifting human/environment interaction patterns based on political economic factors. We conceptualize these environmental/climate changes as expressions of the rise of the Anthropocene as a geochronical era characterized by a global political economy that enables and facilitates an ever-growing human capacity to restructure planetary conditions. In the Anthropocene, a warming planet and other environmental shifts at regional or local scales favor tick dispersal coincident with human occupation and reoccupation of local tick and reservoir species-populated environments. Increases in the incidence of TBDs and the pace of discovery of new tick-borne pathogens has eclipsed the epidemiological, social economic, and political ecological assessment of factors driving the spread of ticks, the diseases they transmit, and the role of adverse disease interactions in elevating the tick-mediated disease burden of human communities. Although "medical anthropologists have paid insufficient attention to zoonotic diseases, recognition of the importance of human/animal relationships is growing because many public health problems have their ultimate origins in animal bodies" (Singer *et al.* 2011: 164). As has been demonstrated with non-ecoparasitic vectors, the adverse health impacts of zoonotic diseases are significantly enhanced through syndemic interaction (Rock *et al.* 2009). In the same fashion, tick-borne syndemics, the nature and distribution of which are just beginning to emerge from existing research around the world, represent a potentially significant and growing set of environmental threats to human health and well-being.

Assessing and effectively responding to these threats is dependent on focused research informed by syndemic theory. Such investigation requires close attention to an array of factors, most or all of which are of anthropological concern, including changes in human impacts on biodiversity as well as environmental and climatic systems, the political economic factors driving these changes in local, regional, or broader settings, the shifting climate/environment forces pushing in-migrating tick and animal host species, the pathogens brought together in coinfections, the biological and other pathways of pathogen and TBD interactions, the health consequences of various kinds of tick-borne pathogen interactions, and the preparedness of health care systems to diagnose and treat tick-borne polyinfection. In this chapter, we have addressed the syndemic consequences of polyinfection caused by pathogen-bearing tick species. This synergy, however, comprises only one aspect of TBD syndemic interaction. Future research should investigate the interaction of TBDs and non-TBD infectious and noninfectious diseases, as these too may constitute significant sources of environmental disease burden on human populations.

REFERENCES

Aasland, A. and Tyldum, G. 2000. *Better or Worse: Living Conditions Developments in Estonia, Latvia and Lithuania 1994–1999.* Oslo: Fafo Institute for Applied Social Science.

Adelson, M.E., Rao, R.-V.S., Tilton, R.C., Cabets, K., Eskow, E., Fein, L., Occi, J.L., and Mordechai, E, 2004. "Prevalence of *Borrelia burgdorferi*, *Bartonella* spp., *Babesia microti*, and *Anaplasma phagocytophila* in *Ixodes scapularis* Ticks Collected in Northern New Jersey." *Journal of Clinical Microbiology*, 42(6): 2799–2801.

Afzelius, A. 1921. *"Erythema chronicum migrans." Acta Dermato-Venereologica (Stockholm)*, 2: 120–125.

Alekseev, A.N., Semenov, A.V., and Dubinina, H.V. 2003. "Evidence of *Babesia microti* Infection in Multi-infected *Ixodes persulcatus* Ticks in Russia." *Experimental and Applied Acarology*, 29: 345–353.

Allan, B.F., Keesing, F., and Ostfeld, R.S. 2003. "Effect of Forest Fragmentation on Lyme Disease Risk." *Conservation Biology*, 171: 267–272.

Amâncio, F.F., Amorim, V.D., Chamone, T.O., de Brito, M.G., Calic, S.B., Leite, A.C., Fraga, G.L., Ferraz, M.L. 2011. ["Epidemiological Characteristics of Brazilian Spotted Fever in Minas Gerais State, Brazil, 2000–2008."] *Cadernos de Saude Publica*, 27(10): 1969–1976. [Article in Portuguese]

Apperson, C.S., Engber, B., Nicholson, W.L., Mead, D.G., Engel, J., Yabsley, M.J., Dail, K., Johnson, J., and Watson, D.W. 2008. "Tick-borne Diseases in North Carolina: Is "*Rickettsia amblyommii*" a Possible Cause of *rickettsiosis* Reported as Rocky Mountain Spotted Fever?" *Vector Borne Zoonotic Diseases*, 8: 597–606.

Baer, H. and Singer, M. 2009. *Global Warming and the Political Ecology of Health.* Walnut Creek, CA: Left Coast Press.

Baer, H. and Singer, M. 2014. *The Anthropology of Climate Change: Can We Make a Difference?* London: Earthscan, Routledge.

Bannwarth, A. 1941. "Chronische lymphocytäre Meningitis, entzündliche Polyneuritis und 'Rheumatismus'. Ein beitrag zum Problem 'Allergie und Nervensystem'." *Archiv für Psychiatrie und Nervenkrankheiten*, 113: 284–376.

Bannwarth, A. 1944. "Zur Klinik und Pathogenese der 'chronischen lymphocytären Meningitis'. *Archiv für Psychiatrie und Nervenkrankheiten*, 117: 161–185, 682–716.

Barker, S.C. and Murrell, A. 2008. "Systematics and Evolution of Ticks with a List of Valid Genus and Species Names." In A.S. Bowman and P.A. Nuttall (Eds.), *Ticks: Biology, Disease and Control* (pp. 1–39). Cambridge: Cambridge University Press.

Belongia, E.A. 2002. "Epidemiology and Impact of Coinfections Acquired from Ixodes Ticks." *Vector-Borne and Zoonotic Diseases*, 2(4): 265–273.

Belongia, E.A., Reed, K.D., Mitchell, P.D., Chyou, P.-H., Mueller-Rizner, N., Finkel, M.F., and Schriefer, M.E. 1999. "Clinical and Epidemiological Features of Early Lyme Disease and Human Granulocytic Ehrlichiosis in Wisconsin." *Clinical Infectious Diseases*, 29: 1472–1477.

Benach, J.L., Coleman, J.L., Habicht, G.S., MacDonald, A., Grunwaldt, E., and Giron, J.A. 1985. "Serological Evidence For Simultaneous Occurrences of Lyme Disease and *Babesiosis*." *Journal of Infectious Diseases*, 152: 473–477.

Benoit, J.B., Yoder, J.A., Lopez-Martinez, G., Elnitsky, M.A., Lee Jr., R.E., and Denlinger, D.L. 2007. "Habitat Requirements of the Seabird Tick, *Ixodes Uriae* (Acari: Ixodidae), from the Antarctic Peninsula in Relation to Water Balance Characteristics of Eggs, Nonfed and Engorged Stages." *Journal of Comparative Physiology B: Biochemical, Systemic, and Environmental Physiology*, 177(2): 205–215.

Berenguer, J., Corraliza, J.A., and Martin, R. 2005. "Rural–Urban Differences in Environmental Concern, Attitudes, and Actions." *European Journal of Psychological Assessment*, 21(2): 128–138.

Boel, M., Carrara, V., Rijken, M., Proux, S., Nacher, M., Pimapanarak, M., Paw, M.M. …, and McGready, R. 2010. "Complex Interactions between Soil-Transmitted Helminths and Malaria in Pregnant Women on the Thai–Burmese Border." *PLoS Neglected Tropical Diseases*, 4(11): e887. doi: 10.1371/journal.pntd.0000887.

Bransfield, R.C. 2007. "*Lyme Disease, Comorbid Tick-Borne Diseases, and Neuropsychiatric Disorders.*" *Psychiatric Times.* http://www.psychiatrictimes.com/articles/lyme-disease-comorbid-tick-borne-diseases-and-neuropsychiatric-disorders (accessed December 11, 2015).

Bröker, M. 2012. "Following a Tick Bite: Double Infections by Tick-Borne Encephalitis Virus and the Spirochete Borrelia and Other Potential Multiple Infections." *Zoonoses and Public Health*, 59: 176–180.

Bulled, N., Singer, M., and Dillingham, R. 2014. "The Syndemics of Childhood Diarrhea: a biosocial perspective on efforts to combat global inequities in diarrhea-related morbidity and mortality." *Global Public Health*, 9(7): 841–853.

Burgdorfer, W., Barbour, A.G., Hayes, S.G., Benach, J.L., Grunwaldt, E., and Davis, J.P. 1982. Lyme Disease – A Tick-borne Spirochetosis?" *Science*, 216: 131–1319.

Bustamente Moreno, J.G. and Pon Méndez, A. 2010. "Actualización en la vigilancia epidemiológica de 'rickettsiosis'." Part I. *Epidemiológia Boletin*, 6: 1–4. [Article in Portuguese]

Cao, W.-C., Zhao, Q.-M., Zhang, P.-H., Yang, H., Wu, Z.-M., Wen, B.-H., Zhang, X.-T., and Habbema, J.D.F. 2003. "Prevalence of *Anaplasma phagocytophila* and *Borrelia burgdorferi* in *Ixodes persulcatus* Ticks from Northeastern China." *American Journal of Tropical Medicine and Hygiene*, 68: 547–550.

CDC (Centers for Disease Control and Prevention). 1996. "Lyme Disease – United States, 1995." *Morbidity and Mortality Weekly Report*, 45: 481–484.

CDC (Centers for Disease Control and Prevention). 2008a. "Provisional Cases of Infrequently Reported Notifiable Diseases (<1,000 cases reported during the preceding year) – United States, week ending January 3, 2008." *Morbidity and Mortality Weekly Report*, 57: 1420.

CDC (Centers for Disease Control and Prevention). 2008b. "Provisional Cases of Selected Notifiable Diseases, United States, weeks ending January 3, 2009 and December 29, 2009." *Morbidity and Mortality Weekly Report*, 57: 1422–1431.

CDC (Centers for Disease Control and Prevention). 2012. "Reported Cases of Lyme disease by Year, United States, 2002–2011." http://www.cdc.gov/lyme/stats/chartstables/casesbyyear.html. (accessed June 2, 2013).

CDC (Centers for Disease Control and Prevention). 2013. "Lyme Disease." http://www.cdc.gov/lyme/stats/ (accessed June 2, 2013).

Chernomas, R. and Hudson, I. 2009. *Social Murder and Other Shortcomings of Conservative Economics*. Winnipeg: Arbeiter Ring Publishing.

Christova, I., Schouls, L., van de Pol, I., Park, J., Panayotov, S., Lefterova, V., Kantardjiev, T., and Dumler, J.S. 2001. "High Prevalence of Granulocytic Ehrlichiae and *Borrelia burgdorferi sensu lato* in *Ixodes ricinus* Ticks from Bulgaria." *Journal of Clinical Microbiology*, 39: 4172–4174.

Cimperman, J., Maraspin, V., Lotrič-Furlan, S., Ružić-Sablijić, E., Avšič-Županc, T., Picken, R.N., and Strle, F. 1998. "Concomitant Infection with Tick-Borne Encephalitis Virus and *Borrelia Burgdorferi Sensu Lato* in Patients with Acute Meningitis or Meningoencephalitis." *Infection*, 26: 160–164.

Coleman, J.L., Levine, D., Thill, C., Kuhlow, C., and Benach, J.L. 2005. "*Babesia microti* and *Borrelia burgdorferi* Follow Independent Courses of Infection in Mice." *Journal of Infectious Diseases*, 192: 1634–1641.

Commins, S.P. and Platts-Mills, T.A.E. 2013. "Tick Bites and Red Meat Allergy." *Current Opinion Allergy Clinical Immunology*, 13(4): 354–359.

Crutzen, P.J. and Schwägerl, C. 2011. "Living in the Anthropocene: Toward a New Global Ethos." *Yale Environment 360*. http://e360.yale.edu/feature/living_in_the_anthropocene_toward_a_new_global_ethos/2363/ (accessed December 12, 2015).

Crutzen, P. and Stoermer, E. 2000. "The 'Anthropocene'." *Global Change Newsletter*, 41: 17–18.

Dahlgren, F.S., Mandel, E.J., Krebs, J.W., Massung, R.F., and McQuiston, J.H. 2011. "Surveillance for Infections with *Ehrlichia chaffeensis* and *Anaplasma phagocyophilum* in the United States, 2000–2007." *American Journal of Tropical Medicine and Hygiene*, 85(1): 124–131.

Dennis, D.T., Nekomoto, T.S., Victor, J.C., Paul, W.S., and Piesman, J. 1998. "Reported Distribution of *Ixodes scapularis* and *Ixodes pacificus* (Acari: Ixodidae) in the United States." *Journal of Medical Entomology*, 35(5): 629–638.

Dennis, D.T. and Piesman, J. 2005. "Overview of Tick-borne Infections of Humans." In J.L. Goodman, D.T. Dennis, and D.E. Sonenshine (Eds.), *Tick-borne Diseases of Humans* (pp. 3–11). Washington, DC: ASM Press.

Dowie, M. 2009. *Conservation Refugees: The Hundred-Year Conflict between Global Conservation and Native Peoples.* Cambridge, MA: The MIT Press.

Dubinina, E.V. and Alekseev, A.N. 1999. ["The Biodiversity Dynamics of the Causative Agents of Diseases Transmitted by Ticks in the Genus *Ixodes*: An Analysis of Multiyear Data."[*Meditsinskaia Parazitologiia*, 2: 13–19. [Article in Russian]

Estrada-Peña, A. 2009. "Tick-borne Pathogens, Transmission Rates and Climate Change." *Frontiers of Bioscience*, 14: 2674–2687.

Estrada-Peña, A., Zatansever, Z., Gargili, A., and Ergonul, O.2010. "The Trend towards Habitat Fragmentation Is the Key Factor Driving the Spread of Crimean-Congo Haemorrhagic Fever." *Epidemiology and Infection*, 138: 1194–1203.

Faber, D. 2009. "Capitalizing on Environmental Crime: A Case Study of the U.S.A. Polluter-industrial Complex in the Age of Globalization." In K. Kangasputa, and I.H. Marshall (Eds.), *Eco-Crime and Justice: Essays on Environmental Crime* (pp. 80–104). Turin: United Nations and Public Information Department, UNICRI.

Farkas, R., Estrada-Peña, P., Jaenson, T.G.T., Pascucci, I., and Madder, M. 2012. "Basic Biology and Geographical Distribution of Tick Species Involved in the Transmission of Animal Pathogens, Including Zoonoses." In M.D. Salma and J. Tarres-Call (Eds.), *Ticks and Tick-borne Diseases: Geographical Distribution and Control Strategies in the Euro-Asia Region* (pp. 6–26). Wallingford, UK: CAB International.

Foster, J.B. 1994. *The Vulnerable Planet: A Short Economic History of the Environment.* New York: Monthly Review Press.

Freudenberg, N., Fahs, M., Galea, S., and Greenberg, A. 2006. "The Impact of New York City's 1975 Fiscal Crisis on the Tuberculosis, HIV, and Homicide Syndemic." *American Journal of Public Health*, 96(3): 424–434.

Fuente, J. de la. 2003. "The Fossil Record and the Origin of Ticks (Acari: Parasitiformes: Ixodida)." *Vector-borne and Zoonotic Diseases*, 29: 331–344.

Ginsberg, H.S. 2008. "Potential Effects of Mixed Infections in Ticks on Transmission Dynamics of Pathogens: Comparative Analysis of Published Records." *Experimental and Applied Acarology*, 46(1–4): 29–41.

Goodman, J.L., Dennis, D.T., and Sonenshine, D.E. (Eds.) 2005. *Tick-Borne Diseases of Humans.* Washington, DC: ASM Press.

Gore, R. 1995. *Green Imperialism: Colonial Expansion, Tropical Island Edens, and the Origins of Environmentalism, 1600–1860.* Cambridge: Cambridge University Press.

Gotteli, N. 2000. "Model Analysis of Species Co-occurrence Patterns." *Ecology*, 81: 2606–2621.

Gray, J.S, Dautel, H., Estrada-Pena, A., Kahl, O., and Lindgren, E. 2009. "Effects of Climate Change on Ticks and Tick-Borne Diseases in Europe." *Interdisciplinary Perspectives on Infectious Diseases*, 1–12.

Grunwaldt, E., Barbour, A.G., and Benach, J.L. 1983. "Simultaneous Occurrence of *babesiosis* and Lyme Disease." *New England Journal of Medicine*, 308: 1166.

Gutman, J.D., Kotton, C.N., and Kratz, A. 2003. "Case Records of the Massachusetts General Hospital. Weekly Clinicopathological Exercises. Case 29-2003. A 60-Year-Old Man with Fever, Rigors, and Sweats." *New England Journal of Medicine*, 349: 1168–1175.

Halos, L., Jamal, T., Maillard, R., Beugnet, F., Le Menach, A., Boulouis, H.-J., and Vayssier-Taussat, M. 2005. "Evidence of *Bartonella* sp. in Questing Adult and Nymphal *Ixodes ricinus* Ticks from France and Co-infection with *Borrelia burgdorferi sensu lato* and *Babesia* sp." *Veterinary Research*, 36: 79–87.

Harkin, T. 2009. *Proceedings of a Regional Workshop to Assess Research and Outreach Needs in Integrated Pest Management to Reduce the Incidence of Tick-borne Diseases in the Southern United States, January 21–23.* Global Communication Center, CDC. Atlanta, Georgia. http://www.sripmc.org/tickworkshop/Tick-borne_Disease_IPM_Workshop_Proceedings.pdf (accessed December 13, 2015).

Hawkinson, D. 2014. "Statement on Bourbon Virus." *Medical Daily.* http://www.medicaldaily.com/bourbon-virus-new-tick-borne-virus-linked-death-kansas-man-315266 (accessed December 13, 2015).

Healy, G.N. 1989. "The Impact of Cultural and Environmental Changes on the Epidemiology and Control of Human Babesiosis." *Transactions of the Royal Society of Tropical Medicine and Hygiene*, 83(Suppl.): 35–38.

Holden, K., Hodzic, E., Feng, S., Freet, K.J., Lefebvre, R.B., and Barthold, S.W. 2005. "Coinfection with *Anaplasma phagocytophilum* alters *Borrelia burgdorferi* Population Distribution in C3H/HeN Mice. *Infection and Immunity*, 73: 3440–3444.

Hoogstraal, H. 1979. "The Epidemiology of Tick-borne Crimean-Congo Hemorrhagic Fever in Asia, Europe and Africa." *Journal of Medical Entomology*, 15(4): 307–407.

Hu, R., Markowski, D., Hyland, K.E., Kelly, C., and Mather, T.N. 1996. "Human Infection with Tick-transmitted *Babesia microti* in Rhode Island: Serologic Evidence and Risk Factor Assessment." *Journal of Spirochetal and Tick-Borne Diseases*, 3(3/4): 135–139.

Jaaskelainen, A.E., Tikkakoski, T., Uzcategui, N.Y., Alekseev, A.N., Vaheri, A., and Vapalahti, O. 2006. "Siberian Subtype Tickborne Encephalitis Virus, Finland." *Emerging Infectious Diseases*, 12: 10.

Jacoby, K. 2006. *Crimes Against Nature: Squatters, Poachers, Thieves, and the Hidden History of American Conservation.* Berkeley, CA: University of California Press.

Jaenson, T.G. T., Jaenson, D.G.E., Eisen, L., Petersson, E., and Lindgren, E. 2012. "Changes in the Geographical Distribution and Abundance of the Tick *Ixodes ricinus* during the Past 30 Years in Sweden." *Parasites and Vectors*, 5: 8.

Jore, S., Viljugrein, H., Hofshagen, M., Brun-Hansen, H., Kristoffersen, A.B., Nygard, K., Brun, E. …, and Ytrehus, B. 2011. "Multi-source Analysis Reveals Latitudinal and Altitudinal Shifts in Range of *Ixodes ricinus* at Its Northern Distribution Limit." *Parasites and Vectors*, 4: 84.

Jore, S. 2013. "The Impact of Climatic Factors upon Zoonotic Diseases – An Epidemiological Investigation." Doctoral dissertation, Norwegian School of Veterinary Sciences, Oslo, Norway.

Keirans, J.E., and Durden, L.A. 2005. "Tick Systematics and Identification." In J.L. Goodman, D.T. Dennis, and D.E. Sonenshine (Eds.), *Tick-borne Diseases of Humans* (pp. 123–140). Washington, DC: ASM Press.

Kolbert, E. 2011." Age of Man." *National Geographic*, March. http://ngm.nationalgeographic.com/2011/03/age-of-man/kolbert-text (accessed December 13 2015).

Krause, P.J., McKay, K., Thompson, C.A., Sikand, V.K., Lentz, R., Lepore, T., Closter, L. …, and Spielman, A. 2002. "Disease-specific Diagnosis of Coinfecting Tickborne Zoonoses: Babesiosis, Human Granulocytic Ehrlichiosis, and Lyme Disease." *Clinical Infectious Diseases*, 34: 1184–1191.

Krause, P.J., Telford III, S.R., Ryan, R., Hurta, A.B., Kwasnik, I., Luger, S., Niederman, J., Gerber, M., Spielman, A. 1991. "Geographical and Temporal Distribution of Babesial Infection in Connecticut." *Journal of Clinical Microbiology*, 29 :1–4.

Krause, P.J., Telford III, S.R., Spielman, A., Sikand, V., Ryan, R., Christianson, D., Burke, G. …, Persing, D.H. 1996. "Concurrent Lyme Disease and *Babesiosis.*

Evidence for Increased Severity and Duration of Illness." *Journal of the American Medical Association*, 275: 1657–1660.

Kristoferitsch W., Stanek, G., and Kunz, C. 1986. "Double Infection with Early Summer Meningoencephalitis Virus and Borrelia burgdorferi." *Deutsche Medizinische Wochenschrift*, 111(22) :861–864.

Lane, R.S. and Quistad, G.B. 1998. "Borreliacidal Factor in the Blood of the Western Fence Lizard (*Sceloporus occidentalis*). *Journal for Parasitology*, 84: 29–34.

Levi, T., Kilpatrick, A.M., Mangel, M., and Wilmers, C.C. 2012. "Deer, Predators, and the Emergence of Lyme Disease." *Proceedings of the National Academy of Sciences*, 109(20): 10942–10947.

Lindgren, E.A., Tälleklint, L., and Polfeldt, T. 2000. "Impact of Climate Change on the Northern Latitude Limit and Population Density Of The Disease-Transmitting European Tick *Ixodes ricinus*." *Environmental Health Perspective*, 108(2): 119–123.

Littleton, J. and Park, J. 2009. "Tuberculosis and Syndemics: Implications for Pacific Health in New Zealand." *Social Science and Medicine*, 69: 1674–1680.

Magnarelli, L.A., Ijdo, J.W., Anderson, J.F., Padula, S.J., Flavell, R.A., and Fikrig, E. 1998. "Human Exposure to a Granulocytic Ehrlichia and Other Tick-borne Agents in Connecticut." *Journal of Clinical Microbiology*, 36: 2823–2827.

Maltezou, H.C., Andonova, L., Andraghetti, R., Bouloy, M., Ergonul, O., Jongejan, F., Kalvatchev, N. ..., and Zeller, H. 2010. "Crimean-Congo Hemorrhagic Fever in Europe: Current Situation Calls for Preparedness." *Eurosurveillance*, 15(10): pii=19504.

Marshall, M. 2013. *Drinking Smoke: The Tobacco Syndemic in Oceania*. Honolulu: University of Hawai'i Press.

Marsters, E. 2013. "A Transnational Syndemic: Cook Islanders and Their Experiences of TB and Diabetes." PhD dissertation, University of Auckland.

Mayer, G. 2010. "Bacteriology." *Rickettsia, Orientia, Anaplasma, Coxiella* and *Bartonella*. Microbiology and Immunology Online Textbook. The Board of Trustees of the University of South Carolina. http://pathmicro.med.sc.edu/mayer/ricketsia.htm (accessed February 22, 2014).

McNeill, W. 1976. *Plagues and Peoples*. Garden City, NY: Anchor Books.

Mendenhall, E. 2012. *Syndemic Suffering: Social Distress, Depression, and Diabetes among Mexican Immigrant Women*. Walnut Creek CA: Left Coast Press.

Mitchel, P.D., Reed, K.D., and Hofkes, J.M. 1996. "Immunoserologic Evidence of Coinfection with *Borrelia burgdorferi*, *Babesia microti*, and Human Granulocytic Ehrlichia Species in Residents of Wisconsin and Minnesota." *Journal of Clinical Microbiology*, 34(3): 724–727.

Moro, M.H., Zegarra-Moro, O.L., Bjornsson, J., Hofmeister, E.K., Bruinsma, E., Germer, J.J., and Persing, D.H. 2002. "Increased Arthritis Severity in Mice Coinfected with *Borrelia burgdorferi* and *Babesia microti*." *Journal of Infectious Diseases*, 186: 428–431.

Muir, J. 1893. *The Mountains of California*. New York: Century.

Munderloh, U. and Timothy Kurtti, T. 2011. "Emerging and Re-Emerging Tick-borne Diseases: New Challenges at the Interface of Human and Animal Health." In *Critical Needs and Gaps in Understanding Prevention, Amelioration and Resolution of Lyme and Other Tick-Borne Diseases: The Short-Term and Long Term Outcomes* (pp. A142–A166). Washington, DC: The National Academies of Sciences Press.

Nadelman, R.B., Horowitz, H.W., Hsieh, T.-C., Wu, J.M., Aguero-Rosenfeld, M.E., Schwartz, I., Nowakowski, J., Varde, S., and Wormser, G.P. 1997. "Simultaneous Human Granulocytic Ehrlichiosis and Lyme Borreliosis." *New England Journal of Medicine*, 337: 27–30.

Nash, L. 2006. *Inescapable Ecologies: A History of Environmental Disease, and Knowledge*. Berkeley, CA: University of California Press.

National Park Service, 2003. John Muir Historic Site. http://www.sierraclub.org/john_muir_exhibit/john_muir_national_historic_site/the_importance_of_john_muir.aspx (accessed February 20, 2014).

Neitzel, D.F., Jarnefeld, J.L., and Sjogren, R.D. 1993. "An *Ixodes scapularis* (deer tick) Distribution Study in the Minneapolis-St. Paul, Minnesota Area." *Bulletin of the Society for Vector Ecology*, 18: 67–73.

Nichter, M. 1992. "Of Ticks, Kings, Spirits, and the Promise of Vaccines." In C.M. Leslie and A. Young (Eds.), *Paths to Asian Medical Knowledge* (pp. 224–253). Berkeley, CA: University of California Press.

Nicolson, G.L., Gan, R., and Haier, J. 2005. "Evidence for *Brucella* spp. and *Mycoplasma* spp. Co-Infections in Blood of Chronic Fatigue Syndrome Patients." *Journal of Chronic Fatigue Syndrome*, 12(2): 5–17.

Nijhof, A.M., Bodaan, C., Postigo, M., Nieuwenhuijs, H., Opsteegh, M., Franssen, L., Jebbink, F., and Jongejan, F. 2007. "Ticks and Associated Pathogens Collected from Domestic Animals in the Netherlands." *Vector-Borne and Zoonotic Diseases*, 7: 585–595.

Norval, R.A., Andrew, H.R., and Yunker, C.E. 1989. "Pheromone-mediation of Host-selection in Bont Ticks (Amblyomma hebraeum Koch)." *Science*, 243: 364–365.

Odum, E.P. 1983. *Basic Ecology*. Philadelphia: Saunders College Publishers.

Oliver, J.H. Jr., Cummins, G.A., and Joiner, M.S. 1993. "Immature *Ixodes scapularis* (Acari: Ixodidae) Parasitizing Lizards from the Southeastern USA." *Journal for Parasitology*, 79(4): 684–689.

Olson, S. and Patz, J. 2011. "Global Environmental Change and Tick Borne Disease incidence." Commissioned Paper for Critical Needs and Gaps in Understanding Prevention, Amelioration, and Resolution of Lyme and Other Tick-Borne Diseases: The Short-Term and Long-Term Outcomes: Workshop Report, pp. A267–A290. Washington, DC: The National Academy of Medicine.

Openshaw, J.J., Swerdlow, D.L., Krebs, J.W.,. Holman, R.C., Mandel, E., Harvey, A., Haberling, D., Massung, R.F., and McQuiston, J.H. 2010. "Rocky Mountain Spotted Fever in the United States, 2000–2007: Interpreting Contemporary Increases in Incidence." *American Journal of Tropical Medicine and Hygiene*, 83: 174–182.

Oxenstierna, S. 2002. "Labor Market Policies." In W. Maciejewski (Ed.), *The Baltic Sea Region: Culture, Politics, Societies* (pp. 651–664). Uppsala: Baltic University Press.

Paddock, C.D., Finley, R.W., Wright, C.S., Robinson, H.N., Schrodt, B.J., Lane, C.C., Ekenna, O. ..., and Eremeeva, M.E. 2008. "*Rickettsia parkeri rickettsiosis* and Its Clinical Distinction from Rocky Mountain Spotted Fever." *Clinical Infectious Diseases*, 47: 1188–1196.

Paddock, C.D. and Telford, S.R. 2011. "Through a Glass Darkly: The Global Incidence of Tick-Borne Diseases." Commissioned Paper for Critical Needs and Gaps in Understanding Prevention, Amelioration, and Resolution of Lyme and Other Tick-Borne Diseases: The Short-Term and Long-Term Outcomes. Workshop Report, pp. 221–266. Washington, DC: The National Academy of Medicine.

Pancholi, P., Kolbert, C.P., Mitchell, P.D., Reed, Jr., K.D., Dumler, J.S., Bakken, J.S., Telford III, S.R., and Persing, D.H. 1995. "*Ixodes dammini* as a Potential Vector of Human Granulocytic Ehrlichiosis." *Journal of Infectious Diseases*, 172: 1007–1012.

Parola, P., Paddock, C.D., and Raoult, D. 2005. "Tick-borne Rickettsioses around the World: Emerging Diseases Challenging Old Concepts." *Clinical Microbiology Reviews*, 18: 719–756.

Pattnaik, P. 2006. "Kyasanur Forest Disease: An Epidemiological View in India." *Reviews in Medical Virology*, 16: 151–165.

Platts-Mills, T.A.E. and Commins, S.P. 2013. "Emerging Antigens Involved in Allergic Responses." *Current Opinion Immunology*, 25(6): 769–774.

Pyramid Communications. 2005. *Building Relationships with Communities of Color.* Washington, DC: The Nature Conservancy.

Randolph, S.E. 2001. "The Shifting Landscape of Tick-Borne Zoonoses: Tick-Borne Encephalitis and Lyme borreliosis in Europe." *Philosophical Transactions of the Royal Society of London*, 356(1411): 1045–1056.

Randolph, S.E. 2004. "Tick Ecology: Processes and Patterns behind the Epidemiological Risk Posed by Ixodid Ticks as Vectors." *Parasitology*, 129: S37–S65.

Randolph, S.E. 2008. "Tick-borne Encephalitis in Central and Eastern Europe: Consequences of Political Transition." *Microbes and Infection*, 10: 209–216.

Randolph, S.E. 2009. "Tick-borne Disease Systems Emerge from the Shadows: The Beauty Lies in Molecular Detail, the Message in Epidemiology." *Parasitology*, 136: 1403–1413.

Randolph, S.E. 2010. "To What Extent Has Climate Change Contributed to the Recent Epidemiology of Tick-Borne Diseases?" *Veterinary Parasitology*, 167: 92–94.

Raoult, D., Broqui, P., and Roux, V. 1996. "A New Spotted Fever Group Rickettsiosis." *Lancet*, 348: 412.

Reis, C., Cote, M., Paul, R.E.L., and Bonnet, S. 2011. "Questing Ticks in Suburban Forest Are Infected by at Least Six Tick-borne Pathogens." *Vector Borne Zoonotic Diseases*, 11(7): 907–916.

Renvoisé, A., Delaunay, P., Blanchouin, E., Cannavo, I., Cua, E., Socolovschi, C., Parola, P., and Raoult, D. 2012. "Urban Family Cluster of Spotted Fever Rickettsiosis Linked to *Rhipicephalus sanguineus* Infected with *Rickettsia conorii* subsp. *caspia* and *Rickettsia massiliae*." *Ticks and Tick Borne Disease*, 3(5–6): 389–392.

Revkin, A. 2008. "Earth is Us." *New York Times*, Dot Earth. http://dotearth.blogs.nytimes.com/2008/01/28/earth-is-us/ (accessed December 13, 2015).

Ricketts, H. 1991. "Some Aspects of Rocky Mountain Spotted Fever as Shown by Recent Investigations." *Reviews of Infectious Diseases*, 13(6): 1227–1240.

Rock, M., Bonnie J. Buntain, Jennifer M. Hatfield, and Benedikt Hallgrímsson, 2009. "Animal–Human Connections, 'One Health,' and the Syndemic Approach to Prevention." *Social Science and Medicine*, 68(6): 991–995.

Scheper-Hughes, N. 1992. *Death Without Weeping: The Violence of Everyday Life in Brazil.* Berkeley: University of California Press.

Schicht, S., Schnieder, T., and Strube, C. 2012. "*Rickettsia* spp. and Coinfections with Other Pathogenic Microorganisms in Hard Ticks from Northern Germany." *Journal of Medical Entomology*, 49(3): 766–771.

Schouls, L.M., Van De Pol, I., Rijpkema, S.G.T., and Schot, C.S. 1999. "Detection and Identification of *Ehrlichia, Borrelia burgdorferi* Sensu Lato, and *Bartonella* Species in Dutch *Ixodes ricinus* Ticks." *Journal of Clinical Microbiology*, 37(7): 2215–2222.

Schulze, T.L., Jordan, R.A., Healy, S.P., and Roegner, V.E. 2013. "Detection of *Babesia microti* and *Borrelia burgdorferi* in Host-seeking *Ixodes scapularis* (Acari: Ixodidae) in Monmouth County, New Jersey." *Journal of Medical Entomology*, 50(2): 379–383.

Scott, W. 2000. *Recent Changes in Social Conditions of Countries in Transition: Eastern Europe, the Baltic States and the Commonwealth of Independent States.* Geneva: United Nations, Research Institute for Social Development.

Shapiro, M.R., Fritz, C.L., Tait, K., Paddock, C.D., Nicholson, W.L., Abramowicz, K.F., Karpahty, S.E. …, and Marina E. Eremeeva, 2010. "*Rickettsia* 364D: A Newly Recognized Cause of Eschar-associated Illness in California." *Clinical Infectious Diseases*, 50: 541–548.

Silveira, S.J. 2004. "The American Environmental Movement: Surviving Through Diversity." *Boston College Environmental Affairs Law Review*, 28(2): 497–532.

Singer, M. 1996. "A Dose of Drugs, A Touch of Violence, A Case of AIDS: Conceptualizing the SAVA Syndemic." *Free Inquiry in Creative Sociology*, 24(2): 99–110.

Singer, M. 2009. *Introduction to Syndemics: A Systems Approach to Public and Community Health*. San Francisco.CA: Jossey-Bass.

Singer, M. 2010. "Pathogen-Pathogen Interaction: A Syndemic Model of Complex Biosocial Processes in Disease." *Virulence*, 1(1): 10–18.

Singer, M. 2011. "Double Jeopardy: Vulnerable Children and the Possible Global Lead Poisoning/Infectious Disease Syndemic." In R. Parker and M. Sommer (Eds.), *International Handbook on Global Health* (pp. 154–161). London: Routledge.

Singer, M. and Bulled, N. in press. "Ectoparasitic Syndemics: Polymicrobial Tick-borne Disease Interactions in a Changing Anthropogenic Landscape." *Medical Anthropology Quarterly*. ISSN 1548–1387.

Singer, M. and Clair, S. 2003. "Syndemics and Public Health: Reconceptualizing Disease in Bio-Social Context." *Medical Anthropology Quarterly*, 17(4): 423–441.

Singer, M., Herring, D.A., Littleton, J., and Rock, M. 2011. "Syndemics in Global Health." In M. Singer and P.I. Erickson (Eds.), *A Companion to Medical Anthropology* (pp. 159–179). San Francisco, CA: Wiley.

Siński, E. 2009. [Effect of Coinfections in *Ixodidae* Ticks on Transmission of Blood Microparasites.] *Wiadomosci Parazytologiczne*, 55(4): 341–347. [Article in Polish]

Skotarczak, B., Rymaszewska, A., Wodecka, B., and Sawczuk, M. 2003. "Molecular Evidence of Coinfection of *Borrelia burgdorferi sensu lato*, Human Granulocytic Ehrlichiosis Agent, and *Babesia microti* in Ticks from Northwestern Poland." *Journal for Parasitology*, 89: 194–196.

Spielman, A., Wilson, M.L., Levine, J.F., and Piesman, J. 1985. "Ecology of *Ixodes dammini*-borne Human Babesiosis and Lyme Disease." *Annual Review of Entomology*, 30: 439–460.

Stall, R., Mills, T.C., Williamson, J., Hart, T., Greenwood, G., Paul, J., Pollack, L. … and A. Catania, 2003. "Association of Co-occurring Psychosocial Health Problems and Increased Vulnerability to HIV/AIDS Among Urban Men Who Have Sex with Men." *American Journal of Public Health*, 93(6): 939–942.

Stanczak, J., Gabre, R.M., Kruminis-Lozowska, W., Racewicz, M., and Kubica-Biernat, B. 2004. "*Ixodes ricinus* as a Vector of *Borrelia burgdorferi sensu lato*, *Anaplasma phagocytophilum* and *Babesia microti* in Urban and Suburban Forests." *Annals of Agricultural and Environmental Medicine*, 11: 109–114.

Steere, A.C., Malawista, S.E., Snydman, D.R., Shope, R.E., Andiman, W.A., Ross, M.R., and Steele, F.M. 1977. "Lyme Arthritis: An Epidemic of Oligoarticular Arthritis in Children and Adults in Three Connecticut Communities." *Arthritis and Rheumatism*, 20: 7–17.

Steere, A.C., Malawista, S.E., Hardin, J.A., Ruddy, S., Askenase, P.W., and Andiman, W.A. 1977. "Erythema Chronicum Migrans and Lyme Arthritis. The Enlarging Clinical Spectrum." *Annals of Internal Medicine*, 86: 685–698.

Steffen, W., Crutzen, P.J., and McNeill, J.R. 2007. "The Anthropocene: Are Humans Now Overwhelming the Great Forces of Nature?" *Ambio*, 36(8): 614–621.

Stevenson, P. 1982. "Capitalism and Inequality: The Negative Consequences for Humanity." *Contemporary Crises*, 6(4): 333–371.

Sumilo, D., Asokliene, L., Bormane, A., Vasilenko, V., Golovljova, I., and Randolph, S.E. 2007. "Climate Change Cannot Explain the Upsurge of Tick-Borne Encephalitis in the Baltics." *PLoS One*, 2(6): e500.

Sun, Y., Liu, G.-P., Yang, L.-W., Xu, R.-M., and Yu, Y.X. 2007. "Multiple Infections of Tick-borne Pathogens in *Ixodes persulcatus* Collected from Forests in Heilongjiang Province." *Acta Parasitology et Medica Entomologica Sinica*, 4: 231–240.

Swanepoel, R., Gill, D., Shepherd, A., Leman, P., Mynhardt, J., and Harvey, S. 1988. "The clinical pathology of Crimean-Congo hemorrhagic fever." *Reviews of Infectious Diseases*, Supplement 4: S794–800.

Swanson, S.J., Neitzel, D., Reed, K.D., and Belongia, E.A. 2006. "Coinfections acquired from *Ixodes* Ticks." *Clinical Microbiology Reviews*, 19(4): 708–727.

Tarlock, A.D. 1993. "City versus Countryside: Environmental Equity in Context." *Fordham Urban Law Journal*, 21(3): 461–494.

Telfer, S., Lambin, X., Birtles, R., Beldomenico, P., Burthe, S., Paterson, S., and Begon, M. 2010. "Species Interactions in a Parasite Community Drive Infection Risk in a Wildlife Population." *Science*, 330: 243–246.

The Center for Diversity and the Environment, 2007. "The Facts." http://www.environmentaldiversity.org/ (accessed February 2, 2014).

The National Academy of Medicine. 2011. *Critical Needs and Gaps in Understanding Prevention, Amelioration, and Resolution of Lyme and Other Tick-Borne Diseases: The Short-Term and Long-Term Outcomes: Workshop Report.* Washington, DC: The National Academy of Medicine.

The Outdoor Foundation, 2012. *Outdoor Recreation: Participant Report.* Boulder, CO: The Outdoor Foundation.

Thomas, V., Anguita, J., Barthold, S.W., and Fikrig, E. 2001. "Coinfection with *Borrelia burgdorferi* and the Agent of Human Granulocytic Ehrlichiosis Alters Murine Immune Responses, Pathogen Burden, and Severity of Lyme Arthritis." *Infection and Immunity.* 69: 3359–3371.

Tokarz, R., Jain, K., Bennett, A., Briese, T., and Lipkin, W.I. 2010. "Assessment of Polymicrobial Infections in Ticks in New York State." *Vector Borne Zoonotic Disease*, 10(3): 217–221.

Václav, R., Ficová, M., Prokop, P., and Betáková, T. 2011. "Associations between Coinfection Prevalence of *Borrelia lusitaniae*, *Anaplasma* sp., and *Rickettsia* sp. in Hard Ticks Feeding on Reptile Hosts." *Microbial Ecology*, 61(2): 245–253.

Wang, T.J., Liang, M.H., Sangha, O., Phillips, C.B., Lew, R.A., Wright, E.A., Berardi, V., Fossel, A.H., and Shadick, N.A. 2000. "Coexposure to *Borrelia burgdorferi* and *Babesia microti* Does Not Worsen the Long-term Outcome of Lyme Disease." *Clinical Infectious Diseases*, 31: 1149–1154.

Wikel, S.K., Ramachandra, R.N., and Bergman, D.K. 1994. "Tick-induced Modulation of the Host Immune Response." *International Journal for Parasitology*, 24(1): 59–66.

Wilson, M.L. 1998. "Distribution and Abundance of *Ixodes scapularis* (Acari: Ixodidae) in North America: Ecological Processes and Spatial Analysis." *Journal of Medical Entomology*, 35: 446–457.

Wilson, M.L. and Spielman, A. 1985. "Seasonal Activity of Immature *Ixodes dammini* (Acari: Ixodidae)." *Journal of Medical Entomology*, 22: 408–414.

Zeidner, N.S., Burkot, T.R., Massung, R., Nicholson, W.L., Dolan, M.C., Rutherford, J.S., Biggerstaff, B.J., and Maupin, G.O. 2000. "Transmission of the Agent of Human Granulocytic Ehrlichiosis by Ixodes spinipalpis Ticks: Evidence of an Enzootic Cycle of Dual Infection with *Borrelia burgdorferi* in Northern Colorado." *Journal of Infectious Diseases*, 182: 616–619.

Index

A Companion to the Anthropology of Environmental Health, First Edition. Edited by Merrill Singer.

www.ingramcontent.com/pod-product-compliance
Lightning Source LLC
Chambersburg PA
CBHW081422030126
37659CB00005B/24
9781118786994